THE WASHINGTON MANUAL™

Cardiology **Subspecialty Consult**

Marty
Grissom

330 - 524 - 3619

THE WASHINGTON MANUAL™

Cardiology `Subspecialty Consult`

Third Edition

Editors

Phillip S. Cuculich, MD

Assistant Professor of Medicine
Department of Internal Medicine
Cardiovascular Division
Washington University School of Medicine
St. Louis, Missouri

Andrew M. Kates, MD

Associate Professor of Medicine
Department of Internal Medicine
Cardiovascular Division
Washington University School of Medicine
St. Louis, Missouri

Series Editors

Thomas M. De Fer, MD

Associate Professor of Internal Medicine
Division of Medical Education
Washington University School of
    Medicine
St. Louis, Missouri

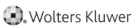
. Wolters Kluwer
Health
Philadelphia · Baltimore · New York · London
Buenos Aires · Hong Kong · Sydney · Tokyo

Executive Editor: Rebecca Gaertner
Senior Product Development Editor: Kristina Oberle
Production Project Manager: Marian Bellus
Marketing Manager: Stephanie Manzo
Senior Manufacturing Manager: Beth Welsh
Design Coordinator: Teresa Mallon
Editorial Coordinator: Katie Sharp
Production Service: Integra Software Services Pvt. Ltd.

Third Edition

© 2014 by Department of Medicine, Washington University School of Medicine

Second Edition, © 2009 by Department of Medicine, Washington University School of Medicine
First Edition, © 2004 by Department of Medicine, Washington University School of Medicine

Printed in China

9 8 7 6 5 4 3 2 1

Library of Congress Cataloging-in-Publication Data

The Washington manual cardiology subspecialty consult / editors, Phillip S. Cuculich, Andrew M. Kates, Thomas M. De Fer. — Third edition.
    p. ; cm. — (Washington manual subspecialty consult series)
   Cardiology subspecialty consult
   Includes bibliographical references and index.
   ISBN 978-1-4511-1422-5
   I. Cuculich, Phillip S., editor of compilation.   II. Kates, Andrew M., editor of compilation.
III. De Fer, Thomas M., editor of compilation.   IV. Title: Cardiology subspecialty consult.   V. Series: Washington manual subspecialty consult series.
   [DNLM: 1. Cardiovascular Diseases—Handbooks.   2. Cardiology—methods—Handbooks. WG 39]
   RC667
   616.1'2—dc23

                                    2014003539

The Washington Manual™ is an intent-to-use mark belonging to Washington University in St. Louis to which international legal protection applies. The mark is used in this publication by LWW under license from Washington University.

Care has been taken to confirm the accuracy of the information present and to describe generally accepted practices. However, the authors, editors, and publisher are not responsible for errors or omissions or for any consequences from application of the information in this book and make no warranty, expressed or implied, with respect to the currency, completeness, or accuracy of the contents of the publication. Application of this information in a particular situation remains the professional responsibility of the practitioner; the clinical treatments described and recommended may not be considered absolute and universal recommendations.

The authors, editors, and publisher have exerted every effort to ensure that drug selection and dosage set forth in this text are in accordance with current recommendations and practice at the time of publication. However, in view of ongoing research, changes in government regulations, and the constant flow of information relating to drug therapy and drug reactions, the reader is urged to check the package insert for each drug for any change in indications and dosage and for added warnings and precautions. This is particularly important when the recommended agent is a new or infrequently employed drug.

Some drugs and medical devices presented in this publication have Food and Drug Administration (FDA) clearance for limited use in restricted research settings. It is the responsibility of health care providers to ascertain the FDA status of each drug or device planned for use in their clinical practice.

We dedicate this book to the many people who influence us: our wives, children, teachers, students, and patients. We thank you for inspiring us, teaching us and keeping us humble.

—PSC & AMK

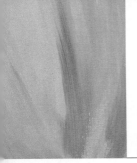

American College of Cardiology/American Heart Association Clinical Practice Guidelines

Rating Scheme for the Strength of the Recommendations

Class I: Conditions for which there is evidence and/or general agreement that a given procedure or treatment is beneficial, useful, and effective.

Class II: Conditions for which there is conflicting evidence and/or a divergence of opinion about the usefulness/efficacy of a procedure or treatment.

    Class IIa: Weight of evidence/opinion is in favor of usefulness/efficacy.

    Class IIb: Usefulness/efficacy is less well established by evidence/opinion.

Class III: Conditions for which there is evidence and/or general agreement that a procedure/treatment is not useful/effective and in some cases may be harmful.

Rating Scheme for the Strength of the Evidence

Level of Evidence A: Data derived from multiple randomized clinical trials or meta-analyses.

Level of Evidence B: Data derived from a single randomized trial or nonrandomized studies.

Level of Evidence C: Only consensus opinion of experts, case studies, or standard-of-care.

Gibbons RJ, Smith S, Antman E. American College of Cardiology/American Heart Association clinical practice guidelines: Part I: where do they come from? *Circulation* 2003;107:2979-2986.

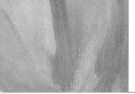

Contributing Authors

Suzanne V. Arnold
Adjunct Assistant Professor of Medicine
Department of Internal Medicine
Cardiovascular Division
Washington University School of Medicine
St. Louis, Missouri

Richard G. Bach
Associate Professor of Medicine
Department of Internal Medicine
Cardiovascular Division
Washington University School of Medicine
St. Louis, Missouri

Alok Bachuwar
Clinical Fellow
Department of Internal Medicine
Cardiovascular Division
Washington University School of Medicine
St. Louis, Missouri

Sudeshna Banerjee
Clinical Fellow
Department of Internal Medicine
Cardiovascular Division
Washington University School of Medicine
St. Louis, Missouri

Preben Bjerregaard
Clinical Fellow
Department of Internal Medicine
Cardiovascular Division
Washington University School of Medicine
St. Louis, Missouri

Elisa A. Bradley
Clinical Fellow
Department of Internal Medicine
Cardiovascular Division
Washington University School of Medicine
St. Louis, Missouri

Alan C. Braverman
Alumni Endowed Professor of
Cardiovascular Diseases in Medicine
Department of Internal Medicine
Cardiovascular Division
Washington University School of Medicine
St. Louis, Missouri

Angela L. Brown
Associate Professor of Medicine
Department of Internal Medicine
Cardiovascular Division
Washington University School of Medicine
St. Louis, Missouri

Ari M. Cedars
Assistant Professor of Medicine
Department of Internal Medicine
Cardiovascular Division
Washington University School of Medicine
St. Louis, Missouri

Murali M. Chakinala
Associate Professor of Medicine
Department of Internal Medicine
Pulmonary Division
Washington University School of Medicine
St. Louis, Missouri

Jane Chen
Associate Professor of Medicine
Department of Internal Medicine
Cardiovascular Division
Washington University School of Medicine
St. Louis, Missouri

Risa M. Cohen
Clinical Fellow
Department of Internal Medicine
Cardiovascular Division
Washington University School of Medicine
St. Louis, Missouri

Daniel H. Cooper
Assistant Professor of Medicine
Department of Internal Medicine
Cardiovascular Division
Washington University School of Medicine
St. Louis, Missouri

Phillip S. Cuculich
Assistant Professor of Medicine
Department of Internal Medicine
Cardiovascular Division
Washington University School of Medicine
St. Louis, Missouri

Jeremiah P. Depta
Clinical Fellow
Department of Internal Medicine
Cardiovascular Division
Washington University School of Medicine
St. Louis, Missouri

Gregory A. Ewald
Associate Professor of Medicine
Department of Internal Medicine
Cardiovascular Division
Washington University School of Medicine
St. Louis, Missouri

Mitchell N. Faddis
Associate Professor of Medicine
Department of Internal Medicine
Cardiovascular Division
Washington University School of Medicine
St. Louis, Missouri

Derrick R. Fansler
Clinical Fellow
Department of Internal Medicine
Cardiovascular Division
Washington University School of Medicine
St. Louis, Missouri

Corey G. Foster
Clinical Fellow
Department of Internal Medicine
Cardiovascular Division
Washington University School of Medicine
St. Louis, Missouri

Marye J. Gleva
Associate Professor of Medicine
Department of Internal Medicine
Cardiovascular Division
Washington University School of Medicine
St. Louis, Missouri

Chirayu Gor
Clinical Fellow
Department of Internal Medicine
Cardiovascular Division
Washington University School of Medicine
St. Louis, Missouri

Robert J. Gropler
Professor of Radiology
Department of Radiology
Nuclear Medicine Division
Washington University School of Medicine
St. Louis, Missouri

Mohammed Hadi
Clinical Fellow
Department of Internal Medicine
Cardiovascular Division
Washington University School of Medicine
St. Louis, Missouri

Ilia G. Halatchev
Clinical Fellow
Department of Internal Medicine
Cardiovascular Division
Washington University School of Medicine
St. Louis, Missouri

Christopher L. Holley
Instructor in Medicine
Department of Internal Medicine
Cardiovascular Division
Washington University School of Medicine
St. Louis, Missouri

Sudhir K. Jain
Associate Professor of Medicine
Department of Internal Medicine
Cardiovascular Division
Washington University School of Medicine
St. Louis, Missouri

Susan M. Joseph
Assistant Professor of Medicine
Department of Internal Medicine
Cardiovascular Division
Washington University School of Medicine
St. Louis, Missouri

Andrew M. Kates
Associate Professor of Medicine
Department of Internal Medicine
Cardiovascular Division
Washington University School of Medicine
St. Louis, Missouri

Mohammad Ali Kizilbash
Assistant Professor of Medicine
Department of Internal Medicine
Cardiovascular Division
Washington University School of Medicine
St. Louis, Missouri

Andrew J. Krainik
Clinical Fellow
Department of Internal Medicine
Cardiovascular Division
Washington University School of Medicine
St. Louis, Missouri

Ronald J. Krone
John E. Simon Scholar in Medicine
Department of Internal Medicine
Cardiovascular Division
Washington University School of Medicine
St. Louis, Missouri

Thomas K. Kurian
Clinical Fellow
Department of Internal Medicine
Cardiovascular Division
Washington University School of Medicine
St. Louis, Missouri

Howard I. Kurz
Professor of Medicine
Department of Internal Medicine
Cardiovascular Division
Washington University School of Medicine
St. Louis, Missouri

Shane J. LaRue
Instructor in Medicine
Department of Internal Medicine
Cardiovascular Division
Washington University School of Medicine
St. Louis, Missouri

John M. Lasala
Professor of Medicine
Department of Internal Medicine
Cardiovascular Division
Washington University School of Medicine
St. Louis, Missouri

Jeffrey M.C. Lau
Clinical Fellow
Department of Internal Medicine
Cardiovascular Division
Washington University School of Medicine
St. Louis, Missouri

Kory J. Lavine
Clinical Fellow
Department of Internal Medicine
Cardiovascular Division
Washington University School of Medicine
St. Louis, Missouri

Jefferson Lee
Clinical Fellow
Department of Internal Medicine
Cardiovascular Division
Washington University School of Medicine
St. Louis, Missouri

C. Huie Lin
Clinical Fellow
Department of Internal Medicine
Cardiovascular Division
Washington University School of Medicine
St. Louis, Missouri

Brian R. Lindman
Assistant Professor Medicine
Department of Internal Medicine
Cardiovascular Division
Washington University School of Medicine
St. Louis, Missouri

Jose A. Madrazo
Assistant Professor of Medicine
Department of Internal Medicine
Cardiovascular Division
Washington University School of Medicine
St. Louis, Missouri

Majesh Makan
Associate Professor of Medicine
Department of Internal Medicine
Cardiovascular Division
Washington University School of Medicine
St. Louis, Missouri

Keith Mankowitz
Associate Professor of Medicine
Department of Internal Medicine
Cardiovascular Division
Washington University School of Medicine
St. Louis, Missouri

Sara C. Martinez
Clinical Fellow
Department of Internal Medicine
Cardiovascular Division
Washington University School of Medicine
St. Louis, Missouri

William J. Nienaber
Clinical Fellow
Department of Internal Medicine
Cardiovascular Division
Washington University School of Medicine
St. Louis, Missouri

Scott M. Nordlicht
Professor of Medicine
Department of Internal Medicine
Cardiovascular Division
Washington University School of Medicine
St. Louis, Missouri

Jiafu Ou
Assistant Professor of Medicine
Department of Internal Medicine
Cardiovascular Division
Washington University School of Medicine
St. Louis, Missouri

Ravi Rasalingam
Assistant Professor of Medicine
Department of Internal Medicine
Cardiovascular Division
Washington University School of Medicine
St. Louis, Missouri

Ashwin Ravichandran
Clinical Fellow
Department of Internal Medicine
Cardiovascular Division
Washington University School of Medicine
St. Louis, Missouri

Craig K. Reiss
Professor of Medicine
Department of Internal Medicine
Cardiovascular Division
Washington University School of Medicine
St. Louis, Missouri

Michael W. Rich
Professor of Medicine
Department of Internal Medicine
Cardiovascular Division
Washington University School of Medicine
St. Louis, Missouri

Mohammed Saghir
Clinical Fellow
Department of Internal Medicine
Cardiovascular Division
Washington University School of Medicine
St. Louis, Missouri

Joel D. Schilling
Assistant Professor of Medicine
Department of Internal Medicine
Cardiovascular Division
Washington University School of Medicine
St. Louis, Missouri

David B. Schwartz
Associate Professor of Medicine
Department of Internal Medicine
Cardiovascular Division
Washington University School of Medicine
St. Louis, Missouri

Kristen Scott-Tillery
Clinical Fellow
Department of Internal Medicine
Cardiovascular Division
Washington University School of Medicine
St. Louis, Missouri

Lynne M. Seacord
Assistant Professor of Medicine
Department of Internal Medicine
Cardiovascular Division
Washington University School of Medicine
St. Louis, Missouri

Jay Shah
Clinical Fellow
Department of Internal Medicine
Cardiovascular Division
Washington University School of Medicine
St. Louis, Missouri

Shimoli Shah
Clinical Fellow
Department of Internal Medicine
Cardiovascular Division
Washington University School of Medicine
St. Louis, Missouri

Shivak Sharma
Clinical Fellow
Department of Internal Medicine
Cardiovascular Division
Washington University School of Medicine
St. Louis, Missouri

Jasvindar Singh
Associate Professor of Medicine
Department of Internal Medicine
Cardiovascular Division
Washington University School of Medicine
St. Louis, Missouri

Timothy W. Smith
Associate Professor of Medicine
Department of Internal Medicine
Cardiovascular Division
Washington University School of Medicine
St. Louis, Missouri

Pablo F. Soto
Clinical Fellow
Department of Internal Medicine
Cardiovascular Division
Washington University School of Medicine
St. Louis, Missouri

Justin M. Vader
Clinical Fellow
Department of Internal Medicine
Cardiovascular Division
Washington University School of Medicine
St. Louis, Missouri

John Verbsky
Clinical Fellow
Department of Internal Medicine
Cardiovascular Division
Washington University School of Medicine
St. Louis, Missouri

Alan N. Weiss
Professor or Medicine
Department of Internal Medicine
Cardiovascular Division
Washington University School of Medicine
St. Louis, Missouri

Michael Yeung
Clinical Fellow
Department of Internal Medicine
Cardiovascular Division
Washington University School of Medicine
St. Louis, Missouri

Alan Zajarias
Assistant Professor of Medicine
Department of Internal Medicine
Cardiovascular Division
Washington University School of Medicine
St. Louis, Missouri

Chairman's Note

I t is a pleasure to present the new edition of *The Washington Manual*™ Subspecialty Consult Series: *Cardiology Subspecialty Consult*. This pocket-size book continues to be a primary reference for medical students, interns, residents, and other practitioners who need ready access to practical clinical information to diagnose and treat patients with a wide variety of disorders. Medical knowledge continues to increase at an astounding rate, which creates a challenge for physicians to keep up with the biomedical discoveries, genetic and genomic information, and novel therapeutics that can positively impact patient outcomes. The *Washington Manual*™ Subspecialty Consult Series addresses this challenge by concisely and practically providing current scientific information for clinicians to aid them in the diagnosis, investigation, and treatment of common medical conditions.

I want to personally thank the authors, which include house officers, fellows, and attendings at Washington University School of Medicine and Barnes-Jewish Hospital. Their commitment to patient care and education are unsurpassed, and their efforts and skill in compiling this manual are evident in the quality of the final product. In particular, I would like to acknowledge our editors, Drs. Phillip S. Cuculich and Andrew M. Kates, and the series editor, Dr. Tom De Fer, who have worked tirelessly to produce another outstanding edition of this manual. I would also like to thank Dr. Melvin Blanchard, Chief of the Division of Medical Education in the Department of Medicine at Washington University School of Medicine, for his advice and guidance. I believe this *Manual* will meet its desired goal of providing practical knowledge that can be directly applied at the bedside and in outpatient settings to improve patient care.

Victoria J. Fraser, MD
Adolphus Busch Professor of Medicine
Chairman, Department of Medicine
Washington University School of Medicine
St. Louis, Missouri

Foreword

Advances in cardiovascular medicine are currently proceeding at a breathtaking pace. As the knowledge base in cardiovascular medicine expands, it becomes increasingly important to condense this new information into a format that honors the traditional approaches to teaching clinical medicine, but is also up to date and readily accessible to busy health care providers. The third edition of *The Washington Manual™ Cardiology Subspecialty Consult* was written with the challenges of the busy practitioner in mind. Each chapter in the third edition was written by a cardiovascular fellow who was paired with an attending physician with considerable clinical expertise. This team approach to writing allowed each chapter to be suffused with real-world approaches to real-world problems that are not only evidence based, but also based on the expertise of seasoned clinicians who have devoted their careers to training the next generation of health care providers. The new edition, which was masterfully edited and organized by Drs. Andy Kates and Phillip Cuculich, has new chapters on the physical exam, heart failure with preserved ejection fraction, and cardiovascular diseases in elderly populations and in women. As with the previous editions, the chapters contain simple easy-to-read figures and flow diagrams coupled with bullet-point lists and countless bold-faced clinical pearls. I believe the third edition of *The Washington Manual™ Cardiology Subspecialty Consult* will be enormously useful as an extremely "readable" resource for health care providers who must provide care for the growing numbers of patients with cardiovascular disease. I am proud to endorse this book, which will ultimately benefit the millions of patients with cardiovascular disease.

Douglas L. Mann, MD
Lewin Chair and Chief, Cardiovascular Division
Professor of Medicine, Cell Biology and Physiology
Cardiologist-in-Chief, Barnes-Jewish Hospital
St. Louis, Missouri

Preface

We, the editors of the third edition of *The Washington Manual™ Cardiology Subspecialty Consult*, wish to thank you for choosing our book as worthy of your time to learn about cardiovascular diseases. There are many excellent resources available to learners, but we hope that as you navigate through these pages, you discover the passion that our authors have harnessed to create this up-to-date and clinically impactful portable text.

We specifically wish to thank the editor of the first edition, Dr. Peter Crawford, who planted the seeds of high-level intellect and compassionate tutelage from which this edition grows. We are most indebted to the marvelous effort of those who contributed to the current edition: house staff, fellows, and attending physicians alike. While we expected excellence from our authors, we were overwhelmed by the high quality of information and clear passion for teaching found in each chapter.

Every chapter of the third edition has been written by a pair of authors: one cardiovascular fellow and one cardiovascular or pulmonary clinician-educator. This pairing embodies the overriding theme of this edition: front-line, middle-of-the-night synthesis and application of up-to-date guidelines, seasoned with expert clinical experience. As with previous editions, we deliberately stress the most useful information as it relates to the patient's diagnosis and treatment with mnemonics, bullet-point lists, bold-faced clinical pearls, and easy-to-read figures. To keep the text thin enough to be portable, guidelines from the American Heart Association and American College of Cardiology are emphasized with journal and online references at the end of each chapter. We strongly encourage reading these current practice recommendations as well as peer-reviewed journals, review articles, and primary textbooks to supplement the material in this handbook.

We are particularly proud of the depth of the specialties in this edition. For example, in an effort to restore the lost art of the cardiovascular physical exam, we asked one of our most gifted master clinicians to author a dedicated chapter on this topic. Additionally, the clinical impact of heart failure with preserved ejection fraction, or diastolic heart failure, has inspired a new chapter for this edition. The continued importance of individualization of medicine inspired dedicated chapters on cardiovascular diseases in elderly populations and in women specifically. These new chapters are coupled with a simplified reorganization of the book, grouping chapters together in the most logical ways.

Now more than ever, it is a thrilling time to be interested in cardiovascular disease. Discovery is happening at a rapid pace, and translating these new discoveries to the patient's bedside happens quickly. More so than decades past, there is a strong interest in providing cost-effective evidence-based cardiology. This process requires a continuous synthesis and evaluation of the most recent clinical trials into daily practice while maintaining diagnostic skills that are at the center of cardiovascular disease management. It is our hope that both the information and the enthusiasm contained in the chapters that follow provide you with the means to meet these challenges and with it become a better teacher, a better learner, and a better physician.

—PSC & AMK

Contents

Approach to the Cardiovascular Consult

Andrew M. Kates

GENERAL PRINCIPLES

- The cardiovascular consultant is unique in medicine, and cardiology may be considered a most rewarding specialty to pursue.
- Consultative cardiology affords the opportunity to integrate physiology with physical examination skills in the setting of rapidly developing procedures and techniques, to practice evidence-based medicine in a constantly advancing technological environment, and above all to make a significant difference in the patient and the patient's family.
- There are many reasons why physicians are asked to see a patient with presumed cardiac problems, including atrial fibrillation, elevated cardiac enzymes, an abnormal stress test, heart failure, tachy- or bradycardia, and so on.
- In approaching the patient with potential cardiac issues, it is helpful to understand **the role of the consultant** in this process—that is, to know what makes a "good," effective consultant. Such a consultant should do the following:
  - Define what the referring physician wants from the consultation.
  - Establish urgency.
  - Investigate for himself or herself ("trust but verify").
  - Address the referring physician's concerns.
  - Make specific and succinct recommendations.
  - Include a problem list.
  - Limit the number of recommendations to fewer than six if possible.
  - Call the referring physician.
  - Make a follow-up visit.
- Not all requests for consultation are expressed in a clear manner.
  - In a teaching hospital, consults may be requested by medical students or junior house officers who are unfamiliar with the patient or the issues regarding the consultation.
  - In a community hospital, it may be a nurse or secretary, with even less information about the patient, who requests the consult.
  - Although there are rules for a "good referral," it is up to the consultant both to determine the reason for the consultation and to assess the patient.
- The aforementioned footprint for effective consultation can be modified to apply specifically to the cardiology consultation.
- Following are **some critical questions** that should be answered as quickly as possible, especially in assessing a patient who may be critically ill:
  - Why is the patient being seen?
  - What is the patient's primary problem (often distinct from the above)?
  - What are his or her vital signs right now?
  - Where is the patient right now (home, clinic, patient testing, emergency department, ward, operating room, holding area, intensive care unit [ICU])?
  - How long has the problem been present?
  - What are the important examination findings?
  - What does the electrocardiogram show?

- To help answer these questions, consider the following issues when the patient is evaluated:
  - What diagnostic study, procedure, or therapeutic (medical or surgical) intervention is appropriate for this patient?
  - How soon does he or she need it?
  - Where does this patient need to be now (e.g., floor, ICU) to best receive care?

DIAGNOSIS

- After the above questions have been answered, **workup and management** can begin. Obviously, the amount of time it takes to complete this process, including the history and physical examination, will vary depending on the answers to the above questions.
- The consultant's ability to determine these parameters will develop with knowledge and experience. We hope that this book will serve as a valuable resource for consultant physicians as they care for patients in the myriad clinical situations likely to be encountered.

TREATMENT

- Depending upon the complexity of the situation, an opinion regarding management of the patient with cardiac issues can be reasonably rendered by house officers on the medical service or consult service, a cardiology fellow in training, an internist or hospitalist in private practice, or a board-certified cardiologist.
- Inherent in providing an opinion, however, is an understanding of one's limitations. Although this book may serve as a thorough, useful review of several areas in cardiology—ranging from common clinical presentations, to acute coronary syndromes, to the many faces of heart failure, as well as issues in electrophysiology, valvular disease, and many places in between—it is by no means a substitute for reading the primary literature, reviewing published guidelines, amassing clinical experience, or undertaking advanced cardiology training. To quote Hippocrates: "As to diseases, make a habit of two things—to help, or at least to do no harm."

SUGGESTED READING

Pearson SD. Principles of generalist-specialist relationships. *J Gen Intern Med* 1999; 14:S13-S20.

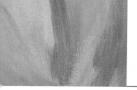

Cardiovascular Physical Examination

2

Justin M. Vader and Alan N. Weiss

GENERAL PRINCIPLES

- The physical examination is fundamental to the assessment and management of patients with known or suspected cardiovascular disease.
- Studies suggests that a physician's physical diagnostic skills have deteriorated over time as the number and scope of diagnostic technologies have increased.
- The purpose of this chapter is to review the importance of physical examination findings in cardiovascular disease and to present the context and evidence for their use.
- Physical findings are rapidly obtained data that may independently have modest effects on disease likelihood, but in aggregate strongly influence clinical diagnosis.

GENERAL PHYSICAL EXAMINATION AND CARDIOVASCULAR DISEASE

- Overall appearance
  - Age, sex, and body habitus are important variables impacting cardiovascular disease risk and significantly influence first impressions of disease likelihood.
  - Findings of generalized distress such as agitation, diaphoresis, and vomiting may suggest states of high sympathetic or vagal tone and may portend worse pathology.
  - Stigmata of past interventions such as prior sternotomy scars, pacemaker or implantable cardioverter defibrillator, vascular access scars, and fistulae are particularly useful in the patient with limited ability to provide history.
  - Cardiovascular pathology is common in a variety of disease syndromes with characteristic examination findings (Table 2-1).
- Ophthalmologic examination
  - A variety of metabolic derangements manifests in corneal, palpebral, and retinal pathology and shares associations with cardiovascular disease.
  - **Corneal arcus** is predictive of cardiovascular disease due mainly via association with increasing age.[1,2]
  - **Xanthelasma palpebrarum** suggests underlying hyperlipidemia.[3]
  - **Diabetic retinopathy**
    - Progression from mild disease with dot-blot hemorrhage, hard exudates, and microaneurysms to moderate disease with "cotton wool" spots to severe disease with neovascularization.
    - There is an independent association between retinopathy, particularly advanced retinopathy, and cardiovascular events,[4] stroke,[5] and heart failure.[6]
  - **Hypertensive retinopathy** is predictive of coronary heart disease. Routine fundoscopy does not appear to be of additional value in the management of chronically hypertensive patients.[7]
- Skin and extremities
  - **Edema**
    - Common but complicated examination finding resulting from the net movement of fluid from the intravascular space to the interstitium.

TABLE 2-1	SYNDROMIC PHYSICAL FINDINGS AND ASSOCIATED CARDIOVASCULAR DISEASE	
Condition	Physical findings	Cardiovascular manifestations
Marfan syndrome	Pectus deformity, arm span > height, legs > torso, pes planus, scoliosis, wrist sign, thumb sign	Bicuspid aortic valve, MVP, aortic aneurysm
Ehlers–Danlos syndrome	Hyperextensible skin, joint hypermobility, atrophic scars, velvety skin, high arching palate	Dysautonomia, MVP, aortic dissection (less than Marfan syndrome)
Loeys–Dietz syndrome	Similar to Marfan plus hypertelorism, bifid uvula	Bicuspid aortic valve, MVP, aortic aneurysm
Turner syndrome	Shield chest, webbed neck, short stature, female	Bicuspid aortic valve, aortic coarctation, anomalous pulmonary venous return
Noonan syndrome	Short stature, pectus excavatum, webbed neck	Pulmonic stenosis, ASD, VSD
LEOPARD syndrome	Multiple lentigines, hypertelorism, short stature, cryptorchidism	Left ventricular hypertrophy, PS, coronary artery dilatation
Fabry disease	Angiokeratomas, corneal clouding, anhidrosis/hyperhidrosis	Hypertension, cardiomyopathy
Down syndrome	Epicanthal fold, small chin, macroglossia, flat nasal bridge, single palmar crease, Brushfield spots	Endocardial cushion defects in 40%, just VSD 30%

MVP, mitral valve prolapse; ASD, atrial septal defect; VSD, ventricular septal defect; PS, pulmonic stenosis.

- May be affected by low-oncotic states, capillary disintegrity, or impaired lymphatic drainage in addition to elevated venous pressures.
- Determine if the jugular pulse suggests elevation of right atrial pressure.
- Assess for stigmata of liver disease, nephrotic syndrome, and venous insufficiency.
- The most common cause of bilateral leg edema is venous insufficiency, affecting 25% to 30% of the general population.[8]
- True anasarca is rare in heart failure.
  ○ Nail bed findings
    - **Capillary refill and nail bed pallor** as an estimate of volume depletion have limited reliability and high interobserver variability in adults.[9]
    - **Digital clubbing** is present in a variety of disorders including cyanotic congenital heart diseases.
      □ Defined by nail fold angle >180°, distal phalangeal depth > proximal depth, and Schamroth sign.
      □ Inspection of all digits for differential signs of clubbing and cyanosis may suggest the presence of vascular abnormalities such as patent ductus arteriosus (PDA).

- ○ Cutaneous manifestations of cardiovascular disease include[10]
  - Janeway lesions, subungual splinter hemorrhages, and Osler nodes of endocarditis
  - Livedo reticularis in cholesterol emboli syndrome
  - Waxy papular rash or "pinch purpura" in amyloidosis
  - Achilles tendon xanthoma in familial hypercholesterolemia
- • Pulmonary examination
  - ○ Respiratory rate and pattern
    - May reflect increased minute ventilation requirements due to metabolic acidosis or a central response to physiologic stress or pain.
    - **Respiratory failure** requiring positive pressure ventilation is not uncommon (3% to 5% of patients) in decompensated heart failure.[11]
    - **Cheyne–Stokes periodic breathing** during sleep is common in congestive heart failure (CHF) with a prevalence of 30% even in well-treated outpatients.[12]
  - ○ Auscultation of the lungs
    - Focused on the search for crackles or wheezes.
    - **Crackles** suggest pulmonary edema and are moderately predictive of heart failure in dyspneic emergency department patients.[13]
    - Cardiogenic pulmonary edema implies a pulmonary capillary wedge pressure (PCWP) of >24 mmHg in acute heart failure or >30 mmHg in chronic heart failure.[14-16]
    - Higher pressures are required to generate pulmonary edema in chronic heart failure due to hypertrophy of lymphatics draining the lungs.[17]
    - **Wheezing** (cardiac asthma) may result from pulmonary edema.[18]
  - ○ Percussion, fremitus, and chest expansion
    - Asymmetry of percussion, tactile fremitus, and chest expansion are useful in detecting **pleural effusions**.[19]
    - Pleural effusions are a common finding in heart failure and may be bilateral or unilateral.
    - Postcardiac injury syndrome with pleural and pericardial effusions may result from myocardial infarction (MI), cardiac surgery, or other cardiac trauma.
- • Abdominal examination
  - ○ Focused on the liver and intra-abdominal vascular structures.
    - **Hepatomegaly** may be the result of chronically elevated right-sided cardiac and central venous pressures.
    - A pulsatile, enlarged liver suggests severe tricuspid regurgitation (TR).
    - **Ascites** may result from passive hepatic congestion in the setting of elevated right-sided pressures or right ventricular (RV) diastolic dysfunction.
    - Cardiac ascites should lead one to consider restrictive or constrictive physiology.

EXAMINATION OF THE ARTERIAL PULSES

- • Pulse characterization
  - ○ Assess pulse contour, timing, strength, volume, size, and symmetry in addition to auscultation for bruits.
  - ○ A basic sequenced approach includes brachial, radial, femoral, popliteal, dorsalis pedis, and posterior tibialis.
  - ○ Changes in the peripheral pulse contour may reflect aortic pathology, changes in cardiac output, or changes in arteriovenous (AV) synchrony (Figure 2-1).
  - ○ **Pulse duration** reflects stroke volume in normal individuals and in patients with heart failure.
    - In heart failure, pulse duration is abbreviated.
    - In aortic stenosis (AS), prolonged ejection reflects worsening severity of stenosis.
    - Slow pulse rise, **pulsus tardus**, in either carotid[20] or radial[21] arteries is suggestive of severe AS.

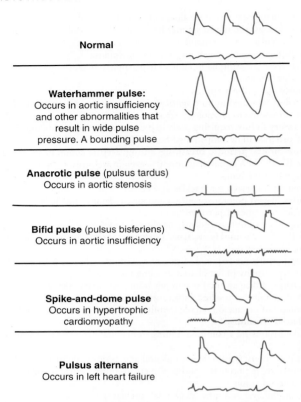

Normal

Waterhammer pulse:
Occurs in aortic insufficiency
and other abnormalities that
result in wide pulse
pressure. A bounding pulse

Anacrotic pulse (pulsus tardus)
Occurs in aortic stenosis

Bifid pulse (pulsus bisferiens)
Occurs in aortic insufficiency

Spike-and-dome pulse
Occurs in hypertrophic
cardiomyopathy

Pulsus alternans
Occurs in left heart failure

FIGURE 2-1. Arterial pulse. (Adapted from Judge RD, Zuidema GD, Fitzgerald FT. *Clinical Diagnosis*, 5th ed. Boston, MA: Little, Brown; 1989:258.)

- **Pulsus alternans** is a common finding in severe left ventricular (LV) dysfunction.
- **Bisferiens (biphasic) pulse** may suggest aortic regurgitation (AR), hypertrophic cardiomyopathy, or sepsis.
- Pulse inequality or pulse delay may be an important clue to aortic or large branch vessel pathology such as aneurysm, dissection, and coarctation.
  - Radial to radial delay suggests subclavian stenosis.
  - Radial to femoral delay suggests aortic coarctation.
- Dorsalis pedis pulses are absent in up to 3% of the population.[22]
- **Allen test** for ulnar artery patency
  - Commonly performed before radial artery cannulation or harvest.
  - Have the patient hold an elevated and clenched fist for 30 seconds with compression applied by the practitioner to the ulnar and radial pulses.
  - After release of the ulnar pulse, this test is 100% sensitive for a nonfunctional ulnar artery if color fails to return at 3 seconds and is most accurate at 5 seconds.[23]
- Abdominal palpation for the presence of an aortic aneurysm. There is good sensitivity for large aneurysms (particularly if >4 cm in size) in patients at risk.[24]

- Arterial bruits
  - Best heard by examination in a quiet room with light pressure on the stethoscope using both diaphragm and bell.
  - **Carotid bruit**
    - Confers a fourfold increase in risk for transient ischemic attack and doubles the risk for both stroke and cardiovascular death.[25,26]
    - Absent in one-third of symptomatic carotid stenosis.[27]
  - **Abdominal bruits**
    - Consider in patients suspected of having renovascular hypertension.
    - Common in normal individuals of all ages.[28]
    - Presence of diastolic *and* systolic bruits is highly specific for renovascular disease.[29]
  - Iliac (periumbilical area), femoral, and popliteal arteries
    - Consider in patients with known or suspected vascular disease.
    - Even in an asymptomatic patient, femoral bruit is suggestive of peripheral vascular disease.[30]

BLOOD PRESSURE MEASUREMENT

- Use proper technique to avoid common errors (Table 2-2).
- Clinically important blood pressure (BP) measurements
  - **Pulsus paradoxus**
    - Greater than 10 mmHg inspiratory decrease in systolic blood pressure (SBP).
    - Inflate the cuff to 20 mmHg above the measured SBP. Decrease pressure very gradually while watching the patient breathe. The pulsus is the difference between pressure where sounds are heard in expiration only and pressure where sounds are heard in both inspiration and expiration.
    - May be observed in a variety of conditions including cardiac tamponade, pericardial constriction (generally effusive–constrictive), myocardial restriction (rare), pulmonary embolus, cardiogenic shock, acute MI, restrictive airways disease, and tension pneumothorax.
    - Pulsus paradoxus >12 mmHg is highly sensitive and moderately specific for **pericardial tamponade** in the setting of pericardial effusion.[31]
  - Pulse pressure (PP) and proportional pulse pressure (PPP)
    - PP reflects the interaction between stroke volume and arterial resistance.
    - PP = SBP – diastolic BP.
    - PPP = PP/SBP.
    - PP is narrow with low stroke volume and in AS.

TABLE 2-2	NKF K/DOQI GUIDELINES FOR BP MEASUREMENT

1. Patient resting 5 minutes in chair with back supported and bare arm at heart level
2. Bladder cuff at least 80% circumference of middle of upper arm
3. Bell of stethoscope 2 cm above antecubital fossa
4. Inflate the cuff to 30 mmHg above palpated SBP. Deflate at 3 mmHg/s.
5. Errors: cuff too small (overestimates BP), cuff too large (underestimates BP), incorrect patient position, rapid cuff deflation, monitor not kept at eye level, inadequate premeasurement rest

SBP, systolic blood pressure; BP, blood pressure.

- PP is wide in high output states (e.g., fever, pregnancy, anemia, thyrotoxicosis, and AV fistula), AR, aortic dissection, and elevated intracranial pressure.
- Narrow PP is associated with worse outcomes in CHF.[32]
- PPP may be used to estimate cardiac index, with a PPP <25% indicating index <2.2 L/m/m^2.[33]
- BP and pulse inequalities
  - Disparate upper extremity BPs are common in the general population with a 20% prevalence of SBP difference >10 mmHg.[34]
  - Obstructive disease is unlikely unless differences are large (>40 mmHg) and consistent.[35]
  - While marked arm–arm or arm–leg differences in BP may be useful in identifying acute aortic dissection, the prevalence in a large registry of dissection was quite low (<20%).[36]
  - Aortic coarctation is an uncommon secondary cause of hypertension in adults. Consider when >20 mmHg differential between arm and leg SBP.

JUGULAR VENOUS PRESSURE ESTIMATES

- Proper technique is essential (Table 2-3).
- May be distinguished from carotid pulsation by
  - Biphasic contour
  - Respiratory and positional variation
  - Disappearance with proximal occlusion
- Distance from the sternal angle to mid-right atrium is 5 cm with the patient at 0 degree and increases to 8–9 cm with partial upright posture.
- Jugular venous pressure (JVP) >3 cm above the sternal angle indicates elevated right atrial pressure.[37]
- External jugular vein examination can be highly reliable even in a critically ill population and may be superior to internal jugular vein observation.[38]
- Conversion of cm H_2O to mmHg is 1.36 to 1.

JUGULAR VENOUS WAVEFORMS

- Waveforms are presented in Figure 2-2.
- Clinically useful in the assessment of a number of conditions including

---

TABLE 2-3	ASSESSING JUGULAR VENOUS PULSE

1. Observe the patient's right internal and external jugular veins by standing on patient's right with tangential light falling across the neck.
2. Rotate patient neck to left 30–45 degrees and avoid over-rotation.
3. Observe rise and fall of venous pulse throughout the respiratory cycle. The height at inspiration estimates right atrial filling pressure.
4. Occlude the venous pulse proximally to differentiate carotid and jugular contours.
5. Move the patient from 0- to 90-degree angle to discern maximal height of venous pulse.
6. External jugular veins may be used if they show respiratory variation and expected venous contour.
7. Right atrial pressure in cm H_2O is estimated by adding 5 cm to height of jugular pulse above the sternal angle of Lewis. Note: 1.36 cm H_2O = 1.0 mmHg.

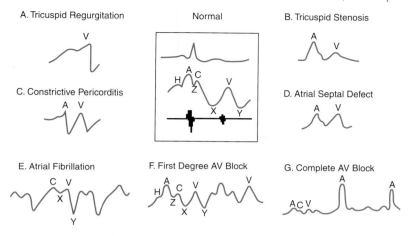

FIGURE 2-2. Pathologic jugular venous waveforms.

- ○ Constriction
- ○ Tamponade
- ○ AV dyssynchrony
- ○ RV infarction
- The basic components of the waveform are
  - ○ A wave: atrial contraction—absent in atrial fibrillation, elevated with decreased RV compliance or tricuspid stenosis, "cannon" in AV dyssynchrony.
  - ○ X descent: atrial diastole—blunted in TR, prominent in tamponade.
  - ○ V wave: atrial venous filling—prominent in TR, and restriction.
  - ○ Y descent: passive ventricular filling—prominent in constriction and restriction, blunted in tamponade.

ABDOMINOJUGULAR (HEPATOJUGULAR) REFLUX

- Hold firm pressure on the right upper quadrant for 15–20 seconds while observing the jugular pulse wave.
- A positive test is defined as >3 cm rise in peak and trough of the wave sustained throughout the period of pressure.
- Manifests in settings where the RV cannot accommodate increased venous return, such as pericardial constriction, restriction, RV infarct, and LV failure with elevated PCWP.
- Highly reproducible, and in dyspneic patients with heart failure, reliably suggests elevated PCWP.[39]

CARDIAC PALPATION

- Place fingertips at left second intercostal space (pulmonary artery), left sternal border (right ventricle), and apex (left ventricle).
- Normal finding: apical impulse is within 10 cm of mid-sternal line, <3 cm in diameter, and duration is <2/3 of systole.
- Noninvasive left ventricular ejection fraction (LVEF) estimate: apical impulse palpation with a nonpalpable S4 and sustained (2/3 systole) apical impulse suggests LVEF <40%.[40]

- Left parasternal heave suggests right ventricular hypertrophy.
- Palpable pulsation in the left second intercostal space suggests pulmonary hypertension.

CARDIAC AUSCULTATION

- Refer to Figure 2-3.
- The stethoscope
  - The diaphragm
    - High-pitched sounds: S1, S2, regurgitant murmurs, and pericardial rubs.
  - The bell
    - Low-pitched sounds: S3, S4, and mitral stenosis (MS).
    - Firm pressure with the bell results in a functional change to the diaphragm.
- Normal heart sounds
  - S1 is produced by vibrations of mitral (M1) and tricuspid (T1) valve closure.
    - Intensity is increased in hypercontractile states, MS, with short PR interval.
    - Intensity is decreased in hypocontractile states, with long PR interval, and in acute AR.
    - Splitting results from late closure of tricuspid valve as in right bundle branch block and atrial septal defect (ASD).
  - S2 is produced by the vibrations of aortic (A2) and pulmonic (P2) valve closure.
    - Aortic pressure normally exceeds pulmonary pressure; thus, A2 precedes P2 and is louder.
    - Increased intensity of A2 is heard in systemic hypertension.
    - Increased intensity of P2 is heard in pulmonary hypertension, accompanied by narrow inspiratory splitting.
    - Decreased S2 intensity may result from AS or pulmonic stenosis (PS).
  - Physiologic splitting of S2: as inspiration causes pulmonary capacitance to increase and LV preload to decrease, A2 occurs earlier and P2 occurs later.

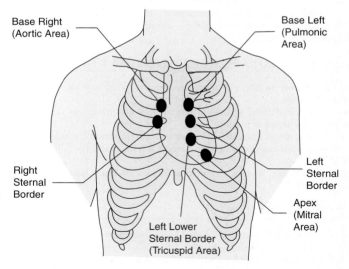

FIGURE 2-3. Cardinal auscultation positions.

- Paradoxical splitting of S2 results when A2 occurs after P2 and inspiration therefore moves these sounds closer together.
    - Causes include left bundle branch block, severe AS, or hypertrophic obstructive cardiomyopathy (HOCM) with left ventricular outflow tract obstruction.
    - Fixed splitting of S2 suggests the presence of an ASD or ventricular pacing.
- Gallops
  - S3 is produced by vibrations from the passive filling phase of ventricular diastole.
    - Left-sided S3 gallops are best heard at the apex using the bell with the patient in left lateral decubitus.
    - Right-sided S3 gallops are best heard at the lower left sternal border upon inspiration.
  - **Physiologically normal S3 may be heard in young, athletic, or pregnant patients**.
  - Left-sided S3
    - Specific for a diagnosis of LV dysfunction and CHF in the acutely ill, dyspneic patient.
    - Confers a worse prognosis in patients with a prior diagnosis of heart failure.[41,42]
    - Indicative of severe regurgitation in the setting of AR, though an absent S3 does not exclude severe AR.[43]
  - Right-sided S3
    - RV dysfunction with high RV filling pressures.
    - May suggest acute pulmonary embolism in the acutely ill patient.
  - S4 is produced by vibrations from the active filling phase of ventricular diastole.
    - Due to decreased ventricular compliance in diastole such as with cardiac hypertrophy.
    - Suggests myocardial ischemia in the setting of acute chest pain.
- Ejection sounds
  - Heard around S1 and results from forceful LV ejection, rapid distension of either aorta or main pulmonary artery, or with doming of either aortic or pulmonic valves.
    - Heard in noncritical and noncalcific stenosis.
    - Pulmonic ejection sounds are unique among right-sided heart tones since they are fainter during inspiration.
- Systolic clicks
  - Result from sudden tensing of elongate atrioventricular valve leaflets and chordae in prolapsed valves.
  - Mitral valve prolapse (MVP)
    - High-pitched sound heard best with the diaphragm at apex or lower left sternal border in mid-to-late systole.
    - Sometimes associated with a murmur of regurgitation.
    - With the strain phase of Valsalva, the click of MVP intensifies and occurs earlier, then softens and occurs later with release.
    - The characteristic click is considered diagnostic for MVP.
    - The presence of a click in the absence of a murmur does not appear to be associated with a worse clinical outcome.[44]
- Murmurs
  - Systolic murmurs may be benign or pathologic. Diastolic murmurs are pathologic.
  - Innocent murmurs[45]
    - Grade 1–2 intensity
    - Left sternal border location
    - Follow a systolic ejection pattern
    - Associated with normal intensity and splitting of S2
    - Associated with no other abnormal sounds or murmurs
    - Echocardiography for evaluation of innocent murmurs not indicated
  - Early systolic murmurs
    - Related to ventricular ejection
    - Differential includes AS, PS, acute MR, outflow tract obstruction

- Aortic stenosis
  - Transmitted to carotids
  - May also be heard as a musical apical (Gallavardin) murmur.
  - Late peaking when associated with decreased intensity of S2 or slow rate of carotid rise.[46]
  - Murmur intensity deceptively reduced in patients with decreased systolic function.
- Pulmonic stenosis
  - Left second intercostal space.
  - Accentuated by inspiration.
  - May be associated with a valve click or other features of right heart hypertrophy or failure.
- HOCM
  - Murmur is less likely to radiate to the carotids.
  - Maneuvers that alter preload and afterload are useful in distinguishing HOCM from AS.
  - Failure of a murmur to accentuate with movement from standing to squatting is suggestive of HOCM.
- Holosystolic murmurs
  - Due to regurgitation across the atrioventricular valves or ventricular septal defect (VSD)
  - Mitral regurgitation
    - Holosystolic when ventricular pressure exceeds atrial pressure throughout systole
    - Radiation to left axilla and back with anterior leaflet disruption
    - Radiation to base with posterior leaflet disruption
    - Murmur intensity is associated with severity of MR[47]
  - TR
    - Low-pitched, sharply defined at lower left sternal border
    - Difficult to detect with coincident MR
    - Inspiratory accentuation
  - VSD
    - Harsh, nonradiating, and associated with a palpable thrill
    - Louder at left sternal border than at apex in acute VSD
    - Decreases in intensity and disappears in late systole as pulmonary hypertension develops[48]
- Late systolic murmurs
  - Variations in MR
- Diastolic clicks and murmurs
  - Mitral stenosis
    - Opening snap in early diastole
    - Brief high-pitched sound using diaphragm at the left sternal border
    - A2 to opening snap interval is not well correlated with valve area.[49]
- Early diastolic murmurs
  - Aortic regurgitation
    - Blowing, decrescendo murmur at the sternal border
    - Accentuated by listening at end expiration with the patient sitting forward
    - Associated systolic flow murmur due to increased stroke volume
    - Late diastolic rumbling murmur at the apex (Austin Flint murmur)
  - Pulmonic regurgitation
    - Similar to the murmur of AR.
    - Distinguished by its accentuation with inspiration

- ○ Late diastolic murmurs
  - Mitral stenosis
    - □ Best heard with the bell at the apex with the patient in lateral decubitus position
    - □ Associated with an opening snap diastolic sound or a loud S1
- ○ Continuous murmurs
  - Most commonly systolic murmurs that carry over into diastole
  - The differential diagnosis includes PDA (pulmonic area), AV fistula, venous hums (e.g., jugular), and vascular stenotic lesions
- ○ Pericardial rub
  - Suggestive of pericarditis
  - "Rough" sounding
  - Characteristically triphasic in patients who are in sinus rhythm, but either biphasic or monophasic in half of the cases[50]
  - Absence of a rub is not sufficient to exclude the diagnosis[51]
- ○ Pericardial knock
  - Easily mistaken for the opening snap of MS
  - Best distinguished by the presence of the jugular venous findings of constrictive pericarditis

A SEQUENTIAL APPROACH

A systematic approach to the physical examination will improve diagnostic yield and accuracy. Such an approach is presented in Table 2-4.

TABLE 2-4	THE SEQUENTIAL APPROACH TO THE CARDIOVASCULAR EXAMINATION
1. Are right-sided cardiac pressures high?	Estimate jugular venous pressure
2. Can the right side handle volume?	Abdominojugular reflux Presence of right-sided S3
3. Is the right ventricle morphologically normal?	RV heave
4. Are pulmonary pressures high?	Loud P2 Narrow split S2 Pulmonary artery tap TR murmur
5. Is left atrial pressure acutely high?	Crackles
6. Is LV function depressed?	Sustained apical impulse Nonpalpable S4 Short pulse duration Soft S1 Presence of S3
7. Is LV compliance impaired?	S4
8. Is systemic vascular resistance high?	Cool extremities

RV, right ventricular; TR, tricuspid regurgitation; LV, left ventricular.

REFERENCES

1. Fernandez AB, Keyes MJ, Penciana M, et al. Relation of corneal arcus to cardiovascular disease (from the Framingham Heart Study data set). *Am J Cardiol* 2009;103(1):64-66.
2. Fernándeza A, Sorokina A, Thompson PD. Corneal arcus as coronary artery disease risk factor. *Atherosclerosis* 2007;193:235-240.
3. Özdöl S, Şahin S, Tokgözoğlu L. Xanthelasma palpebrarum and its relation to atherosclerotic risk factors and lipoprotein (a). *Int J Dermatol* 2008;47:785-789.
4. Cheung N, Wang JJ, Klein R, et al. Diabetic retinopathy and the risk of coronary heart disease: the Atherosclerosis Risk in Communities Study. *Diabetes Care* 2007;30:1742-1746.
5. Cheung N, Rogers S, Couper DJ, et al. Is diabetic retinopathy an independent risk factor for ischemic stroke? *Stroke* 2007;38:398-401.
6. Cheung N, Wang JJ, Rogers SL, et al. Diabetic retinopathy and risk of heart failure. *J Am Coll Cardiol* 2008;51:1573-1578.
7. van den Born BJ, Hulsman CA, Hoekstra JB, et al. Value of routine funduscopy in patients with hypertension: systematic review. *BMJ* 2005;331:73-77.
8. Blankfield RP, Finkelhor RS, Alexander JJ, et al. Etiology and diagnosis of bilateral leg edema in primary care. *Am J Med* 1998;105:192-197.
9. Lewin J, Maconochie I. Capillary refill time in adults. *Emerg Med J* 2008;25:325-326.
10. Uliasz A, Lebwohl M. Cutaneous manifestations of cardiovascular diseases. *Clin Dermatol* 2008;26:243-254.
11. Fonarow GC, Heywood JT, Heidenreich PA, et al. Temporal trends in clinical characteristics, treatments, and outcomes for heart failure hospitalizations, 2002 to 2004: findings from Acute Decompensated Heart Failure National Registry (ADHERE). *Am Heart J* 2007;153:1021-1028.
12. Hagenah G, Beil D. Prevalence of Cheyne–Stokes respiration in modern treated congestive heart failure. *Sleep Breath* 2009;13:181-185.
13. Wang CS, FitzGerald JM, Schulzer M, et al. Does this patient in the emergency department have congestive heart failure? *JAMA* 2005;294:1944-56.
14. Mueller HS, Chatterjee K, Davis KB, et al. Present use of bedside right heart catheterization in patients with cardiac disease. *J Am Coll Cardiol* 1998;32:P840-P864.
15. Sprung CL, Rackow EC, Fein IA, et al. The spectrum of pulmonary edema: differentiation of cardiogenic, intermediate and non-cardiogenic forms of pulmonary edema. *Am Rev Respir Dis* 1981;124:718-722.
16. McHugh TJ, Forrester J, Adler L, et al. Pulmonary vascular congestion in acute myocardial infarction: hemodynamic and radiologic correlations. *Ann Intern Med* 1972;76:29-33.
17. Dumont AE, Clauss RH, Reed GE, et al. Lymph drainage in patients with congestive heart failure. Comparison with findings in hepatic cirrhosis. *N Engl J Med* 1963;269:949-952.
18. Jorge S, Becquemin MH, Delerme S, et al. Cardiac asthma in elderly patients: incidence, clinical presentation and outcome. *BMC Cardiovasc Disord* 2007;7:16.
19. Diaz-Guzman E, Budev MM. Accuracy of the physical examination in evaluating pleural effusion. *Clev Clin J Med* 2008;75:297-303.
20. Aronow WS, Kronzon I. Correlation of prevalence and severity of valvular aortic stenosis determined by continuous-wave Doppler echocardiography with physical signs of aortic stenosis in patients aged 62 to 100 years with aortic systolic ejection murmurs. *Am J Cardiol* 1987;60:399-401.
21. Yoshioka N, Fujita Y, Yasukawa T, et al. Do radial arterial pressure curves have diagnostic validity for identify severe aortic stenosis? *J Anesth* 2010;24:7-10.
22. Chavatzas D. Revision of the incidence of congenital absence of dorsalis pedis artery by an ultrasonic technique. *Anat Rec* 1974;178:289-290.
23. Jarvis MA, Jarvis CL, Jones PR, et al. Reliability of Allen's test in selection of patients for radial artery harvest. *Ann Thorac Surg* 2000;70:1362-1365.
24. Lederle FA, Simel D. Does this patient have abdominal aortic aneurysm? *JAMA* 1999;281:77-82.
25. Pickett CA, Jackson JL, Hemann BA, et al. Carotid bruits and cerebrovascular disease risk: a meta-analysis. *Stroke* 2010;41:2295-2302.
26. Pickett CA, Jackson JL, Hemann BA, et al. Carotid bruits as a prognostic indicator of cardiovascular death and myocardial infarction: a meta-analysis. *Lancet* 2008;371:1587-1594.
27. NASCET Collaborators. Beneficial effect of carotid endarterectomy in symptomatic patients with high-grade carotid stenosis. *N Engl J Med* 1991;325:445-453.

28. Rivin AU. Abdominal vascular sounds. *JAMA* 1972;221:688-690.
29. Grim CE, Luft FC, Weinberger MH, et al. Sensitivity and specificity of screening tests for renal vascular hypertension. *Ann Intern Med* 1979;91:617-622.
30. Criqui MH, Fronek A, Klauber MR, et al. The sensitivity, specificity, and predictive value of traditional clinical evaluation of peripheral arterial disease: results from noninvasive testing in a defined population. *Circulation* 1985;71:516-522.
31. Curtiss EI, Reddy PS, Uretsky BF, et al. Pulsus paradoxus: definition and relation to the severity of cardiac tamponade. *Am Heart J* 1988;115:391-398.
32. Petrie CJ, Voors AA, van Veldhuisen DJ. Low pulse pressure is an independent predictor of mortality and morbidity in non ischaemic, but not in ischaemic advanced heart failure patients. *Int J Cardiol* 2009;131:336-344.
33. Stevenson LW, Perloff JK. The limited reliability of physical signs for estimating hemodynamics in chronic heart failure. *JAMA* 1989;261:884-888.
34. Clark CE, Campbell JL, Evans PH, et al. Prevalence and clinical implications of the inter-arm blood pressure difference: a systematic review. *J Hum Hypertens* 2006;20:923-931.
35. Eguchi K, Yacoub M, Jhalani J, et al. Consistency of blood pressure differences between the left and right arms. *Arch Intern Med* 2007;167:388-393.
36. Hagan PG, Nienaber, Isselbacher EM, et al. The International Registry of Acute Aortic Dissection (IRAD): new insights into an old disease. *JAMA* 2000;283:897-903.
37. Seth R, Magner P, Matzinger F, et al. How far is the sternal angle from the mid-right atrium? *J Gen Intern Med* 2002;17:852-856.
38. Vinayak AG, Levitt J, Gehlbach B, et al. Usefulness of the external jugular vein examination in detecting abnormal central venous pressure in critically ill patients. *Arch Intern Med* 2006;166:2132-2137.
39. Wiese J. The abdominojugular reflux sign. *Am J Med.* 2000;109:59-61.
40. Ranganathan N, Juma Z, Sivaciyan V. The apical impulse in coronary heart disease. *Clin Cardiol* 1985;8:20-33.
41. Drazner MH, Rame JE, Stevenson LW, et al. Prognostic importance of elevated jugular venous pressure and a third heart sound in patients with heart failure. *N Engl J Med* 2001;345:574-581.
42. Wang CS, FitzGerald JM, Schulzer M, et al. Does this dyspneic patient in the emergency department have congestive heart failure? *JAMA* 2005;294:1944-1956.
43. Tribouilloy CM, Enriquez-Sarano M, Mohty D, et al. Pathophysiologic determinants of third heart sounds: a prospective clinical and Doppler echocardiographic study. *Am J Med* 2001;111:96-102.
44. Etchells E, Bell C, Robb K. Does this patient have an abnormal systolic murmur? *JAMA* 1997;277:564-571.
45. American College of Cardiology; American Heart Association Task Force on Practice Guidelines. ACC/AHA 2006 guidelines for the management of patients with valvular heart disease: a report of the American College of Cardiology/American Heart Association Task Force on Practice Guidelines. *J Am Coll Cardiol* 2006;48:e1-e148.
46. Aronow WS, Kronzon I. Correlation of prevalence and severity of valvular aortic stenosis determined by continuous-wave Doppler echocardiography with physical signs of aortic stenosis in patients aged 62 to 100 years with aortic systolic ejection murmurs. *Am J Cardiol* 1987;60:399-401.
47. Desjardins VA, Enriquez-Sarano M, Tajik AJ, et al. Intensity of murmurs correlates with severity of valvular regurgitation. *Am J Med* 1996;100:149-156.
48. Bleifer S, Donoso E, Grishman A. The auscultatory and phonocardiographic signs of ventricular septal defects. *Am J Cardiol* 1960;5:191-198.
49. Ebringer R, Pitt A, Anderson ST. Haemodynamic factors influencing opening snap interval in mitral stenosis. *Br Heart J* 1970;32:350-354.
50. Spodick DH. Pericardial rub. Prospective, multiple observer investigation of pericardial friction in 100 patients. *Am J Cardiol* 1975;35:357-362.
51. Zayas R, Anguita M, Torres F, et al. Incidence of specific etiology and role of methods for specific etiologic diagnosis of primary acute pericarditis. *Am J Cardiol* 1995;75:378-382.

Basic Electrocardiography   3

Phillip S. Cuculich and John Verbsky

GENERAL PRINCIPLES

- In general, the electrocardiogram (ECG) may be the single most important and widely used test in the hospital, yet ECG interpretation is usually poorly taught in medical school. There are large gaps in time between each lesson, and ECG basics may never be taught that well in the first place. This chapter is not meant to bridge those gaps of to be a complete guide to ECG reading. It is an "in the trenches" practical guide to coming close to a diagnosis, with the ultimate goal of helping you with high-pressure ECG analysis at 2 AM on call.
- Three very important pieces of advice will serve you well:
  - **Practice, practice, practice.** Invest in a book of unknown ECG tracings with answers. Do online tutorials. Look at ECGs from patients on a cardiology service. Avoid the gaps in time that plagued your learning in medical school.
  - **Same way every time.** By using the same approach with every ECG, you will become efficient and accurate. More importantly, you will be less likely to miss subtle diagnoses.
  - **Keep a file** of interesting ECGs. By collecting interesting ECGs, you maintain a sense of interest and vigilance. You will begin to recognize certain patterns of disease. Additionally, it will help to have the collection when you are asked to give a conference on short notice.

DIAGNOSIS

The Practical Five-Step Method: Rate, Rhythm, Axis, Intervals, Injury

- **Rate: Give a Number**
  - Two useful, easy methods of determining the ventricular rate include
    - Rely on the computer and look in the upper-left-hand corner of the ECG (risky, but often correct).
    - Memorize the R-R interval distance chant: **"300, 150, 100, 75, 60, 50 ... ."** If the distance between two QRS complexes is four big boxes, the ventricular rate is (chant silently: 300, 150, 100) **75** beats per minute (bpm).
    - Common numbers to know:
      - □ 60 to 100 bpm: sinus rhythm.
      - □ 40 to 60 bpm: junctional escape rhythm.
      - □ 35 bpm: ventricular escape rhythm.
      - □ 150 bpm: atrial flutter with 2:1 conduction.
- **Rhythm: Sinus or Otherwise?** (Figure 3-1)
  - Let us think about the physiology of one normal sinus beat. The impulse starts from the sinus node and depolarizes both atria (forming the P wave) and then activates the atrioventricular (AV) node, and after some time (this time represents the PR interval), the ventricle depolarizes in a coordinated fashion, using the His-Purkinje system (forming the QRS complex). When determining the rhythm on an ECG, your eyes should follow the same path as the heartbeat: P wave ... PR interval ... QRS complex.

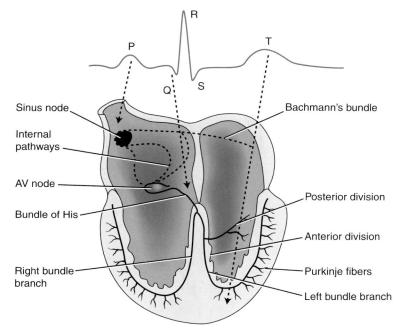

FIGURE 3-1. Rhythm: ECG components of a single sinus beat with anatomic correlation. The P wave reflects atrial activation from the sinus node. The PR interval is the time during which the signal is passing through the AV node. The narrow QRS complex represents the coordinated ventricular activation through the His-Purkinje system. The T wave signifies ventricular repolarization.

- ○ A normal sinus P wave is regularly occurring. There should be one P wave for every QRS (one for one).
- ○ Significant variation in P-wave regularity or shape can imply causes such as an ectopic atrial tachycardia or multifocal atrial tachycardia. Absence of a P wave usually means atrial fibrillation, although atrial standstill can occur with severe hyperkalemia.
- ○ The PR interval represents conduction through the AV node. If the PR interval is changing, some type of AV block is often to blame.
- ○ A narrow QRS (<120 milliseconds, three small boxes) implies that the ventricle is being activated through the AV node. A QRS should follow every P wave. If the QRS is wide (>120 milliseconds), it may be that there is slow conduction in the ventricle (left bundle branch block [LBBB] or right bundle branch block [RBBB] or idioventricular conduction delay) or that the beat is coming from the ventricle, such as a premature ventricular contraction or ventricular tachycardia. Figure 3-1 links these concepts visually with the anatomy of the heart for a better understanding. Determination of the rhythm should rely on the simple concept of the physiology of a heartbeat and not on rote memorization.
- • **Axis: Up in Lead I, Up in Lead II** (Figure 3-2)
  - ○ "Axis" is the major direction of the heart's depolarization. Normal direction is inferior and to the patient's left (−30 degrees to +90 degrees).

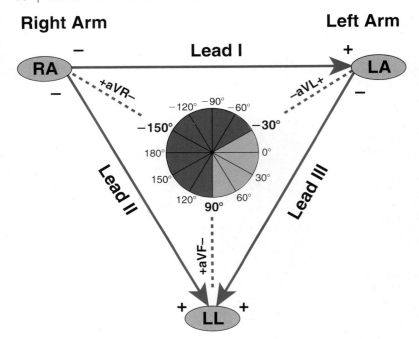

FIGURE 3-2. Axis: Einthoven triangle and normal QRS axis (–30 degrees to + 90 degrees). (From Yanowitz FG, Alan E. Lindsay ECG Learning Center. University of Utah: Intermountain Healthcare, with permission. http://library.med.utah.edu/kw/ecg.)

- ○ Determining if an axis is normal requires looking in two leads: lead I and lead II. In Figure 3-2, lead I runs across the top of the diagram, from the patient's right to his/her left. If the QRS is predominantly positive in lead I, the electrical signal is heading in the direction of lead I or toward the patient's left (anywhere from –90 degrees to +90 degrees). In the same way, we can look at lead II. If it is predominantly positive, we know that the electrical signal is heading in the direction of lead II or leftward and inferior (anywhere from –30 degrees to 150 degrees).
- ○ If the QRS is positive in **both** lead I and lead II, the axis must be in the area where the two leads overlap, which is the normal axis between –30 degrees and +90 degrees (Figure 3-2).
- ○ If the QRS is mostly up in lead I and down in lead II, what is the axis? Well, the signal is moving from the patient's right to his/her left, but now in the opposite direction of lead II. This puts the axis between –30 degrees and –90 degrees, so the answer is left axis deviation (LAD). How about if the QRS is down in lead I and up in lead II? Answer: It is between +90 degrees and +150 degrees or right axis deviation (RAD).
- **Intervals: Shape and Width** (Figure 3-3)
  - ○ P waves: Looking for **left atrial enlargement** (LAE) in V1 (normal is biphasic, and abnormal has a large negative component) and right atrial enlargement (RAE) in lead II (two little boxes wide by two little boxes tall ... 2 × 2 in lead II).
  - ○ PR interval: A normal PR interval is 200 milliseconds (five little boxes).

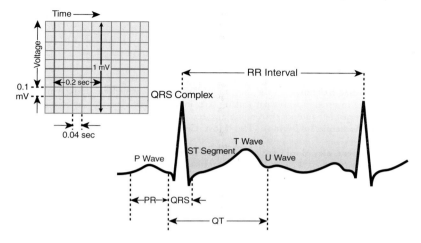

FIGURE 3-3. Intervals: Defining the intervals and segments on the ECG and identifying specific pathology to look for in each interval or segment. (From Yanowitz, FG. Alan E. Lindsay ECG Learning Center. University of Utah: Intermountain Healthcare, with permission. http://library.med.utah.edu/kw/ecg.) **P wave size:** Look for atrial enlargement (LAE in V1, RAE in lead II). **PR interval:** Look for AV block (PR >200 milliseconds) or ventricular pre-excitation (PR <40 milliseconds). **QRS size:** Large voltage suggests LVH, and small voltage suggests pericardial effusion. **QRS interval:** Wide QRS (>120 milliseconds) signifies a poorly coordinated beat due to LBBB, RBBB, IVCD, or ventricular beats. **QT interval:** LQT intervals can be due to many causes, including "hypos," "antis," congenital syndromes, intracerebral hemorrhage, or cardiac ischemia (see text).

- If the PR interval is long, varies between beats, or does not conduct to every QRS complex, some form of **AV block** is to blame.
- A short PR interval (<40 milliseconds) suggests the presence of an accessory AV connection, known as **Wolff-Parkinson-White (WPW) syndrome**.
  ○ **QRS** interval (width) and QRS height:
    - Width: Normally QRS width ranges between 80 and 120 milliseconds. If it is >120 milliseconds, see above (LBBB, RBBB, intraventricular conduction delay [IVCD], ventricular in origin).
    - Height: **Left ventricular hypertrophy** (LVH) can give large voltages. There are many criteria for determining LVH, but a commonly used one adds the depth of lead V1 with the height of leads V5 or V6 (>35 mV is LVH). Small voltages (<5 mV in the limb leads, <10 mV in the precordial leads) can happen when a poorly conductive material gets between the heart and the ECG lead, such as air (hyperinflated lungs in chronic obstructive pulmonary disease), water (pericardial effusion), or fat.
  ○ **QT interval**: The QT interval should be corrected for the underlying heart rate by using the formula QTc = QT (milliseconds)/square root of R-R interval (seconds).
    - Normal QTc is 440 milliseconds for men and 460 milliseconds for women. The ECG machine generally does a good job of measuring and calculating this for you. However, especially in situations where prolonged QTc may be a concern, there is no substitute for determining the QT interval yourself.

- Long QT (LQT) is associated with torsade de pointes, a potentially lethal ventricular rhythm. The five causes of LQT can be grouped into:
  - **Hypos**: hypokalemia, hypomagnesemia, hypothermia.
  - **Antis**: antibiotics, antiarrhythmics, antihistamines, antipsychotics.
  - **Congenital**: LQT syndromes (see Chapter 20).
  - **Intracerebral hemorrhage**: diffuse, deep, symmetric, large inverted T waves.
  - **Cardiac ischemia**: "in the form of Wellen's waves," which are deep, symmetric, large inverted T waves particularly seen in V1 to V3, classically associated with proximal left anterior descending disease.
- **Injury (Ischemia/Infarction): The Most Common Reason to Order an ECG** (Figure 3-4)
  - **ST-segment elevation:** classically described in acute myocardial infarction (MI), although it can be seen in LVH, pericarditis, and ventricular aneurysms. Note that ST elevation is best termed an **acute injury pattern** until Q waves (see below) have developed. The criteria for MI require >1 mm elevation in two contiguous limb leads or >2 mm in two contiguous precordial leads.

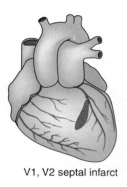

V1, V2 septal infarct

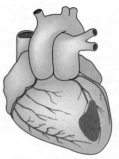

V3, V4 anterior infarct

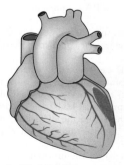

I. aVL, V5, V6 lateral infarct

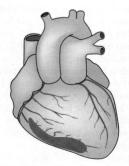

II, III aVF inferior infarct

FIGURE 3-4. Injury: ECG leads and coronary artery distributions. ST-segment elevations in specific leads reflect a myocardial injury (infarction or ischemia) in certain anatomic locations, as shown.

- ○ **ST-segment depression**: classically described with myocardial ischemia, although it can be seen in LVH, digoxin toxicity, and WPW syndrome. ST depressions can represent ST elevations on the opposite side of the heart, known as reciprocal changes.
- ○ **T-wave inversions**: nonspecific, though Wellen's waves are more suspicious for ischemia.
- ○ **Q waves**: signify a prior infarct that has subsequently developed scar.
- ○ The distribution of the particular findings should be noted, as changes consistent throughout a specific coronary artery territory are more likely to indicate a true ischemic finding (Figure 3-4).
  - ▪ Inferior (usually right coronary artery territory): leads II, III, aVF.
  - ▪ Anterior (usually left anterior descending territory): leads V2 to V4.
  - ▪ Lateral (usually left circumflex artery territory): leads V5 to V6, I, aVL.
- • **Put It All Together**
  - ○ When you are initially learning how to read an ECG, talk out loud and say what you see.
  - ○ **Rate/Rhythm/Axis**: "The rate is (300, 150, 100) about 75 and the rhythm is sinus. Axis is up in I and down in II, so LAD."
  - ○ **Intervals**: "P waves are normal in shape, so there's no atrial enlargement. PR interval is 220 milliseconds, so it is a first-degree AV block. QRS is 100 milliseconds, which is normal. No LVH. QTc interval is 410 milliseconds, which is normal."
  - ○ **Injury**: "I do not see any ST elevation or depressions, but there are Q waves in II, III, and aVF, so probably an old inferior myocardial infarct."
  - ○ Practice will make perfect, so this chapter concludes with several unknown ECG tracing (Figures 3-5 through 3-8 with answers). Please try out the *rate, rhythm, axis, interval, injury* method.

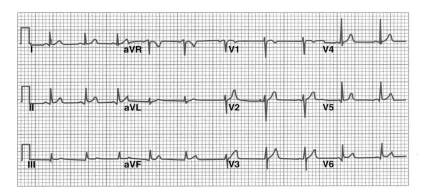

FIGURE 3-5. ECG for interpretation. (From Yanowitz, FG. Alan E. Lindsay ECG Learning Center. University of Utah: Intermountain Healthcare, with permission. http://library.med.utah.edu/kw/ecg.) **Rate:** 75 beats per minute. **Rhythm:** Sinus (seen best in V1 or lead II). **Axis:** Normal (up in lead I and lead II). **Intervals:** P waves normal; PR interval normal (<200 milliseconds, five small boxes); QRS normal (<120 milliseconds, three small boxes wide); no LVH; QT interval normal. **Injury**: No significant ST elevations or depressions. **Putting it together:** Normal ECG.

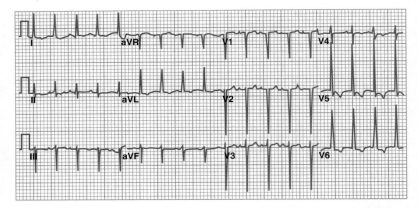

FIGURE 3-6. ECG for interpretation. (From Yanowitz, FG. Alan E. Lindsay ECG Learning Center. University of Utah: Intermountain Healthcare, with permission. http://library.med.utah.edu/kw/ecg). **Rate**: 80 beats per minute. **Rhythm**: Sinus (lead V1). **Axis**: Positive in lead I and II. **Intervals**: P waves are biphasic with a large negative component. QRS narrow. QT interval is prolonged. **Injury**: No significant ST elevations or depressions. **Putting it all together**: Normal sinus rhythm with LAE and a prolonged QT interval.

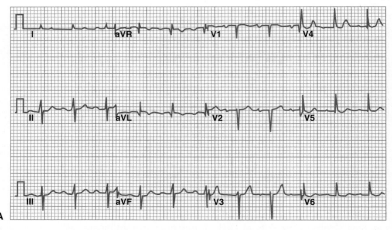

A

FIGURE 3-7. ECG for interpretation. (From Yanowitz FG, Alan E. Lindsay ECG Learning Center. University of Utah: Intermountain Healthcare, with permission. http://library.med.utah.edu/kw/ecg.) **Rate**: 44 beats per minute. **Rhythm**: Sinus. **Axis**: Normal axis. **Intervals**: PR interval is prolonged (first-degree AV block). Normal QRS size and width. Prolonged QT interval. **Injury**: No significant ST elevation or depression. **Putting it all together**: Sinus bradycardia with first-degree AV block and a prolonged QT interval.

Lead II

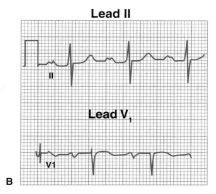

B

FIGURE 3-7. (*Continued*)

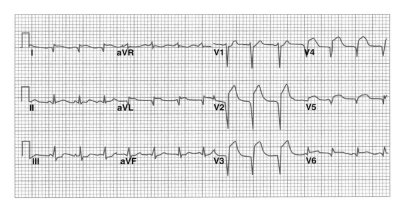

FIGURE 3-8. ECG for interpretation. (From Yanowitz FG, Alan E. Lindsay ECG Learning Center. University of Utah: Intermountain Healthcare, with permission. http://library.med.utah.edu/kw/ecg.) **Rate**: 80 beats per minute. **Rhythm**: Sinus. **Axis**: RAD (down in lead I, up in lead II). **Intervals**: Normal P waves and PR interval. QRS normal height and width. QT interval prolonged. **Injury**: ST elevations in leads V2 to V6 and leads I and aVL. ST depressions in leads III and aVF. Q waves in leads V2 to V6 and leads I and aVL. **Putting it all together**: Anterior–lateral ST-segment MI.

SUGGESTED READINGS

Dubin D. *Rapid Interpretation of EKGs*, 6th ed. Tampa, FL: Cover Publishing; 2000.

O'Keefe JH, Hammill S. *The ECG Criteria Book*, 2nd ed. Royal Oak, MI: Physician's Press; 2002.

Surawicz B, Knilans T, eds. *Chou's Electrocardiography in Clinical Practice*, 5th ed. Philadelphia, PA: Saunders; 2001.

Yanowitz, FG. Alan E. *Lindsay ECG Learning Center*. http://library.med.utah.edu/kw/ecg. Last accessed 15 May 2013.

Evaluation of Acute Chest Pain

4

Christopher L. Holley

GENERAL PRINCIPLES

- Acute presentations of chest pain represent a wide spectrum of disease, from benign to life-threatening conditions. As such, the initial evaluation must focus on ruling out **the five most common life-threatening conditions** that present acutely with chest pain:
  - Acute coronary syndrome (ACS), including acute myocardial infarction (AMI)
  - Aortic dissection
  - Pulmonary embolism (PE)
  - Cardiac tamponade
  - Tension pneumothorax
- In following with Dr. W. Proctor Harvey's "five-fingered" approach to cardiac diagnosis, the accurate and rapid triage of patients with chest pain includes **focused history, directed physical examination, electrocardiogram (ECG), chest X-ray (CXR), and appropriate laboratory studies**.
- General appearance should be assessed immediately to identify patients who are critically ill. Patients who are pale, diaphoretic, anxious, and ill-appearing require immediate attention, including hemodynamic assessment, ECG, and CXR. Hemodynamically unstable patients should be evaluated and stabilized per the advanced cardiac life support protocol.

Definition

- The words "chest pain" may be a patient's specific symptomatic complaint (e.g., "I am having chest pain"), but they are more broadly used by health care providers in reference to a variety of presentations involving complaints of discomfort in the chest region.
- Much of the uncertainty in this term comes from the fact that patients have a broad interpretation of what constitutes the "chest" (patients often include the upper abdomen) and how they describe their discomfort (which may not include the word "pain").

Epidemiology

- Chest pain accounts for 9% to 10% of adult noninjury emergency department (ED) visits every year (5.5 million visits for 2007–2008). Of those visits, 13% of presentations were diagnosed as ACS, but up to 54% of ED visits chest pain can be classified as "serious cardiovascular disease" (including ACS, AMI, PE, and heart failure).[1]
- Chest pain accounts for a smaller percent of outpatient visits (1% to 2%), and the majority of etiologies in that setting are musculoskeletal or gastrointestinal (GI).[2]

DIAGNOSIS

Clinical Presentation

History

- Emphasis should be placed on **rapidly and accurately characterizing the current episode of chest pain**.
- A simple, ECG-related mnemonic of "PQRST" can provide the framework for a focused history: presentation, quality, radiation, symptoms, and timing (Table 4-1). This method

TABLE 4-1	**RAPID CHARACTERIZATION OF CHEST PAIN ("PQRST")**

	Questions and considerations	LR for AMI
P = Presentation	"Are you having pain right now?" Ongoing pain requires especially rapid diagnosis and treatment. "What were you doing when the pain started?" (exercise/stressful situation vs. resting/sleeping)	Exertional pain: LR = 2.4
Q = Quality	"How would you describe the pain?" Classic description of ischemic pain is "pressure," while "sharp" (knifelike) pain is less likely to be ischemia; if known coronary artery disease, is this pain worse than the patient's typical angina or same as prior MI? Is the pain pleuritic, positional, or reproducible on palpation? ("3 P's")	"Pressure": LR = 1.3 Worse than patient's typical angina, or similar to prior AMI: LR = 1.8 "Sharp": LR = 0.3 **P**leuritic, **p**ositional, or reproducible on **p**alpation: LR = 0.3
R = Radiation	"Point to where the pain is." "Does it go anywhere else?" Pain radiating to shoulders or arms is more likely to be ischemic; think about aortic dissection with pain radiating to the back	Right arm or shoulder: LR = 4.73 Both arms or shoulders: LR = 4.1 Left arm only: LR = 2.3
S = Symptoms	"When you were having the pain, did you feel sick to your stomach, sweaty, or short of breath?" ("3 S's")	Nausea or vomiting: LR = 1.9 Diaphoresis: LR = 2
T = Timing	"How long did the pain last?" Seconds, minutes, hours, days? Single or multiple episodes? Fleeting CP is rarely ischemic. Classic ischemia pattern is crescendo over several minutes (2–10 minutes for angina pectoris, 10–30 minutes for unstable angina); for sudden onset of maximal pain, think aortic dissection; pain >30 minutes is either MI (infarction, not just ischemia) or nonischemic (most often GI/esophageal)	Pain that is **not** of sudden onset lowers likelihood of aortic dissection, negative LR = 0.3

Confounders: diabetes, women, and elderly patients (reduced accuracy of diagnosis).

LRs from Klompas[3] and Swap and Nagurney.[4]

LR, likelihood ratio; AMI, acute myocardial infarction; CP, cerebral palsy; MI, myocardial infarction; GI, gastrointestinal.

uses evidence-based medicine to elicit aspects of the history that can raise (or lower) your suspicion for a presentation of AMI.

- **High-risk features for AMI include** exertional chest pressure radiating to shoulders/ arms, with associated nausea, vomiting, diaphoresis, or worse than the patient's typical angina (or similar to prior AMI pain). The absence of these features does not reduce the likelihood of AMI.
- Findings that have a lower risk for AMI include pain that is "sharp" (stabbing), pleuritic, positional, or reproducible on palpation.
- Confounding features that reduce the accuracy of diagnosing ACS include diabetes, female sex, and advanced age.
- Be sure also to remember that while ACS is the most common life-threatening presentation of chest pain, it is not the only presentation that requires urgent attention. Certain aspects of the history will help you recognize patients at high risk for other chest pain etiologies. For example, the likelihood of aortic dissection is increased with an abrupt onset of maximally intense pain, while the likelihood of acute PE is increased in patients with prior venous thromboembolism, malignancy, and recent surgery or immobilization.

Physical Examination

- Based on the information obtained in the history, the directed examination should be used to confirm or refute a suspected diagnosis or at least narrow the differential diagnosis list.
- Much like the focused history, a directed examination should rapidly and accurately characterize the chest pain and screen for life-threatening findings. Most of the few minutes spent examining the patient should be focused on the cardiovascular and pulmonary examinations.
- Clinical pearls for a chest pain–directed examination are listed in Table 4-2.

TABLE 4-2	CHEST PAIN–DIRECTED PHYSICAL EXAMINATION WITH SPECIFIC CLINICAL PEARLS
Blood pressure	• Check both arms, especially if considering aortic dissection
	• Severe hypertension and hypotension require urgent intervention
	• Pulsus paradoxus: drop of >10 mmHg in SBP at end inspiration (tamponade)
Jugular veins	• Start with patient reclined at 45 degrees. Patients with significantly elevated JVP may need to be sitting up at 90 degrees before the jugular venous pulse can be seen
	• Hepatojugular reflux: sustained distention of jugular veins with pressure on abdomen (heart failure)
	• Kussmaul sign: elevation (or lack of decrease) in JVP with inspiration (constriction)
Carotid arteries	• Palpation for stroke volume: normal carotid upstroke unlikely in severe LV dysfunction or AS
	• Pulsus parvus et tardus: weak and late pulse (AS)

TABLE 4-2	CHEST PAIN–DIRECTED PHYSICAL EXAMINATION WITH SPECIFIC CLINICAL PEARLS (*Continued*)
Palpation	• Laterally displaced PMI (dilated LV) • RV heave (right-sided heart failure)
Heart sounds	• S3 (heart failure) • S4 (HTN and/or heart failure; never heard with atrial fibrillation) • Friction rub (pericarditis)
Murmurs	• Acute AR or MR may not have a murmur • AS: Crescendo–decrescendo systolic murmur, loudest at RUSB, commonly with radiation to the carotids when severe • AR: diastolic murmur; always pathologic (endocarditis, dissection) • MR: systolic blowing murmur loudest at apex (ischemia, LV dilation) • VSD: harsh, loud holosystolic murmur (3–8 days after septal MI)
Pulmonary	• Crackles/rales (atelectasis, pneumonia, pulmonary edema) • Wheezing (usually bronchospasm, but sometimes heart failure) • Absent breath sounds with tracheal deviation away from affected side (tension pneumothorax) • Decreased breath sounds, dullness to percussion (pneumonia and/or pleural effusion)
Musculoskeletal	• Pain that is reproducible on examination is rarely cardiac in nature • Dermatomal rash with pain (herpes zoster)
Abdominal	• Hepatomegaly, pulsatile liver, and ascites (heart failure) • Epigastric pain with palpation (PUD or pancreatitis) • RUQ pain (cholecystitis)
Extremities	• Cool extremities (poor cardiac output or occlusive ischemic event if unilateral) • Pitting edema (volume overload)

SBP, systolic blood pressure; JVP, jugular venous pressure; LV, left ventricular; AS, aortic stenosis; PMI, point of maximum impulse; RV, right ventricular; HTN, hypertension; AR, aortic regurgitation; MR, mitral regurgitation; MI, myocardial infarction; RUSB, right upper sternal border; PUD, peptic ulcer disease; RUQ, right upper quadrant; VSD, ventricular septal defect.

Differential Diagnosis

- The differential diagnosis of acute chest pain should begin with consideration of life-threatening conditions, as noted previously: ACS, aortic dissection, PE, cardiac tamponade, and tension pneumothorax.
- When it is clear that the patient is at lower risk and does not have a life-threatening condition, a broader differential diagnosis should include:
  - Cardiac: stable angina, pericarditis, coronary vasospasm, and decompensated heart failure.
  - Pulmonary: pneumonia, pleuritis, and chronic obstructive pulmonary disease.
  - GI: gastroesophageal reflux disease, peptic ulcer disease, esophagitis, pancreatitis, and cholecystitis.
  - Neuromusculoskeletal: costochondritis, injury of the pectoralis or intercostal muscle, and herpes zoster.
  - Psychiatric: panic attack, anxiety disorder, and chronic pain syndromes.

Diagnostic Testing

- The ECG is the most critical diagnostic test when evaluating acute chest pain—it is rapid and can be diagnostic for detecting ACS. It should be completed within 10 minutes for patients presenting to the ED with chest pain.
- The CXR is also rapid, is readily available, and gives useful information that can help diagnose the other potentially life-threatening causes of chest pain.
- Serum cardiac biomarker (troponin, creatinine kinase fraction) levels are also a critical aspect of the evaluation, but may take up to an hour to be reported by the laboratory.

Laboratories

- If there is concern for ACS, serum **cardiac biomarker** levels should be measured.
- At our institution, initial troponin levels are drawn at the time when the patient presents for evaluation. Because the elevation of serum troponin lags behind an ischemic event by at least several hours, a repeat troponin should be obtained 6–12 hours after the onset of pain. **Two negative tests 8 hours apart are usually sufficient to rule out a myocardial infarction (MI).**
- Conversely, **a single positive troponin in the appropriate clinical setting is sufficient to make the diagnosis of AMI**.
- Because troponin levels stay elevated for several days after an infarct, they are less useful with recurrent chest pain in the days after an initial infarction. In that case, Creatine kinase-MB fraction (CK-MB) or myoglobin levels are useful for diagnosing reinfarction in patients with a recent MI. They both have a shorter serum half-life than troponin and will therefore rise and fall with recurrent ischemic episodes.
- For patients with a high-risk presentation for ACS, additional blood work should include complete blood count, basic metabolic profile, international normalized ratio, and partial thromboplastin time (in anticipation of systemic anticoagulation and possible cardiac catheterization thrombolytic therapy). For patients with a low to intermediate pretest risk of PE, a negative D-dimer is associated with a very low likelihood of PE. If a GI etiology is suspected, appropriate serum tests should be obtained (such as amylase/lipase and liver function tests).

Electrocardiography

- The ECG is of utmost importance in the evaluation of chest pain and should be completed within 10 minutes for patients presenting to the ED with chest pain. For the acutely ill patient, it is prudent to quickly review the ECG prior to completing the history and physical examination.

TABLE 4-3	ECG FINDINGS RELEVANT TO EVALUATION OF CHEST PAIN
ST-segment elevations	• Any ST elevation in the patient with chest pain is suspicious. • Typical ischemic ST elevation has a convex ("tombstone") appearance in two or more adjacent leads with reciprocal ST depressions. • Diffuse ST elevations with PR depression and/or ST depression in aVR suggest pericarditis in the appropriate clinical scenario.
New LBBB	• ST elevation "equivalent" in the appropriate clinical scenario.
ST-segment depression	• Flat or down-sloping ST depressions are concerning for ischemia. • Specificity of ST depression for ischemia is significantly lower in patients with evidence of prior MI (Q waves) or baseline ST abnormalities.
T-wave inversions	• Not specific, but may be first indicator of ischemia.
S1Q3T3	• S wave in I, Q wave and inverted T wave in III: can be seen with PE or right heart strain.

ECG, electrocardiogram; LBBB, left bundle branch block; MI, myocardial infarction; PE, pulmonary embolism.

• ECG findings that should not be missed are outlined in Table 4-3 and further discussed in Chapters 2 and 18. **A normal ECG does not rule out ACS. ST elevations do not always indicate AMI.**
• Prior ECGs for comparison are invaluable.
• If ischemia is a concern, serial ECGs are useful to look for evolving changes.
• Suspicion for a right ventricular infarct should be investigated with right-sided precordial leads, and suspicion for a posterior infarct should prompt evaluation with posterior chest leads.

Imaging
• The **CXR** complements the ECG by screening for many of the life-threatening conditions that the ECG fails to identify. These include:
   ○ Aortic dissection (widened mediastinum)
   ○ Heart failure (pulmonary edema)
   ○ Pericardial effusion (enlargement of the heart shadow)
   ○ Pneumothorax (free air in the thorax, usually at the apices in an upright patient)
   ○ Pulmonary infiltrates (pneumonia)
   ○ PE (Hampton hump: peripherally based, wedge-shaped infarction)
   ○ GI perforation (free air beneath the diaphragm)
• Suspected aortic dissection should be confirmed with appropriate imaging (transesophageal echocardiography, computed tomography [CT], or magnetic resonance imaging).
• Suspected PE can be evaluated by CT angiography or ventilation/perfusion (V/Q) scan.

- Coronary CT angiography may be useful in the ED for the evaluation of chest pain when the primary concern is ACS, if there are no signs of ischemia on ECG and if the initial troponin is not positive.[5]

Diagnostic Procedures

- Cardiac catheterization should be performed emergently for patients presenting with apparent ST-segment elevation myocardial infarction (STEMI).
- For presentations of non-STEMI ACS, medical therapy should be started immediately (see Chapter 11). Diagnostic cardiac catheterization may be delayed if necessary in accordance with guidelines.
- Patients presenting with PE should undergo venous ultrasonography of the lower extremities to evaluate for venous thrombus.

TREATMENT

- If one of the five most common life-threatening causes of chest pain is identified, an emergent treatment plan should be enacted:
  - STEMI requires rapid reestablishment of coronary blood flow (intravenous thrombolytic therapy or percutaneous coronary intervention) (see Chapter 12). Non-STEMI ACS should be initially treated medically, including aspirin, thienopyridine, statin, and systemic anticoagulation (see Chapter 11).
  - Cardiac tamponade is managed with pericardiocentesis (see Chapters 8 and 17).
  - Type A aortic dissections require emergent surgical consultation and repair (see Chapter 29).
  - Tension pneumothorax requires immediate needle decompression followed by chest tube placement.
  - PE should be treated with systemic anticoagulation unless contraindicated. Thrombolytic therapy should be reserved for patients with hemodynamic compromise.
- Other diagnoses should also be managed with the appropriate standard of care.

REFERENCES

1. Bhuiya FA, Pitts SR, McCaig LF. Emergency department visits for chest pain and abdominal pain: United States, 1999–2008. *NCHS Data Brief* 2010;43:1-8.
2. Cayley WE Jr. Diagnosing the cause of chest pain. *Am Fam Physician* 2005;72:2012-2021.
3. Klompas M. Does this patient have an acute thoracic aortic dissection? *JAMA* 2002;287: 2262-2272.
4. Swap CJ, Nagurney JT. Value and limitations of chest pain history in the evaluation of patients with suspected acute coronary syndromes. *JAMA* 2005;294:2623-2629.
5. Hoffman U, Truong QA, Schoenfeld DA, et al. Coronary CT angiography versus standard evaluation in acute chest pain. *N Engl J Med* 2012;367:299-308.

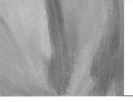

Evaluation of Acute Heart Failure

Kory J. Lavine and Joel D. Schilling

GENERAL PRINCIPLES

- Heart failure (HF) is a common clinical syndrome with significant morbidity and mortality. Early detection can lead to initiation of appropriate lifesaving and symptom-reducing therapies.
- Ischemic cardiomyopathy (ICM) is the most common cause of HF with reduced left ventricular (LV) ejection fraction. Hypertension, diabetes, obesity, and coronary artery disease (CAD) play a contributory role in HF with preserved systolic function (PSF).
- The three primary objectives of the history and physical examination are to (1) identify the cause of HF, (2) assess the progression and severity of the illness, and (3) assess volume status.
- A mnemonic for the causes of HF decompensation is "Patients who are frequently admitted for HF exacerbations often VANISH."
- To guide treatment decisions, the physician's goal is to classify the patient as having one of three common clinical phenotypes: (1) "flash" pulmonary edema with hypertension (HTN), (2) slowly progressive fluid accumulation, or (3) a low-output state.

Definition

- HF is a clinical syndrome characterized by dyspnea, exercise intolerance, and fluid retention in the setting of abnormal cardiac function.
- Pathophysiologically, HF is defined as the inability of the heart to maintain adequate systemic perfusion at normal cardiac chamber pressures.
- As a consequence, patients with HF require higher intracardiac filling pressures to successfully maintain cardiac output. Overactivation of this compensatory mechanism leads to excessive fluid retention and manifests clinically with pulmonary and/or peripheral edema.

Classification

- Patients with HF can be broadly classified into four groups based on their clinical presentation:
  - Warm and dry (well-compensated HF)
  - Warm and wet (congested without evidence of low cardiac output)
  - Cold and dry (low output without congestion)
  - Cold and wet (low output with congestion, highest risk population)
- Patients presenting with acute HF can also be classified by whether their signs and symptoms are predominantly left HF (dyspnea, orthopnea, pulmonary edema), right HF (venous distention, abdominal distention/ascites, edema), or a combination of both.
- LV failure can be further subdivided based on the presence of either systolic or diastolic dysfunction (i.e., HF with reduced systolic function vs. HF with PSF).
- Patients who present with HF should be categorized as new-onset cardiomyopathy or an exacerbation of chronic LV dysfunction.
- Chronic HF is further categorized based on the New York Heart Association (NYHA) functional class and American Heart Association (AHA) disease stage (see Chapters 14 and 15).

Epidemiology

- HF is one of the fastest growing cardiovascular diagnoses in the United States.
- More than 5 million people in the United States currently have HF, with an estimated 550,000 new diagnoses each year. There are over 1 million hospitalizations for HF annually, at a cost exceeding $33 billion.[1,2]
- Despite significant advancements in the management of HF, the mortality remains high; once a patient is hospitalized for HF, the 1- and 5-year death rates are approximately 30% and 50%, respectively.
- About 50% of patients who are hospitalized for HF prove to have PSF.[3]
- Approximately 75% of patients with acute decompensated HF have a prior history of HF.

Etiology

- Considering the etiology of cardiac dysfunction, it is useful to subdivide patients into two groups: (1) HF patients with abnormal systolic function and (2) HF patients with PSF.
- These two patient populations represent distinct disease processes often with differing underlying pathophysiology and clinical presentations.
  - Among patients with abnormal systolic function (ejection fraction ≤40%), approximately two-thirds will have an ICM. This generally results from prior myocardial infarction (MI).
  - The causes of nonischemic cardiomyopathy in patients with systolic dysfunction are more varied and are shown in Table 5-1.
- HF-PSF is most commonly associated with HTN, diabetes mellitus (DM), obesity, and occasionally CAD (about 25%). Rare causes of HF with PSF include infiltrative cardiomyopathies, hypertrophic cardiomyopathy, and Fabry disease.
  - HF-PSF is more common in females and patients >65 years of age.
  - Atrial fibrillation (AF) and chronic renal insufficiency are frequent comorbidities in this patient population.

Pathophysiology

- HF is associated with **compensatory activation of the renin–angiotensin and sympathetic nervous systems** as a means of maintaining cardiac output in the setting of abnormal myocardial function.
- Although initially adaptive, over time **these neurohumoral responses lead to excessive fluid retention and elevated vascular resistance**. Together, these processes raise intracardiac filling pressures and account for the signs and symptoms of decompensated HF.

Risk Factors

- There are a multitude of risk factors for the development and progression of HF. Common risk factors include CAD, HTN, DM, and renal dysfunction. Exposure to cardiotoxins such as chemotherapeutic drugs (i.e., anthracyclines), alcohol, and illicit drugs (i.e., cocaine) can also increase the risk of developing HF. Recent data suggest that depression, obesity, and obstructive sleep apnea may also play an important role.
- In addition, there are several risk factors associated with decompensation in patients with chronic HF. A helpful mnemonic is "Patients who are frequently hospitalized for HF eventually VANISH."
  - **V**alvular disease
  - **A**rrhythmia (AF)
  - **N**oncompliance (medications, diet)
  - **I**schemia or infection
  - **S**ubstance abuse
  - **H**ypertension

TABLE 5-1	COMMON ETIOLOGIES OF HF
Systolic HF	**HF with PSF**
CAD	HTN
HTN	Diabetes
Myocarditis:	CAD
Infectious	
Autoimmune	
Toxin-induced:	Infiltrative:
Alcohol	Amyloid
Cocaine	Sarcoid
Amphetamines	Hemochromatosis
Chemotherapies	Hypertrophic cardiomyopathy
Genetic	High-output:
Cardiac-specific:	Arteriovenous malformation
ARVCI/D	Arteriovenous fistula
Generalized myopathies:	Hyperthyroidism
Duchenne or Becker muscular dystrophy	Anemia
Diabetes	Constrictive
Postpartum	Idiopathic cardiac fibrosis
Tachycardia-induced	
Idiopathic	

HF, heart failure; PSF, preserved systolic function; CAD, coronary artery disease; HTN, hypertension; ARVCI/D, arrhythmogenic right ventricular cardiomyopathy/dysplasia.

Associated Conditions

- Anemia, hypothyroidism/hyperthyroidism, DM, and renal dysfunction are common comorbidities in patients with HF. In general, they pretend a poorer prognosis independent of the type or etiology of the cardiomyopathy. It is currently unknown whether correction of anemia and abnormal thyroid improves outcomes.
- HF may also be associated with underlying systemic illnesses. In the case of HF-PSF examples include DM, HTN, multiple myeloma with amyloidosis, and sarcoidosis. In addition, both HF-PSF and HF with reduced systolic function can be seen with acromegaly, hemochromatosis, and autoimmune diseases (rheumatoid arthritis, scleroderma, antiphospholipid syndrome, and lupus). In some cases, treatment of these underlying disease processes may slow the progression of the cardiomyopathy.

DIAGNOSIS

Clinical Presentation

- The clinical presentations of HF are highly variable and range from acute respiratory or circulatory compromise to gradual worsening of dyspnea on exertion. In general, patients with HF can be divided into three basic presentations:
  - Flash or acute pulmonary edema with HTN
  - Slowly progressive fluid accumulation
  - Low cardiac output state

- The most dramatic presentation is acute or flash pulmonary edema (FPE). Frequently, these patients have a rapid onset of symptoms and elevated blood pressure. The problem is usually not significant volume overload, but instead **volume redistribution secondary to increased vascular tone (afterload) and poor LV relaxation**. This can be seen in HF patients with either normal or reduced systolic function. The acute management of these patients should focus on the use of vasodilators rather than diuretics (see Table 5-2).
- The patient with slowly progressive fluid accumulation most commonly has chronic systolic dysfunction and is typified by normal to mildly elevated blood pressures and signs or symptoms of slowly progressive fluid accumulation. These patients have dyspnea on exertion, paroxysmal nocturnal dyspnea (PND), orthopnea, lower extremity edema, and weight gain. The use of IV diuretics combined with afterload reduction is generally very effective in the treatment of these patients.
- The third, and least common presentation, is the patient with a low cardiac output state. These patients may be either normotensive or hypotensive. They often have evidence of end-organ hypoperfusion (prerenal azotemia, cool extremities, poor energy level, and confusion). Careful questioning may reveal evidence of mesenteric ischemia and cardiac cachexia. These patients often require admission to the ICU for placement of a pulmonary artery catheter (Swan-Ganz catheter [SGC]) and/or inotropic support. In patients with refractory shock despite inotropes, mechanical circulatory support should be instituted.
- The management of patients with each of these clinical presentations is unique and discussed in detail in Chapters 14 and 15.

History

- There are three primary objectives of the history when interviewing a patient with HF:
  - To identify etiology of HF and/or factors contributing to disease decompensation.
  - To assess progression and severity of illness.
  - To assess volume status.
- It is important to identify factors that may have contributed to the etiology of the HF. For patients with a first presentation of HF, questioning should probe the likelihood of ischemic heart disease (e.g., history of MI, chest pain, risk factors), myocarditis or viral cardiomyopathy (e.g., recent viral illness or upper respiratory symptoms, rheumatologic disease history or symptoms), genetic cardiomyopathy (e.g., family history of HF or sudden death), toxic cardiomyopathy (e.g., alcohol or drug abuse, history of chemotherapy), and peripartum cardiomyopathy (e.g., recent pregnancy). In addition, the presence of HTN and/or diabetes should be elicited.
- For patients with a known cardiomyopathy presenting with an acute decompensation, it is important to **identify the potential triggers of the exacerbation** (see Risk Factors).
- The second critical area to assess in patients with new-onset or established HF is their **current functional status** and the rate of decline in their activity level. Important questions to ask include what they can do before becoming short of breath currently (How far can they walk? How many flights of stairs can they climb?) and how this compares with what they were able to do 6 to 12 months prior. The answers to these questions allow patients to be categorized into an NYHA functional class and an AHA HF stage (see Chapters 14 and 15), which helps direct therapy and assess prognosis.
- The third important issue to address with the history is the patient's **volume status**. The inability to lie flat (**orthopnea**) and waking up at night short of breath (**PND**) **are very suggestive of volume overload in patients with chronic HF**. In addition, changes in body weight should always be discussed with the patient, as increased weight often signifies fluid retention even in the absence of other congestive symptoms. Other manifestations of increased fluid volume include abdominal bloating and/or right upper quadrant pain and lower extremity edema.

TABLE 5-2 PRESENTATION AND INITIAL MANAGEMENT OF HF

	Warm and dry	Flash pulmonary edema	Warm and wet	Cool and wet	Cool and dry
History	Exertional dyspnea, minimal orthopnea, PND; Minimal edema	Sudden onset dyspnea, minimal orthopnea, PND; Minimal edema	Exertional dyspnea, orthopnea, PND; Edema	Fatigue, dyspnea at rest, orthopnea, PND; Edema	Fatigue, orthostasis, minimal orthopnea, PND; Mild edema
Physical examination	Minimal JVD; No crackles; Minimal edema; Normal pulses	HTN, JVD; Prominent crackles; Minimal edema; Normal pulses	JVD/HJR; Crackle; Edema; Normal pulses	JVD/HJR; Crackles; Edema; Weak pulses	Hypotension, minimal JVD; Minimal crackles; Minimal edema; Weak pulses
Laboratory	Normal/mildly increased BNP	Increased BNP	Increased BNP	Increased BNP, Cr, AST, ALT	Increased Cr, AST, ALT, acidosis
Imaging	Clear lung fields	Pulmonary edema	Pulmonary edema	Pulmonary edema	Minimal pulmonary edema
PA catheter	CI >2 L/min normal PCWP	CI >2 L/min elevated PCWP	CI >2 L/min elevated PCWP	CI <2 L/min elevated PCWP	CI <2 L/min normal PCWP
Management	β-Blocker and ACEi/ARB	Vasodilator therapy (NTG, nesiritide)	Diuretics and afterload reduction	Inotropes, diuretics	Inotropes, IVF if PCWP <12 mmHg

HF, heart failure; FPE, flash pulmonary edema; PND, paroxysmal nocturnal dyspnea; JVD, jugular venous distention; HTN, hypertension; HJR, hepatojugular reflux; BNP, brain natriuretic protein; Cr, creatinine; AST, aspartate aminotransferase; ALT, alanine aminotransferase; PCWP, pulmonary capillary wedge pressure; CI, cardiac index; ACEi, angiotensin-converting enzyme inhibitor; ARB, angiotensin II receptor blocker; NTG, nitroglycerin; IVF, intravenous fluids.

- Additional information regarding excessive fatigue, postprandial abdominal discomfort, and orthostasis particularly after administration of HF medicines may aid in identifying patients with low cardiac output. It is important to note that a significant number of patients may report symptoms associated with low cardiac output in the absence of congestion.

Physical Examination

- The primary function of the physical examination in patients with HF is to assess volume status. The examination findings should allow the patient to be characterized as hypovolemic, euvolemic, or volume-overloaded (see Chapter 2). This determination helps to guide treatment and assess the response to therapy (Table 5-2).
- In addition, the physical examination can also provide important clues as to the etiology of cardiac dysfunction. For example, the presence of a murmur or a pericardial knock may indicate a primary valvular process or pericardial constriction, respectively.
- When examining a patient, it is important to recognize that the clinical manifestations of volume overload in HF can be highly variable. The physical examination is a critical component of volume assessment; however, there are several notable limitations of common physical examination findings.
  - The presence of jugular venous distention (JVD) and/or hepatojugular reflux (HJR) is the most specific and reliable physical examination indicator of volume overload (approximately 80% sensitive) and is best assessed with a penlight and the patient positioned at about 45 degrees.[4,5] The jugular venous pulse can be distinguished from carotid pulsations by the biphasic appearance of the latter. Of note, elevated neck veins can also be seen with pulmonary HTN, severe tricuspid regurgitation, and pericardial diseases such as tamponade and constriction.
  - Pulmonary crackles may be present on lung examination and indicate fluid extravasation into the alveoli due to elevated left ventricular end-diastolic pressure (LVEDP). This examination finding is often mistakenly considered mandatory for the diagnosis of decompensated HF. In reality, crackles signify either rapid increases in LVEDP or severe volume overload; they are present in only about 20% to 50% of HF patients with elevated filling pressures.[5] In patients with chronic cardiomyopathy, the gradual increase in LVEDP is compensated for by increased pulmonary lymphatic drainage; thus, crackles are often a late sign of decompensation.
  - Lower extremity edema is another marker of fluid overload when present; however, the sensitivity for predicting elevated filling pressures is relatively poor. In addition, patients can have predominantly abdominal congestive symptoms without any evidence of peripheral or pulmonary edema.
- Other examination findings suggest systolic dysfunction and volume overload, a diffuse and laterally displaced point of maximum impulse, an S3 gallop, a mitral regurgitation murmur at the apex, diminished carotid upstrokes, ascites, and pulsatile hepatomegaly.
- Signs of low cardiac output include cool extremities, fluctuating mental status, orthostasis, resting sinus tachycardia, narrow pulse pressure, and weak pulses. Some patients may have pulsus alternans (alternating intensity of peripheral pulsus despite sinus rhythm), a sign of profoundly low cardiac output.

Diagnostic Criteria

- HF is a clinical diagnosis based on history, physical examination findings, and chest radiography (CXR). Although there are no universally agreed upon diagnostic criteria for HF, the Framingham criteria are reasonable. The diagnosis requires two major or one major and two minor criteria.
  - **Major criteria**: PND, JVD, crackles, cardiomegaly, pulmonary edema, S3, HJR, weight loss with diuresis (>4.5 lb).

○ **Minor criteria**: LE edema, nocturnal cough, dyspnea on exertion, hepatomegaly, pleural effusions, tachycardia, decrease in vital capacity.
• The diagnosis of HF is further supported by laboratory values and imaging studies. These include elevated brain natriuretic peptide (BNP) and an abnormal cardiac echocardiogram (see below).

Differential Diagnosis

• It is important to consider other acute diseases that can mimic the presentation of HF with dyspnea, elevated neck veins, and lower extremity edema (i.e., pulmonary HTN, pulmonary embolism, and pericardial diseases [constriction and tamponade]).
• Pulmonary inflammatory diseases, progressive pleural effusions, significant anemia, hypothyroidism, and some systemic neurologic disorders can also present with progressive exertional dyspnea and should remain on the differential diagnosis list if a cardiac cause of the symptoms cannot be found.

Diagnostic Testing

See Figure 5-1.

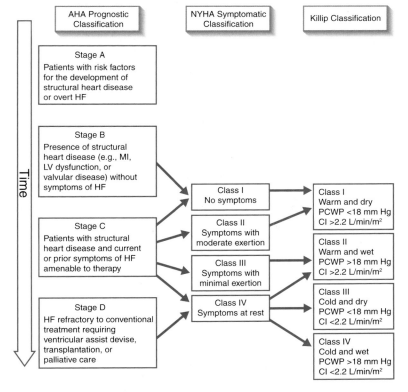

FIGURE 5-1. Classification of heart failure. (Modified from McBride BF, White CM. Acute decompensated heart failure: a contemporary approach to pharmacotherapeutic management. *Pharmacotherapy* 2003;23:997-1020, with permission.)

Laboratories
- BNP and amino-terminal pro-BNP are the most useful biomarkers in diagnosing HF. These natriuretic peptides are released from the heart in response to mechanical stretch and are indicators of volume overload.
  - The normal range for BNP is <100 pg/mL and for pro-BNP is <125 pg/mL. There can be significant fluctuations in level based on age, gender, renal dysfunction (increases level), and obesity (reduces level). In general, levels >200 pg/mL in a symptomatic patient are suggestive of HF.
  - Renal dysfunction strongly influences BNP and pro-BNP levels. Elevated levels over the patient's baseline (if known) may be suggestive of HF. Measuring levels in patients on dialysis is not reliable; however, elevated BNP levels are still predictive of mortality in this patient population.
  - Persistent elevations in BNP and pro-BNP after optimization of volume status identify a population of HF patients at higher risk for morbidity and mortality.
  - The use of BNP and pro-BNP to monitor the response to diuretic therapy may be a helpful strategy to optimize HF treatment. These biomarkers may also be useful if questions arise regarding the effectiveness of diuresis.
- The presence of hyponatremia, elevated creatinine/blood urea nitrogen, and elevated liver enzymes identify high-risk patients. These findings signify the presence of poor cardiac output and/or severe volume overload and independently pretend an unfavorable prognosis.
- Persistently elevated troponin levels can be seen in a subset of both ischemic and nonischemic HF patients and are associated with a worse prognosis.
- Additional laboratory values that may be useful include identifying the presence of anemia, thyroid abnormalities, dyslipidemia, diabetes, and markers of infection.

Electrocardiography
- The electrocardiography (ECG) may provide diagnostic information regarding the etiology of a patient's cardiomyopathy or point to a cause of decompensation in chronic HF patients. Examples include Q-waves characteristic of prior MI, ST segment abnormalities suggestive of ongoing ischemia, or cardiac arrhythmias (i.e., AF/flutter).
- Both ECG and telemetry monitoring may also aid in the detection of cardiac arrhythmias that are relevant to the patient's presentation.
- QRS width and the presence of a left bundle branch block help to identify patients who may favorably respond to cardiac resynchronization therapy.

Imaging
- CXR can help in the diagnosis of HF and in the assessment of volume status. Signs of HF decompensation include pulmonary congestion (perihilar fullness and pulmonary vascular redistribution), pulmonary edema, Kerley B lines, and pleural effusions. However, the absence of pulmonary vascular redistribution or pulmonary edema on CXR does not exclude the diagnosis of HF. The CXR can also help evaluate for other causes of dyspnea such as emphysema, pneumonia, and pneumothorax.
- The echocardiogram is the diagnostic modality of choice for the diagnosis and characterization of HF. It is useful for the assessment of both systolic and diastolic ventricular dysfunction. Echocardiography also provides a detailed structural and functional analysis of valvular heart disease as well as the assessment of congenital malformations, cardiac chamber dynamics, and pericardial diseases. Echocardiography is also useful for assessing the response to HF therapies.
- Cardiac MRI (CMR) is an emerging technology that is increasingly utilized in the assessment of new-onset cardiomyopathies. In addition to characterization of structural heart disease, CMR serves as a powerful tool to help define the etiology of cardiac dysfunction. The presence and pattern of delayed gadolinium enhancement aid in the noninvasive

diagnosis of specific cardiomyopathies, including ischemic, amyloid, sarcoid, hypertrophic, and myocarditis.

- In patients with ICM who have high-grade coronary lesions, a myocardial viability study can be useful to determine the benefit of revascularization. There are several types of viability imaging studies including thallium rest/redistribution, dobutamine echocardiography, positron emission tomography, and MRI. The choice of modality should be driven by the institutional expertise.

Diagnostic Procedures

- Cardiac catheterization is the gold standard for invasive assessment of CAD and cardiac hemodynamics.
  - Given the high prevalence of CAD in patients with reduced LV function, coronary angiography is recommended for the majority of patients with new-onset cardiomyopathy to evaluate the extent of CAD.
  - In patients with a high ischemic burden and viable myocardium, revascularization can improve cardiac function and survival.
  - It is reasonable to consider noninvasive stress testing in patients at very low risk for CAD.
- Right heart catheterization with an SGC allows the measurement of intracardiac filling pressures and cardiac output, thereby providing information regarding volume status, pulmonary artery pressure, cardiac output, and the presence of an intracardiac shunt.
  - Right heart catheterization is particularly beneficial for monitoring cardiac performance in patients with cardiogenic shock requiring either inotropic or mechanical support.
  - SGC is not necessary for the management of routine HF decompensation; however, it is appropriate to consider for patients not responding to medical therapy or those with signs of reduced cardiac output.
- Simultaneous right and left cardiac catheterization can be useful in patients with suspected constrictive pericarditis or valvular cardiomyopathy to aid in diagnosis and treatment options.

REFERENCES

1. Rosamond W, Flegal K, Friday G, et al. Heart disease and stroke statistics—2007 update: a report of the American Heart Association Statistics Committee and Stroke Statistics Committee. *Circulation* 2007;115:e69-e171.
2. Chan PS, Soto G, Jones PG, et al. Patient health status and costs in heart failure: insights from the eplerenone post-acute myocardial infarction heart failure efficacy and survival study (EPHESUS). *Circulation* 2009;119:398-407.
3. Yancy CW, Lopatin M, Stevenson LW, et al. Clinical presentation, management, and in-hospital outcomes of patients admitted with acute decompensated heart failure with preserved systolic function: a report from the Acute Decompensated Heart Failure National Registry (ADHERE) Database. *J Am Coll Cardiol* 2006;47:76-84.
4. Cook DJ, Simel DL. The rational clinical examination: does this patient have abnormal central venous pressure? *JAMA* 1996;275:630-634.
5. Butman SM, Ewy GW, Standen, JR, et al. Bedside cardiovascular examination in patients with severe chronic heart failure: importance of rest or inducible jugular venous distension. *J Am Coll Cardiol* 1993;22:968-974.

Approach to Syncope 6

Christopher L. Holley, Daniel H. Cooper, and Scott M. Nordlicht

GENERAL PRINCIPLES

- The evaluation of syncope can be daunting as there are a myriad of circumstances that can cause or mimic this common clinical problem.
- It is a presentation that requires a consistent approach with realization that we often will never know with certainty the original precipitating etiology.
- Our role as consultants is to help risk stratify these patients for future events via diagnostic testing, as appropriate, and to recommend therapy to prevent recurrences and reduce the risk of injury or death.

Definition

- The term "syncope" should be applied to situations where there is
  - Temporary, transient loss of consciousness (TLOC)
  - Complete and, typically, rapid recovery
  - Global cerebral hypoperfusion as the final common pathway regardless of etiology
- Otherwise, the episode should be referred to as "TLOC" so as to include nonsyncopal etiologies in the differential diagnosis (Table 6-1).

Epidemiology

- The lifetime incidence of syncope is 30% to 50%.[1-3]
- It accounts for 3% to 5% of emergency room visits and 1% to 6% of hospital admissions. Many more cases of syncope are not reported.[4]
- Large population data showed a rate of 6.2 per 1,000 person-years, with an increasing incidence in the elderly.[5] For institutionalized patients over the age of 70, the incidence is as high as 23% over 10 years.[6]

Etiology

- Syncope first must be differentiated from nonsyncopal events involving real or apparent TLOC, such as seizures and falls (Table 6-1).
- Further subdivision of true syncope is based on specific pathophysiologic etiologies that include the following four general categories (Table 6-2) in descending order of frequency:
  - Neurally mediated (reflex) syncope
  - Orthostatic syncope
  - Primary cardiac arrhythmias
  - Structural cardiac or cardiopulmonary disease

DIAGNOSIS

Clinical Presentation

- Initial evaluation of syncope utilizes the history, physical examination, and electrocardiogram (ECG) to classify presumed causes and identify patients who are at high

TABLE 6-1	CAUSES OF NONSYNCOPAL TLOC
No loss of consciousness	**Partial or complete loss of consciousness**
Falls	Epilepsy
Cataplexy/drop attacks	Intoxication
Psychogenic pseudosyncope	Metabolic disorders (hypoglycemia and hypoxemia)
TIA, CAD	TIA, vertebrobasilar disease

TLOC, transient loss of consciousness; CAD, carotid artery disease; TIA, transient ischemic attack.

TABLE 6-2	CLASSIFICATION AND CLASSIC PRESENTATIONS OF SYNCOPE
Types of syncope	**Classic presentations**
Reflex (neurally mediated)	Combination of reflex bradycardia and vasodilation, most common cause of syncope
Vasovagal	Precipitated by emotional stress, prolonged standing, and association with nausea
Carotid sinus	Precipitated by carotid artery manipulation
Situational	Related to micturition, defecation, or coughing
Orthostatic hypotension	Posture changes result in symptoms and/or a drop in systolic blood pressure >20 mmHg
Volume depletion	Heat exposure, poor intake, diuretic use
Autonomic failure	Parkinson disease, diabetes
Drug-induced	Nitrates, α-blockers, clonidine, other antihypertensives
Cardiac arrhythmia	Insufficient cardiac output to meet systemic demands due to either bradycardia or tachycardia
	Often preceded by palpitations
Sinus node dysfunction	Symptomatic bradycardia, sick sinus syndrome with AF
AV conduction disease	β-Blockers, calcium channel blockers, Lenègre disease
Tachycardias	SVT or VT
Long-QT	Congenital and/or drug-induced

(Continued)

TABLE 6-2	CLASSIFICATION AND CLASSIC PRESENTATIONS OF SYNCOPE (*Continued*)
Types of syncope	**Classic presentations**
	Current use of certain antiarrhythmic, antihistamine, antibiotic, antipsychotic, antidepressant medications
Cardiopulmonary disease	Insufficient cardiac output to meet systemic demands due to abnormalities in the structure or function of the heart
	Clues include known cardiac disease, exertional syncope, family history of sudden death, and syncope while supine
Valvular heart disease	Severe aortic stenosis
Acute ischemia/infarction	Particularly right ventricular infarct
HCM	Often exercise-induced syncope
Pulmonary hypertension or embolism	Acute decrease in LV filling
Vascular steal	Subclavian steal syndrome, with increased arterial blood flow to upper extremity causing a reversal of blood flow in the Circle of Willis

AF, atrial fibrillation; AV, atrioventricular; SVT, supraventricular tachycardia; VT, ventricular tachycardia; HCM, hypertrophic cardiomyopathy; LV, left ventricular.

risk for death. There are three key questions that need to be answered with the initial evaluation:
  ○ Is loss of consciousness attributable to syncope or not?
  ○ Is heart disease present or not?
  ○ Are there important clinical features in the history that suggest the diagnosis?
• In addition, consideration of inpatient versus outpatient evaluation should depend on comorbidities and initial findings. In general, patients with the following should be admitted to avoid delay and adverse outcomes:
  ○ Elderly (age > 65 years)
  ○ Known structural heart disease
  ○ Symptoms suggestive of primary cardiac syncope
  ○ Abnormal ECG
  ○ Severe orthostatic hypotension
  ○ Focal neurological deficits
  ○ Family history of sudden death
  ○ Exertional syncope
  ○ Syncope causing severe injury
  ○ Syncope while driving

History

- Often, the diagnosis of syncope is evident from the history.
- Aspects of the history that need to be explored in order to aid diagnosis and further categorize the event include a prodrome **before** the attack, **eyewitness** accounts during the event, the patient's recollection immediately **after** the attack, **circumstances** that may have played a causative role in the event, and general questions about the patient's medical **history**.
- A helpful mnemonic is, "I passed out on the BEACH" (Table 6-3).
- **For patients with recognizable reflex or orthostatic syncope that occurs infrequently or as an isolated episode, no further workup is necessary.** These patients generally have a good prognosis and can be managed as outpatients with treatments listed below.
- **In patients with a suspected cardiac etiology, an inpatient cardiac evaluation is warranted.**

Physical Examination

- The examination should include assessment of orthostatic vital signs and careful neurologic, pulmonary, and cardiovascular assessment.
  - Proper orthostatic vital signs include
    - Blood pressure (BP) checked (both arms) after the patient lies supine for at least 5 minutes
    - BP measured 3 minutes after standing
    - Orthostasis = 20-mmHg decrease in systolic BP and/or 10-mmHg decrease in diastolic BP and/or 10-bpm increase in heart rate (HR)
  - Cardiovascular findings that may point to cardiogenic syncope include
    - Arrhythmias (tachyarrhythmias, bradyarrhythmias, and irregularity)
    - Murmurs (especially aortic stenosis or hypertrophic obstructive cardiomyopathy)
    - Evidence for heart failure (S3, S4, edema, and elevated JVD)
  - Neurologic findings are often absent, but might include evidence of autonomic neuropathy (e.g., inappropriate sweating, lack of HR variability, extreme orthostatic BP changes).

TABLE 6-3	ESSENTIAL QUESTIONS TO EVALUATE HISTORY OF SYNCOPE
Before	Nausea, vomiting, feeling cold, sweating, dizziness, visual changes
Eyewitness	Duration of transient loss of consciousness, movements (tonic, clonic, other), description of patient falling
After	Confusion, muscle aches, incontinence, nausea, vomiting, sweating, pallor
Circumstances	Position (supine, standing), activity (rest, exercise, rising to stand, cough, urination), possible precipitants (fear, pain, prolonged standing)
History	Prior syncopal episodes, known cardiac, neurologic, or metabolic disease, known history or symptoms of obstructive sleep apnea medications (including over the counter), alcohol or illicit drug use, family history of sudden cardiac death

- A firm massage at the carotid artery bifurcation for 5 to 10 seconds may reproduce symptoms, particularly in the elderly.
  - This maneuver can be performed safely at the bedside with the patient lying recumbent on telemetry monitoring and appropriate bradycardia treatments available.
  - The test is considered positive if it results in a ventricular pause of >3 seconds.
  - Neurologic complications are rare (<0.5%), but the procedure should be avoided in patients with known carotid disease, carotid bruits, or a recent transient ischemic attack (TIA)/cerebrovascular accident.

Diagnostic Testing

- Given the broad differential, the syncope evaluation is notorious for triggering extensive, multimodality diagnostic testing.
- The 2006 American Heart Association (AHA)/American College of Cardiology (ACC) algorithm for cardiac evaluation of syncope is outlined in Figure 6-1.[7]

Electrocardiography

Specific abnormalities to look for on ECG include
- Evidence of sinus node dysfunction
- Evidence of atrioventricular conduction abnormalities
- Tachyarrhythmias (supraventricular tachycardia [SVT], ventricular tachycardia [VT], atrial fibrillation [AF])
- Evidence of ventricular preexcitation (delta waves)
- Evidence of underlying structural heart disease includes
  - Q waves suggestive of prior myocardial infection
  - Wide QRS (>120 milliseconds)
  - Left ventricular hypertrophy pattern suggestive of hypertrophic cardiomyopathy (HCM)
  - Anterior precordial T-wave inversions and/or epsilon waves suggestive of arrhythmogenic right ventricular dysplasia (ARVD)
- Evidence of channelopathy:
  - Long or short QT.
  - Right bundle branch block with down-sloping ST elevation and T-wave inversion in V1–V3 (Brugada pattern).

Imaging

- The expanded cardiac evaluation includes an **echocardiogram, exercise testing, and an ischemic evaluation**.
  - In appropriate patients, an exercise stress echo would be sufficient to complete all three aspects of testing (baseline imaging followed by exercise protocol and stress imaging).
  - The echocardiogram alone may be diagnostic in cases of valvular heart disease, cardiomyopathy, or congenital heart disease.
  - Exercise testing is preferable to pharmacologic stress and should be symptom-limited.
  - Noninvasive testing for ischemia should be followed by **cardiac catheterization** if there is an evidence of ischemia or previously unrecognized infarction.
- Cardiac magnetic resonance imaging or computed tomography may be helpful in the evaluation of structural heart disease, including HCM, ARVD, or coronary anomalies.
- If an arrhythmic cause is suspected, but not evident on the initial workup or on expanded cardiac evaluation, **ambulatory cardiac rhythm monitoring** can be achieved via one of the following modalities[8]:
  - Holter monitor (24 to 48 hours of continuous recording)
  - Event recorder (1 month of patient-activated or patient-triggered recordings to temporally correlate with symptoms)
  - Mobile Continuous Outpatient Telemetry (MCOT) for up to one month of continuous monitoring
  - Implantable loop recorder (years of continuous recording)

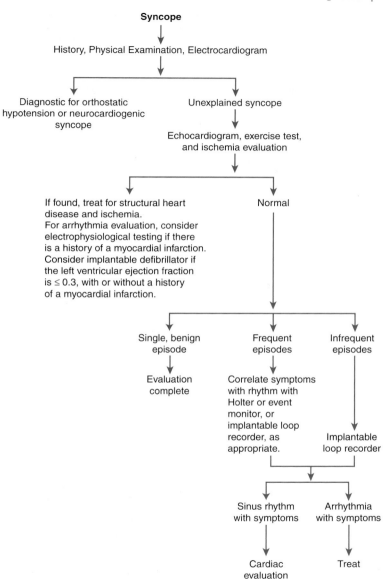

FIGURE 6-1. Algorithm for the evaluation of syncope. (Modified from American Heart Association/American College of Cardiology Foundation. AHA/ACCF scientific statement on the evaluation of syncope. *Circulation* 2006;113:316.)

- ◦ The choice of monitoring is dependent on the frequency of symptoms and type of suspected arrhythmia. Even in a highly selected population, the diagnostic yield of ambulatory cardiac monitoring is relatively low.
- **Tilt table testing** has been used traditionally as a diagnostic tool to characterize a patient's hemodynamic response to controlled postural change from supine to upright state to aid in the diagnosis of a reflex-mediated (neurocardiogenic) syncope.
  - ◦ Physiologically, there is a large volume shift during repositioning, with 500 to 1000 mL of blood moving from the thorax to the distensible venous system below the diaphragm within the first 10 seconds.
  - ◦ The hydrostatic pressures created by the upright position result in a similar volume of fluid moving to the interstitial space within 10 minutes.
  - ◦ Autonomic vasoconstriction is the key reflex to counter this orthostatic stress, and failure of the vasoconstriction mechanism at any point may result in syncope.
  - ◦ An under-filled right ventricle will trigger a strong vagal response, leading to bradycardia and hypotension
  - ◦ Results are classified as primarily vasodepressor, cardioinhibitory, or mixed.
  - ◦ Unfortunately, **the test has a low sensitivity and reproducibility**. It is our institutional bias that a tilt table test adds very little to a thorough history, physical examination, and standard cardiac workup of syncope.
- **Electrophysiology studies (EPS)** can be useful in selected patients. Indications for EPS include
  - ◦ Abnormal ECG suggesting conduction system cause
  - ◦ Syncope during exertion or while supine or in the presence of structural heart disease
  - ◦ Syncope with associated palpitations
  - ◦ Family history of sudden death
  - ◦ To define/ablate identified arrhythmias in patients with high-risk occupations

TREATMENT

- Treatment of syncope can be broadly defined as **preventing recurrences** and **reducing the risk of injury or death**.
- In general, this is tailored to treat the suspected underlying etiology of the syncope.
- Various approaches to treating the four etiologies of syncope are shown in Table 6-4.

Medications

- The most common pharmacologic options for preventing venous pooling and aiding intravascular volume expansion include
  - ◦ **Midodrine** (2.5 to 10 mg by mouth (PO) three times a day)[9,10]
    - ▪ Peripheral α-agonist causing both arterial and venous constriction
    - ▪ Adverse effects: paresthesias, piloerection, pruritus, and supine hypertension
    - ▪ Avoid in patients with carotid artery disease (CAD), peripheral arterial disease, and acute renal failure
    - ▪ The only drug shown effective in trials for orthostatic hypotension and reflex-mediated syncope
  - ◦ **Fludrocortisone** (start 0.1 mg PO daily, can increase by 0.1 mg weekly to maximum of 1.0 mg PO daily)
    - ▪ Synthetic mineralocorticoid causing sodium retention and volume expansion
    - ▪ Adverse effects: hypertension, peripheral edema, and hypokalemia[11]
    - ▪ An ongoing randomized control trial (POST II) is investigating effectiveness in reflex syncope[12]
  - ◦ β-Blockers are often prescribed for syncope, though trials do not support this practice.[13]

TABLE 6-4	TAILORED TREATMENT OF SYNCOPE
Reflex	Avoid precipitants (prolonged standing, overheating); adequate hydration; isometric muscle contraction during prodrome to abort episodes; cardiac pacing for carotid sinus syncope with bradycardia; compression stockings; salt supplementation; fludrocortisone; midodrine
Orthostatic	Adequate hydration; eliminate offending drugs; stand slowly; support stockings; consider salt supplementation, fludrocortisone, or midodrine
Arrhythmia	Cardiac pacing for sinus node dysfunction or high-degree AV block; discontinue QT-prolonging drugs; ICD for documented VT without correctable cause; endocardial ablation procedure in select patients
Cardiopulmonary	Correction of underlying disorder (valve replacement, revascularization); ICD for syncope with EF <35% even in the absence of documented arrhythmia (presumed VT)

AV, atrioventricular; ICD, implantable cardioverter/defibrillator; VT, ventricular tachycardia; EF, ejection fraction.

Other Nonpharmacologic Therapies

- For reflex syncope, effective treatment may be as simple as avoiding syncopal precipitants.
- When such precipitants cannot be avoided, coping strategies can be helpful. Isometric muscle contractions can improve venous return and abort frank syncope in patients with a recognizable prodrome.

Lifestyle/Risk Modification

- Driving restrictions should be discussed in patients with unexplained syncope when appropriate.
- Recommendations currently vary depending on etiology, underlying disease, type of license held (private versus commercial), and adequacy of treatment.
- If cause of syncope is an active cardiac arrhythmia, patients should be instructed not to drive until successful treatment has been initiated and the patient has received permission from the treating physician.
- In general, in patients with a serious episode of syncope that is not clearly due to a reversible etiology, guidelines recommend driving restriction for 3 to 6 syncope-free months. Also, federal law and variable state law pertinent to licensure in these individuals exist and should be consulted when applicable.

OUTCOME/PROGNOSIS

- One-third of the patients with syncope will have a recurrent event within 3 years.
- Select subgroups of patients with noncardiac syncope who have an excellent prognosis. Young, otherwise healthy individuals with a normal ECG and without identifiable heart disease have essentially no increased risk of death relative to the population at large.

- Reflex syncope is associated with no increase in mortality risk.
- Syncope from orthostatic hypotension has an excellent prognosis if the underlying abnormality is easily identified and treated.
- In contrast, syncope with an identifiable cardiac etiology carries a higher risk of mortality, particularly in patients with advanced heart failure. Mortality approaches 45% at 1 year for patients with syncope and left ventricular (LV) ejection fraction <20%.[14]

REFERENCES

1. Kenny RA, Bhangu J, King-Kallimanis BL. Epidemiology of syncope/collapse in younger and older Western patient populations. *Prog Cardiovasc Dis* 2013;55:357-363.
2. Ganzeboom KS, Mairuhu G, Reitsma JB, et al. Lifetime cumulative incidence of syncope in the general population: a study of 549 Dutch subjects aged 35-60 years. *J Cariovasc Electrophysiol* 2006;17:1172-1176.
3. Manolis AS, Linzer M, Salem D, Estes NA, 3rd. Syncope: current diagnostic evaluation and management. *Ann Intern Med* 1990;112:850-863.
4. Shen WK, Decker WW, Smars PA, et al. Syncope Evaluation in the Emergency Department Study (SEEDS): a multidisciplinary approach to syncope management. *Circulation* 2004;110: 3636-3645.
5. Soteriades ES, Evans JC, Larson MG, et al. Incidence and prognosis of syncope. *N Engl J Med* 2002;347:878-885.
6. Lipsitz LA, Wei JY, Rowe JW. Syncope in an elderly, institutionalised population. prevalence, incidence, and associated risk. *Q J Med* 1985;55:45-54.
7. Strickberger SA, Benson DW, Biaggioni I, et al. AHA/ACCF Scientific Statement on the evaluation of syncope: from the American Heart Association Councils on Clinical Cardiology, Cardiovascular Nursing, Cardiovascular Disease in the Young, and Stroke, and the Quality of Care and Outcomes Research Interdisciplinary Working Group; and the American College of Cardiology Foundation: in collaboration with the Heart Rhythm Society: endorsed by the American Autonomic Society. *Circulation* 2006;113:316-327.
8. Subbiah R, Gula LJ, Klein GJ, et al. Syncope: review of monitoring modalities. *Curr Cardiol Rev* 2008;4:41-48.
9. Low PA, Gilden JL, Freeman R, et al. Efficacy of midodrine vs placebo in neurogenic orthostatic hypotension. A randomized, double-blind multicenter study. Midodrine Study Group. *JAMA* 1997;277:1046-1051.
10. Wright RA, Kaufmann HC, Perera R, et al. A double-blind, dose-response study of midodrine in neurogenic orthostatic hypotension. *Neurology* 1998;51:120-124.
11. Chobanian AV, Volicer L, Tifft CP, et al. Mineralocorticoid-induced hypertension in patients with orthostatic hypotension. *N Engl J Med* 1979;301:68-73.
12. Raj SR, Rose S, Ritchie D, et al.; POST II Investigators. The Second Prevention of Syncope Trial (POST II)—a randomized clinical trial of fludrocortisone for the prevention of neurally mediated syncope: rationale and study design. *Am Heart J* 2006;151:1186.e11-17.
13. Sheldon R, Connolly S, Rose, et al. POST Investigators. Prevention of Syncope Trial (POST): a randomized, placebo-controlled study of metoprolol in the prevention of vasovagal syncope. *Circulation* 2006;113:1164-1170.
14. Middlekauff HR, Stevenson WG, Stevenson LW, et al. Syncope in advanced heart failure: high risk of sudden death regardless of origin of syncope. *J Am Coll Cardiol* 1993;21:110-116.

Cardiovascular Emergencies

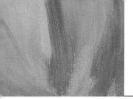

7

Sara C. Martinez and Phillip S. Cuculich

- Cardiovascular emergencies require urgent care by a cardiovascular care team and treatment in an intensive care unit (ICU) or emergency department setting after initial stabilization.
- Topics presented in this chapter include symptomatic bradycardia, symptomatic tachycardia, ST-segment elevation myocardial infarction (STEMI), late complications of a myocardial infarction (MI), cardiac tamponade, hypertensive emergencies, cardiogenic shock including acute decompensated heart failure (ADHF), and cardiac device malfunctions.
- This chapter is meant as a hands-on, rapid checklist to help manage patients with the above cardiovascular emergencies. Detailed discussion of each disease can be found elsewhere in this book.

Symptomatic Bradycardia

GENERAL PRINCIPLES

- Asking yourself the "Five S" questions to a SSSSSlow heart rate can quickly help organize your diagnostic thoughts and action plans: Is the patient "**Stable**"?, What are the "**Symptoms**"?, Where is the "**Source**"?, How do I "**Speed**" up the Heart?, and Should I "**Set up**" for a pacemaker?
- Advanced Cardiac Life Support (ACLS) guidelines for symptomatic bradycardia are provided in Figure 7-1.[1]
- Ensure that the patient has adequate intravenous (IV) access and oxygenation. Call for a code cart. Additionally, external pads should be placed on the patient and connected to a monitor with transcutaneous pacing capacity.

DIAGNOSIS

- Bradycardia in an adult is defined as a resting heart rate less than 60 beats per minute (bpm); however, it is rarely symptomatic unless less than 50 bpm. Correlate a palpated pulse with an electrocardiogram (ECG). **Asymptomatic bradycardia does not require emergent treatment**.
- Symptomatic bradycardia at rest or with hypotension or syncope requires immediate attention to the circulation, airway, and breathing and initiation of basic life support if appropriate.
- A brief review of the rhythm strip or ECG is important to determine whether the bradycardia originates above or below the atrioventricular (AV) node.
- Advanced AV block (type II second- or third-degree AV block) is unlikely to respond to the increased atrial heart rates that atropine provides and will likely need urgent pacing.
- Ventricular escape bradycardia is unstable and requires preparation for urgent pacing.

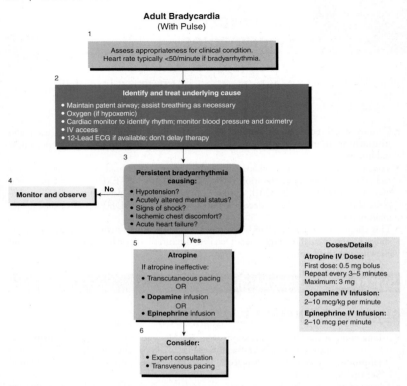

FIGURE 7-1. ACLS algorithm for management of bradycardia. (From Neumar RW, Otto CW, Link MS, et al. Part 8: adult advanced cardiovascular life support: 2010 American Heart Association Guidelines for Cardiopulmonary Resuscitation and Emergency Cardiovascular Care. *Circulation* 2010;122:S729-S767, with permission.)

TREATMENT

Medications

- **Atropine**: 0.5–1.0 mg IV. Doses can be repeated every 3 to 5 minutes. The **exception** to using atropine is type II second-degree AV block, which may be worsened by atropine. Atropine may be given through an endotracheal tube (1 to 2 mg diluted to a total not to exceed 10 mL of sterile water or normal saline) if IV access is not available.
- **Dopamine**: 2 to 10 μg/kg/minute IV to keep systolic blood pressure (SBP) >90 mmHg.
- **Epinephrine**: 2 to 10 μg/minute IV to keep SBP >90 mmHg.

Other Nonpharmacologic Therapies

Transcutaneous Pacing

- Place pads on the anterior and posterior chest walls. Initially, begin pacing at the highest output. Rapidly reduce the output until ventricular capture is lost and then

increase the output until regular capture is seen. If hypotension is not severe, sedate the patient.
• Prepare for transvenous pacing (see Chapter 8).

SPECIAL CONSIDERATIONS

• Check a daily portable chest radiograph on patients with temporary pacemakers, as pacing wires may migrate.
• The patient who exhibits rising hypertension, bradycardia, and erratic breathing (Cushing triad) merits an immediate head computed tomography (CT) and neurosurgical consult, as this implies severely increased intracranial pressure (ICP).

Symptomatic Tachycardia

GENERAL PRINCIPLES

• Similar to the assessment of the patient with bradycardia, the first question to ask yourself is, "Is this person stable?" Check the palpable pulse, blood pressure (BP), and oxygen saturation. If the patient is pulseless or clinically unstable, proceed to defibrillation as described in the "Clinically Unstable" heading in this section and ACLS guidelines for tachycardia in Figure 7-2.[1]

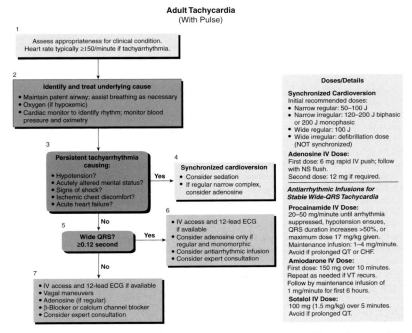

FIGURE 7-2. ACLS algorithm for management of tachycardia. (From Neumar RW, Otto CW, Link MS, et al. Part 8: adult advanced cardiovascular life support: 2010 American Heart Association Guidelines for Cardiopulmonary Resuscitation and Emergency Cardiovascular Care. *Circulation* 2010;122:S729-S767, with permission.)

- Ensure adequate IV access and oxygenation and call for a crash cart.
- Analysis of the ECG dictates management of the clinically stable patient.
- Heart rate typically defined as greater than 150 bpm in an adult.

DIAGNOSIS

Narrow QRS Complex Tachycardias

- Supraventricular tachycardia (SVT) with a QRS complex <120-millisecond duration on ECG.
- The most common SVTs in order of frequency are
  - Sinus tachycardia
  - Atrial fibrillation
  - Atrial flutter
  - AV nodal reentry tachycardia (AVNRT)
  - AV reentry tachycardia (AVRT, accessory pathway-mediated)
  - Atrial tachycardia (ectopic and reentrant)
  - Multifocal atrial tachycardia
  - Junctional tachycardia
- Narrow QRS complex arrhythmias are further diagnosed and often treated by slowing the conduction through the AV node. This can demonstrate the underlying atrial rhythm without large ventricular QRS complexes obscuring the rhythm (atrial fibrillation, flutter, and ectopic atrial tachycardia). Additionally, slowing AV node conduction can halt the tachycardia if it is dependent on the AV node as part of the tachycardia circuit (AVNRT and AVRT).

Wide QRS Complex Tachycardia

- QRS duration ≥120 milliseconds:
  - Ventricular tachycardia (VT)
  - SVT with aberrancy
  - Preexcited tachycardias (Wolff-Parkinson-White syndrome)
  - Ventricular pacemaker
- Typically, wide QRS complex tachycardias are more challenging by requiring a working diagnosis before the treatment plan is executed. Treatment of VT is different from SVT with aberrancy or preexcited tachycardia.
- The following points suggest VT as the cause:
  - Known structural disease: Patients with coronary disease or ventricular dysfunction are more likely to have VT as the cause of wide complex tachycardia.
  - Change in QRS morphology: A major change in QRS morphology and/or a shift in axis in comparison with a prior ECG suggests VT.
  - VA dissociation
  - Fusion/capture beats
  - Positive or negative concordance of QRS in ECG leads V1 to V6
- ECG 201 has additional criteria to aid in determining the rhythm of a wide complex tachycardia (see Chapter 23).

TREATMENT

Clinically Unstable

- **Patients who are pulseless or clinically unstable with tachycardia require immediate defibrillation with unsynchronized high-energy shocks** (200 J, 300 J, 360 J) followed by appropriate C-A-B attention of ACLS, focusing on high-quality cardiopulmonary resuscitation compressions.

- **Amiodarone** (300 mg IV once, repeat at 150 mg IV once) should be given for continued pulseless VT.
- **Epinephrine** 1 mg IV/IO should be given every 3 to 5 minutes.
- Vasopressin 40 units IV/IO can also be given.
- Maximum output shocks should continue every 30 to 60 seconds if the VT/ventricular fibrillation (VF) continues.
- Calcium and bicarbonate should be administered if hyperkalemia is suspected.

Clinically Stable

Narrow QRS Complex Tachycardia

- AV node slowing can be achieved by **increasing vagal tone** with a carotid sinus massage; however, this should be avoided in patients with known carotid artery disease (CAD).
- **Adenosine** can be rapidly pushed (6 to 12 mg) IV with a flush. Ideally, have a continuous 12-lead ECG printing as a "rhythm strip," while adenosine is given. If possible, warn the patient about a flushing sensation and possible coughing.

Wide QRS Complex Tachycardia

- **Monomorphic VT**: Amiodarone (150 mg IV over 10 minutes, followed by 1 mg/minute continuous infusion for 6 hours and then 0.5 mg/minute continuous infusion for the next 18 hours) should be used. Alternative options include procainamide or sotalol. If the patient becomes unstable or the VT persists, a synchronized defibrillation shock should be considered with sedation.
- In the absence of contraindications, the general order of medical treatment for **recurrent VT** (VT storm) is (1) IV amiodarone, (2) IV and oral β-blockers, (3) IV lidocaine, (4) IV and oral benzodiazepine, and (5) general anesthesia and endotracheal intubation. Electrophysiologic study with catheter ablation may play a role for treating VT. Selective sympathetic denervation (spinal anesthesia and stellate ganglion surgery) and ventricular support devices (intraaortic balloon pump [IABP] or left ventricular assist device [LVAD]) have a role in refractory cases.
- **Polymorphic VT**: This can become unstable quickly. A prolonged QT interval in sinus rhythm should raise the concern of torsades de pointes. Immediate treatment should include administering 4 g IV magnesium, overdrive pacing, or IV isoproterenol at 5 μg/minute IV infusion. Amiodarone (150 mg IV over 10 minutes) may be helpful, particularly if the QT interval is normal at baseline. Underlying medications or overdoses should be investigated.
- Persistent **torsades de pointes** requires defibrillation.

SPECIAL CONSIDERATIONS

- Patients with a prolonged QT interval at their baseline should have their medications reviewed for QT prolonging agents.
- Patients who are started on an antiarrhythmic medication should have continuous telemetry monitoring and periodic 12-lead ECGs. Class 3 antiarrhythmics (amiodarone and sotalol) can prolong the QT interval. Class 1 antiarrhythmics can prolong the QRS complex.
- For patients on IV lidocaine, there should be frequent neurologic checks and serum lidocaine levels should be checked to avoid toxicity.

ST-Segment Elevation Myocardial Infarction

- "Time is muscle!" is the overriding theme of countless clinical studies regarding a STEMI, meaning that early successful coronary reperfusion strategies lead to improved short- and long-term outcomes.

- IV thrombolytic medication and/or percutaneous coronary intervention may achieve reperfusion in appropriate patients.
- A detailed discussion can be found in Chapter 12 including benchmark goals and treatment algorithms.

Late Complications of Myocardial Infarction

GENERAL PRINCIPLES

- These consist of ischemic, mechanical, arrhythmic, inflammatory, or thrombotic events occurring after a prior MI.
- Postinfarction complications rates have fallen dramatically since the advent of early reperfusion strategies.
- Patients with large infarction, silent infarction, late presentation, delayed, or incomplete reperfusion remain at a high risk for life-threatening late complications of MI.

DIAGNOSIS

- An **urgent bedside echocardiogram** cannot be overemphasized for the rapid diagnosis of many late complications of MIs.
- The mnemonic "**FEAR A MI**" is a logical way to remember and respect the following potentially life-threatening complications while caring for a patient in the ICU:
  - **Failure**: Left ventricular (LV) dysfunction is the single most powerful predictor of survival following an MI. Clinical symptoms of heart failure are more likely in patients with large infarcts, advanced age, and/or diabetes. Treatment for post-MI systolic heart failure can be found in Chapters 5 and 14.
  - **Effusion and Tamponade**: Post-MI effusions are rarely life-threatening and can be from inflammatory or hemorrhagic causes. If tamponade physiology is present, consider hemorrhagic effusion from a ventricular rupture (see "Cardiac Tamponade" below).
  - **Arrhythmia**: Infarction-specific arrhythmias include the following:
    - **Accelerated idioventricular rhythm** (AIVR) is considered a reperfusion rhythm, as it is often seen immediately after a successful reperfusion. It is characterized by a relatively slow ventricular rate (80 to 110 bpm).
    - **VT** is often the terminal rhythm in the periinfarct time period and is associated with increased mortality when it occurs in the first 48 hours of hospitalization.
    - In contrast, **nonsustained VT** is not associated with an increased risk of death during the index hospitalization or over the first year after infarction.
    - MI can cause a block at any level of the conduction system.
    - In general, **proximal (AV nodal)** conduction disease is associated with an infarct of the right coronary artery. This type of heart block often reverse with time.
    - **Distal (infranodal)** conduction disease is frequently associated with a large left anterior descending (LAD)/septal infarct and is longer lasting and potentially life-threatening.
  - **Rupture:**
    - Ventricular rupture is often a striking and life-threatening clinical presentation. The rupture can be in the ventricular freewall, ventricular septum, or papillary muscle.
    - Clinical suspicion, the timely use of echocardiography, and a pulmonary artery catheter (PAC) are essential for prompt diagnosis of this serious complication.
  - **Aneurysm:** True LV aneurysms complicate less than 5% of acute infarctions, but are associated with a considerably lower survival rate.

○ The characteristic ECG findings of LV aneurysm are Q waves with persistent ST elevations, though the diagnosis is best confirmed with a noninvasive imaging study.
○ A pseudoaneurysm, distinct from an aneurysm, can be thought of as a contained rupture. It is most often seen with an inferior MI and the treatment is urgent surgery. Both surgical and medical treatments carry a very high mortality.
- **Recurrent ischemia/reinfarction:** The complaint of chest pain after an MI may represent recurrent ischemia from incomplete revascularization. Ischemia recurs in 20% to 30% of patients receiving thrombolytic therapy and up to 10% of patients after percutaneous revascularization. Serial cardiac biomarkers and ECG can help identify at-risk patients.

TREATMENT

- No treatment is warranted for **AIVR** when it is combined with a clinical scenario of reperfusion.
- Transient **proximal AV block** often does not warrant immediate temporary pacemaker placement. One exception is AV block in the setting of RV infarction, where restoration of AV synchrony can improve RV filling and thus cardiac output.
- **Distal AV block** is frequently associated with an LAD/septal infarct and is longer lasting and potentially life-threatening. Immediate **pacing efforts** should be pursued.
- **Ventricular rupture requires emergent surgical consultation**.
- Normally, antianginal medications (nitrates and β-blockers) can control symptoms of recurrent ischemia.
- Reinfarction due to stent thrombosis usually has a dramatic presentation with severe anginal pain refractory to medical therapy and evolving ST elevations on ECG. These findings warrant additional prompt revascularization efforts.

Cardiac Tamponade

GENERAL PRINCIPLES

- Cardiac tamponade is compression of the cardiac chambers by a pericardial effusion mechanically inhibiting their proper filling.
- The presence of a pericardial effusion does not necessarily mean that tamponade physiology is present.
- Detailed discussion on the etiology, pathophysiology, and nonemergent management of pericardial effusion is presented in Chapter 17.

DIAGNOSIS

- Characterized by the following parameters:
  ○ Elevation of intrapericardial pressure
  ○ Limitation of RV diastolic filling
  ○ Reduction of LV stroke volume and cardiac output
- Cardiac tamponade is a **clinical diagnosis** associated with relative hypotension.
- History can reveal a potential cause and rate of fluid accumulation.
- Pertinent physical examination findings include altered mental status, hypotension, tachycardia, jugular venous distension, and pulsus paradoxus.[2]
- Supporting diagnostic information can be obtained by evaluating an ECG for low voltage and electrical alternans and a chest x-ray (CXR) for a water bottle–shaped heart.
- Echocardiography: distinguishing features on a transthoracic echocardiogram:

- Pericardial effusion
- RV diastolic collapse
- Right atrial notching
- Tricuspid and mitral valve inflow variation in Doppler velocities of >40% and >25%, respectively
- Dilated inferior vena cava

TREATMENT

- **Initial medical management:**
  - **Volume expansion**: Initial management consists of increasing preload with IV fluids.
  - **BP**: Maintain BP with norepinephrine and dobutamine as needed.
  - Avoid vasodilators and diuretics.
  - The decision to drain the pericardial fluid, as well as the method (surgical or percutaneous) and timing (emergent or elective) of the procedure, should be individualized to each patient taking into account the acuity of the patient's condition, availability of trained personnel, and etiology of the effusion.
- **Pericardiocentesis:**
  - Pericardiocentesis is a potentially life-threatening procedure, which should be performed by trained personnel with hemodynamic monitoring and echocardiographic guidance whenever possible.
  - Blind percutaneous pericardiocentesis may be needed to stabilize a hemodynamically unstable patient.
  - Use a "pericardiocentesis kit" if possible, which allows for a rapid procedure with appropriate supplies.
  - Insert the 8-cm, 19-gauge blunt tipped needle attached to a syringe through the subxiphoid region.
  - Direct the tip posteriorly toward the patient's left shoulder and slowly advance the needle at a 30-degree angle to the body with gentle aspiration.
  - Attaching an ECG electrode to the pericardiocentesis needle may aid in avoiding myocardial puncture. Electrical activity will be seen on the monitor when the needle contacts ventricular myocardium.
  - Aspiration of clear, serous fluid may be from the pericardium or pleural effusion. Aspiration of bloody fluid may be from the pericardium or the right ventricle.
  - Removal of 50 to 100 mL of pericardial fluid should cause a hemodynamic improvement if tamponade is the cause of the hypotension

Hypertensive Emergency

GENERAL PRINCIPLES

- Severe hypertension affects the renal (elevated serum creatinine and hematuria), cardiovascular (angina, heart failure, and aortic dissection), and neurologic (headache, mental status changes, vision alterations from retinal damage, and papilledema) systems.
- **Hypertensive emergency** is the presence of end-organ damage from elevated BP necessitating rapid reduction by using IV medications.
- In contrast, **hypertensive urgency** can be treated with oral medications with the goal of BP reduction over the course of days.

DIAGNOSIS

- Elevated BP recordings, often with SBP >200 and diastolic blood pressure (DBP) >120 mmHg.

- End-organ damage can manifest with physical examination findings of an abnormal neurologic examination, pulmonary edema, or discrepant BP readings from each arm, suggestive of an aortic dissection.

TREATMENT

- A reasonable and safe goal for hypertensive emergency is to reduce **the mean arterial pressure (MAP) by 20% to 25% within a few hours.**
- A larger reduction in BP in the first few hours may worsen end-organ damage, particularly in the brain.
- Exceptions include aortic dissection, LV failure, and pulmonary edema, in which BP should be reduced quickly and to a lower target BP.
- Placement of an arterial line should be strongly considered for the most accurate BP measurement.
- Specific antihypertensive medications should be adjusted for the situation.
- Commonly used first-line IV agents include
  - **Sodium nitroprusside**: A rapid arterial and venous dilator. IV dosing starts at 0.25 µg/kg/minute and is titrated every 5 minutes to a maximum of 10 µg/kg/minute. Thiocyanate toxicity is an uncommon side effect and occurs with prolonged infusions (days) in patients with hepatic or renal insufficiency.
  - **Labetalol**: An α-antagonist and nonselective β-antagonist with partial β-2 agonist quality. Labetalol can be given as bolus doses of 20 to 40 mg IV every 10 to 15 minutes or with an infusion of 0.5 to 2 mg/minute. Relative contraindications to labetalol include heart failure, bradycardia, AV conduction block, and chronic obstructive pulmonary disease.
  - **Esmolol**: A rapidly acting, β-1-selective agent with a short half-life. Similar relative contraindications to labetalol.
  - **Nitroglycerin (NTG)**: A weak systemic arterial dilator but should be considered when managing hypertension associated with CAD. The usual initial dose is 5 to 15 µg/minute and can be titrated every 5 minutes to goal BP or onset of headache (common side effect). NTG has a rapid onset and offset of action.
  - **Hydralazine**: A direct arterial vasodilator. A starting dose of 10 to 20 mg IV may be given. The onset of action is 10 to 30 minutes. Hydralazine causes a reflex tachycardia and is contraindicated in myocardial ischemia and aortic dissection.
  - **Fenoldopam**: A selective dopamine (D1) receptor partial agonist also improves renal perfusion.[3,4] It may be particularly beneficial for those with accompanying renal dysfunction. The IV dosage is 0.1–1 µg/kg/minute starting at 0.025 to 0.3 µg/kg/minute, increasing by 0.05 to 0.1 µg/kg/minute every 15 minutes. Fenoldopam should be avoided in patients with increased intraocular pressure.

SPECIAL CONSIDERATIONS

- Reversible causes of severe, medical refractory hypertension are warranted for patients who present with hypertensive urgency/emergency. These include blood tests for hyperaldosteronism and a noninvasive scan for renal artery stenosis.
- **Hypertensive encephalopathy**:
  - Agents of choice are nitroprusside or labetalol.
  - Central nervous system depressants, such as clonidine, should be avoided.
  - Antiepileptics may help patients with seizures and lower BP.
- **Cerebrovascular injury**:
  - **The need to maintain cerebral perfusion pressure outweighs the acute need to lower BP.**

- Cerebral perfusion pressure (MAP–ICP) should be kept >70 mmHg if ICP monitoring is available.
- Acute stroke or intracranial hemorrhage:
  - BP >230/140 mmHg: Nitroprusside is agent of choice.
  - BP 180–230/140–105 mmHg: Labetalol, esmolol, or other easily titratable IV antihypertensive.
  - BP <180/105: Defer hypertensive management.
- **Aortic dissection**:
  - Type A dissection: Patients should be referred for emergent surgical correction and aggressively treated with antihypertensives.
  - Type B dissection: Treated with antihypertensives. Labetalol or esmolol should be started initially to lower heart rate, followed by nitroprusside if necessary. See Chapter 29 for a detailed approach to aortic dissection.
- **LV failure with pulmonary edema**:
  - Rapid reduction in BP should be achieved with a nitrate or NTG.
  - Small doses of loop diuretics are often effective.
- **Myocardial ischemia:**
  - IV NTG will improve coronary blood flow, decrease LV preload, and moderately decrease systemic arterial pressure.
  - β-Blockers should be added to decrease heart rate and BP.
- **Preeclampsia and eclampsia:**
  - Methyldopa, a centrally acting α-blocker, is the drug of choice for hypertension in pregnancy due to large experience in this setting.
  - IV labetalol may also be used with appropriate fetal monitoring.
  - Angiotensin converting enzyme (ACE) inhibitors are contraindicated in pregnancy.
- **Pheochromocytoma** may present with a markedly elevated BP, profound sweating, marked tachycardia, pallor, and numbness/coldness/tingling in the extremities.
  - **Phentolamine**, 5 to 10 mg IV, is the drug of choice and should be repeated as needed.
  - Nitroprusside may be added if necessary.
  - A β-blocker should be added only after phentolamine to avoid unopposed α-adrenergic activity. Of note, labetalol (α-blocker and nonselective β-blocker) and clonidine interfere with catecholamine assays used in the diagnosis of pheochromocytoma, so they should be held before the diagnosis is made.
- **Cocaine-related hypertensive emergency** can be treated with **benzodiazepines**.
  - Severe hypertension should be treated with nondihydropyridine calcium channel blockers (e.g., IV diltiazem), NTG, nitroprusside, or phentolamine.
  - β-Blockers should be avoided given the risk of unopposed α-adrenergic activity, although labetalol, which has α-antagonist activity, may be used.

Cardiogenic Shock

GENERAL PRINCIPLES

- A logical algorithm for the assessment and treatment of ADHF is presented in Figures 5-1 and 14-2.
- Approximately 6% to 8% of patients with acute coronary syndrome will develop cardiogenic shock during hospitalization, most often due to a STEMI.[5,6]
- Objective measures of shock include mental status, urine output, and arterial and venous oxygenation. Other secondary markers that are helpful include BP, heart rate, PAC values, serum creatinine, and liver enzymes.

Definition

- Patients with the highest immediate mortality (>50%) are those with cardiogenic shock: a low-output state with signs and symptoms of organ underperfusion.
- The patient has typical LV pump failure as the cause of cardiogenic shock if the SBP is <90 mmHg and the cardiac index is <2.2 L/minute/m².

Etiology

- **The most common cause is an extensive MI**, which severely and acutely compromises LV function.
- Less common causes include RV infarction and mechanical complications, such as papillary muscle dysfunction or rupture, ventricular septal rupture, and free wall rupture.

Risk Factors

- Risk factors for developing shock include older age, diabetes, anterior infarct, history of previous MI, peripheral vascular disease, decreased LV ejection fraction, and larger infarct.
- Underlying cardiomyopathy is a common cause.

DIAGNOSIS

Clinical Presentation

- Patients with cardiogenic shock are profoundly hypotensive, peripherally vasoconstricted (cool to touch), anuric, and often have altered mental status.
- Pulses are diminished and rapid. Cardiac examination may reveal tachycardia with the presence of an S3 and/or S4.
- Pay close attention to systolic murmurs indicative of a ventricular septal defect (VSD) or papillary muscle rupture.
- Jugular venous distention and pulmonary rales may also be present.

Diagnostic Testing

- May show arterial hypoxia, elevated creatinine, and lactic acidosis.
- CXR may reveal evidence of pulmonary congestion.
- Bedside echocardiography gives rapid information regarding LV systolic function and mechanical complications, including acute VSD, severe mitral regurgitation, free wall rupture, and tamponade.
- Placement of a PAC is appropriate in this setting and allows for differentiation of LV and RV infarction, mechanical complication, and volume depletion.
- In addition, a PAC will guide treatment when starting inotropes and/or giving volume repletion (see Chapter 8).

TREATMENT

Immediate Management

- **Oxygen**: Maintain O₂ saturation above 90% if possible. Intubation may be necessary, but be prepared for the further hypotension that results from the sedation and decreased cardiac filling with positive pressure ventilation.
- **Medications**: Discontinue β-blockers and vasodilators immediately.
- **IV fluids**: Goal pulmonary capillary wedge pressure (PCWP) is approximately 18 mmHg. Patients with low PCWP will benefit from gentle hydration. Patients with pulmonary edema or elevated PCWP will often benefit from diuresis with IV furosemide. Be vigilant for hypotension related to the diuresis.

- **Inotropes and vasopressors**: Vasopressor medications are useful in the management of cardiogenic shock but should be titrated with PAC guidance.
  - If SBP is <70 mmHg, start norepinephrine at 2 μg/minute and titrate to 20 μg/minute to achieve a mean arterial pressure of 70 mmHg.
  - If SBP is 70 to 90 mmHg, start dopamine. At 2 to 5 μg/kg/minute, dopamine increases cardiac output and renal blood flow through β- and dopamine-specific receptors, respectively. At 5–20 μg/kg/minute, dopamine has a-adrenergic stimulation leading to vasoconstriction.
  - With SBP >90 mmHg, dobutamine is the preferred agent. Dobutamine is started at 2.5 μg/kg/minute and slowly titrated to effect (usual maximum dose is 10 μg/kg/minute). The phosphodiesterase inhibitor milrinone acts as an inotrope and vasodilator and may be used if other agents prove ineffective.

Advanced Support

- Advanced percutaneous or surgically implanted therapeutic options have been developed for cardiogenic shock, due to the high incidence of morbidity and mortality from irreversible organ damage secondary to pump failure.
- It is reasonable to consider transferring the patient to a facility capable of advanced therapies for cardiogenic shock.
- Therapeutic interventions and devices include
  - **Coronary reperfusion**: Several trials have examined the benefit of revascularization (percutaneously or surgically) or medical treatment in patients with cardiogenic shock. The SHOCK trial prospectively examined patients who developed cardiogenic shock within 36 hours of acute MI and compared revascularization with aggressive medical management.[7] Although there was no mortality benefit at 30 days, there were significant mortality benefits at 6 months and 1 year with early revascularization. Younger patients (≤75 years) showed greater benefit with revascularization, whereas older patients had better outcomes with medical management.
  - **Intra Aortic Balloon Pump (IABP) and percutaneous Left Ventricular Assist Device (LVAD):** Placed by an interventional cardiologist, and an IABP reduces afterload, increases coronary perfusion, augments DBP, and promotes a slight increase in cardiac output.[8-10] See Chapter 8 for further discussion of IABP and percutaneous LVAD.

SPECIAL CONSIDERATIONS

- Patients with long-standing heart failure may eventually decline to a point where β-blockers, ACE inhibitors, and vasodilators need to be decreased or stopped. Refer to Chapters 14 and 15 for heart failure management.
- Patients with **LVAD cannot** receive compressions in resuscitative efforts. If a patient with an LVAD presents in duress, it is helpful to obtain the power, flow, and pulse indices if possible while arranging for transfer to an LVAD center. Because these patients are at an increased risk for bleeding, a STAT complete blood count and international normalized ratio (INR) should be obtained and corrected to a hemoglobin of 10 g/dL and INR between 1.5 and 2.0.
- Patients with an orthotopic **heart transplant** developing cardiogenic shock should be managed as above and transferred to a heart transplant center. A concerning cause of a failing transplanted heart is rejection, which often requires an endomyocardial biopsy to prove and medication adjustments to treat. If time allows, a brief transthoracic echocardiogram with myocardial tissue Doppler imaging may provide valuable information regarding valvular and contractile function.

Cardiac Device Emergencies (Pacemakers and Defibrillators)

GENERAL PRINCIPLES

There are two types of cardiac emergencies for patients with cardiac devices:
- Pacemaker malfunction in a patient who is pacemaker-dependent, that is, with underlying symptomatic bradycardia or asystole in the absence of pacing.
- Multiple internal cardioverter defibrillator (ICD) shocks in a patient with a defibrillator.

DIAGNOSIS

- **Identify the device.** Patients with cardiac devices are asked to carry an identification card, which gives the information regarding the type of device and device manufacturer.
- **Identify the rhythm.** A 12-lead ECG can rapidly determine the patient's rhythm and the response of the cardiac device.
- A pacemaker may either fail to sense a beat or fail to capture the heart with a pacing output. This can become an emergency if the patient has underlying symptomatic bradycardia or asystole without effective pacing.
- Two or more ICD shocks in the span of 24 hours is generally considered concerning. This may be due to either appropriate shocks for recurrent ventricular arrhythmia, shocks for an SVT with a fast ventricular rate, or inappropriate ICD sensing, which is most commonly due to a lead fracture or migration.

TREATMENT

- Device interrogation and chest X-ray can often help identify the problematic heart rhythm or device programming/function. Further treatment is tailored toward the arrhythmia or device settings.
- If the patient has symptomatic bradycardia, treatment should focus on maintaining a reasonable heart rate (see "Symptomatic Bradycardia" section).
- If the patient is receiving inappropriate ICD shocks, a medical magnet may be placed over the pulse generator, which suspends ICD therapy, but not pacing.

SPECIAL CONSIDERATIONS

- Regular cardiac device checkups can monitor for changes in lead performance, which can herald lead failure.
- Wireless home monitoring is available for many newer cardiac devices and has been shown to quickly identify important clinically actionable events.
- Medical treatment and/or catheter ablation of tachyarrhythmias can often prevent future ICD shocks.

REFERENCES

1. Neumar RW, Otto CW, Link MS, et al. Part 8: adult advanced cardiovascular life support: 2010 American Heart Association Guidelines for Cardiopulmonary Resuscitation and Emergency Cardiovascular Care. *Circulation* 2010;122:S729-S767.
2. Roy CL, Minor MA, Brookhart MA, et al. Does this patient with a pericardial effusion have cardiac tamponade? *JAMA* 2007;297:1810-1818.

3. Tumlin JA, Dunbar LM, Oparil S, et al. Fenoldopam, a dopamine agonist, for hypertensive emergency: a multicenter randomized trial. Fenoldopam Study Group. *Acad Emerg Med* 2000;7:653-663.

4. Murphy MB, Murray C, Shorten GD. Fenoldopam: a selective peripheral dopamine-receptor agonist for the treatment of severe hypertension. *N Engl J Med* 2001;345:1548-1557.

5. Jeger RV, Radovanovic D, Hunziker PR, et al. Ten-year trends in the incidence and treatment of cardiogenic shock. *Ann Intern Med* 2008;149:618-626.

6. Goldberg RJ, Spencer FA, Gore JM, et al. Thirty-year trends (1975 to 2005) in the magnitude of, management of, and hospital death rates associated with cardiogenic shock in patients with acute myocardial infarction: a population-based perspective. *Circulation* 2009;119:1211-1219.

7. Hochman JS, Sleeper LA, Webb JG, et al. Early revascularization in acute myocardial infarction complicated by cardiogenic shock. SHOCK Investigators. Should we emergently revascularize occluded coronaries for cardiogenic shock. *N Engl J Med* 1999;341:625-634.

8. Thiele J, Schuler G, Neumann FJ, et al. Intraaortic balloon counterpulsation in acute myocardial infarction complicated by cardiogenic shock: design and rationale of the Intraaortic Balloon Pump in Cardiogenic Shock II (IABP-SHOCK II) trial. *Am Heart J* 2012;163:938-945.

9. Barron HV, Every NR, Parsons LS, et al. Investigators in the National Registry of Myocardial Infarction 2. *Am Heart J* 2001;14:933-939.

10. Sjauw KD, Engström AD, Vis MM, et al. A systematic review and meta-analysis of intra-aortic balloon pump therapy in ST-elevation myocardial infarction: should we change the guidelines? *Eur Heart J* 2009;30:459-468.

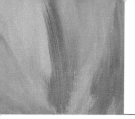

Procedures in Cardiovascular Critical Care

8

C. Huie Lin and Alan Zajarias

Management of cardiovascular issues in the critically ill patient is complex, but extremely important. Altered ventricular filling, poor myocardial perfusion, cardiac dysrhythmias, and severe valvular lesions all can complicate management. With appropriate patient selection and when performed in a timely manner, the invasive procedures described in this chapter may help guide treatment or stabilize the critically ill patient. As with all invasive procedures, however, understanding of appropriate indications, technique, interpretation of results, and troubleshooting are essential to success. The following five procedures will be discussed in this chapter:
- Pulmonary artery (PA; Swan-Ganz) catheterization
- Temporary transvenous pacing
- Pericardiocentesis
- Intraaortic balloon pump (IABP)
- Percutaneous ventricular assist device (VAD)

Pulmonary Artery (Swan-Ganz) Catheterization

GENERAL PRINCIPLES

- Today PA catheterization has become both an essential and controversial procedure in the management of critically ill patients; the technique is invasive with the risk of complications, and it is inherently diagnostic, not therapeutic.[1-5]
- Nonetheless, a PA catheterization may provide valuable information regarding right heart pressures, cardiac output (CO), left and right heart filling pressures, systemic and pulmonary vascular resistance, and shunt quantification.
- In particular, the PA catheterization can assist in identifying the etiology of shock or the driving deficiency in resuscitation of complex shock (Table 8-1).[6]

DIAGNOSIS

Diagnostic Testing

- **Choice of venous access site** should be determined on a case-by-case basis according to the risks and benefits of each location in an individual patient.
  - In general, the left subclavian and the right internal jugular vein approaches take advantage of the natural curvature of the catheter and allow easiest passage of the catheter into the PA.
  - Femoral access can be used but requires fluoroscopic guidance to place and is associated with higher risks of deep venous thrombosis and infection.
  - Modified Seldinger technique is used for placement of a 7-Fr or 8-Fr introducer (also called a sheath).

TABLE 8-1	SHOCK: ETIOLOGY-DEPENDENT HEMODYNAMICS			
Etiology of shock	PCWP	RAP	CO	SVR
Cardiogenic	High	High	Low	High
Septic	Low	Low	High/ normal	Low
Pulmonary embolism/ pulmonary HTN	Normal	High	Low	High/ normal
Hypovolemic	Low	Low	Low	High

PCWP, pulmonary capillary wedge pressure; RAP, right arterial pressure; CO, cardiac output; SVR, systemic vascular resistance; HTN, hypertension.

- **Balloon insertion**: With the balloon inflated, the progress of the catheter as it is advanced can be monitored and recorded by the characteristic pressure waveforms of each of the right-sided chambers (Figure 8-1).
  - Once advanced to the wedged position, the balloon is deflated to reacquire the PA tracing. If pulmonary capillary wedge pressure (PCWP) persists despite deflation of the balloon, the catheter may need to be withdrawn until the PA tracing is seen.
  - The balloon should then be **slowly** reinflated, and the volume of air required to wedge should be recorded and used for subsequent wedge measurements.
  - Fluoroscopic guidance can be used to facilitate balloon insertion, particularly for patients with indwelling cardiac devices.
- **Confirm location**: Once position of the catheter is stabilized by suture, a chest radiograph (CXR) should be performed to confirm the position of the PA catheter and to evaluate for pneumothorax if subclavian or internal jugular approach was used.
  - Ideally, the catheter tip should be in zone III of the lung, where arterial pressure exceeds venous and alveolar pressures, thereby creating a column of blood to the left atrium.
  - **To minimize risk, the balloon should be kept in the deflated position unless a PCWP measurement is being made.**
- **Pressure measurement and waveforms**
  - To complete a full diagnostic study, pressures should be noted and recorded in each of the right-sided chambers as the catheter is advanced; nominal hemodynamic values are listed in Table 8-2.
  - Interpretation of hemodynamics must include evaluation for errors in pressure measurements such as inaccurate zero referencing of the manometer, overdamping of the waveform due to air in the line, and underdamping with a noisy tracing.
- **Right atrial tracing** (Figure 8-1)
  - Right atrial systole follows the P wave on the electrocardiogram (ECG) and produces the *a* **wave** of the right atrial pressure tracing. With atrial relaxation, there is a decline in the pressure, known as the *x* **descent**.
  - Filling of the right atrium from the venous circulation and retrograde movement of the tricuspid valve annulus during right ventricular (RV) systole produces the *v* **wave**. As the tricuspid valve opens, blood from the right atrium empties into the RV, causing a decline in the right atrial pressure and producing the *y* **descent**.

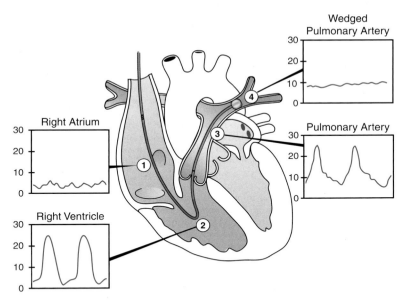

FIGURE 8-1. Pressure tracing exhibited in the various chambers and positions during right-heart catheterization. (From Marino PL. *The ICU Book,* 2nd ed. Philadelphia, PA: Lippincott Williams & Wilkins; 1997:157.)

TABLE 8-2	NORMAL HEMODYNAMIC VALUES
CI (L/min/m^2)	2.6–4.2
PCWP (mmHg)	6–12
PA (mmHg)	16–30/3–12
Mean	10–16
RV (mmHg)	16–30/0–8
RA (mmHg)	0–8
SVR (dynes/sec/cm^{-5})	700–1,600
PVR (dynes/sec/cm^{-5})	20–130

CI, cardiac index; PCWP, pulmonary capillary wedge pressure; PA, pulmonary artery; RV, right ventricle; RA, right atrium; SVR, systemic vascular resistance; PVR, pulmonary vascular resistance.

- ○ The pressure of the peak *a* wave is higher than that of the peak *v* wave, except in the setting of significant tricuspid regurgitation.
- **RV tracing**
  - ○ RV systole follows the QRS complex, which gives rise to a rapidly increasing systolic pressure waveform.
  - ○ With ventricular relaxation, the pressure waveform declines and reaches a nadir.
- **PA tracing**
  - ○ The normal PA pressure consists of a systolic wave that coincides with RV systole. The decline in the pressure wave is usually interrupted by the **dicrotic notch**, which corresponds to pulmonic valve closure.
  - ○ The nadir of the decline represents the end-diastolic arterial pressure.
- **Pulmonary capillary wedge tracing**: The pressure obtained is a transmitted left atrial pressure, and an *a* wave, an *x* descent, a *v* wave, and a *y* descent can be seen, corresponding to the left atrial systole, relaxation, filling, and emptying, respectively.
- **CO**
  - ○ CO is reported as liters per minute, whereas the cardiac index (CI) is the CO normalized to body surface area. Two common methods of measuring CO are the **Fick method** and the **thermodilution (TD) technique.**
  - ○ The **Fick method** is based on the concept that oxygen extraction in the body is inversely related to CO. Oxygen extraction can be determined by the arteriovenous oxygen (AVO_2) difference, and this relationship is expressed by the following equation:

$$CO \ (L/minute) = \frac{O_2 \ consumption \ (mL/minute)}{AVO_2 \ difference \ (mL/L)}$$

  - ■ O_2 consumption is either assumed or estimated from a nomogram based up age and gender of the patient.
  - ■ In practice, a mixed venous oxygen saturation sample is drawn from the PA, and an arterial oxygen saturation sample is drawn from either the aorta (SAO_2) or other arterial bed, and a hemoglobin level is fed into the following equation:

$$CO \ (L/minute) = \frac{O_2 consumption \ (mL/minute)}{13.6 \times (SAO_2 - PAO_2) \times Hemogloblin \ (g/dL)}$$

  - ■ The constant 13.6 represents the oxygen-carrying capacity of hemoglobin. The Fick method **is most accurate for patients with a low CO and least accurate in patients with a high CO or significant shunts.**
  - ○ To determine CO by the **TD technique**, a known amount of indicator (10 cc of cold saline) is injected into the right atrium, and the rate of dilution is measured by a thermistor at the distal tip of the catheter in the PA.
    - ■ A time–concentration curve is generated, and the area under the curve corresponds to the CO.
    - ■ Three to five measurements are made, and the mean CO is taken.
    - ■ This method does require the use of a catheter with a proximal right atrium (RA) port and a distal thermistor, referred to as a TD catheter.
    - ■ This technique is inexpensive, is easy to perform, and does not require arterial sampling; **however, certain conditions may render the results unreliable, such as tricuspid regurgitation, pulmonic regurgitation, and intracardiac shunts and low CO.**

- **Vascular resistance**
  - The resistance of a vascular bed is calculated by dividing the pressure gradient across the bed by the flow through it.
  - **Systemic vascular resistance (SVR)** is determined by the following formula:

$$SVC = \frac{(\text{Mean arterial pressure} - \text{Mean RA pressure})}{CO}$$

  - Increased SVR is usually present in patients with systemic hypertension and may be seen in patients with low a CO and compensatory vasoconstriction.
  - Reduced SVR is seen with inappropriately increased CO (e.g., sepsis, arteriovenous [AV] fistulas, anemia, fever, and thyrotoxicosis).
  - **Pulmonary vascular resistance (PVR)** is calculated by the following formula:

$$PVR = \frac{(\text{Mean PA pressure} - \text{Mean PCWP})}{CO}$$

Elevated PVR can be seen in pulmonary hypertension, pulmonary diseases, or Eisenmenger syndrome.
- **Shunt calculation:** The magnitude and direction of an intracardiac shunt can be calculated by oximetry, using the following equation:

$$\frac{\dot{Q}p}{\dot{Q}s} = \frac{(SAO_2 - MVO_2)}{(PVO_2 - PAO_2)}$$

  - $\dot{Q}p$ is pulmonary blood flow, $\dot{Q}s$ is systemic blood flow, SAO_2 is systemic arterial oxygen saturation, MVO_2 is mixed venous oxygen saturation, PVO_2 is pulmonary venous oxygen saturation, and PAO_2 is pulmonary arterial oxygen saturation.

  - MVO_2 is usually equal to the PAO_2 unless there is an atrial or ventricular level shunt and/or congenital anomaly, in which case the MVO_2 can be calculated by the Flamm correction:

$$MVO_2 = [(3 \times SVCO_2) + (IVCO_2)]/4$$

  - $SVCO_2$ is the oxygen saturation of the superior vena cava and $IVCO_2$ is that of the inferior vena cava (IVC).
  - The PVO_2 can be drawn from the catheter tip in the wedge position (carefully!), although a true PVO_2 should be drawn from the left atrium. A $\dot{Q}p/\dot{Q}s > 1$ suggests a net left-to-right shunt, and < 1 is a right-to-left shunt.

COMPLICATIONS

- While PA catheterization can be a relatively straightforward procedure, the risk of complications can include the following:
  - Air embolism
  - Endocarditis/sepsis
  - PA rupture
  - Bleeding/hemoptysis
  - Cardiac tamponade/perforation

- ○ Pulmonary infarction
- ○ Right bundle branch block (complete heart block if there is an underlying left bundle branch block)
- ○ Pneumothorax (if the superior approach is used)
- ○ Sustained ventricular arrhythmias
- ○ Thromboembolism
- As with all procedures, careful planning, technique, and supervision will decrease the likelihood of complications.

Temporary Transvenous Pacing

GENERAL PRINCIPLES

- Bradyarrhythmias can be caused by intrinsic disease of the conduction system or by extrinsic factors acting on the conduction system (see Chapter 24).
- Indications for the insertion of a temporary pacemaker and the clinical situations for its use are shown in Table 8-3.[7,8]
- It is important to note that the location of a myocardial infarct has a large influence on the prognosis and treatment of conduction disease.
  - ○ In general, proximal (AV nodal) conduction disease is associated with an infarct of the RCA. This causes a transient AV block and often does not warrant immediate placement of a temporary pacemaker.
  - ○ One exception is AV block in the setting of RV infarction, where restoration of AV synchrony can improve RV filling and thus CO.

TABLE 8-3	COMMON INDICATIONS FOR TRANSVENOUS TEMPORARY PACING
Condition	**Setting**
Third-degree AV block	Symptomatic congenital complete heart block
	Symptomatic acquired complete heart block
	Postoperative symptomatic complete heart block
Second-degree AV block	Symptomatic Mobitz I or II AV block
Acute MI	Symptomatic bradycardia
	High-grade AV block (trifascicular block)
	Complete AV block in setting of anterior MI
Sinus node dysfunction	Symptomatic bradyarrhythmias
Tachycardia prevention/treatment	Bradycardia-dependent arrhythmias

AV, atrioventricular; MI, myocardial infarction.

○ Distal (infranodal) conduction disease is frequently associated with a left anterior descending/septal infarct and is more lasting and life-threatening. Immediate pacing efforts should be pursued.

DIAGNOSIS

Diagnostic Testing

- Transvenous pacing involves the insertion of a pacing catheter, typically into the right ventricle to directly stimulate the myocardium.
- Briefly, a percutaneous entry site is chosen, usually the right internal jugular vein or the femoral vein.
- Left-sided central veins should be left uncontaminated if possible, since, if a permanent pacer is required, they are the preferred sites of access.
- The modified Seldinger technique allows the placement of a 6-Fr introducer sheath.
- A bipolar pacing lead is introduced into the RV under the aid of a balloon-tipped catheter, which allows easy flotation of the pacing wire to the apex of the RV.
- Alternative ways to assure proper placement of the bipolar pacing lead include fluoroscopy (most common), catheter tip electrogram, and ECG rhythm strip during pacemaker stimulation.
- The lead is attached to a pacing generator after confirmation of placement by fluoroscopy or CXR.
- A prosthetic tricuspid valve is a relative contraindication to placement of a transvenous pacer. The femoral vein should not be used if the patient has an IVC filter in place.
- The pacing generator's **sensitivity** may be set on demand (synchronous) mode or fixed (asynchronous) mode.
  - ○ In **demand mode**, the lead "senses" the heart's intrinsic electrical activity; in the absence of conduction, the pulse generator delivers an impulse at a preset adjustable voltage.
  - ○ **Fixed (asynchronous) mode** delivers a set amount of impulses per time, regardless of the underlying native conduction.
- A **pacing threshold** must be established; this is defined as the least amount of current (in milliamperes) necessary to depolarize or capture the ventricle.
  - ○ The threshold gives the operator an idea of the proximity of the pacing lead to the ventricular wall. Therefore, the lower the threshold, the closer the pacing wire is to the ventricular wall. The optimal pacing threshold is <1 milliampere. The voltage delivered by the pulse generator is usually set at least 2 milliamperes above the pacing threshold.
  - ○ The threshold should be checked twice daily; if the threshold is >2 milliamperes, the patient should be restricted to bed rest and repositioning of the lead should be considered.
- The **set rate** depends on the clinical scenario. Usually, it is set at 40 to 50 beats per minute (bpm) as a backup to the intrinsic heart rate unless the CO is very low. For tachyarrhythmia prevention, pacing is usually set at approximately 100 bpm until the underlying predisposition is corrected.

COMPLICATIONS

- Complications include the following:
  - ○ Pneumothorax
  - ○ Myocardial perforation

- ○ Bleeding
- ○ Ventricular ectopy/nonsustained ventricular tachycardia
- ○ Thromboembolism
- ○ Infection
- **Failure to capture** is illustrated on the rhythm strip as pacer spikes that do not initiate capture (i.e., there is no ventricular depolarization).
  - ○ This is most likely due to displacement of the lead, which means that the pacing threshold will have increased beyond the voltage delivered by the pulse generator.
  - ○ The generator voltage should be increased immediately until an appropriate pacing is seen, and the lead should be repositioned.
  - ○ **Other reasons for failure to pace** include fracture of the lead or an overly sensitive pacing generator that detects impulses traveling from the chest muscles that inhibit the pulse generator. This can be corrected by reducing the sensitivity of the pulse generator or pacing in a fixed (asynchronous) mode.
- **Diaphragmatic pacing** is a complication associated with a high preset voltage; as a result, the phrenic nerve is stimulated through the wall of the RV. It also may indicate a perforation of the RV wall, with the lead stimulating the diaphragm directly. Beware of a patient hiccupping at a rate identical to the pacer rate.

Pericardiocentesis

GENERAL PRINCIPLES

- In either circumstance, timely diagnosis and treatment of tamponade are crucial, and the index of suspicion should be high in the setting of refractory shock.[9]
- Hypotension resulting from cardiac tamponade can be an acute event resulting from trauma, perforation, or myocardial infarction (MI) or can be insidious in the setting of metastatic cancer or infection.
- Transthoracic echocardiography (TTE) and chest computed tomography can diagnose the presence of a pericardial effusion, but cardiac tamponade remains a clinical diagnosis.
- Identifying **signs of impending decompensation** such as Beck triad (muffled heart sounds, jugular venous distention, and low blood pressure), shortness of breath, pulsus paradoxus, and tachycardia should prompt the clinician for expedient bedside echo and plan for pericardiocentesis.[10]

DIAGNOSIS

Diagnostic Testing
- **Preparation**
  - ○ If time allows, TTE should be prepared at bedside.
  - ○ The probe should be placed 1 to 2 cm on the patient's left of the xiphoid process. From this position, the depth and extent of the pericardial fluid can be estimated, and the angle of approach can be identified. This position should be marked and the angle noted, after which the entire chest should be prepped and draped in sterile fashion.
  - ○ If an assistant is available, the apical four-chamber view should be acquired on the TTE to guide the procedure.

- **Access**
  - ○ Although a preprepared pericardiocentesis kit is preferable, emergent pericardiocentesis can be performed using basic equipment.
  - ○ Pericardiocentesis can be performed by a subxiphoid, apical, or parasternal approach.
  - ○ Once prepped and draped, the site (1 to 2 cm to the patient's left of the xiphoid process) should be anesthetized using a 21-G and/or 25-G needle and 1% to 2% lidocaine. Care should be taken to anesthetize up to the lowest rib.
  - ○ The 18-G access needle (9 to 15 cm depending on the size of the patient) should then be introduced into the skin with the stylet still in place, directed toward the left shoulder. The access needle should then be advanced at an about 15-degree angle to touch the lowest rib.
  - ○ The stylet can then be removed and replaced with a 10-mL syringe containing 2 to 3 mL of lidocaine. With negative pressure applied through the syringe, the needle should be "walked" down to a position immediately deep to the rib.
  - ○ As this is done, 0.5 to 1 mL of lidocaine can be given to continue anesthetizing the track and maintain a clear needle. The position of the needle will not be well visualized on TTE.
- Echocardiographic confirmation
  - ○ Once the pericardium is punctured and fluid is freely drawn into the 10-mL syringe, agitated saline should be injected through the needle.
  - ○ Saline contrast in the pericardial space documented by TTE will confirm appropriate positioning. If bubbles are seen in the RV instead, the needle should be slowly withdrawn, and additional agitated saline injected to evaluate the position until the study confirms pericardial position of the needle.
  - ○ RV needle punctures rarely cause continuous bleeding into the pericardium, unless pulmonary hypertension, coagulopathy, or thrombocytopenia is present.
- **Drain placement**
  - ○ If position in the pericardial space is confirmed, a 0.035-inch J-tip wire should be advanced through the access needle into the pericardial space.
  - ○ Over the needle, a scalpel nick should be made to open the skin in preparation for placement of a drain.
  - ○ The needle should then be removed and a vessel dilator matching the drain size (6 Fr to 8.5 Fr) should be advanced and rotated carefully to dilate the skin and soft tissue tract.
  - ○ This can then be exchanged for the drain. Our preference is to manually drain the fluid by aspirating through a 60-mL syringe connected to a drainage bag via a three-way stopcock.
  - ○ Appropriate drainage should be confirmed by TTE as well as improvement in vital signs and symptoms. Once manual drainage no longer produces fluid, the drain secured to the skin via suture and connected to a Jackson-Pratt drain.
  - ○ Follow-up TTE should be performed daily to confirm adequate drainage.
- Laboratory studies of the pericardial fluid should be tailored to the patient's clinical scenario; however, basic studies should include pH, cytology, gram stain and culture, and acid-fast stain.
- If the decision is made to transition to surgical pericardial window, a pericardial biopsy can be sent for histologic analysis.

COMPLICATIONS

Complications of pericardiocentesis include the following:
- RV puncture
- Coronary artery puncture

- Pneumothorax
- Bleeding
- Enterotomy
- Infection

Intra-Aortic Balloon Pump

GENERAL PRINCIPLES

- IABP, developed in 1960s, was the first mechanical hemodynamic support device that could be placed at bedside.
  - Currently it remains a mainstay in initial therapy of cardiogenic shock or refractory ischemia as it provides improvements in the myocardial O_2 supply/demand ratio and some circulatory support.
  - Because of its simplicity in concept, ease of insertion, and long clinical track record, the IABP continues to be the most widely used mechanical cardiac support device.
- The IABP exerts its hemodynamic effects through counterpulsation. The balloon rapidly inflates during diastole and deflates during systole. The inflation and deflation provide two specific hemodynamic effects:
  - **Diastolic augmentation**: Inflation of the balloon after aortic valve closure increases diastolic pressure, increasing coronary perfusion pressure.
  - **Systolic unloading**: Deflation of the balloon before the opening of the aortic valve removes effective aortic volume decreases afterload, decreasing left ventricle (LV) myocardial O_2 requirements.
- **Indications** for IABP support include the following:
  - Cardiogenic shock: acute MI, acute mitral regurgitation, ventricular septal defect, myocarditis, stress-induced cardiomyopathy (takotsubo cardiomyopathy), or drug toxicity[11-13]
  - Unstable angina
  - Prophylaxis in the setting of high-risk coronary artery intervention[14,15]
  - Severe symptomatic aortic stenosis, especially when associated with heart failure
  - Severe multivessel or left main coronary artery disease requiring urgent cardiac or noncardiac surgery

DIAGNOSIS

Diagnostic Testing

- Prior to insertion, clinical data on the patient should be reviewed for evidence of **contraindications** to IABP support.
  - Significant aortic regurgitation
  - Abdominal aortic aneurysm
  - Aortic dissection
  - Septicemia
  - Uncontrolled bleeding
  - Severe bilateral peripheral vascular disease (including bilateral femoropopliteal bypass grafts)
  - Significant iliac tortuosity

- **Access**
  - ○ As with the placement of any intravascular device, the patient should be fastidiously prepped and draped in a sterile fashion.
  - ○ Percutaneous access to the common femoral artery is obtained using the modified Seldinger technique, often with the use of a micropuncture set.
  - ○ We commonly perform an ipsilateral iliofemoral angiogram by hand injection to rule out significant peripheral arterial disease and confirm that the arterial system can accommodate the device.
  - ○ While some IABP systems are now sheathless, we generally place a 7.5-Fr or 8-Fr sheath in order to ensure secure access.
- **Placement**
  - ○ The appropriate-sized balloon pump kit (based on patient height) should be prepared.
  - ○ While IABP systems differ, most are placed with the use of a 0.025-inch guidewire placed in the IABP catheter itself, allowing atraumatic introduction of the catheter into the sheath and up to the thoracic aorta.
  - ○ Under fluoroscopy, the radiopaque tip of the catheter can be advanced to midpoint of the aortic knob and the guidewire removed.
  - ○ The IABP system may then be activated and filled with helium per protocol. Confirmation of placement and full expansion of the balloon should be performed using fluoroscopy, while the patient remains prepped.
  - ○ In emergent situations, the procedure can be done at the bedside without the aid of fluoroscopy.
  - ○ Systemic **anticoagulation** should then be initiated (most commonly intravenous heparin infusion).
- **Management**
  - ○ Confirmation by CXR of IABP tip position just below the aortic arch (distal to the left subclavian artery) is essential.
  - ○ Daily monitoring while the IABP is in place should consist of the following: (1) distal lower extremity pulse examination, (2) left radial pulse examination (to ensure that the left subclavian remains unobstructed), (3) platelet count (thrombocytopenia), (4) CXR for position, and (5) timing of inflation and deflation.
  - ○ To optimize IABP support, timing of the balloon inflation and deflation is of utmost importance (Table 8-4).
    - ■ Although modern IABP consoles perform autotiming algorithms via ECG trigger, manual timing adjustments may still be required.
    - ■ Evaluation of timing is best performed by printing a tracing at 1:2 inflation ratio such that one support cycle and one unsupported cycle can be evaluated side by side (Figure 8-2).
    - ■ Balloon inflation should coincide with the dicrotic notch on the arterial waveform.
    - ■ Balloon deflation should immediately precede LV contraction on the arterial waveform. Practically, this can be timed by maximizing the nadir of the "V".
  - ○ The following four scenarios should be avoided by careful adjustment of timing when feasible:
    - ■ **Late balloon inflation**: Balloon inflates **late** if the inflation curve occurs after the dicrotic notch (late after the aortic valve closes). In this situation, diastolic augmentation is reduced, which translates into reduced improvement in coronary perfusion.
    - ■ **Early balloon inflation**: Balloon inflates **before** the aortic valve closes, increasing afterload and increasing myocardial oxygen consumption. This can be a potentially dangerous situation.

| TABLE 8-4 | IABP TERMINOLOGY |

Terminology (at a 1:2 pumping rate)	Effects
Peak systolic pressure	Systolic pressure without activity related to the balloon pump
Inflation point	Point on the arterial pressure tracing where balloon inflation originates, just after the dicrotic notch
Peak diastolic pressure	Augmented increase in diastolic pressure that occurs when the balloon inflation displaces aortic blood volume due to counterpulsation
Balloon aortic end-diastolic pressure	Lowest pressure in the aorta, reflecting balloon deflation
Assisted peak systolic pressure	Systolic peak that reflects the afterload reduction produced by the balloon pump
Dicrotic notch	Landmark on the downslope of the arterial pressure waveform that signals aortic valve closure and the beginning of diastole

IABP, Intraaortic balloon pump.

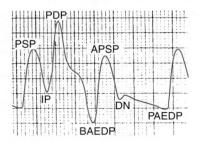

FIGURE 8-2. Normal arterial waveform with IABP set at 1:2 pulsation (with every other beat, the balloon inflates, and deflates). APSP, assisted peak systolic pressure; BAEDP, balloon aortic end-diastolic pressure; DN, dicrotic notch; IP, inflation point; PAEDP, patient aortic end-diastolic pressure; PDP, peak diastolic pressure; PSP, peak systolic pressure. (From Sorrentino M, Feldman T. Techniques for IABP timing, use, and discontinuance. *J Crit Illn* 1992;7:597-604.)

- **Early balloon deflation**: Balloon deflates **before** isovolumetric contraction, and the aorta refills with blood before ventricular ejection. This decreases the benefit of systolic unloading, removing the potential benefit of decreasing myocardial oxygen consumption.
- **Late balloon deflation**: Balloon deflates **late** after the aortic valve opens; afterload is again increased, again increasing myocardial oxygen consumption.

COMPLICATIONS

- **Thrombocytopenia** may occur due to mechanical destruction by the balloon pump or related to heparin anticoagulation.
  - Commonly, the platelet count should begin to rebound by the fourth day.
  - However, if profound thrombocytopenia persists, other sources such as heparin-induced thrombotic thrombocytopenia and continued mechanical destruction should be considered.
- **Limb ischemia** is related to simple mechanical obstruction by the balloon catheter at the insertion site. Balloon removal generally alleviates the problem.
- Iatrogenic retrograde **arterial dissection** may occur as a result of wire advancement into a false channel or via dissection by balloon inflation and usually presents with a severe back pain.
- **Cholesterol embolization** usually manifests as bilateral, painful, cold, mottled limbs (livedo reticularis) with associated eosinophilia, eosinophiluria, and thrombocytopenia as well as renal failure secondary to cholesterol emboli.
- Embolic **cerebrovascular accident** may occur if the IABP's central lumen has been flushed vigorously due to thrombus formation. Therefore, the central lumen of the IABP should not be used as a source of arterial blood.
- **Sepsis** can occur as a result of prolonged support and foreign body infection.
- **Balloon rupture** occurs due to calcification in the aorta. The ruptured balloon may produce thrombus within the balloon, making percutaneous removal impossible and requiring consultation from a vascular surgeon. Rarely, balloon rupture may be associated with helium embolization.

Percutaneous Ventricular Assist Device

GENERAL PRINCIPLES

- The advent of the percutaneous left VAD has revolutionized the care of patients with impending or confirmed cardiogenic shock.[16]
- For decades, hemodynamic support was limited to the IABP (as described above), extracorporeal membrane oxygenation, or surgical implantation of left VAD, each with significant limitations.
- The Tandem Heart System (CardiacAssist Inc., Pittsburgh, http://www.cardiacassist .com/TandemHeart, last accessed 5/21/13) and Impella systems (Abiomed, Danvers, http://www.abiomed.com/, last accessed 5/21/13) have allowed relatively rapid and effective (up to 5 L/minute) hemodynamic support by percutaneous methods.
- Technical aspects of placement of these devices are beyond the scope of this chapter; however, an overview of these devices is discussed. See Table 14-3 for further detail.

DIAGNOSIS

Diagnostic Testing

- Impella 2.5
  - The Impella 2.5 system is fully percutaneous.
  - Both Impella devices consist of a one-piece catheter with microaxial pump; the inlet is placed in the LV, and the outlet is placed in the ascending aorta.
  - The device can deliver a maximum 2.5 to 2.6 L/minute support for 5 minutes, but continuous use can only be maintained at 2.1 to 2.5 L/minute.

- The use of this device is contraindicated in the setting of significant aortic regurgitation.
- Placement of the catheter is performed by standard modified Seldinger technique in the common femoral artery. Angiography of the external iliac and femoral system is recommended to confirm that the arterial system can accommodate the 13-Fr sheath and Impella catheter.
- After initial access is obtained, the included 13-Fr sheath is placed, and a diagnostic catheter and wire are used to cross the aortic valve. The included 0.018-inch wire is then advanced through the diagnostic catheter into the LV, and the diagnostic catheter is removed.
- The Impella catheter is then advanced over the 0.018-inch wire to the LV, and the pump console is initiated.
- Once placed, monitoring the position of the catheter is an important component of managing the patient. Daily blood counts, pulse examination, chest radiography, and position by console monitoring should be performed.
- Approved usage of the Impella 2.5 is for 6 hours, although off-label use over the course of a longer period of time may be required.

- **Impella 5.0**
  - The Impella 5.0 is functionally similar to the 2.5 model; however, access for the catheter must be obtained by surgical cutdown as the microaxial pump housing is 21 Fr in diameter.
  - Our practice has been to obtain percutaneous access on the contralateral side to perform iliofemoral angiography to confirm that the arterial system can accommodate the catheter.
  - In addition, placement of the Impella 5.0 is performed in a hybrid operating suite as general anesthesia and surgical support is required. Otherwise, once surgical cutdown to the common femoral artery has been obtained, delivery of the Impella 5.0 is similar to that of the Impella 2.5.
  - Approved usage of the device is limited to 6 hours; however, extended periods of support have been reported without significant complications.

- **Tandem Heart**
  - The Tandem Heart System differs in concept from the Impella system in several ways:
    - First, the pump is extracorporeal, consisting of a centrifugal pump with a spinning rotor supported by hydrodynamic fluid bearing lubricated by constant heparinized saline infusion.
    - Second, the inflow cannula is placed in the left atrium from venous access via transseptal puncture.
    - Third, the outflow cannula is placed in the femoral artery. Importantly, although the manufacturer suggests that percutaneous arterial access can be used, the bore of the femoral artery cannula frequently requires the use of surgical cutdown.
  - As a result of these differences in access, the Tandem Heart can be technically more challenging to place, especially as transseptal puncture may be a technique that is unfamiliar to some operators.
  - Nevertheless, the Tandem Heart System offers several advantages.
    - The system can provide definitive full support and maintain continuous output of 5.0 L/minute.
    - Location of the inflow cannula in the left atrium may be advantageous in the setting of a ventricular septal rupture after MI, as placement of an inflow cannula in the LV may promote right-to-left shunt and further cyanosis.
    - Tandem Heart is approved for use up to 14 days.

- As with all hemodynamic support, a critical element in the management of the patient is a decision with regard to goals of care.
- While some patients may be candidates for heart transplant or surgically implanted VAD destination therapy and others may have self-limited cardiomyopathy, some patients may not have a clear clinical end point.
- The decision to place a percutaneous VAD, irrespective of access site, should be accompanied by a definitive care plan. Nevertheless, ventricular support must be provided in a timely manner, and the first signs of cardiogenic systemic hypoperfusion should prompt consideration of mechanical assistance.

COMPLICATIONS

Complications due to percutaneous VAD therapy include the following:
- Hemolysis
- Disseminated intravascular coagulation
- Lower extremity ischemia
- Infection
- Ventricular arrhythmias

REFERENCES

1. Ivanov R, Allen J, Calvin JE. The incidence of major morbidity in critically ill patients managed with pulmonary artery catheters: a meta-analysis: *Crit Care Med* 2000;28:615-619.
2. Shah MR, Hasselblad V, Stevenson LW, et al. Impact of the pulmonary artery catheter in critically ill patients: meta-analysis of randomized clinical trials: *JAMA* 2005;294:1664-1670.
3. Vincent JL, Pinsky MR, Sprung CL, et al. The pulmonary artery catheter: in medio virtus: *Crit Care Med* 2008;36:3093-3096.
4. Bethlehem C, Groenwold FM, Butler H, et al. The impact of a pulmonary-artery-catheter-based protocol on fluid and catecholamine administration in early sepsis: *Crit Care Res Pract* 2012;2012:161879. doi:10.1155/2012/161879. Epub 2012 Feb 21.
5. Rajaram SS, Desai NK, Kalra A, et al. Pulmonary artery catheters for adult patient in intensive care: *Cochrane Database Syst Rev* 2013;2:CD003408.
6. Marino PL. *The ICU Book*, 2nd ed. Philadelphia, PA: Lippincott Williams & Wilkins; 1997:157.
7. Epstein AE, DiMarco JP, Ellenbogen KA, et al. ACC/AHA/HRS 2008 guidelines for device-based therapy of cardiac rhythm abnormalities: *Circulation* 2008;117:e305-e408.
8. Epstein AE, DiMarco JP, Ellenbogen KA, et al. 2012 ACCF/AHA/HRS focused update incorporated into the ACCF/AHA/HRS 2008 guidelines for device-based therapy of cardiac rhythm abnormalities: *Circulation* 2013;127:e283-e352.
9. Spodick DH. Acute cardiac tamponade: *N Engl J Med* 2003;349:684-690.
10. Roy CL, Minor MA, Brookhart MA, et al. Does this patient with a pericardial effusion have cardiac tamponade? *JAMA* 2007;297:1810-1818.
11. Barron HV, Every NR, Parsons LS, et al. Investigators in the National Registry of Myocardial Infarction 2: *Am Heart J* 2001;14:933-939.
12. Sjauw KD, Engström AD, Vis MM, et al. A systematic review and meta-analysis of intra-aortic balloon pump therapy in ST-elevation myocardial infarction: should we change the guidelines? *Eur Heart J* 2009;30:459-468.
13. Thiele J, Schuler G, Neumann FJ, et al. Intraaortic balloon counterpulsation in acute myocardial infarction complicated by cardiogenic shock: design and rationale of the Intraaortic Balloon Pump in Cardiogenic Shock II (IABP-SHOCK II) trial: *Am Heart J* 2012;163:938-945.

14. Mishra S, Chu WW, Torguson R, et al. Role of prophylactic intra-aortic balloon pump in high-risk patients undergoing percutaneous coronary intervention: *Am J Cardiol* 2006;98:608-612.

15. Perera D, Stables R, Clayton T, et al. Long-term mortality data from the balloon pump-assisted coronary intervention study (BCIS-1): a randomized, controlled trial of elective balloon counterpulsation during high-risk percutaneous coronary intervention: *Circulation* 2013;127:207-212.

16. Kar B, Basra SS, Shah NR, et al. Percutaneous circulatory support in cardiogenic shock: interventional bridge to recovery: *Circulation* 2012;125:1809-1817.

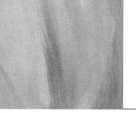

The Cardiac Patient Undergoing Noncardiac Surgery

9

Corey G. Foster and Lynne M. Seacord

GENERAL PRINCIPLES

- Evaluation of the patient with known or suspected cardiovascular disease undergoing noncardiac surgery is one of the most common reasons for cardiac consultation.
- The role of the consultant is to determine the stability of the patient's cardiovascular status and whether the patient is in best medical condition within the context of the surgical illness.
- Cardiac "clearance" is not the purpose, and the use of this term is strongly discouraged. Rather, risk assessment and optimization are the goals and should include discussions with the surgeon, anesthesiologist, and other physicians, when appropriate.
- In 2007, the American College of Cardiology (ACC) and the American Heart Association (AHA) published joint guidelines that provide updated recommendations for this purpose (Figure 9-1).[1]

Classification

- Preoperative cardiac evaluation considers both the nature of the surgery and the clinical characteristics of the patient.
- In the setting of a surgical emergency, preoperative evaluation may be limited to a rapid assessment including vital signs, volume status, hematocrit, electrolytes, renal function, and electrocardiogram (ECG). Only the most essential tests and interventions are appropriate until the acute surgical emergency is resolved.
- Under less urgent circumstances, preoperative cardiac evaluation may lead to a variety of responses, some of which may result in postponement or cancellation of an elective procedure. The algorithm for perioperative cardiac evaluation and care is shown in Figure 9-1.[1]

Risk Factors

- The level of risk of the surgery is considered. For low-risk surgery, no preoperative testing is needed. Risk for specific types of surgery is shown in Table 9-1.[1]
- For intermediate- and high-risk elective surgeries, the algorithm in Figure 9-1 is applied.[1] The first question asked is whether the patient has an active cardiac condition (Figure 9-1, step 2).[1] If such a high-risk condition is present, elective surgery is postponed until diagnosis and treatment of this condition is complete. These conditions include
  - Unstable coronary syndromes
  - Unstable or severe angina (Canadian Cardiovascular Society class III or IV)
  - Recent myocardial infarction (MI) (7–30 days)
  - Decompensated heart failure
  - Significant arrhythmias (including symptomatic bradycardia, Class IIb or III AV block, atrial fibrillation not rate-controlled, and new ventricular tachycardia)
  - Severe stenotic valvular disease, that is, aortic stenosis (mean gradient >40 mm, aortic valve area <1.0 cm^2 or symptomatic) or symptomatic mitral stenosis

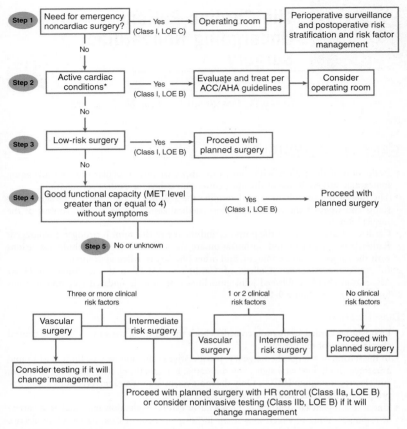

FIGURE 9-1. Algorithm for cardiac evaluation and management. (From Fleisher LA, Beckman JA, Brown KA, et al. ACC/AHA 2007 guidelines on perioperative cardiovascular evaluation and care for noncardiac surgery: *J Am Coll Cardiol* 2007;50: e159-e241.)

DIAGNOSIS

Clinical Presentation

- If no active cardiac condition is present, the patient's functional capacity must be carefully assessed (Figure 9-1, steps 4 and 5).[1]
- The patient's functional status is a reliable predictor of both perioperative and long-term cardiac risk. Functional status based on different activities is shown in Table 9-2.[1]
- Patients who can complete 4 METs are at relatively low risk for perioperative complications, even if they have other cardiac risks.
- If the patient is unable to complete 4 METs of activity without symptoms, other clinical risks must be considered, including the following:
  - History of ischemic heart disease
  - History of compensated or prior heart failure
  - History of cerebrovascular disease

TABLE 9-1	RISK STRATIFICATION BASED ON THE TYPE OF SURGERY[a]

Risk stratification	Procedure examples
Vascular (reported cardiac risk often >5%)	Aortic and other major vascular surgery Peripheral vascular surgery
Intermediate (reported cardiac risk generally 1–5%)	Intraperitoneal and intrathoracic surgery Carotid endarterectomy Head and neck surgery Orthopedic surgery Prostate surgery
Low[b] (reported cardiac risk generally <1%)	Endoscopic procedures Superficial procedure Cataract surgery Breast surgery Ambulatory surgery

[a]Combined incidence of cardiac death and nonfatal MI.

[b]These procedures do not generally require further preoperative cardiac testing.

TABLE 9-2	ESTIMATION OF FUNCTIONAL STATUS

Energy	Activity	Energy	Activity
1 MET	Take care of yourself Eat, dress, use the toilet Walk indoors around the house Walk 1–2 blocks on level ground at 2–3 mph (3.2–4.8 kph)	**4 METs**	Climb a flight of stairs or walk up a hill Walk on level ground at 4 mph (6.4 kph) Run a short distance
4 METs	Do light work around the house like dusting or washing dishes		Do heavy work around the house like scrubbing floors or lifting or moving heavy furniture Moderate recreational activities like golf, bowling, dancing, doubles tennis, or throwing a baseball or football
		>10 METs	Strenuous sports like swimming, singles tennis, football, basketball, or skiing

MET, metabolic equivalent; mph, miles per hour; kph, kilometers per hour.

(Modified from Fleisher LA, Beckman JA, Brown KA, et al. ACC/AHA 2007 guidelines on perioperative cardiovascular evaluation and care for noncardiac surgery. *J Am Coll Cardiol* 2007;50:e159-e241.)

  ○ Diabetes mellitus
  ○ Renal insufficiency
- If the patient has one or more of these risk factors, the clinician may consider further diagnostic testing prior to surgery (Figure 9-1, step 5).[1]

Diagnostic Testing

- If the patient is unable to complete 4 METs of activity without symptoms and has other clinical risks, one may consider further diagnostic testing prior to surgery (Figure 9-1, step 5).[1]
- Before pursuing preoperative testing, one must **consider the consequences of positive study results and their implication for subsequent revascularization**, particularly percutaneous intervention (PCI). As stressed in the guidelines, preoperative tests should be recommended only if the information obtained will result in a change in the surgical procedure performed, a change in medical therapy or monitoring during or after surgery, or a postponement of surgery until the cardiac condition can be corrected or stabilized.
- **There are little controlled data suggesting that preoperative revascularization in an asymptomatic individual lowers surgical risks**. See Other Nonpharmacologic Therapies under Medications.

TREATMENT

Medications

First Line

- **β-Blockers**
  ○ Perioperative β-blockade has been advocated to reduce the perioperative risk in patients undergoing intermediate- or high-risk surgery in which revascularization is not planned.
  ○ Since the publication of the 2007 update, there has been a burgeoning body of evidence evaluating the safety and efficacy of this strategy.
    ▪ The Perioperative Ischemic Evaluation Trial randomly assigned patients to receive extended-release metoprolol succinate at a fixed dose of 100 mg or placebo, starting 2 to 4 hours before surgery and continuing for 30 days, with a primary composite end point of cardiovascular death, nonfatal MI, and nonfatal cardiac arrest.[2] The results suggested a clear reduction in MI and a decrease in both coronary revascularization and atrial fibrillation with β-blocker, but an accompanying increase in death and stroke and an increase in hypotension and bradycardia. Critics have charged that the large fixed dose predisposed subjects to hypotension and poorer outcomes.
    ▪ In contrast, the Dutch Echocardiographic Cardiac Risk Evaluation Applying Stress Echo Study Group (DECREASE-IV) randomized patients scheduled for elective noncardiac surgery to bisoprolol, with or without a statin, versus placebo.[3] Bisoprolol was started preoperatively at a low dose and titrated to a heart rate of 50–70 bpm. Those randomized to bisoprolol had a lower incidence of cardiac death and nonfatal MI, without an increased incidence of perioperative stroke or mortality. The validity of these findings have been called into question. In light of this controversy, the ACC and AHA issued a focused update on the topic of perioperative β-blockade as an addendum to the guidelines.[4] Specific recommendations are shown in Table 9-3.[4,5]

Second Line

- **Dual antiplatelet therapy**
  ○ Noncardiac surgery is associated with a proinflammatory and prothrombotic state, increasing the potential risk of thrombosis, particularly for coronary artery stents.
  ○ Dual antiplatelet therapy with aspirin and a thienopyridine has been shown to reduce cardiac events after coronary stenting.

TABLE 9-3 INDICATIONS FOR β-BLOCKER THERAPY

Surgery	No clinical risk factors	Single clinical risk factor	Coronary heart disease or high cardiac risk	Patients currently taking β-blockers
Vascular	Class IIb, level of evidence: B	Class IIb, level of evidence: C	Patients found to have myocardial ischemia on pre-operative testing: class IIa, level of evidence: B Patients without ischemia or no previous test: class IIa, level of evidence: B Patients with ≥1 CRF[a]: class IIa, level of evidence: C	Class I, level of evidence: C
Intermediate risk	…	Class IIb, level of evidence: C	Class IIa, level of evidence: B	Class I, level of evidence: C
Low risk	…	…	…	Class I, level of evidence: C

[a]Clinical risk factors: history of ischemic heart disease, history of congestive heart failure, history of stroke or transient ischemic attack, history of insulin-requiring diabetes, chronic kidney disease (creatinine > 2 mg/dL).

○ Premature discontinuation of a thienopyridine after PCI carries a substantial risk of acute stent thrombosis, which in turn confers a high mortality rate. This risk is increased in patients with a previous history of stent thrombosis and those who have high-risk coronary stent locations.

○ **Dual antiplatelet therapy is recommended for 30 days after PCI with a bare metal stent and for 1 year after PCI with a drug-eluting stent.**[6] It is recommended that patients not receive elective surgery during this period.

○ There is no safe substitution for a thienopyridine in patients in whom this is indicated.

○ To minimize the risk of surgical bleeding, discontinuation of thienopyridine treatment for a minimum of 5–7 days is recommended prior to noncardiac surgery.

○ **Current guidelines recommend continuing aspirin throughout the perioperative period** in the patient who has had any type of previous coronary revascularization unless there is a major contraindication.

○ Patients undergoing noncardiac surgery within 4–6 weeks of stent placement have been found to have extremely high rates of stent thrombosis, MI, and death.[7] If PCI is clinically indicated before a noncardiac surgical procedure, the current clinical bias is toward the placement of a bare metal stent and a delay in the procedure for the week after the thienopyridine is discontinued. However, the influence of stent type and period of risk still are not well defined.

Other Nonpharmacologic Therapies

• Preoperative revascularization with PCI

○ In the Coronary Artery Revascularization Prophylaxis trial, over 250 patients were randomized to revascularization or no revascularization.[8] All patients had multiple clinical risk factors, and 75% of the patients had moderate to large ischemic burden on stress imaging. Results showed no significant difference between groups in regard to the primary end points of death or MI at either 30-day or 2.7-year follow-up.

○ The Dutch Echocardiographic Cardiac Risk Evaluation Applying Stress Echo Study Group (DECREASE-V) identified over 100 patients scheduled for major vascular surgery who had both three or more clinical risk factors and extensive ischemia on stress imaging studies.[9] These patients were randomized to receive either revascularization or optimal β-blocker therapy, titrated preoperatively to a target heart rate control of less than 65 beats/minute. No difference was observed in the rate of 30-day all-cause death or nonfatal MI between the revascularization and β-blocker groups. In addition, there were no significant outcome differences observed between groups at 1 year.

• In contrast, a strategy of routine preoperative coronary angiography and subsequent selective PCI provided better long-term survival and event-free survival for patients undergoing abdominal aortic surgery when compared with a strategy of selective coronary angiography and PCI performed only after preoperative noninvasive testing showed significant ischemia.[10] Both groups received β-blockers targeted to a heart rate of <65 bpm. There was a trend toward better periprocedural outcomes with routine revascularization, although this did not reach significance. Longer-term (>20 month) outcomes were significantly improved by revascularization.

MONITORING/FOLLOW-UP

• Despite advances in preoperative risk assessment, medical therapy, and surgical and anesthetic techniques, cardiovascular complications continue to be among the most common and treatable adverse consequences of noncardiac surgery. Patients who have a symptomatic MI after surgery have a marked increase in their risk of death.[11] Thus, the consultant's role should continue after risk assessment to the postoperative setting for all but the lowest risk patients.

- Perioperative MI can be documented by assessing clinical symptoms, serial ECGs, and cardiac-specific biomarkers before and after surgery. Because of the improved sensitivity of current cardiac-specific biomarkers, perioperative MI is diagnosed with greater frequency than previously.[12]
- Many perioperative conditions causing increased ventricular wall stress can result in troponin elevations, including heart failure, hypotension, sepsis, and pulmonary embolism. Routine measurement of troponin in the perioperative setting is more likely to identify patients without acute MI, especially in the absence of ischemic symptoms and EKG changes. The role of revascularization in patients with an elevated troponin level but no other manifestation of MI remains unclear.
- Routine surveillance for acute coronary syndromes with routine ECG and cardiac serum biomarkers is unnecessary in clinically low-risk patients undergoing low-risk operative procedures. In addition, **the routine use of serial troponin measurement is not well established even in patients undergoing intermediate- to high-risk procedures**. In patients with clinically suspected ischemia or those with ECG evidence of ischemia or infarction, serial ECGs and troponin measurements are indicated.

REFERENCES

1. Fleisher LA, Beckman JA, Brown KA, et al. ACC/AHA 2007 guidelines on perioperative cardiovascular evaluation and care for noncardiac surgery: *J Am Coll Cardiol* 2007;50:e159-e241.
2. POISE Study Group. Effects of extended-release metoprolol succinate in patients undergoing non-cardiac surgery (POISE trial): a randomised controlled trial: *Lancet* 2008;371:1839-1847.
3. Dunkelgrun M, Boersma E, Schouten O, et al. Bisoprolol and Fluvastatin for the reduction of perioperative cardiac mortality and myocardial infarction in intermediate-risk patients undergoing noncardiovascular surgery: a randomized controlled trial (DECREASE-IV): *Ann Surg* 2009;249;921-926.
4. Fleischmann K, Beckman J, Buller C, et al. 2009 ACCF/AHA focused update on perioperative beta blockade: *J Am Coll Cardiol* 2009;54:2102-2128.
5. Lee TH, Marcantonio, ER, Mangione CM, et al. Derivation and prospective validation of a simple index for prediction of cardiac risk of major non cardiac surgery: *Circulation* 1999;100:1043-1049.
6. Grines CL, Bonow RO, Casey DE Jr, et al. Prevention of premature discontinuation of dual antiplatelet therapy in patients with coronary artery stents: *Circulation* 2007;115:813-818.
7. Riddell JW, Chiche L, Plaud B, et al. Coronary stents and noncardiac surgery: *Circulation* 2007;116:e378-e382.
8. McFalls EO, Ward HB, Moritz TE, et al. Coronary-artery revascularization before elective major vascular surgery: *N Engl J Med* 2004;351:2795-2804.
9. Poldermans D, Schouten O, Vidakovic R, et al. A clinical randomized trial to evaluate the safety of a noninvasive approach in high-risk patients undergoing major vascular surgery: The DECREASE-V Pilot Study: *J Am Coll Cardiol* 2007;49:1763-1769.
10. Monaco M, Stassano P, Di Tommaso L, et al. Systemic strategy of prophylactic coronary angiography improves long-term outcome after major vascular surgery in medium- to high-risk patients: a prospective, randomized study: *J Am Coll Cardiol* 2009;54:989-996.
11. Mangano, DT, Goldman, L. Preoperative assessment of patients with known or suspected coronary disease: *N Eng J Med* 1995;333:1750-1756.
12. Landesberg G, Mosseri M, Shatz V, et al. Cardiac troponin after major vascular surgery: the role of perioperative ischemia, preoperative thallium scanning, and coronary revascularization: *J Am Coll Cardiol* 2004;44:569-575.

Stable Angina

10

Sara C. Martinez and David B. Schwartz

GENERAL PRINCIPLES

Definition

- Angina is a symptom of myocardial ischemia, most commonly caused by coronary artery disease (CAD).
  - Typical angina is (1) substernal chest discomfort with a characteristic quality and duration that is (2) precipitated by stress and (3) relieved by rest or nitroglycerin.
  - Atypical angina meets two of the above criteria.
  - Noncardiac chest pain meets one or none of the above criteria.
- Anginal equivalent symptoms vary from patient to patient but may include exertional dyspnea, fatigue or weakness, diaphoresis, dizziness, nausea, and syncope.
- Women (more often than men) may experience atypical angina symptoms such as epigastric discomfort or other symptoms that represent their anginal equivalent.
- Diabetic patients may experience anginal equivalent symptoms (e.g., epigastric distress), rather than classic chest discomfort.

Classification

- The Canadian Classification of Angina is commonly employed to stratify patients in terms of severity. Anginal symptoms are precipitated by
  - Class I: Strenuous activity
  - Class II: Moderate activity, such as walking more than one flight of stairs
  - Class III: Mild activity, such as walking less than one flight of stairs
  - Class IV: Any activity. Symptoms may also occur at rest.
- The severity of angina is not directly proportional to the degree of angiographic stenosis of the diseased coronary artery (or arteries).
- More severe angina does correlate with an increased short-term risk of death or nonfatal myocardial infarction (MI).

Epidemiology

- Approximately 15 million Americans have coronary heart disease (CHD).
- Despite the well-documented decline in cardiovascular mortality, ischemic heart disease remains the leading single cause of death in the United States.
- CHD is responsible for nearly one of every five deaths.

Pathophysiology

- Stable angina most often results from fixed coronary lesions that produce a mismatch of myocardial oxygen supply and demand with increasing cardiac workload.
- Determinants of myocardial oxygen demand include heart rate (HR), afterload or systemic vascular resistance, myocardial wall stress (measured by preload), and myocardial contractility.
- A fixed stenosis of an epicardial coronary artery, usually >70% of the original luminal diameter of the vessel, is sufficient to limit blood flow distal to the lesion.

- The presence of CAD can predispose patients to heart failure, cardiac arrhythmias, and sudden cardiac death.

Risk Factors
- Tobacco abuse
- Hypertension
- Diabetes
- Metabolic syndrome
- See also Chapter 13

DIAGNOSIS

Clinical Presentation

History
- A thorough history can often yield an accurate diagnosis in a patient presenting with chest discomfort (Table 10-1).[1-3]
- Focusing on the nature of symptoms as well as other information (risk factors and past history) will help to risk stratify the patient and provide an appropriate pretest probability of CAD.
- Pertinent information about the chest discomfort includes
  - Location
  - Character/quality of the discomfort
  - Setting
  - Duration
  - Severity
  - Associated symptoms
  - Exacerbating and attenuating factors
- Diabetic patients may not experience any anginal symptoms despite having ischemic cardiac disease.

TABLE 10-1	PRETEST LIKELIHOOD (%) OF CORONARY ARTERY DISEASE IN SYMPTOMATIC PATIENTS ACCORDING TO AGE AND SEX					
	Nonanginal chest pain		Atypical angina		Typical angina	
Age (years)	Men	Women	Men	Women	Men	Women
30–39	4	2	34	12	76	26
40–49	13	3	51	22	87	55
50–59	20	7	65	31	93	73
60–69	27	14	72	51	94	86

From Fihn SD, Gardin JM, Abrams J, et al. 2012 ACCF/AHA/ACP/AATS/PCNA/SCAI/STS guideline for the diagnosis and management of patients with stable ischemic heart disease. *Circulation* 2012;126:e354-e471.

- Social history including tobacco use in the past and present as well as (total pack-years of use) and drug use (cocaine or other stimulants).
- Assessment of functional status
  - Sedentary patient may not exert themselves enough to experience angina.
  - Alternatively, patients who are relatively inactive may be limiting their activity due to anginal symptoms.

Physical Examination

As with the history, the physical examination is a key component in the evaluation of the patient with suspected coronary disease. A focused examination must include

- Vital signs (including blood pressure readings in both arms, HR, and oxygen saturation)
- Head, ears, eyes, nose, and throat: corneal arcus senilis, xanthelasma, and diagonal earlobe crease (Frank sign)
- Neck: carotid artery bruits
- Lungs: rales (if present during an episode of chest pain may suggest pulmonary edema secondary to ischemia)
- Cardiac: murmurs (suggestive of stenotic or regurgitant valvular disease), S3 or S4 gallops, and friction rubs. Assess the position, size, and characteristics of the precordial impulse
- Abdomen: listen for bruits (aortic or renal arteries), pulsatile mass (abdominal aortic aneurysm)
- Extremities: strength of the peripheral pulses (femoral, dorsalis pedis, posterior tibialis, etc.), listen for femoral artery bruits, peripheral edema, or signs of vascular insufficiency.

Differential Diagnosis

- Congenital cardiac anomalies
- Myocardial bridge
- Coronary arteritis
- Coronary artery ectasia
- Radiation arteriopathy
- Cocaine
- Aortic stenosis
- Hypertrophic cardiomyopathy
- Prinzmetal (variant) angina. Coronary artery spasm may be provoked during cardiac catheterization by the infusion of dopamine, acetylcholine, or ergonovine.
- Syndrome X
- Other cardiac causes
  - Myocardial disease—chronic heart failure (thought secondary to myocardial stretch), myocarditis, reversible left ventricular (LV) dysfunction related to stress (takotsubo)
  - Pericardial disease: pericarditis
  - Vasculature: aortic dissection
- Other noncardiac causes (Table 10-2)

Diagnostic Testing

The initial evaluation of the patient with cardiac disease can be tailored to the level of clinical suspicion for CHD and the degree of symptoms experienced by the patient.

Laboratories

- Biochemical markers including a complete blood count, fasting glucose, and lipid profile should be obtained in all patients with suspected CHD, with an added troponin in acute coronary syndrome (ACS) presentations.
- Elevated baseline C-reactive protein, lipoprotein(a), and homocysteine levels are associated with an increased risk of CAD and can be evaluated in those patients in whom standard cardiac risk factors are absent and an alternative explanation for CAD is sought.

TABLE 10-2 NONCARDIAC CAUSES OF CHEST PAIN

Pulmonary:
Pulmonary embolism or
  pulmonary hypertension
Lung parenchyma: pneumonia or
  pneumothorax
Pleural tissue: pleuritis or pleural
  effusion
Gastrointestinal:
Gastroesophageal reflux disease
Esophageal spasm or abnormal
  motility
Achalasia
Esophagitis
Esophageal rupture (Boerhaave
  syndrome)
Peptic ulcer disease
Pancreatitis
Cholecystitis

Urologic:
Nephrolithiasis
Pyelonephritis
Dermatologic:
Herpes zoster
Musculoskeletal:
Costochondritis
Rib fractures
Rheumatoid arthritis
Psoriatic arthritis
Fibromyalgia
Psychiatric:
Anxiety disorder
Panic disorder
Somatoform disorders
Delusional disorder

Electrocardiography
- **A normal rest electrocardiogram (ECG) does not exclude the presence of CAD.**
- The following ECG abnormalities increase the likelihood of a cardiac etiology in patients with stable angina:
  - Pathologic Q waves (>0.4 mV and greater than 25% of the corresponding R wave) consistent with a prior MI
  - Resting ST-segment depression
  - T-wave inversion
  - LV hypertrophy (LVH)

Imaging
A chest radiograph should be obtained if there is an evidence of congestive heart failure, valvular disease, or aortic disease, or if an abnormal cardiac impulse is noted on physical examination.

Diagnostic Procedures
Exercise Stress Testing
- Exercise stress testing (without imaging) provides functional information and allows risk stratification in patients with suspected angina.
- The Bruce protocol is most commonly used, consisting of 3-minute stages of increasing treadmill speed and incline.
- Monitor for appropriate physiologic response to exercise with blood pressure and HR measurements during the walk and into the recovery period.
- Question for the presence of anginal symptoms.
- Monitor throughout the study to evaluate for ischemic changes.
- The **Duke treadmill score** (DTS) provides prognostic information.
  - DTS = minutes exercise – [5 × maximum ST-segment deviation (mm)] – [4 × anginal score]).
  - Angina score is defined as 0 (no angina), 1 (nonlimiting anginal symptoms), or 2 (angina requiring termination of the test).

TABLE 10-3	SURVIVAL ACCORDING TO RISK GROUPS BASED ON DUKE TREADMILL SCORES		
Risk group (score)	Percentage of total	4-year survival (%)	Annual mortality (%)
Low ($\geq$+5)	62	99	0.25
Moderate (–10 to +4)	34	95	1.25
High (<–10)	4	79	5.0

Modified from Mark DB, Shaw L, Harrell FE Jr, et al. Prognostic value of a treadmill exercise score in outpatients with suspected coronary artery disease. *N Engl J Med* 1991;325:849-853.

- ○ Scores of >(+)5, (–)10 to (+)4, and <(–)11 are associated with low, moderate, and high risk, respectively, of subsequent cardiovascular events (Table 10-3).[4]
- Exercise sufficient to increase the HR to 85% of maximum predicted heart rate (MPHR = 220 – age) is necessary for optimal sensitivity.
- Medications such as β-blockers, calcium channel blockers (CCBs) (verapamil and diltiazem), and nitrates should be discontinued in patients prior to performing stress tests when looking for new ischemia. These medications can be continued if the stress test is performed to optimize medical therapy.
- Exercise stress testing has a sensitivity and specificity of approximately 75%.
- The specificity of the test is adversely affected by the presence of resting ECG abnormalities, inability to exercise, or medication use, which may prohibit attaining 85% of the MPHR (e.g., β-blockers).
- A positive stress test indicative of severe CHD is defined with the presence of any of the following:
  - ○ New ST-segment depression at the start of exercise
  - ○ New ST-segment depression >2 mm in multiple leads
  - ○ Hypotensive response to exercise
  - ○ Development of heart failure or sustained ventricular arrhythmia during the study
  - ○ Prolonged interval after exercise (>5 minutes) before ischemic changes return to baseline
- Patients with a markedly positive stress test should undergo cardiac catheterization to be evaluated for coronary revascularization options.
- Exercise stress testing is **contraindicated** for patients with the following:
  - ○ Acute MI:
    - ■ A submaximal or symptom-limited stress test may be performed in stabilized patients after 48 hours.
    - ■ A standard stress test may be performed after 4 to 6 weeks.
  - ○ Unstable angina not previously stabilized by medical therapy
  - ○ Cardiac arrhythmias causing symptoms or hemodynamic compromise
  - ○ Symptomatic severe aortic stenosis
  - ○ Symptomatic heart failure
  - ○ Acute pulmonary embolus, myocarditis, pericarditis, and aortic dissection

Cardiac Stress Testing with Imaging

- Stress testing with imaging is an appropriate initial diagnostic study in those patients in the following categories:

- ○ Evidence of pre-excitation (Wolff-Parkinson-White syndrome)
- ○ LVH
- ○ Left bundle branch block (LBBB)
- ○ Ventricular pacing
- ○ Resting ST- and T-wave changes (intrinsic or due to digoxin therapy)
- **Stress myocardial perfusion imaging** (see Chapter 30)
  - ○ Imaging with thallium-201 (^{201}Tl) or technetium-99m (^{99}mTc) sestamibi has been reported to increase sensitivity for detection of CAD to 80% and specificity to 80% to 90%.
  - ○ Stress perfusion imaging allows the diagnosis and localization of areas of ischemia, the determination of ejection fraction, and the distinction between ischemic and infracted tissue (viability).
- **Pharmacologic stress testing**
  - ○ There are three vasodilator agents used in stress testing: dipyridamole, adenosine, and regadenoson.
  - ○ **Adenosine** causes coronary vasodilation through A2A receptors.
    - There will be a greater vasodilation in normal coronary blood vessels than in ischemic myocardial regions.
    - Undesirable effects of adenosine are mediated through its activation of the A1 (atrioventricular [AV] block), A2B (peripheral vasodilation), and A3 (bronchospasm) receptors.
  - ○ **Regadenoson** is another vasodilator; however, it has much high avidity for the A2A receptor and less for the A1, A2B, and A3 receptors. Thus, its side effect profile is less than that of adenosine.
  - ○ Methylxanthines (i.e., caffeine, theophylline, and theobromine) are competitive inhibitors of this effect, which requires withholding methylxanthines prior to testing.
  - ○ Aminophylline 50 mg to 250 mg IV is used to reverse the bronchospastic effect of the vasodilator agents.
  - ○ **Indications** for the use of adenosine stress testing are the same as for exercise stress testing AND when the patient has the following conditions:
    - Inability to perform adequate exercise (i.e., due to pulmonary, peripheral vascular disease, musculoskeletal or mental conditions)
    - Baseline ECG abnormalities such as LBBB, ventricular preexcitation, and permanent ventricular pacing
    - Risk stratification of clinically stable patients into low- and high-risk groups very early after acute MI (more than 1 day) or presentation with a presumptive ACS
  - ○ **Contraindications** for adenosine stress testing include
    - Asthmatic patients with active wheezing should not undergo adenosine stress testing.
    - Adequately controlled asthma is not a contraindication.
    - Bronchospasm
    - Second- or third-degree AV block without a pacemaker or sick sinus syndrome
    - Systolic blood pressure <90 mmHg
    - Recent use of dipyridamole, dipyridamole-containing medications (e.g., Aggrenox)
    - Methylxanthines such as aminophylline, caffeine, and theobromine block within 12 hours of testing
    - Known hypersensitivity to adenosine
    - Acute MI or ACS
  - ○ Relative contraindications for adenosine stress testing include profound sinus bradycardia (HRs <40 bpm).
  - ○ Common side effects of adenosine[5]:
    - Flushing (35% to 40%)
    - Chest pain (25% to 30%) which is not specific for CHD
    - Dyspnea (20%)

- Dizziness (7%)
- Nausea (5%)
- Symptomatic hypotension (5%)
  ○ Indications and contraindications for regadenoson stress testing are the same as that for adenosine.
    - Little evidence exists for the safe use of regadenoson in patients with bronchospasm.
    - Common side effects of regadenoson include shortness of breath, flushing, and headache.
    - Less common side effects include chest pain, dizziness, nausea, and abdominal discomfort.
- **Exercise stress echocardiography**:
  ○ Stress echo can be performed to aid in the evaluation of CAD in a patient with anginal symptoms (see Chapter 31).
  ○ Compared with standard exercise treadmill testing, stress echocardiography provides an additional clinical value for detecting and localizing myocardial ischemia and visualizing structure and function.
  ○ When the patient cannot exercise to the optimal level (>85% MPHR) or in other specified circumstances (see above), pharmacologic stress testing with dobutamine may be preferable.
- Stress testing with cardiac magnetic resonance imaging and positron emission tomography: These newer imaging modalities have shown promise in the noninvasive evaluation of CAD (see Chapter 32).

Stress Testing in Specific Populations

- Stress testing **after MI**:
  ○ A submaximal study performed 2 to 7 days after acute MI or a maximal exercise stress test 4 to 6 weeks after MI aids in determining the patient's ischemic burden and provides prognostic information.
  ○ A treadmill stress test after acute MI, either with or without revascularization, helps guide recommendations for a cardiac rehabilitation program.
  ○ Vasodilator-mediated stress testing with thallium-201 (^{201}Tl) or technetium-99m (^{99}mTc) sestamibi imaging may be performed within 48 hours of an acute MI in clinically stable patients.
- Stress testing in patients with **established CHD**
  ○ The routine use of stress testing in asymptomatic patients after percutaneous or surgical revascularization remains controversial.
  ○ Stress testing in patients who are >5 years from coronary artery bypass grafting (CABG) and/or >2 years from percutaneous coronary intervention (PCI) in whom revascularization is reasonable.
  ○ Stress testing should be performed in conjunction with an imaging modality (nuclear or echocardiographic) to increase the sensitivity of the test and to localize any area of ischemia that may exist.
- Stress testing in **women**
  ○ The use of exercise testing in women presents difficulties that are not experienced in men (see Chapter 38).
  ○ These difficulties reflect the differences between men and women regarding the prevalence of CAD and the sensitivity and specificity of exercise testing.
- Stress testing in **elderly**
  ○ Exercise testing poses additional problems in the elderly as functional capacity in these patients is often compromised from muscle weakness and deconditioning (see Chapter 36).
  ○ Pharmacologic testing is encouraged in this population.

Coronary Angiography

- Coronary angiography or cardiac catheterization is considered the "gold standard" technique for diagnosing CAD (see Chapter 34).
- **Indications**:
  - Known or suspected angina with a markedly positive stress test.
  - Survived sudden cardiac death (e.g., ventricular tachycardia).
  - High pretest probability of left main or three-vessel CAD or for those whose occupation requires a definitive diagnosis.
  - Recent stress test is nondiagnostic and for individuals who are unable to undergo noninvasive testing.
  - In selected patients with recurrent hospitalizations for chest pain or those with an overriding desire for a definite diagnosis and an intermediate or high pretest probability of CAD.
  - Patients with angina who are suspected of having a nonatherosclerotic cause of ischemia (e.g., coronary anomaly, coronary dissection, and radiation vasculopathy).
- **Coronary angiography is not indicated (class III indication) for stable angina responding to medical therapy or patients with asymptomatic disease.**
- New technologies are available to assist in the invasive diagnosis of CAD (see Chapter 34):
  - Intravascular ultrasound
  - Doppler flow wire for fractional flow reserve

TREATMENT

- The goal of treatment or patients with stable angina is to reduce symptoms of ischemia.
- Both pharmacologic therapy and revascularization are important options which should be considered in addition to diet and lifestyle modifications.[3,6,7]
- One approach to guide the treatment of patients with ischemic heart disease is the "ABCDE" mnemonic: **A**ntiplatelet therapy, **B**lood pressure control/β-blocker, **C**holesterol lowering/cigarette cessation, **D**iabetes control/diet and weight loss, **E**xercise/ejection fraction.

Medication

- The purpose of medication therapy is to
  - Reduce myocardial oxygen demand
  - Improve myocardial oxygen supply
  - Treat cardiac risk factors (e.g., hypertension, diabetes, and obesity)
  - Control exacerbating factors (valvular stenosis and anemia) that may precipitate ischemia
- **Aspirin**:
  - The use of aspirin in patients with stable angina has been shown to reduce cardiovascular events by 33%.
  - In asymptomatic patients in the Physician's Health Study, aspirin (325 mg every other day) decreased the incidence of MI by 44% over a 5-year period.[8]
  - Clopidogrel (75 mg/day) can be used in patients who are allergic to or intolerant of aspirin.[9]
  - Both aspirin and clopidogrel can be used in patients with severe CAD, although with an increased risk of bleeding.[10]
  - Consultation with an allergist should be considered for the patient suspected of having aspirin allergy.
- **β-Blockers:**
  - β-Blockers should be considered initial therapy of symptomatic CAD among patients with a history of prior MI.

- ○ Effective in controlling angina by decreasing HR, contractility, and blood pressure. Additionally, the reduction in HR also allows for increased diastolic filling time and may increase coronary perfusion.
  - ▪ The dose can be adjusted to result in a resting HR of 50 to 60 beats per minute (bpm).
  - ▪ In patients with persistent angina, a target HR <50 bpm is warranted, provided that no symptoms are associated with the bradycardia and that heart block does not develop.
  - ▪ With moderate exercise (two flights of stairs), the HR should be <90 bpm.
- ○ Use is contraindicated in patients with severe bronchospasm, significant AV block, marked resting bradycardia, or decompensated heart failure.
- ○ β-Blocking agents with β-1 selectivity (such as metoprolol and atenolol) are preferable in patients with asthma, chronic obstructive pulmonary disease (COPD), insulin-dependent diabetes, or peripheral vascular disease.
- ○ Permanent pacemaker placement may be indicated in patients for whom excessive β-blockade results in symptomatic bradycardia but is otherwise warranted.
- ○ Titration of β-blocker dosing should occur over 6 to 12 weeks.
- ○ Should be weaned over a 2- to 3-week period if side effects warrant discontinuation of β-blockers to prevent worsening angina or precipitation of an ischemic event.
- **CCB**
  - ○ CCB may be used in lieu of β-blockers when contraindicated or not tolerated owing to significant adverse effects.
  - ○ CCBs are also used in conjunction with β-blockers if the latter alone are not fully effective at relieving anginal symptoms.
  - ○ CCBs decrease systemic vascular resistance and blood pressure, resulting in a decrease in myocardial oxygen demand.
  - ○ They reduce the transmembrane flux of calcium and thereby decrease coronary vascular resistance and increase coronary blood flow, thus increasing myocardial oxygen supply. This is the principal mechanism of benefit in vasospastic angina.
  - ○ CCBs may also decrease contractility (negative inotropic effects), which can decrease myocardial oxygen demand.
  - ○ Some CCBs (the nondihydropyridines) decrease HR (negative chronotropy) or decrease conduction through the AV node, thereby reducing myocardial oxygen demand.
  - ○ Use of short-acting dihydropyridines (e.g., nifedipine) should be avoided because of their potential to increase the risk of adverse cardiac events.
- **Nitrates**
  - ○ Nitrates are endothelium-independent vasodilators.
  - ○ They reduce myocardial oxygen demand by decreasing blood pressure, thereby decreasing afterload and decreasing preload through venodilation.
  - ○ They dilate epicardial coronary arteries and increase myocardial oxygen supply.
  - ○ Long-acting formulations for chronic use or sublingual preparations for acute anginal symptoms can be used as adjuncts to baseline therapy with β-blockers or CCBs or both.
  - ○ Sublingual preparations can be used at the first indication of angina or prophylactically before engaging in activities that are known to precipitate angina.
    - ▪ Patients should seek prompt medical attention if angina occurs at rest or fails to respond to the third sublingual dose.
    - ▪ The patient should take the medication while seated because of possible side effects of hypotension.
  - ○ Nitrate tolerance, resulting in reduced therapeutic response, may occur with all nitrate preparations. The institution of a nitrate-free period of 10 to 12 hours can enhance treatment efficacy.
  - ○ The benefits of nitrate therapy may be offset by the detrimental long-term effects of reactive oxygen species generated by these agents.

- **Ranolazine**
  - Mechanism of action providing angina relief is unclear; however, it appears to have an effect on the function of cardiomyocyte sodium ion channels.[11,12]
  - It has shown benefit in providing symptomatic relief of angina independent of effects on HR or blood pressure.[13-15]
- **Angiotensin converting enzyme (ACE) inhibitors**
  - A reduction in exercise-induced myocardial ischemia has been reported with the addition of an ACE inhibitor in patients with stable angina with optimal β-blockade and normal LV function.[16-19] However, not all trials have shown a benefit.[20]
  - The potential benefit is thought to be independent of blood pressure effects.
- **Cholesterol-lowering agents**
  - Multiple agents including statins, fibrates, bile acid sequestrants, and niacin have been shown to reduce recurrent events and improve overall outcome in patients with established CAD.
  - The most studied of these agents are the 3-hydroxy-3-methyl-glutaryl-CoA reductase or HMG Co-A reductase inhibitors (statins).
  - Some evidence suggests that statins exert beneficial (pleiotropic) effects on endothelial function, independent of their effects on LDL levels.[21,22] However, a 2005 meta-analysis has suggested otherwise.[23]
- Miscellaneous
  - Chelation therapy and acupuncture have not been found to be effective in relieving symptoms and are not recommended for the treatment of chronic stable angina.[24] The results of the high controversial NIH sponsored Trial to Assess Chelation Therapy were published in 2013.[25] Although the results suggested benefit of chelation therapy, the reliability of the trial and its results have been heavily criticized.[26]
  - Although atherosclerotic disease is considered an inflammatory-mediated process, the use of antibiotics has not been shown to reduce clinical events due to CAD.[27]

Other Nonpharmacologic Therapies

- Medical therapy with at least two and preferably three classes of antianginal agents should be attempted before the treatment is considered a failure.
- Patients who are refractory to medical therapy should be assessed with coronary angiography if the anatomy has not already been defined.
- **PCI**:
  - Catheter-based revascularization is ideal for candidates for PCI who have angina, are <75 years old, have single- or two-vessel CAD, have normal LV function, and do not have diabetes.
  - Stents are deployed after percutaneous transluminal coronary angioplasty (PTCA) for most lesions warranting percutaneous revascularization as long-term patency rates and overall outcomes are improved compared with PTCA alone.
  - Patients enrolled in the COURAGE trial had stable angina and were randomized to either PCI with optimal medical therapy or optimal medical therapy alone and followed for a median of 4.6 years.[28,29]
    - PCI did not reduce the risk of death, MI, or other major cardiovascular events over the course of the trial.
    - Its merits mention that <10% of screened patients were enrolled, a substantial number of patients crossed over into the PCI arm, and a relatively small percentage of patients received drug-eluting stents.
    - As the decision is made regarding PCI versus medical management, a discussion of data is appropriate.
  - The risks of elective PCI include <1% mortality, a 2% to 5% rate of nonfatal MI, and <1% need for emergent CABG for an unsuccessful procedure.

- ○ Coronary artery dissection often can be repaired with multiple stents but may necessitate bypass surgery
- **CABG**
  - ○ CABG is optimal for patients at a high risk for cardiac mortality, including those with (1) left main disease, (2) two- or three-vessel disease involving the proximal left anterior descending artery and LV dysfunction, and (3) diabetes and multivessel coronary disease with LV dysfunction.[30,31]
  - ○ The risk of surgery includes 1% to 3% mortality, a 5% to 10% incidence of perioperative MI, a small risk of perioperative stroke or cognitive dysfunction, and a 10% to 20% risk of vein graft failure in the first year, along with added mortality and complications from comorbid factors.
  - ○ Approximately 75% of patients remain free of recurrent angina or adverse cardiac events at 5 years of follow-up.
  - ○ The use of internal mammary artery grafts is associated with 85% graft patency at 10 years, compared with 60% for saphenous vein grafts.[32]
  - ○ The 1-year patency of radial artery grafts has not been shown to be superior to saphenous vein grafts; however, medium-term (1 to 5 years) patency and long-term (>5 years) patency were superior for radial grafts in a meta-analysis.[33,34]
  - ○ After 10 years of follow-up, 50% of patients develop recurrent angina or other adverse cardiac events related to late vein graft failure or progression of native CAD.
  - ○ Two US trials (the multicenter BARI[35] and the single-center EAST[36]) evaluated PTCA versus CABG in patients with multivessel disease. The results of these trials at approximately 5 years showed that early and late survival rates are equivalent for PTCA and CABG groups. However, **subgroup analysis showed a clear survival benefit with CABG for diabetics and for patients with severe multivessel disease**.
- Alternate therapies
  - ○ Transmyocardial laser revascularization has been delivered by percutaneous technique (yttrium–aluminum–garnet [YAG] laser) and by epicardial surgical techniques (CO_2 or YAG laser).
    - ■ The percutaneous approach has not been approved by the U.S. Food and Drug Administration.
    - ■ A thoracotomy approach is used to deliver a series of transmural endomyocardial channels.
    - ■ Surgical transmyocardial laser revascularization has been shown to improve symptoms in patients with stable angina, although the mechanism responsible is controversial.[37-41] On the other hand, not all trials have shown a benefit.[42,43]
    - ■ The data on whether exercise capacity is improved are conflicting, and no benefit has been demonstrated in terms of increasing myocardial perfusion or reducing mortality.
  - ○ Enhanced external counterpulsation (EECP) is a nonpharmacologic technique for which 1 to 2 hours/day, five times a week for 7 weeks of treatment in patients with chronic stable angina and a positive stress test was shown to decrease the frequency of angina and increase the time to exercise-induced ischemia.
    - ■ Treatment improves anginal symptoms in approximately 75% to 80% of patients.[44,45]
    - ■ Additional clinical trial data are required before EECP can be definitively recommended.
  - ○ Chelation therapy is not indicated in the treatment of angina.

FOLLOW-UP

- Changes in the patient's anginal complaints can often be treated with titration or adjustment of the antianginal regimen.
- Reassessment with a stress test (likely in conjunction with an imaging modality) or a cardiac catheterization is warranted for the patient with significant change in anginal

complaints (frequency, severity, or time to onset with activity), or the symptoms are not sufficiently responsive to adjustments in medical therapy. Revascularization (either percutaneous or surgical) should be considered if the anatomy is amenable.

REFERENCES

1. Diamond GA, Forrester JS. Analysis of probability as an aid in the clinical diagnosis of coronary artery disease: *N Engl J Med* 1979;300;1350-1358.
2. Chaitman BR, Bourassa MG, Davis K, et al. Angiographic prevalence of high-risk coronary artery disease in patient subsets (CASS): *Circulation* 1981;64:360-367.
3. Fihn SD, Gardin JM, Abrams J, et al. 2012 ACCF/AHA/ACP/AATS/PCNA/SCAI/STS guideline for the diagnosis and management of patients with stable ischemic heart disease: *Circulation* 2012;126:e354-e471.
4. Mark DB, Shaw L, Harrell FE Jr, et al. Prognostic value of a treadmill exercise score in outpatients with suspected coronary artery disease: *N Engl J Med* 1991;325:849-853.
5. Henzlova MJ, Cergueira MD, Mahmarian JJ, et al. Stress protocols and tracers: *J Nucl Cardiol* 2006;13:e80-e90.
6. Abrams J. Chronic stable angina: *N Engl J Med* 2005;352:2524-2533.
7. Boden WE, O'Rourke RA, Teo KK, et al. Optimal medical therapy with or without PCI for stable coronary disease: *N Engl J Med* 2007;356:1503-1516.
8. Steering Committee of the Physicians' Health Study Research Group. Final report on the aspirin component of the ongoing Physicians' Health Study: *N Engl J Med* 1989;321:129-135.
9. CAPRIE Steering Committee. A randomized, blinded trial of clopidogrel versus aspirin in patients at risk of ischemic events: *Lancet* 1996;348:1329-1339.
10. Squizzato A, Keller T, Romualdi E, et al. Clopidogrel plus aspirin versus aspirin alone for preventing cardiovascular disease: *Cochrane Database Syst Rev* 2011;1:CD005158.
11. Beyder A, Strege PR, Reyes S, et al. Ranolazine decreases mechanosensitivity of the voltage-gated sodium ion channel Na(v)1.5: a novel mechanism of drug action: *Circulation* 2012;125:2698-2706.
12. Stone PH, Chaitman BR, Stocke K, et al. The anti-ischemic mechanism of action of ranolazine in stable ischemic heart disease: *J Am Coll Cardiol* 2010;56:934-942.
13. Chaitman BR, Pepine CJ, Parker JO, et al. Effects of ranolazine with atenolol, amlodipine, or diltiazem on exercise tolerance and angina frequency in patients with severe chronic angina: a randomized controlled trial: *JAMA* 2004;291:309-316.
14. Chaitman BR, Skettino SL, Parker JO, et al. Anti-ischemic effects and long-term survival during ranolazine monotherapy in patients with chronic severe angina: *J Am Coll Cardiol* 2004;43:1375-1382.
15. Stone PH, Gratsiansky NA, Blokhin A, et al. Antianginal efficacy of ranolazine when added to treatment with amlodipine: the ERICA (Efficacy of Ranolazine in Chronic Angina) trial: *J Am Coll Cardiol* 2006;48:566-575.
16. van den Heuvel AF, Dunselman PH, Kingma T, et al. Reduction of exercise-induced myocardial ischemia during add-on treatment with the angiotensin-converting enzyme inhibitor enalapril in patients with normal left ventricular function and optimal beta blockade: *J Am Coll Cardiol* 2001;37:470-474.
17. Kaski JC, Rosano G, Gavrielides S, et al. Effects of angiotensin-converting enzyme inhibition on exercise-induced angina and ST segment depression in patients with microvascular angina: *J Am Coll Cardiol* 1994;23:652-657.
18. Fox KM, Bertrand M, Ferrari R, et al. Efficacy of perindopril, in reduction of cardiovascular events among patients with stable coronary artery disease: randomized, double-blind, placebo-controlled, multicentre trial (the EUROPA study): *Lancet* 2003;362:782-788.
19. Yusuf S, Sleight P, Pogue J, et al. Effects of an angiotensin-converting-enzyme inhibitor, ramipril, on cardiovascular events in high-risk patients (HOPE): *N Engl J Med* 2000;342:145-153.
20. Braunwald E, Domanski M, Fowler S, et al. Angiotensin-converting-enzyme inhibition in stable coronary artery disease: *N Engl J Med* 2004;351:2058-2068.
21. Liao JK. Effects of statins on 3-hydroxy-3-methylglutaryl coenzyme a reductase inhibition beyond low-density lipoprotein cholesterol: *Am J Cardiol* 2005;96:24F-33F.
22. Liao JK, Laufs U. Pleiotropic effects of statins: *Annu Rev Pharmacol Toxicol* 2005;45:89-118.

23. Robinson JG, Smith B, Maheshwari N, et al. Pleiotropic effects of statins: benefit beyond cholesterol reduction? A meta-regression analysis: *J Am coll Cardiol* 2005;46:1855-1862.

24. Ernst E. Chelation therapy for coronary heart disease: an overview of all clinical investigations: *Am Heart J* 2000;140:139-141.

25. Lamas GA, Goertz C, Boineau R, et al. Effect of disodium EDTA chelation regimen on cardiovascular events in patients with previous myocardial infarction: the TACT randomized trial: *JAMA* 2013;309:1241-1250.

26. Nissen SE. Concerns about reliability in the Trial to Assess Chelation Therapy (TACT): *JAMA* 2013;309:1293-1294.

27. Andraws R, Berger JS, Brown DL. Effects of antibiotic therapy on outcomes of patients with coronary artery disease: a meta-analysis of randomized controlled trials: *JAMA* 2005;293:2641-2647.

28. Boden WE, O'Rourke RA, Teo KK, et al. COURAGE Trial Research Group. Optimal medical therapy with or without PCI for stable coronary disease: *N Engl J Med* 2007;356:1503-1516.

29. Weintraub WS, Spertus JA, Kolm P, et al. Effect of PCI on quality of life in patients with stable coronary disease: *New Engl J Med.* 2008;359:677-687.

30. Yusuf S, Zucker D, Peduzzi P, et al. Effect of coronary artery bypass graft surgery on survival: overview of 10-year results from randomized trials by the Coronary Artery Bypass Graft Surgery Trialists Collaboration: *Lancet* 1994;344:563-570.

31. Hannan EL, et al. Long-term outcomes of coronary-artery bypass grafting versus stent implantation: *N Engl J Med* 2005;352:2174-2183.

32. Goldman S, Zadina K, Moritz T, et al. Long-term patency of saphenous vein and left internal mammary artery grafts after coronary artery bypass surgery: results from a Department of Veterans Affairs Cooperative Study: *J Am Coll Cardiol* 2004;44:214-2156.

33. Athanasiou T, Saso S, Rao C, et al. Radial artery versus saphenous vein conduits for coronary artery bypass surgery: forty years of competition—which conduit offers better patency? A systematic review and meta-analysis: *Eur J Cardiothorac Surg* 2011;40:208-220.

34. Goldman S, Sethi GK, Holman W, et al. Radial artery grafts vs saphenous vein grafts in coronary artery bypass surgery: a randomized trial: *JAMA* 2011;305:167-174.

35. The Bypass Angioplasty Revascularization Investigators (BARI). Comparison of coronary bypass surgery with angioplasty in patients with multi-vessel disease: *N Engl J Med* 1996;335:217-225.

36. King SB 3rd, Kosinski AS, Guyton RA, et al. Eight-year mortality in the Emory Angioplasty versus Surgery Trial (EAST): *J Am Coll Cardiol* 2000;35:1116-1121.

37. Allen KB, Dowling RD, Angell WW, et al. Transmyocardial revascularization: 5-year follow-up of a prospective, randomized multicenter trial: *Ann Throc Surg* 2004;77:1228-1234.

38. Allen KB, Dowling RD, Schuch DR, et al. Adjunctive transmyocardial revascularization: five-year follow-up of a prospective, randomized trial: *Ann Thorac Surg* 2004;78:458-465.

39. Aaberge L, Rootwelt K, Blomhoff S, et al. Continued symptomatic improvement three to five years after transmyocardial revascularization with CO_2 laser: a late clinical follow-up of the Norwegian Randomized trial with transmyocardial revascularization: *J Am Coll Cardiol* 2005;39:1588-1593.

40. Allen KB, Dowling RD, Fudge TL, et al. Comparison of transmyocardial revascularization with medical therapy in patients with refractory angina: *N Engl J Med* 1999;341:1029-1036.

41. Burkhoff D, Schmidt S, Schulman SP, et al. Transmyocardial laser revascularisation compared with continued medical therapy for treatment of refractory angina pectoris: a prospective randomised trial. ATLANTIC Investigators. Angina Treatments-Lasers and Normal Therapies in Comparison: *Lancet* 1999;354:885-890.

42. Schofield PM, Sharples LD, Caine N, et al. Transmyocardial laser revascularisation in patients with refractory angina: a randomised controlled trial. *Lancet* 1999;353:519-524.

43. Nägele H, Stubbe HM, Nienaber C, Rödiger W. Results of transmyocardial laser revascularization in non-revascularizable coronary artery disease after 3 years follow-up: *Eur Heart J* 1998;19:1525-1530.

44. Lawson WE, Hui JC, Lang G. Treatment benefit in the enhanced external counterpulsation consortium: *Cardiology* 2000;94:31-35.

45. Soran O, Kennard ED, Kfoury AG, et al.; IEPR Investigators. Two-year clinical outcomes after enhanced external counterpulsation (EECP) therapy in patients with refractory angina pectoris and left ventricular dysfunction (report from The International EECP Patient Registry): *Am J Cardiol* 2006;97:17-20.

Acute Coronary Syndromes

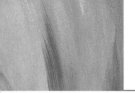

Jeremiah P. Depta and Richard G. Bach

Acute Coronary Syndromes

GENERAL PRINCIPLES

- Acute coronary syndromes (ACS) represent a group of specific clinical conditions resulting from myocardial ischemia or myocardial infarction (MI) related most often to atherothrombotic coronary obstruction.
- For practical purposes, ACS can be divided into ST-segment elevation ACS (STE-ACS, or more commonly, ST-segment elevation MI [STEMI]) and non–ST-segment elevation ACS (NSTE-ACS), which includes both non–ST-segment elevation MI (NSTEMI) and unstable angina (UA). Notably, the clinical presentation and symptoms may be similar for these syndromes.
- The primary goals of treatment in NSTE-ACS are to relieve and/or limit ischemia, prevent infarction or reinfarction, and improve outcomes.

Definitions

- STEMI (see Chapter 12) is diagnosed in an appropriate clinical setting with the finding of ≥1 mm (0.1 mV) ST elevation in at least two contiguous leads of an electrocardiogram (ECG) associated with cardiac biomarker elevation.
- NSTE-ACS is diagnosed in an appropriate clinical setting when such an event is associated with an ECG that does not show ST-segment elevation. ECG may show ST depression or T-wave abnormalities, but may also be normal, with (NSTEMI) or without (UA) myocardial necrosis demonstrated by cardiac biomarker elevation.[1]
- The current universal definition for acute myocardial infarction (AMI) adopted by the European Society of Cardiology/American College of Cardiology Foundation/American Heart Association/World Health Foundation Task Force defines AMI as evidence of myocardial necrosis in the appropriate clinical setting meeting any of the following criteria[2]: elevated cardiac biomarkers, preferably serum troponin, with at least one value >99% of the upper reference limit (URL) with one of the following:
  - Ischemic symptoms
  - New ischemic ECG changes (new ST-T wave changes or new left bundle branch block)
  - New pathologic Q waves
  - Evidence of new infarction by cardiac imaging
  - Intracoronary thrombus noted on angiography or autopsy

Classification

NSTE-ACS can be subdivided into UA and NSTEMI based on the absence or presence, respectively, of myocardial necrosis (i.e., elevated cardiac biomarkers).

Epidemiology

- In 2012, approximately 785,000 Americans presented with new ACS, and approximately 475,000 had recurrent ACS.[3]
- The average age at first AMI for men is 65 years and for women is 70 years.[3]
- Every 25 seconds, an American will suffer from ACS, and every minute, one American will die from AMI.[3]
- One out of every six deaths in the United States is attributable to ACS.[3]
- In-hospital mortality is similar between STEMI and NSTEMI patients.[4]
- One-year mortality is higher for NSTEMI patients compared with STEMI patients.[4]
- Mortality from ACS has declined dramatically with the advent of evidence-based therapies, but up to 25% of patients do not receive optimal medical therapy for ACS, resulting in a significant increase in mortality in those patients.[5]

Etiology

- The underlying cause of myocardial ischemia in NSTE-ACS results from a mismatch between myocardial oxygen supply and demand. Several mechanisms responsible but not mutually exclusive for this mismatch include[1]
  - **Coronary atherothrombosis** associated with coronary artery plaque rupture or erosion (see "Pathophysiology" below).
  - **Coronary vasospasm** resulting from focal vasoconstriction of an epicardial coronary vessel related to hypercontractility of vascular smooth muscle with or without microvascular derangement (e.g., endothelial dysfunction).
  - Other mechanical obstructions to coronary blood flow (e.g., thromboembolism and spontaneous coronary dissection).
  - Secondary NSTE-ACS resulting from
    - Reduced coronary blood flow (e.g., hypotension)
    - Increased myocardial oxygen demand (e.g., tachycardia and thyrotoxicosis)
    - Reduced myocardial oxygen delivery (e.g., anemia and hypoxia)

Pathophysiology

- NSTE-ACS/UA typically results from severe narrowing and/or transient occlusion of a coronary artery:
  - The majority of cases of NSTE-ACS are due to a **critical decrease in coronary blood supply via partial occlusion of the affected vessel**.
  - This is distinct from most STEMI, which is due to a sudden obstruction of coronary blood supply due to total occlusion of the affected vessel.
- Coronary occlusion typically results from atherothrombosis at vulnerable plaques, which may involve
  - Ruptured atherosclerotic plaque
  - Plaque erosion or ulceration
- Coronary atherothrombosis involves platelet-mediated thrombosis at sites of plaque rupture, ulceration, or erosion and occurs by exposure of the subendothelium to the bloodstream that initiates a cascade of events culminating in local thrombus formation.[6]

Risk Factors

- The traditional major risk factors for the development of coronary artery disease (CAD) include hypertension, hyperlipidemia, smoking, diabetes, and a family history of premature CAD.
- Each patient presenting with NSTE-ACS should undergo a thorough assessment of CAD risk factors to initiate appropriate secondary prevention.

DIAGNOSIS

- NSTE-ACS is a clinical diagnosis based on the patient history, physical examination, ECG, and cardiac biomarkers.
- Rapid identification of ACS allows for timely risk stratification and initiation of appropriate therapies.

Clinical Presentation

History

- The symptoms associated with NSTE-ACS are highly variable and can include
  - Chest pressure or heaviness with or without radiation to the arm(s), back, shoulder(s), neck, or jaw; at times, discomfort may be located solely in the arm(s), back, shoulder(s), neck, or jaw.
  - Indigestion or heartburn
  - Nausea and/or vomiting with or without epigastric discomfort
  - Shortness of breath or dyspnea on exertion
  - Weakness, dizziness, light-headedness, or loss of consciousness
- Physicians should recognize that **up to half of the MIs may be silent.**[7]
- Symptoms that typically differentiate NSTE-ACS from chronic stable angina include
  - Chest discomfort that occurs at rest lasting >20 minutes.
  - Chest discomfort developing with increased severity, frequency, or duration
  - Chest discomfort occurring with less exertion
  - New-onset exertional angina of <2-month duration that limits physical activity
  - Angina that severely limits normal physical activity (i.e., angina with walking 1 to 2 blocks or a single flight of stairs)
- Symptoms that are **unlikely to be associated with NSTE-ACS** include[1]
  - Pleuritic pain
  - Pain localized to middle or lower abdominal region
  - Pain localized with one finger
  - Reproducible pain with movement or palpation
  - Pain lasting a few seconds
  - Pain radiating to the lower extremities
  - However, the **presence of atypical symptoms does not exclude the possibility of ACS**.

Physical Examination

- The physical examination in patients with NSTE-ACS is rarely specific or sensitive.
- May be helpful to support considering alternative diagnoses
- Assess for signs/symptoms of heart failure and/or shock which include
  - Extra heart sounds (S3)
  - Elevated jugular venous pressure
  - Pulmonary rales
  - Peripheral edema
  - Hypotension
  - Cyanosis
  - Cool or clammy extremities
- Awareness of the complications of AMI is important, as certain physical examination finding may be present at the time of diagnosis or complicate the course of NSTE-ACS (see Chapter 12).

Diagnostic Criteria

NSTE-ACS is a clinical diagnosis that is based on
- History of symptoms compatible with myocardial ischemia, as described above
- An ECG that may be supportive if showing ST-segment depression and/or T-wave inversion or transient nondiagnostic ST elevation (but that may also be within normal limits)
- Assessment of cardiac biomarkers

Differential Diagnosis

- Cardiovascular: acute pericarditis, myocarditis, cardiac tamponade, aortic dissection, aortic stenosis, hypertrophic obstructive cardiomyopathy (HOCM), or congestive heart failure
- Pulmonary: pulmonary embolism, pneumothorax, pneumonia, asthma, or chronic obstructive pulmonary disease
- Gastrointestinal (GI): esophageal spasm, esophagitis, reflux disease, peptic ulcer disease, gastritis, or cholecystitis
- Psychiatric: anxiety disorders
- Musculoskeletal: muscle sprain/strain, costochondritis, rib fracture, painful lower rib syndrome, fibromyalgia, inflammatory arthropathies, SAPHO syndrome (i.e., synovitis, acne, pustulosis, hyperostosis, and osteitis), sickle cell disease, and malignancy

Diagnostic Testing

Laboratories

- Serial measurements of **cardiac biomarkers** should be obtained on presentation and repeated every 6 to 8 hours.
- Creatine kinase (CK-MB) is present in both skeletal and myocardial muscle cells.
  - No longer considered as sensitive or specific a test for diagnosing ACS as cardiac troponins (see below).
  - Aids in the timing of myocardial injury when symptoms are ambiguous.
  - CK-MB isoenzyme is readily detectable in the blood of normal subjects at low levels, and elevated levels can occur with damage to both skeletal and cardiac muscle cells.
  - Usually present within 4 to 6 hours after injury with peak level attained in approximately 10 to 18 hours.
  - Due to its short half-life, CK-MB is **very useful for assessing recurrent postinfarct ischemic events**, because a fall and subsequent rise suggest reinfarction.
  - **Useful marker when checked serially after percutaneous coronary intervention (PCI)**, as significant rises in CK-MB may be used to diagnose periprocedural MI.
- Cardiac troponins (troponins T and I) are highly specific and sensitive markers of myocardial necrosis.
  - Usually undetectable in normal individuals
  - Detected **as early as 2 hours** after myocardial damage
  - Peak levels occur 8 to 12 hours after the event and **can remain elevated for up to 14 days**.
  - Cardiac troponin may be elevated in several other cardiac and noncardiac conditions:
    - After direct cardiac injury (e.g., defibrillator discharges, cardiac surgery or ablation, cardiac contusion, and myopericarditis), stress-induced (takotsubo) cardiomyopathy, or hypertensive urgency/emergency.
    - Noncardiac conditions (e.g., pulmonary embolism, acute and chronic renal disease).
    - Healthy subjects after extreme endurance events (e.g., marathons).
    - Newer, ultrasensitive assays for serum troponin show enhanced sensitivity and are currently undergoing further study regarding specificity.

- **B-type natriuretic peptide** has been shown to predict subsequent mortality in the setting of NSTE-ACS.[8]

Electrocardiography

Approximately 50% of the patients with NSTE-ACS present with significant ECG abnormalities, including[2]
- ST-segment depression ≥0.5 mm in two contiguous leads
- T-wave inversion ≥1 mm in two contiguous leads with prominent R wave or R/S ratio >1
- Symmetric T-wave inversions of >2 mm across the precordium are fairly specific for myocardial ischemia and worrisome for a lesion located in the proximal left anterior descending (LAD) artery.
- Nonspecific ST-segment changes or T-wave inversions

Diagnostic Testing

Coronary Angiography

- **Coronary angiography** is useful in providing detailed diagnostic information about the patients with symptoms of NSTE-ACS.
- **Indicated for patients who undergo the initial invasive strategy** (see "Early Invasive versus Initial Conservative Strategy" below).
- Women and nonwhites are less likely to have significant angiographic epicardial disease (see Chapter 38). The pathophysiology of ACS in these patients may involve microvascular disease, although this remains under investigation.

Noninvasive Stress Testing

Exercise or pharmacologic stress testing with an imaging modality (either echocardiography or myocardial perfusion) can be used to risk stratify patients with relatively low-risk ACS.

Newer Imaging Modalities

- Cardiac computed tomographic angiography (CCTA) and cardiac magnetic resonance imaging (CMR) have been used to assess low-risk populations, although its precise role is currently under study (see Chapter 32).
- CCTA may be useful in excluding obstructive CAD in symptomatic patients with a low pretest probability for disease, especially patients with a negative ECG and cardiac markers.
- CMR can allow cardiac functional assessment, perfusion imaging (adenosine or dobutamine), and myocardial viability testing at the expense of prolonged study times, patient claustrophobia, and problems with certain metallic implants (e.g., pacemakers/defibrillators).
- These modalities are still being evaluated and are currently being studied in large trials of patients with ACS.

TREATMENT

Risk Stratification
- Risk stratification allows tailoring of evidence-based diagnostic and therapeutic interventions based on the patient's risk for adverse outcomes.
- Rapidly assess the risk for adverse ischemic and bleeding outcomes.
- The Thrombolysis In Myocardial Infarction (TIMI) risk score can differentiate patients' risk based on criteria that predict the likelihood of death, MI, or urgent revascularization (Table 11-1).[9]
- Higher TIMI risk score has been shown to correlate with poorer outcomes (Figure 11-1).

TABLE 11-1 CALCULATING TIMI RISK SCORE

Each positive risk factor is worth one point. Points are added together to determine the TIMI risk score (maximum 7).

Risk factors:

- Age >65 years (1 point)
- Known CAD (>50% stenosis) (1 point)
- Severe anginal symptoms (>2 episodes of chest pain in last 24 hours) (1 point)
- ST deviation on admission ECG (1 point)
- Elevated serum cardiac markers (1 point)
- Use of ASA in the 7 days before presentation (1 point)
- ≥3 risk factors for CAD (1 point)
  - Family history
  - Diabetes
  - Hypertension
  - Dyslipidemia
  - Current smoker

TIMI, thrombolysis in myocardial infarction; CAD, coronary artery disease; ECG, electrocardiogram; ASA, aspirin.

Data from Antman EM, Cohen M, Bernink PJ, et al. The TIMI risk score for unstable angina/non-ST elevation MI: a method for prognostication and therapeutic decision making. *JAMA* 2000;284:835-842.

Bleeding Risk Assessment

- Bleeding in the setting of NSTE-ACS is associated with worse clinical outcomes.[10]
- All patients with NSTE-ACS should be assessed for their risk of bleeding when deciding therapeutic strategies.
- The CRUSADE bleeding score (ranges from 1 to 100) is a validated risk score for NSTE-ACS that determines a patient's baseline risk of in-hospital bleeding.[10] The rate of bleeding for those with a very low risk (≤20) is 3.1%, low risk (21 to 30) 5.5%, moderate risk (31 to 40) 8.6%, high risk (41 to 50) 11.9%, and very high risk (>50) 19.5%.[10]
- A simplified score calculator is available online (http://www.crusadebleedingscore.org, last accessed 5/29/13).[10]

Early Invasive versus Initial Conservative Strategy

- For NSTE-ACS, evidence-based initial management as recommended in the ACC/AHA practice guidelines involves selection of an early invasive or initial conservative strategy (Figure 11-2).[1]
- In the early invasive strategy, patients undergo diagnostic coronary angiography with intent to revascularize significant CAD when indicated.

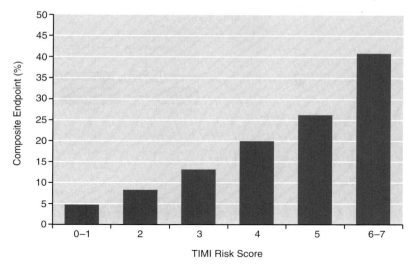

FIGURE 11-1. Rate of death, MI, or urgent revascularization at 14 days from the TIMI 11B and ESSENCE trials according to TIMI risk score. TIMI, thrombolysis in myocardial infarction. (Data from Antman EM, Cohen M, Bernink PJ, et al. The TIMI risk score for unstable angina/non-ST elevation MI: a method for prognostication and therapeutic decision making. *JAMA* 2000;284:835-842.)

- **Patient for whom the invasive strategy is prefered**[1]:
  - Recurrent chest pain despite maximal medical therapy
  - Elevated cardiac biomarkers
  - New ST-segment depression
  - Signs of heart failure
  - New or worsening mitral regurgitation
  - Hemodynamic instability
  - Sustained ventricular tachycardia
  - Prior coronary artery bypass grafting (CABG)
  - High risk score (e.g., TIMI 5–7)
  - PCI within 6 months
  - Reduced left ventricular ejection fraction (LVEF)
- Patients with refractory rest angina despite maximal medical therapy, hemodynamic compromise, or rhythm instability should be referred for immediate angiography.
- **In the initial conservative strategy, the patient may be treated with medical therapy followed by diagnostic testing** (stress testing with or without imaging) performed prior to discharge.
- **Patient for whom the conservative strategy is prefered**[1]:
  - Low risk score (e.g., TIMI 0–2)
  - Patient or physician preference
  - Risk of revascularization outweighs benefits
- For those patients who undergo noninvasive diagnostic testing, coronary angiography should be performed in patients whose LVEF <40% or have an intermediate- or high-risk stress test.[1]

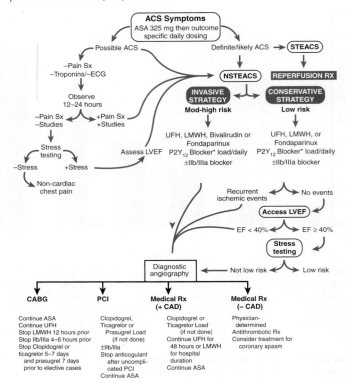

FIGURE 11-2. Management of ACS. *Clopidogrel or ticagrelor may be given when there is a reasonable certainty that the patient will not require CABG. Otherwise, it may be given after diagnostic angiography. Prasugrel may be selected for patients undergoing PCI, but should be avoided in patients with a history of stroke or TIA, the elderly (age ≥75 years), those with weight less than 60 kg, and those with higher bleeding risk. ACS, acute coronary syndrome; STEACS, ST-elevation acute coronary syndrome; NSTEACS, non–ST-elevation acute coronary syndrome; Rx, treatment; Sx, symptoms; UFH, unfractionated heparin; LMWH, low-molecular-weight heparin; IIb/IIIa, glycoprotein IIb/IIIa inhibitor; LVEF, left ventricular ejection fraction; CAD, coronary artery disease; CABG, coronary artery bypass grafting; PCI, percutaneous coronary intervention. (Data from Anderson JL, Adams CD, Antman EM, et al. ACC/AHA 2007 Guidelines for the management of patients with unstable angina/non-ST-elevation myocardial infarction. *J Am Coll Cardiol* 2007;50:e1-e157.)

Medications

- All patients should receive medical management directed at relieving ischemia and reducing the risk for adverse cardiac events.
- The primary goals of pharmacotherapy in NSTE-ACS are:
  - To rapidly limit ischemia and control chest pain with antiischemic and analgesic medications
  - To reduce further thrombus formation and disease progression with an appropriate antithrombotic therapy using antiplatelet and anticoagulation therapies

Antiischemic Therapy

- Antiischemic therapy focuses on improving the balance of oxygen supply and demand.
- Bed rest/monitoring:
  - Limit activity to bed/chair rest to reduce myocardial oxygen demand
  - Continuous ECG/telemetry monitoring
- Oxygen:
  - Oxygen during the first 6 hours of NSTE-ACS
  - All patients with an arterial oxygen saturation <90% or presenting with cyanosis or respiratory distress
- **Nitrates**:
  - Nitroglycerin (NTG) acts as a vasodilator on both the systemic (i.e., reducing myocardial oxygen demand) and coronary circulation (i.e., increasing coronary blood flow).
  - Initial dose is sublingual (SL) NTG 0.4-mg tablets or spray every 5 minutes, up to 3 doses. Intravenous (IV) NTG initiated at a dose of at least 10 μg/minute for[1]:
    - Chest pain that is refractory to SL NTG
    - Elevated blood pressure (BP)
    - Heart failure symptoms
  - Titrate by 10 μg/minute or greater increments every 5 minutes until the patient is chest pain free or hypotension (systolic blood pressure [SBP] <100 mmHg) prevents further increases in dose.
  - There is no maximum dose, but 200 μg/minute may be considered high enough to warrant additional therapy
  - Nitrates are generally contraindicated with[1]
    - SBP <90 mmHg heart rate (HR) <50 or >100 beats per minute (bpm)
    - Used a phosphodiesterase inhibitor within 24 hours of sildenafil or 48 hours of tadalafil
    - Timing for administration of nitrates with vardenafil is unknown and thus should be avoided
  - Nitrates should be used with caution in certain cardiac conditions that may be highly preload dependent[1]
    - Inferior MI with right ventricular infarct physiology
    - Severe aortic stenosis
    - HOCM with significant left ventricular outflow tract obstruction
    - Cardiac tamponade
    - Restrictive cardiomyopathy
  - Patients should generally be discharged with either SL or spray NTG for prn use for anginal symptoms.
- **β-Blockers:**
  - β-Blockers have a proven benefit on mortality for patients with AMI.[1]
  - **Oral β-blocker therapy should be initiated within the first 24 hours** for patients who do not have contraindications (see below).
  - For appropriate patients, treatment may be initiated with metoprolol 5 mg IV every 5 minutes times 3 doses to a target HR of 50 to 60 bpm while maintaining SBP >100 mmHg.
  - After the IV bolus(es) or in patients without active chest pain, start oral (by mouth [PO]) metoprolol, 25 to 50 mg every 6 hours, or atenolol, 50 to 100 mg daily.
  - As needed, IV bolus(es) may be repeated for patients with recurrent chest pain.
  - β-Blockers are contraindicated and may be harmful in patients with[1]
    - Signs of heart failure
    - Evidence of a low cardiac output
    - Increased risk of cardiogenic shock (age >70 years, SBP <120 mmHg, HR <60 bpm, or sinus tachycardia >120 bpm)

- PR interval >0.24 seconds
- Second- or third-degree heart block
- Active asthma or reactive airway disease
- **Calcium channel blockers** (CCBs):
  - **Considered for use in patients who have a contraindication to β-blockers.**[1]
  - Nondihydropyridines (e.g., verapamil or diltiazem) may be used in the absence of severe heart failure.
  - Nondihydropyridine CCB can be used as a third-line agent in patients continuing to have chest pain in the setting of adequate β-blockade and nitrates.
  - **No data have shown significant mortality benefit with the use of CCB.**
  - Extended release dihydropyridines (e.g., amlodipine) may be used when clinically indicated.
  - **Short-acting dihydropyridines**, such as nifedipine, are associated with an increased risk of death when used without β-blockade in the setting of NSTE-ACS and are **contraindicated**.
- **Morphine**:
  - Recommended for patients with persistent chest pain despite nitrates.[1]
  - Improve myocardial oxygen demand by reducing preload and sympathetic drive, due to its analgesic and anxiolytic properties.
  - Dosed in 2- to 4-mg IV boluses with repeated doses as needed.
  - Care should be exercised as morphine can mask symptoms that may indicate a need for intervention and can also lead to hypotension and respiratory depression. No clinical trial data have documented a reduction in adverse outcomes with morphine in the setting of NSTE-ACS.
  - Naloxone 0.4 to 2 mg IV in 2- to 3-minute intervals (maximum 10 mg) can be given to acutely reverse its effects in the setting of overdosage.

Antithrombotic Therapy

- Antithrombotic therapy is essential to reduce further thrombus formation and major adverse cardiac events (MACEs), including death, MI, and stroke.
- Therapy may be tailored to each patient's individual risk.
- **All patients should receive anticoagulation plus antiplatelet therapy.**
- Anticoagulation:
  - Anticoagulant therapy should be initiated as soon as possible after presentation for patients without contraindications.
  - Four antithrombin agents are available and recommended by ACC/AHA practice guidelines for the treatment of NSTE-ACS.
  - Agents may act at different levels of the coagulation cascade to prevent thrombin generation.
  - Currently, the following agents can be considered with variable selection potentially based on the type of management strategy[1]:
    - Early invasive: unfractionated heparin (UFH), enoxaparin, fondaparinux, or bivalirudin[1]
    - Initial conservative: UFH, enoxaparin, and fondaparinux
- **Unfractionated heparin**:
  - UFH acts by binding antithrombin III (ATIII), which in turn binds to and inactivates thrombin (factor II), factor IXa, and factor Xa.
  - IV UFH should be administered with a recommended loading bolus of 60 units (U)/kg (maximum 4,000 U) followed by a continuous infusion of 12 U/kg (maximum 1,000 U/hour).
  - The dose should be adjusted to maintain activated partial thromboplastin time of 1.5 to 2 times the URL.
  - The duration of therapy may be determined by the management strategy[1]:
    - Uncomplicated PCI: typically discontinue therapy after PCI

- Complicated PCI: at the discretion of the interventional cardiologist
- Conservative therapy: 48-hour duration
  - In cases of overdosage or refractory, life-threatening bleeding, to reverse the anticoagulant action of UFH, protamine sulfate can be given (1 mg protamine sulfate IV for every 100 U of active heparin).
  - Except for rare situations, protamine sulfate should be avoided in patients with NSTE-ACS.
  - Heparin-induced thrombocytopenia (HIT) is a serious complication of heparin (unfractionated and less frequently low molecular weight) therapy.
- **Low-molecular-weight heparins** (LMWHs):
  - LMWHs are obtained by shortening the polysaccharide tail on the heparin molecule.
  - Advantages over UFH include better bioavailability, subcutaneous (SQ) dosing, predictable anticoagulant activity that does not require laboratory monitoring, less-frequent type II HIT (<1%), and lower overall cost.
  - Disadvantages include a long half-life that can make emergent catheterization or PCI more complicated and an inability to effectively reverse its effects in the setting of refractory bleeding (i.e., only partly reversed with protamine sulfate).
  - For patients with NSTE-ACS of age <75 years, enoxaparin may be administered at a dose of 30 mg IV bolus followed 15 minutes later by 1 mg/kg SQ q12h (or q24h if CrCl <30 mL/minute).[1]
  - For patients ≥75 years, then omit IV bolus and administer 0.75 mg/kg SQ q12h (or 1 mg/kg SQ q24h if CrCl <30 mL/minute).
  - Enoxaparin is typically discontinued after uncomplicated PCI. For patients managed conservatively, it may have benefit to continue for the duration of hospitalization.[1]
- **Fondaparinux**:
  - Synthetic polysaccharide that contains the same pentasaccharide sequence found in UFH and LMWH.
  - Binds ATIII to predictably inhibit factor Xa without inhibiting thrombin.
  - Lacks the necessary domain to complex with PF4, which decreases the risk of HIT.
  - Administered as 2.5 mg SQ daily
  - Discontinued after uncomplicated PCI or may be continued for the duration of the hospitalization in patients managed conservatively
  - Based on OASIS trials, compared with enoxaparin, fondaparinux appeared to reduce the risk of bleeding but should not be the sole anticoagulant to support PCI due to an increased risk of catheter-related thombosis.[11,12]
- **Direct thrombin inhibitors**:
  - Include hirudin, lepirudin (recombinant hirudin), and bivalirudin. Bivalirudin has class I recommendation for NSTE-ACS in ACC/AHA practice guidelines.
  - Act by directly binding to and inactivating thrombin.
  - If chosen as an initial medical therapy, bivalirudin is administered as 0.1 mg/kg IV bolus and then 0.25 mg/kg/hour.
  - For patients undergoing PCI, bivalirudin is administered as 0.75 mg/kg IV bolus followed by 1.75 mg/kg/hour to continue for 4 hours after PCI.
  - Dosage adjustment is required in patients with CrCl <30 mL/minute or those on dialysis.
  - Bivalirudin may be considered for patients at an increased risk for bleeding undergoing invasive management—based on the results of the ACUITY trial that showed a significant reduction in major bleeding with similar efficacy in ACS patients compared with heparin combined with a glycoprotein (GP) IIb/IIIa inhibitors.[13]

Antiplatelet therapy

- **Aspirin (ASA)**:
  - Give ASA 162 to 325 mg immediately by emergency medical services or on arrival to the emergency department (ED), unless a history of serious intolerance or contraindication.

○ Continued for at least 1 month after bare metal stent (BMS) or 3 to 6 months after drug-eluting stent (DES). Then, ASA 75 to 162 mg should be continued indefinitely.

○ If a patient is allergic to ASA therapy, then consultation with an allergist for possible desensitization is recommended.

- **Adenosine diphosphate P2Y$_{12}$ receptor antagonists**:
  ○ Four oral antagonists of the P2Y$_{12}$ receptor are currently available for treatment: clopidogrel, prasugrel, ticlopidine, and ticagrelor.

  ○ **Patients treated conservatively should receive an ADP P2Y$_{12}$ antagonist (as part of dual antiplatelet therapy with ASA) for up to 1 year.**[14]

  ○ **Patients who undergo PCI should receive dual antiplatelet therapy including an ADP P2Y$_{12}$ antagonist for at least 1 year and possibly beyond in patients with DES.**[12,14,15]

  ○ **Clopidogrel**:
    ▪ Clopidogrel is given as a loading dose of 600 mg PO followed by 75 mg PO daily.[14]
    ▪ Prodrug that requires metabolic conversion to its active metabolite via cytochrome P450 (CYP) isoenzymes in the liver; genetic variability in certain isoenzymes (e.g., CYP2C19) and drug–drug interactions that affect isoenzyme activity can affect the degree of platelet inhibition from clopidogrel. The clinical implications of these observations are currently under intense study.
    ▪ Clopidogrel is generally well tolerated, but cases of thrombotic thrombocytopenic purpura (TTP) have rarely been observed.
    ▪ The CURRENT-OASIS-7 trial demonstrated a reduction in MACE at 30 days with a slight increase in major bleeding in higher-risk NSTE-ACS patients who underwent PCI and received a 600-mg loading dose of clopidogrel followed by 150 mg daily for 1 week then 75 mg daily compared with patients receiving a 300 mg loading dose of clopidogrel then 75 mg daily.[16]
    ▪ For patients undergoing PCI, a loading dose of 600 mg is preferred prior to or at the time of PCI. As mentioned above, for select patients, this may be followed by 150 mg daily for 6 days and then 75 mg daily for at least 1 year.[14]
    ▪ Routine platelet function and genetic testing to determine the platelet inhibitory response to clopidogrel are not recommended and should only be considered in patients at a high risk for poor clinical outcomes and if the results will alter management.[12,14]
    ▪ In patients with established high on-treatment platelet reactivity, alternative agents such as prasugrel and ticagrelor should be considered.[12]

  ○ **Prasugrel**:
    ▪ Prasugrel is a more potent and rapid inhibitor of the P2Y$_{12}$ receptor compared with clopidogrel or ticlopidine.[6]
    ▪ **It should be restricted to patients undergoing PCI.**[14]
    ▪ It is administered as a 60-mg PO loading dose for patients at the time of or up to 1 hour after PCI and then 10 mg PO daily thereafter.[14]
    ▪ In the TRITON-TIMI-38 trial, prasugrel reduced MACE by 19% in ACS patients undergoing PCI who received prasugrel (60-mg loading dose followed by 10 mg daily) compared with clopidogrel (300-mg loading dose followed by 75 mg daily) at the expense of increasing the risk of major bleeding.[17]
    ▪ Prasugrel is **absolutely contraindicated in patients with a history of stroke/TIA**.[14]
    ▪ It should be used with caution in patients whose body weight is <60 kg or who have an increased risk of bleeding, where a maintenance dose of 5 mg daily may be considered.[14]
    ▪ In patients aged ≥75 years, prasugrel is generally not recommended except in high-risk situations (e.g., diabetes or prior MI).[14]
    ▪ Of note, it is recommended that clopidogrel be withheld for at least 5 days and prasugrel for 7 days prior to surgery for patients requiring CABG for revascularization.[14,15]

- **Ticlopidine**:
  - Ticlopidine be used in the setting of an allergy to clopidogrel and contraindication to prasugrel or ticagrelor.
  - With use, there is a significant risk of neutropenia and a small risk of TTP.[6]
  - It is administered as a 500-mg PO loading dose followed by 250 mg PO daily.[6]
- **Ticagrelor**:
  - Ticagrelor is a nonthienopyridine antagonist of the platelet $P2Y_{12}$ receptor.
  - It is reversible and short-acting agent, with a half-life of 7 to 9 hours.
  - It is administered as a 180-mg PO loading dose followed 12 hours later by 90 mg PO twice daily.
  - The PLATO trial demonstrated a 16% reduction in major cardiac events with ticagrelor compared with clopidogrel in ACS patients; however, it was associated with a slightly increased rate of non-CABG major bleeding.[18]
  - It may be theoretically useful given its shorter half-life regarding concerns for delaying CABG in patients whose coronary anatomy has not yet been defined, but this remains speculative and the package insert recommends withholding ticagrelor for 5 days prior to major surgery.
  - When ticagrelor is used, the recommended daily maintenance dose of aspirin is 81 mg.[14]
- **GP IIb/IIIa inhibitors**:
  - GP IIb/IIIa platelet receptors bind fibrinogen and other ligands, mediating the final common pathway for platelet aggregation.
  - **The addition of a GP IIb/IIIa inhibitors to dual antiplatelet therapy** (i.e., aspirin and ADP $P2Y_{12}$ antagonist) **should be considered in the patients who are not at high risk for bleeding** and have[1,12,14]
    - High-risk features including positive troponins, diabetes mellitus, and significant ST-segment depression
    - Refractory ischemia despite maximal medical therapy
    - Delay to angiography >48 hours
  - Recent experience suggests that GP IIb/IIIa inhibitors may be omitted if a patient does not have high-risk features and has received a loading dose of $P2Y_{12}$ antagonist[12,14]
  - GP IIb/IIIa inhibitors should not be initiated prior to PCI in patients on dual antiplatelet therapy who are at low risk (TIMI risk score <2) or at high risk for bleeding.[14]
  - Thrombocytopenia, which can be severe, is an uncommon, but well-described complication of all these agents (more common with abciximab) and should prompt discontinuation of the drug.
  - **Eptifibatide** mimics a peptide sequence on fibrinogen that has a high affinity for the fibrinogen-binding sites for the GP IIb/IIIa receptor.
  - **Tirofiban** is a nonpeptide synthetic derivative of tyrosine that also has a high affinity for the fibrinogen-binding sites for the GP IIb/IIIa receptor.
    - Tirofiban is administered with a loading bolus of 0.4 µg/kg per minute over 30 minutes, followed by a maintenance infusion of 0.1 µg/kg per minute. Both bolus and infusion doses should be decreased by 50% in patients with a CrCl of <30 mL/minute.[1]
    - Eptifibatide and tirofiban are renally eliminated, dosages should be renally adjusted, and both are contraindicated in patients with very severe renal insufficiency and dialysis patients.
    - The half-lives of both are 2 to 3 hours and platelet aggregation returns to normal within 8 to 12 hours after discontinuation of the either drug.
    - The duration of therapy in NSTE-ACS is variable and may continue until 18 to 24 hours after PCI.
    - For patients managed via the conservative strategy, duration is left to the physicians' discretion, though it should be noted that the duration of treatment in major studies was typically 72 to 96 hours.[1]

- Eptifibatide is given with a loading bolus of 180 µg/kg (maximum 22.6 mg) over 2 minutes, followed by a maintenance infusion at 2 µg/kg/minute (maximum 15 mg/hour). If a patient's CrCl is <50 mL/minute, then the maintenance infusion is decreased to 1 µg/kg/minute (maximum 7.5 mg/hour).
  - Tirofiban is administered with a loading bolus of 0.4 µg/kg per minute over 30 minutes, followed by a maintenance infusion of 0.1 µg/kg per minute. Both bolus and infusion doses should be decreased by 50% in patients with a CrCl of <30 mL/minute.
  - **Abciximab** is a humanized chimeric murine monoclonal antibody Fab fragment with affinity for the human GP IIb/IIIa receptor.
    - Abciximab has a plasma half-life of 10 to 30 minutes but longer biologic half-life due to avid binding to platelet receptors; platelet aggregation generally returns to normal roughly 24 to 48 hours after discontinuation.
    - **Abciximab should only be used in patients in whom PCI is planned**, due to an increased risk of mortality associated with upstream use in conservatively managed NSTE-ACS patients in the GUSTO IV-ACS trial.[19]
    - Abciximab is given as a loading dose of 0.25 mg/kg IV bolus and then 0.125 µg/kg/minute (maximum 10 µg/minute) up to 12 hours after PCI.

Additional Secondary Prevention
- Secondary prevention is discussed in detail in Chapter 13.
- **Angiotensin converting enzyme (ACE) inhibitors and angiotensin receptor blockers (ARBs):**
  - **Should be initiated within the first 24 hours in patients with an LVEF <40% or with signs of heart failure.**[1]
  - ARB may be used in ACE inhibitor-intolerant patients.
  - Consider for patients with LVEF <40% or without signs of heart failure, especially for those patients with preexisting hypertension.
  - Because of the potential for harm, an IV ACE inhibitor should be used with caution in the first 24 hours, except in cases of uncontrolled hypertension.
- Aldosterone receptor blockers:
  - May be considered in the early recovery phase after ACS in patients who are tolerating therapeutic doses of an ACE inhibitor and have[1]
    - Diabetes mellitus
    - Signs of congestive heart failure
    - LVEF <40%
  - In the absence of renal dysfunction (CrCl <30 mL/minute) or hyperkalemia, spironolactone or eplerenone may be considered.
  - When initiating therapy, it is important to follow potassium levels closely—baseline, 1 week, 1 month, and then every 3 months.
- **Lipid-lowering therapy:**
  - All patients should have a fasting lipid panel within 24 hours of presentation.[1]
  - Hydroxymethylglutaryl-coenzyme A reductase inhibitors **(statins) should be initiated in all patients who do not have a contraindication regardless of a patient's baseline low-density lipoprotein** (LDL).[1]
  - Goal LDL is <100 mg/dL and an optional goal is <70 mg/dL.
  - In the PROVE IT-TIMI 22 trial, high-dose statin therapy (atorvastatin 80 mg daily) decreased MACE in ACS patients compared with moderate-dose statin therapy (pravastatin 40 mg daily).[20]
- Proton pump inhibitors (PPIs):
  - PPI should be considered in patients requiring dual antiplatelet therapy who have an indication for therapy, a history of GI bleeding, or a risk of GI bleeding.[12,21]
  - In observational studies, an association between PPI use and increased adverse cardiovascular events for patients receiving clopidogrel has raised concerns regarding

an interaction between PPIs and clopidogrel, resulting from reduced platelet inhibition due to an effect of PPIs on CYP enzyme activity.
  - This observation was not confirmed in the prospective, randomized COGENT trial where PPIs did show significant benefit in reducing GI-related adverse events for patients receiving clopidogrel.[22]
- Oral anticoagulation:
  - Triple therapy with aspirin, ADP P2Y 12 antagonist, and warfarin (note: experience with dabigatran, rivaroxaban, or apixaban is very limited) may be considered for patients who require an oral anticoagulant for a separate medical indication (e.g., atrial fibrillation, LV systolic dysfunction, large anterior MI, and venous thromboembolism) and have undergone PCI.[12,14] However, this strategy is associated with an **increased risk of serious bleeding**.[14]
  - For patients requiring warfarin and dual antiplatelet therapy, the dosage of aspirin should not exceed 75 to 81 mg daily, and the therapeutic range of warfarin should be maintained to a goal international normalized ratio of no greater than 2 to 2.5.[12,14]
- Fibrinolytics (thrombolytics): There has been no benefit observed and even a possibility of increased risk of adverse outcome for patients with NSTE-ACS treated with fibrinolytic therapy; therefore, they are contraindicated.[1]
- Nonsteroidal antiinflammatory agents (NSAIDs):
  - Both nonselective cyclooxygenase (COX) inhibitors and COX-2 inhibitors (except ASA) are associated with an increased risk of death, reinfarction, myocardial rupture, hypertension, and heart failure in large meta-analyses.[1]
  - They are contraindicated during hospitalization for NSTE-ACS.
  - Acetaminophen, low-dose opiates, and nonacetylated salicylates are acceptable alternatives for treating chronic musculoskeletal pain in patients with NSTE-ACS.
  - A nonselective COX inhibitor (e.g., naproxen) is reasonable if the above therapies are insufficient.

Other Nonpharmacologic Therapies

- Hemodynamic support:
  - Intra-aortic balloon counterpulsation (IABP) or percutaneous left ventricular assist device (LVAD) (Impella 2.5, Cardiac Power [CP], or 5.0) may be considered in any patient with ACS with[1]:
    - Refractory ischemic symptoms despite maximal medical therapy
    - Hemodynamic compromise
    - Mechanical complications of MI (e.g., acute mitral regurgitation)
  - Percutaneous LVADs have superior hemodynamic support compared with IABP in patients with cardiogenic shock secondary to AMI but have not yet been adequately tested in large-scale clinical trials of ACS patients.[23]
- Blood transfusion:
  - Theoretically, increasing blood hemoglobin concentration in patients who are anemic should improve oxygen-carrying capacity and improve myocardial oxygen supply.
  - However, observational studies have linked transfusion of stored blood to future adverse outcomes, and there remains uncertainty regarding the appropriate indications or threshold hemoglobin value that should trigger transfusion therapy.
  - Transfusion of patients with ACS to a hemoglobin >10 mg/dL or hematocrit $>30\%$ has been recommended but based on limited data regarding benefit.

Surgical Management

- When considering potential revascularization strategies, patients with left main or multivessel disease may be risk stratified using the **SYNTAX score** (Society of Thoracic Surgeons and Synergy between Percutaneous Coronary Intervention with TAXUS and Cardiac Surgery).[12]

- Revascularization by CABG may be indicated for ACS patients with[1]:
  - Unprotected left main disease, although PCI is now considered an acceptable alternative in uncomplicated left main disease, especially in patients with a SYNTAX score <22.[12,15]
  - Three-vessel disease (CABG may be preferred if SYNTAX >2 and good surgical candidate), especially in the setting of impaired LV function
  - Two-vessel disease with proximal LAD involvement
  - Diabetic patients with multivessel CAD including LAD disease

Lifestyle/Risk Modification

- Secondary prevention is discussed in detail in Chapter 13.
- Smoking cessation:
  - All patients should be assessed for current use and desire to quit.
  - Cessation and reduction of environmental exposure is advised for all patients.
  - Pharmacotherapy is useful and should be considered for any patient starting cessation.
- BP control:
  - Patients should be aggressively treated to a goal BP of <140/90.
  - Medications with BP lowering activity that are used to treat NSTE-ACS should be maximized before adding additional BP lowering agents.
- Weight management:
  - Body mass index (BMI) should be assessed during the hospitalization and at each subsequent visit.
  - Goal BMI is 18.6 to 24.9 kg/m^2.
  - For patients who initiate weight loss therapy, a reasonable goal is reduction in weight by 10% over a period of several months.
- Physical activity:
  - All patients should be encouraged to perform moderate aerobic activity for 30 to 60 minutes 5 to 7 times per week.[1]
  - Weight training can be incorporated 2 days out of each week.
  - **Daily walking can begin immediately upon discharge**.
  - Sexual activity can be resumed 7 to 10 days after discharge.
- Cardiac rehabilitation:
  - **All patients should be referred for cardiac rehabilitation**.[1,12]
  - Cardiac rehabilitation can reduce mortality following ACS by as much as 27%, but as few as 16% of patients are referred for rehabilitation.

Cocaine-/Methamphetamine-Associated Myocardial Infarction

GENERAL PRINCIPLES

- An estimated 25 million Americans have used cocaine that is the most common illicit drug used in patients seeking medical attention in the ED.[24]
- Cocaine-induced angina is likely secondary to increased myocardial oxygen demand from[24]:
  - Increased BP, HR, and contractility
  - Vasoconstriction/vasospasm of epicardial vessels
  - Increased platelet aggregation
  - Accelerated atherosclerosis thereby increasing the risk of coronary thrombosis
- The risk of MI is increased by a factor of 24 immediately after cocaine use.[24]
- The incidence of ACS after methamphetamines is unclear, but the pathophysiology is considered likely similar to that of cocaine abuse.

DIAGNOSIS

- Patients with cocaine-induced chest pain should undergo the same diagnostic considerations as other patients with symptoms of NSTE-ACS.
- Diagnostic angiography with intent to perform PCI should be considered for all patients with persistent new ST-elevation or new ST-depression or T-wave changes despite NTG and CCB therapy.[1]

TREATMENT

- Treatment algorithm is modified:
  - All patients should still receive **ASA**.
  - SL or IV **nitrates** should also be given, especially in those with ST-segment or T-wave changes.[1]
  - **CCB**, such as IV diltiazem, can be used to reduce myocardial oxygen demand.
  - **β-Blockers are contraindicated**, as they can lead to unopposed α-mediated vasoconstriction and worsen myocardial ischemia. **One arguable exception is labetalol**, which has both β- and α-blocking properties, and may be administered to patients with SBP >100 mmHg or HR >100 bpm, provided they have been given NTG or CCB 1 hour prior to administration.[1]
  - **Benzodiazepines** are also as an anxiolytic and to reduce ischemia.
  - Even in the setting of vasospasm, many patients may still have luminal thrombosis or plaque rupture requiring PCI.
  - BMS may be preferred in patients with potentially high risk of noncompliance.
  - For patients who cannot undergo coronary angiography, fibrinolytic therapy can be used in patients presenting with persistent ST elevation despite NTG and CCB therapy.[1]
- Patients with methamphetamine-induced ACS should be treated similar to patients with cocaine-induced angina.

REFERENCES

1. Anderson JL, Adams CD, Antman EM, et al. ACC/AHA 2007 Guidelines for the management of patients with unstable angina/non-ST-elevation myocardial infarction: *J Am Coll Cardiol* 2007;50:e1-e157.
2. Thygesen K, Alpert JS, Jaffe AS, et al. Third universal definition of myocardial infarction: *Circulation* 2012;126:2020-2035.
3. Roger VL, Go AS, Lloyd-Jones D, et al. Heart disease and stroke statistics—2012 update: a report from the American Heart Association: *Circulation* 2012;125;e2-e220.
4. Montalescot G, Dallongeville J, Van Belle E, et al. STEMI and NSTEMI: are they so different? 1 year outcomes in acute myocardial infarction as defined by the ESC/ACC definition (the OPERA registry): *Eur Heart J* 2007;28:1409-1417.
5. Peterson ED, Roe MT, Mulgund J, et al. Association between hospital process performance and outcomes among patients with acute coronary syndromes: *JAMA* 2006;295:1912-1920.
6. Depta JP, Bhatt DL. Aspirin and platelet adenosine diphosphate receptor antagonists in acute coronary syndromes and percutaneous coronary intervention: role in therapy and strategies to overcome resistance: *Am J of Cardiovasc Drugs* 2008;8:91-112.
7. Kannel WB. Silent myocardial ischemia and infarction: insights from the Framingham Study: *Cardiol Clin* 1986;4:583-591.
8. Galvani M, Ottani F, Oltrona L, et al. N-terminal pro-brain natriuretic peptide on admission has prognostic value across the whole spectrum of acute coronary syndromes: *Circulation* 2004;110:128-134.
9. Antman EM, Cohen M, Bernink PJ, et al. The TIMI risk score for unstable angina/non-ST elevation MI: a method for prognostication and therapeutic decision making: *JAMA* 2000;284:835-842.
10. Subherwal S, Bach RG, Chen AY, et al. Baseline risk of major bleeding in non-ST-segment-elevation myocardial infarction: the CRUSADE (Can Rapid risk stratification of Unstable angina

patients Suppress ADverse outcomes with Early implementation of the ACC/AHA Guidelines) Bleeding Score: *Circulation* 2009;119:1873-1882.

11. Yusuf S, Mehta SR, Chrolavicius S, et al. Comparison of fondaparinux and enoxaparin in acute coronary syndromes: *N Engl J Med* 2006;354:1464-1476.

12. Levine GN, Bates ER, Blankenship JC, et al. 2011 ACCF/AHA/SCAI Guideline for percutaneous coronary intervention: *Circulation* 2011;124:e574-e651.

13. Stone GW, White HD, Ohman EM, et al. Bivalirudin in patients with acute coronary syndromes undergoing percutaneous coronary intervention: a subgroup analysis from the Acute Catheterization and Urgent Intervention Triage strategy (ACUITY) trial: *Lancet* 2007;369:907-919.

14. Jneid H, Anderson JL, Wright RS, et al. 2012 ACCF/AHA focused update of the Guideline for the management of patients with unstable angina/non-ST-elevation myocardial infarction: *J Am Coll Cardiol* 2012;60:645-681.

15. Kushner FG, Hand M, Smith SC, et al. 2009 focused updates: ACC/AHA guidelines for the management of patients with ST-elevation myocardial infarction and ACC/AHA/SCAI guidelines on percutaneous coronary intervention: *J Am Coll Cardiol* 2009;54:2205-2241.

16. Mehta SR, Bassand JP, Chrolavicius S, et al. Dose comparisons of clopidogrel and aspirin in acute coronary syndromes: *N Engl J Med* 2010;363:930-942.

17. Wiviott SD, Braunwald E, McCabe CH, et al. Prasugrel versus clopidogrel in patients with acute coronary syndromes: *N Engl J Med* 2007;357:2001-2015.

18. Wallentin L, Becker RC, Budaj A, et al. Ticagrelor versus clopidogrel in patients with acute coronary syndromes: *N Engl J Med* 2009;361:1045-1057.

19. Simoons ML. Effect of glycoprotein IIb/IIIa receptor blocker abciximab on outcome in patients with acute coronary syndromes without early coronary revascularisation: the GUSTO IV-ACS randomised trial: *Lancet.* 2001;357:1915-1924.

20. Cannon CP, Braunwald E, McCabe CH, et al. Intensive versus moderate lipid lowering with statins after acute coronary syndromes: *N Engl J Med* 2004;350:1495-1504.

21. Abraham NS, Hlatky MA, Antman EM, et al. ACCF/ACG/AHA 2010 expert consensus document on the concomitant use of proton pump inhibitors and thienopyridines: a focused update of the ACCF/ACG/AHA 2008 expert consensus document on reducing the gastrointestinal risks of antiplatelet therapy and NSAID use: *J Am Coll Cardiol* 2010;56:2051-2066.

22. Bhatt DL, Cryer BL, Contant CF, et al. Clopidogrel with or without omeprazole in coronary artery disease: *N Engl J Med* 2010;363:1909-1917.

23. Seyfarth M, Sibbing D, Bauer I, et al. A randomized clinical trial to evaluate the safety and efficacy of a percutaneous left ventricular assist device versus intra-aortic balloon pumping for treatment of cardiogenic shock caused by myocardial infarction: *J Am Coll Cardiol* 2008;52:1584-1588.

24. Lange RA, Hillis LD. Cardiovascular complications of cocaine use: *N Engl J Med* 2001;345:351-358.

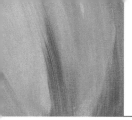

Acute ST-Segment Elevation Myocardial Infarction

12

Michael Yeung, Sudeshna Banerjee, and Howard I. Kurz

GENERAL PRINCIPLES

- ST-segment elevation myocardial infarction (STEMI) represents **a pathophysiologic process among the acute coronary syndromes (ACS) that is different from that of unstable angina and non–ST-segment elevation myocardial infarction** (UA/NSTEMI).
- The therapeutic paradigm for STEMI mandates a rapid decision regarding reperfusion.
- Time to reperfusion (i.e., "door to balloon" or "door to needle") is an important component of these therapies and has become a major benchmark for institutional quality of cardiovascular care.

Definition

- Pathologic definition: **myocyte cell death,** usually due to prolonged myocardial ischemia
- Clinical definition of myocardial infarction (MI) that has been established by the World Health Organization, American Heart Association, European Society of Cardiology, and American College of Cardiology (WHO/AHA/ESC/ACC) requires **the rise and/or fall of cardiac biomarkers for myocardial necrosis in addition to one of the following**[1]:
  - Ischemic symptoms
  - Electrocardiogram (ECG) changes consistent with ischemia or pathologic Q waves
  - Confirmation of infarction on imaging
  - Autopsy evidence of myocardial cell death is also sufficient.
- STEMI can be differentiated clinically from NSTEMI by the presence of specific ECG changes (i.e., ST elevation, new left bundle branch block [LBBB]).

Classification

- The designation of STEMI includes not only classic ST elevation but also new or presumably new LBBB.
- The descriptors "Q wave" and "non-Q wave MI" have lost favor because the majority of STEMIs are Q-wave MIs.
- A consensus statement by the ACC/AHA/ESC/WHF published in 2012 refines and broadens the classification of MI and includes categories based on procedure-associated MIs, demand ischemia, and sudden cardiac death.[1]

Epidemiology

- An estimated 500,000 patients in the United States will suffer a STEMI annually.
- A significant proportion of these patients will die from sudden cardiac death due to ventricular arrhythmia prior to arriving at the hospital.
- The success of the medical community's concerted efforts has led to a 26% reduction in mortality since 1990.

- Overall survival rates across the majority of US centers are >90%.
- However, the death rate remains high among the subgroup of patients who develop cardiogenic shock or other mechanical complications of STEMI, with mortality in excess of 50%.

Etiology

- Any condition or event that results in interruption of coronary flow sufficient to cause myocardial cell death can lead to MI.
- Usually results from an **acute change in a preexisting coronary plaque** that leads to activation of thrombotic mediators and subsequent clot formation with obstruction to blood flow.
- Although there is a spectrum in terms of the degree of artery obstruction and cell death, it is the significant or complete coronary occlusion, which leads to STEMI.
- Other conditions that can lead to STEMI include
  ○ Severe coronary vasospasm
  ○ Embolization
  ○ Spontaneous coronary dissection
  ○ These conditions should be considered in the patient whose clinical findings suggest a process other than acute plaque rupture

Pathophysiology

- Most commonly due to coronary artery occlusion by thrombus, which often forms in situ at the site of an atheromatous plaque.
- The mechanisms involved vary by age and gender.
  ○ **Plaque rupture** causes the majority of events in men and older women.
  ○ **Plaque erosion** is a more common mechanism in younger women.
- Involves mild-to-moderate immature plaques (i.e., those that do not significantly impede coronary flow at baseline) with thin fibrous caps and lipid-rich cores that rupture in the acute setting of inflammation, shear forces, and local rheologic factors.
- This initiates a sequence of platelet aggregation, fibrin deposition, and vasoconstriction, forming the classic **fibrin-rich red thrombus**, which completely occludes the involved artery, predisposing to STEMI.
- Left untreated, the mortality rate of uncomplicated STEMI can exceed 30%.
- Mechanical complications are more common when a STEMI is untreated.
- In addition, the heart undergoes the detrimental process of remodeling.

DIAGNOSIS

Clinical Presentation

- Patients presenting with a suspected ACS should undergo rapid evaluation.
- A focused history, physical, and ECG interpretation should be performed within 10 minutes of arrival in the emergency department to allow for timely reperfusion when appropriate.

History

- Quickly acquire adequate historical information in the setting of diagnostic ECG changes to initiate treatment and mobilize, when appropriate, the team for percutaneous revascularization.
- Chest discomfort is the most common symptom.
  ○ Typically progressive, substernal to left-sided, and often similar in quality to typical angina.
  ○ Usually intense and prolonged, lasting more than 20 to 30 minutes.
  ○ Unlike UA/NSTEMI, rest and nitroglycerin usually do not provide significant relief.

- Review absolute and relative contraindications to thrombolytic therapy (Table 12-1), which are intended as recommendation for clinical decision making, but other contraindications may be present and decisions must be made on a case-by-case basis.[2]
- Review issues regarding primary percutaneous coronary intervention (PCI), including allergy to contrast agents, issues relating to vascular access (peripheral vessel disease or previous peripheral revascularization procedures), previous cardiac catheterizations and complications, history of renal dysfunction, central nervous system disease, pregnancy, or bleeding diathesis.
- Traditional risk factors are weak predictors of the likelihood of acute infarction as the presenting etiology.

TABLE 12-1	CONTRAINDICATIONS TO THROMBOLYTIC THERAPY

Absolute contraindications

  Any prior intracranial hemorrhage

  Known structural cerebral vascular lesion (e.g., arteriovenous malformation)

  Known intracranial malignancy (primary or metastatic)

  Ischemic stroke within 3 months EXCEPT acute ischemic stroke within 4.5 hours

  Suspected aortic dissection

  Active bleeding or bleeding diathesis (excludes menstruation)

  Significant closed-head or facial trauma within 3 months

  Severe uncontrolled hypertension that is unresponsive to emergent treatment

  If using streptokinase, having received streptokinase within the last 6 months

Relative contraindications

  Severe uncontrolled hypertension on presentation (SBP >180 mmHg or DBP >110 mmHg)

  History of severe, poorly controlled chronic hypertension

  History of prior ischemic stroke >3 months; dementia or known intracranial pathology not covered in absolute contraindications

  Traumatic or prolonged (>10 minutes) CPR or major surgery (<3 weeks)

  Recent internal bleeding (within 2–4 weeks)

  Noncompressible vascular punctures

  Pregnancy

  Active peptic ulcer

  Oral anticoagulant use

SBP, systolic blood pressure; DBP, diastolic blood pressure; CPR, cardiopulmonary resuscitation.

Modified from O'Gara PT, Kushner FG, Ascheim DD, et al. 2013 ACCF/AHA guideline for the management of ST-elevation myocardial infarction. *Circulation* 2013;127:e362-e425.

Physical Examination
- Important in determining other potential sources of chest pain, assessing prognosis, and establishing a baseline that will aid in the early recognition of complications.
- The goal is to determine hemodynamic stability, the presence of cardiogenic pulmonary edema, or mechanical complications of MI (papillary muscle dysfunction, free wall rupture, and ventricular septal defect [VSD]) and exclude other etiologies of acute chest discomfort.
- Should include assessment of vital signs and oxygenation with bilateral blood pressures as well as jugular venous pressure; pulmonary examination for pulmonary edema; cardiac examination for arrhythmia, murmurs, gallops, or friction rub; vascular examination for evidence of peripheral vascular disease and pulse deficits; and neurologic examination (especially prior to the administration of thrombolytics).

Differential Diagnosis
- The inherent risks of both thrombolytic therapy and primary PCI mandate that alternative diagnoses be considered in patients with chest pain.
- In particular, administration of thrombolytic agents in certain conditions, such as aortic dissection, may lead to death.
- In the situation when the diagnosis is uncertain, primary PCI offers a distinct advantage as the initial reperfusion strategy.
- Differential diagnosis of chest pain:
  - Life-threatening: aortic dissection, pulmonary embolus, perforated ulcer, tension pneumothorax, and Boerhaave syndrome (esophageal rupture with mediastinitis).
  - Other cardiac and noncardiac causes: pericarditis, myocarditis, vasospastic angina, gastroesophageal reflux disease, esophageal spasm, costochondritis, pleurisy, peptic ulcer disease, panic attack, biliary or pancreatic pain, cervical disc or neuropathic pain, and somatization and psychogenic pain disorder.
- Differential diagnosis of ST elevation on ECG: pericarditis, pulmonary embolism, aortic dissection with coronary artery involvement, normal variant, early repolarization, left ventricular (LV) hypertrophy with strain, Brugada syndrome, myocarditis, hyperkalemia, bundle branch block, Prinzmetal angina, hypertrophic cardiomyopathy, and aortic dissection.

Risk Stratification
- Multiple proven risk assessment tools utilize information obtained during the history, physical examination, and diagnostic evaluation, which provide an estimate of 30-day mortality following AMI.
- The **Killip classification** uses bedside physical examination findings including an S3 gallop, pulmonary congestion, and cardiogenic shock (Table 12-2).[3]
- The **Forrester classification** uses hemodynamic monitoring of cardiac index and pulmonary capillary wedge pressure (PCWP) (Table 12-3).[4]
- The most recent prognostic system, the **thrombolysis in myocardial infarction (TIMI) risk score** (Table 12-4), combines history and examination findings in patients with STEMI treated with thrombolytics.[5]
- This is a different risk score than that used for risk stratification in the setting of UA/NSTEMI.

Diagnostic Testing
Laboratories
- **Cardiac biomarkers** are important in the diagnosis and prognosis of STEMI but have a limited role in the initial decision-making process.

TABLE 12-2 KILLIP CLASSIFICATION IN ACUTE MI

Class	Definition	Mortality (%)
I	No CHF	6
II	S3 and/or basilar rales	17
III	Pulmonary edema	30–40
IV	Cardiogenic shock	60–80

MI, myocardial infarction; CHF, congestive heart failure signs.

Modified from Killip T 3rd, Kimball JT. Treatment of myocardial infarction in a coronary care unit. A two-year experience with 250 patients. *Am J Cardiol* 1967;20:457-464.

TABLE 12-3 FORRESTER CLASSIFICATION SYSTEM FOR ACUTE MI

Class	Cardiac index (L/minute/m²)	PCWP (mmHg)	Mortality (%)
I	≥2.2	<18	3
II	≥2.2	≥18	9
III	<2.2	<18	23
IV	<2.2	≥18	51

MI, myocardial infarction; PCWP, pulmonary capillary wedge pressure.

Data from Forrester JS, Diamond G, Chatterjee K, Swan HJ. Medical therapy of acute myocardial infarction by application of hemodynamic subsets (first of two parts). *N Engl J Med* 1976;295:1356-1362.

- Markers used for determining the presence of myocardial necrosis—including creatine kinase MB, troponin, and myoglobin—are discussed in detail in Chapter 11.
- Standard laboratory evaluation should include a basic metabolic profile, magnesium level, liver function, lipid profile, complete blood count, and coagulation studies.

Electrocardiogram
- The ECG should be performed and interpreted within 10 minutes of presentation (Table 12-5).
- The ECG should be repeated every 20 to 30 minutes for up to 4 hours if the patient has persistent symptoms when there is clinical suspicion for AMI, but the ECG is nondiagnostic.
- Hyperacute T waves, seen as either tall or deeply inverted T waves, may be an early sign of AMI that warrants close monitoring.
- Recognition of the limitations of the ECG in AMI is also important as up to 10% of patients with an acute STEMI may have a normal ECG as certain myocardial segments

TABLE 12-4	TIMI RISK SCORE FOR STEMI
Risk factor (weight)	**Risk score/30-day mortality (%)**
Age 65–74 years (2 points)	0 (0.8)
Age ≥75 years (3 points)	1 (1.6)
DM, HTN, or angina (1 point)	2 (2.2)
SBP <100 (3 points)	3 (4.4)
Heart rate >100 (2 points)	4 (7.3)
Killip classification II–IV (2 points)	5 (12.4)
Weight <67 kg (1 point)	6 (16.1)
Anterior STE or LBBB (1 point)	7 (23.4)
Time to treatment >4 hours (1 point)	8 (26.8)
Risk score = total points (0–14)	>8 (35.9)

STEMI, ST-elevation myocardial infraction; DM, diabetes mellitus; HTN, hypertension; SBP, systolic blood pressure; STE, ST-segment elevation; LBBB, left bundle branch block.

Modified from Morrow DA, Antman EM, Charlesworth A, et al. TIMI risk score for ST-elevation myocardial infarction: a convenient, bedside, clinical score for risk assessment at presentation. *Circulation* 2000;102:2031-2037.

TABLE 12-5	ANATOMIC DISTRIBUTION BASED ON ECG LEADS	
Leads	**Myocardium**	**Coronary artery**
I, aVL	High lateral wall	Diagonal or proximal LCx
V5 to V6	Lateral wall	LCx
V1 to V2	Septal	Proximal LAD
V2 to V4	Anterior wall	LAD
II, III, aVF	Inferior	RCA or LCX

ECG, electrocardiogram; LCx, left circumflex; LAD, left anterior descending; RCA, right coronary artery.

of the left ventricle are not adequately represented, particularly the posterior and lateral walls, which are supplied by the left circumflex artery.
- **ECG criteria for diagnosis of STEMI:**
  ○ ≥1 mm (0.1 mV) of ST-segment elevation (STE) in two or more contiguous limb leads, or
  ○ 2 mm in two contiguous precordial leads for men and 1.5 mm in two precordial leads for women
- The location (Table 12-5) and degree of STE determine the occluded anatomy and prognosis and can alert the physician to potential complications of MI.

- Special considerations:
  - ○ The presence of a **new LBBB** in the setting of acute chest symptoms suggests occlusion of the proximal left anterior descending (LAD).
  - ○ Patients presenting with this finding should be managed in the same manner as the patient with a classic STEMI.
  - ○ In the setting of an old LBBB or an RV-paced rhythm, an acute injury pattern may be supported by the **Sgarbossa criteria**[6]:
    - ▪ STE ≥1 mm in the presence of a positive QRS complex (ST elevation is concordant with QRS).
    - ▪ ST-segment depression ≥1 mm in lead V1, V2, or V3.
    - ▪ STE ≥5 mm in the presence of a negative QRS complex (ST elevation is discordant with QRS).
  - ○ **Posterior MI** is an entity that is often unrecognized and should be suspected by the clinician in the setting of inferior or lateral wall infarct. Isolated posterior MI is uncommon.
    - ▪ The "reverse mirror test" is useful to demonstrate that the ST-segment depression in leads V1 to V3 is actually ST elevations in the posterior wall.
    - ▪ The prominent R waves in these leads represent posterior Q waves.
    - ▪ Inferoposterior and posterolateral MIs typically involve the right coronary artery (RCA) or obtuse marginal branch of the left circumflex coronary artery (LCx), respectively.
    - ▪ Posterior leads (V7 to V9) may be placed to help distinguish posterior MI from anterior ischemia or reciprocal depression in all patients presenting with ST depression in leads V1 to V3.
  - ○ ST elevation in the inferior leads should always prompt a right-sided ECG to assess for **right ventricular (RV) infarction**. ST elevation in leads V3R and V4R suggests RV involvement.
    - ▪ RV infarction should also be suspected on a standard 12-lead ECG when there is STE in V1 along with changes indicating inferior MI.
    - ▪ The finding of ST elevation in lead III greater than in lead II also suggests RV infarct.
    - ▪ Proximal RCA lesions typically involve the RV, as RV marginal branches arise early from the RCA.
    - ▪ Although the principle for the revascularization of RV infarct is the same for other STEMIs, other aspects of treatment are unique, including maintenance of adequate preload and the cautious use of nitrate and β-blocker therapy to avoid hypotension.
  - ○ ST segments in **pericarditis** normalize before there is T-wave inversion, whereas the T waves invert before ST normalization in STEMI.
    - ▪ STE in pericarditis is typically diffuse, does not correlate with a particular vascular territory, and does not exhibit reciprocal ST depressions.
    - ▪ PR-segment depression in acute pericarditis may also differentiate these two conditions (see Chapter 17).
    - ▪ Pericarditis may present later in the course of AMI and should be differentiated from recurrent ischemia or stent thrombosis.

Imaging

- A standard portable **chest radiograph** (CXR) should be included in the initial evaluation protocol.
  - ○ Pulmonary edema on CXR has important prognostic and therapeutic implications.
  - ○ Should be reviewed for mediastinal widening, suggesting acute aortic dissection, prior to initiating thrombolytic therapy.
  - ○ If clinical suspicion is high; however, normal mediastinal width does not exclude dissection.

- The evaluation of a patient with chest pain in the setting of a nondiagnostic ECG (i.e., LBBB of unknown duration, paced rhythm) may be aided by an **echocardiogram**. Segmental wall motion abnormalities suggest myocardial ischemia or infarction, assuming no baseline wall motion abnormalities and can help localize the territory at risk.

TREATMENT

- All medical centers should establish a STEMI protocol that utilizes evidence-based therapies.
- When primary PCI is unavailable, standard protocols regarding the choice of thrombolytic therapy versus rapid transport to a primary PCI facility should be in place.[2]

Early Adjunctive Therapy

- Medications used for treatment of patients with STEMI are similar to those with NSTEMI/UA. See Chapter 11 for detailed discussion of these agents. Situations where the use of the drugs differs between the conditions are discussed in this chapter.
- Medications used for adjunctive therapy for STEMI include
  - Non-enteric coated **aspirin**
  - **Clopidogrel** should be substituted for patients with a true or suspected aspirin allergy.
  - **β-Blockers:**
    - Metoprolol, 5 mg IV every 5 minutes, three doses as tolerated, followed by oral metoprolol, up to 50 mg every 6 hours as blood pressure and heart rate permit.
    - Should be withheld in patients with signs of heart failure or cardiogenic shock until they have been stabilized.
  - Supplemental **oxygen**: The administration of supplemental oxygen should be guided by pulse oximetry and is indicated for the first 6 hours following AMI or longer if the oxygen saturation is <92%.
  - **Morphine**:
    - Provides analgesia for ischemic cardiac pain, produces a favorable hemodynamic effect, and reduces myocardial O_2 consumption.
    - Can be given as doses of 2–4 mg IV and repeated every 10 minutes until pain is relieved or hypotension occurs.
  - **Magnesium**: Indicated when plasma magnesium level is documented to be less than 2.0 mg or in the setting of torsades de pointes.
  - Unfractionated heparin has less supportive evidence than low-molecular-weight heparin, but can be given as an adjunct to fibrinolytic therapy.
  - **Low-molecular-weight heparin**:
    - Enoxaparin with full-dose tenecteplase significantly improved the composite end point of mortality, in-hospital reinfarction, and in-hospital refractory ischemia, with a similar safety profile in the ASSENT-3 trial.[7]
    - Local preference of the PCI laboratory should be considered, as many institutions are not equipped to monitor therapeutic effect on factor Xa activity in the catheterization laboratory.
  - **Direct thrombin inhibitors**:
    - Bivalirudin demonstrated reduction in major bleeding, reinfarction, cardiac mortality, and all-cause mortality in AMI patients undergoing angioplasty when compared to UFH plus GIIb/IIIa inhibitors in the HORIZONS-AMI study.[8]
    - Major bleeding, all-cause mortality, and cardiac mortality, which were significantly lower in bivalirudin patients at 1 year, remained lower at 3 years.
    - Increased early stent thrombosis can be overcome by plavix loading at the time of the intervention.

- ◦ **Glycoprotein IIb/IIIa inhibitors**:
  - ▪ In the setting of primary PCI, the RAPPORT trial showed that the use of abciximab along with primary PTCA significantly reduced the incidence of death, MI, and urgent revascularization at 30 days for patients presenting with AMI.[9]
  - ▪ GIIb/IIIa **inhibitors are not recommended in conjunction with thrombolytic therapy**.

Reperfusion

- Reperfusion is most beneficial for patients who are treated early in the course of their MI.
- The optimal reperfusion strategy should be center-specific, with consideration of available resources. An algorithm to aid in the decision-making process is shown in Figure 12-1.[2] Although most of the protocols in place are based on door-to-balloon time, symptom-to-balloon time is the most important predictor of myocardial salvage.

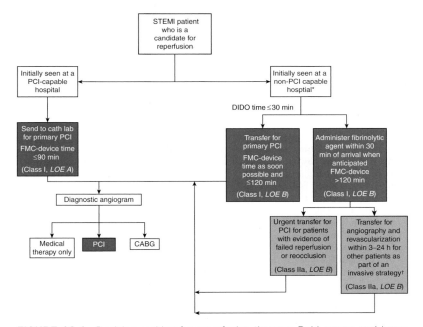

FIGURE 12-1. Decision making for reperfusion therapy. Bold arrows and boxes are the preferred strategies. Performance of PCI is dictated by an anatomically appropriate culprit stenosis. *Patients with cardiogenic shock or severe heart failure initially seen at a non–PCI-capable hospital should be transferred for cardiac catheterization and revascularization as soon as possible, irrespective of time delay from MI onset. †Angiography and revascularization should not be performed within the first 2 to 3 hours after administration of fibrinolytic therapy. CABG, coronary artery bypass graft; DIDO, door-in–door-out; FMC, first medical contact; LOE, level of evidence; MI, myocardial infarction; PCI, percutaneous coronary intervention; STEMI, ST-elevation myocardial infarction. (From O'Gara PT, Kushner FG, Ascheim DD, et al. 2013 ACCF/AHA guideline for the management of ST-elevation myocardial infarction. *Circulation* 2013;127:e362-e425, with permission.)

- **Primary PCI is the preferred reperfusion strategy when door-to-balloon time is <90 minutes and is most important for myocardial salvage when symptoms are ongoing for less than 90 minutes.**[2]
  - The opportunity for myocardial salvage is the greatest in the first 3 hours following vessel occlusion.
  - Patients who present with MI symptoms >12 hours and <24 hours after pain onset should be considered for reperfusion, particularly in the setting of continued ischemia suggested by STE, persistent symptoms, recurrent ischemia, LV dysfunction, and widespread ECG changes. Patients with prior MI, percutaneous revascularization, or coronary artery bypass grafting (CABG) may also be considered.
  - In facilities without PCI capability, the choice of whether to give thrombolytics or transport is based on the duration of symptoms, the time needed to transport, and the clinical condition.
- **Thrombolytic therapy** should be given to patients if presentation is less than 3 hours from symptom onset and if no contraindications are present when transport to a PCI facility is more than 30 minutes (door-to-balloon time/door-to-needle time >60 minutes).
  - If primary PCI is not available, thrombolytic therapy should be given to patients presenting up to 12 to 24 hours with ongoing symptoms if no contraindications are present.
  - Transfer for PCI should generally be considered if symptom duration is more than 3 hours, Killip class is III or greater, or the diagnosis is uncertain.
  - Either transport or thrombolytics are appropriate if symptom onset is more than 3 hours and transport takes more than 1 hour.
  - The administration of thrombolytic therapy to patients greater than 24 hours after symptom onset is contraindicated.

Primary PCI

- Primary PCI is the preferred therapy if performed in a timely fashion (door-to-balloon time <90 minutes) by individuals skilled in the procedure (>75 PCIs per year, of which 11 are STEMIs) and in high-volume centers (>400 PCIs per year, of which >36 are primary PCIs for STEMI per year).[10]
- It results in increased early efficacy in opening occluded arteries when compared with thrombolytics, which is associated with improved survival.
- It is also indicated in patients who present with cardiogenic shock, who have contraindications to thrombolytics, or whose diagnosis is uncertain.
- If significant left main stenosis is found, there should be consideration of emergent CABG. Stenting of the left main may also be considered if the patient is not a candidate for CABG or if the anatomy is suitable for PCI.
- Percutaneous intervention on the non–infarct-related artery in the setting of an AMI should not be performed unless compelling indications exist, which include cardiogenic shock or uncertainty of the infarct-related vessel.

Rescue PCI

- Thrombolytic therapy fails to achieve coronary artery patency in 15% to 50% of patients. Rescue (salvage) PCI is appropriate for patients who have received thrombolytic therapy but have
  - Ongoing symptoms and persistent STE (>50% of original degree of elevation) 90 minutes after administration.
  - Patients with cardiogenic shock, congestive heart failure (CHF), refractory arrhythmias, and particularly those with large anterior MIs.
  - CABG is indicated in the setting of failed PCI in patients with ongoing signs and symptoms of ischemia or in patients whose coronary anatomy is not suitable for PCI.
- Early trials evaluating the role of routine PCI after thrombolysis did not show an improvement in mortality or reinfarction when compared to conservative, ischemia-driven

management primarily because the benefits were offset by the higher rate of bleeding complications.

Facilitated PCI

- Facilitated PCI refers to administration of pharmacologic therapy to establish flow prior to planned PCI. This typically occurs within 2 hours of drug administration.
- A variety of regimens have been used, which lead to either worse outcomes or no benefit as compared with primary PCI.
- **This approach is not recommended**.

Thrombolytic/Fibrinolytic Therapy

- The terms "thrombolytic" and "fibrinolytic" are used somewhat interchangeably.
- The benefits of early (<12 hours) thrombolytic therapy are well established in the medical literature, with pooled data from the FTT Collaborative Group displaying an 18% relative reduction in mortality.[11] When given early following onset of symptoms, thrombolytics can be very effective.
- There is the greatest potential for significant myocardial salvage within the first 3 hours following symptoms.
- Thrombolytics have not been shown to be effective in vein grafts. Thus, if a patient post CABG presents with a STEMI, the preferred mode of reperfusion is PCI.
- The absolute and relative contraindications for thrombolytic therapy are shown in Table 12-1.[2]
- Various thrombolytic agents are available and have similar efficacy. These medications vary in the rate of administration. Details are shown in Table 12-6.[2]
- **Bleeding risk**:
  - The most common and potentially serious side effect of fibrinolytic therapy is bleeding, with intracranial hemorrhage being the most severe.
  - Risks associated with intracerebral hemorrhage (ICH) include the following: age ≥75 years, female sex, African–American race, prior stroke, SBP ≥160 mmHg, use of tissue plasminogen activator (tPA) rather than other agents, International Normalized Ratio (INR) >4, and PT >24 seconds.[12,13]
  - With none or one of these factors, the risk of ICH is 0.7%; with ≥5 the risk goes up to 4.11%.[12]

Later Evaluation and Treatment

- All patients must be monitored in the intensive care unit for at least 24 hours following STEMI.
- Continuous telemetry monitoring, preferably with display of one of the leads involved in STE, to monitor for recurrent ischemia and arrhythmias.
- Daily evaluation should include assessment for recurrent anginal and heart failure symptoms, physical examination for new murmurs or evidence of heart failure, and a daily ECG.
- Most patients can safely be transferred to a step-down unit in 24 hours with telemetry monitoring in the absence of any further problems.

COMPLICATIONS

Cardiogenic Shock (Figure 12.2)

- Cardiogenic shock is an infrequent but serious complication of STEMI.
- It occurs within the first 48 hours after symptom onset, particularly with large anterior infarcts.

TABLE 12-6 THROMBOLYTIC AGENTS

	Streptokinase[a]	Alteplase (tPA)	Reteplase (rPA)	Tenecteplase (TNK-tPA)
Dose	1.5 MU over 30–60 minutes	Up to 100 mg in 90 minutes (based on weight)[b]	10 U × 2 each over 2 minutes	30–50 mg based on weight[c]
Bolus administration	No	No	Yes	Yes
Antigenic	Yes	No	No	No
Allergic reactions (hypotension most common)	Yes	No	No	No
Systemic fibrinogen depletion	Marked	Mild	Moderate	Minimal
Patency rates (90-minute TIMI grade 2–3 flow)	60–68%	73–84%	84%	85%
Cost per dose (U.S. $, average wholesale price)		$6,712.54 for 100 mg	$5,211.86 for 2 10.4 unit vials	$4,571.78 for 50 mg

[a]Not available in the United States.

[b]Bolus 15 mg, infusion 0.75 mg/kg times 30 minutes (maximum 50 mg), then 0.5 mg/kg not to exceed 35 mg over the next 60 minutes to an overall maximum of 100 mg.

[c]Thirty milligrams for weight <60 kg; 35 mg for 60–69 kg; 40 mg for 70–79 mg; 45 mg for 80–89 kg; 50 mg for 90 kg or more.

Modified from O'Gara PT, Kushner FG, Ascheim DD, et al. 2013 ACCF/AHA guideline for the management of ST-elevation myocardial infarction. *Circulation* 2013;127:e362-e425.

Emergency revascularization with either PCI or CABG is recommended in suitable patients with cardiogenic shock due to pump failure after STEMI irrespective of the time delay from MI onset.

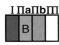

In the absence of contraindications, fibrinolytic therapy should be administered to patients with STEMI and cardiogenic shock who are unsuitable candidates for either PCI or CABG.

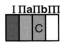

The use of intra-aortic balloon pump counterpulsation can be useful for patients with cardiogenic shock after STEMI who do not quickly stabilize with pharmacological.

Alternative LV assist devices for circulatory support may be considered in patients with refractory cardiogenic shock.

FIGURE 12-2. Management of complicated STEMI. (From: Kushner F, et al. 2009 Focused updates: ACC/AHA Guidelines for the Management of Patients With ST-Elevation Myocardial Infarct (Updating the 2004 Guideline and 2007 Focused Update) and ACC/AHA/SCAI Guidelines on Percutaneous Coronary Intervention (Updating the 2005 Guideline and 2007 Focused Update); available at www.acc.org.)

- • The SHOCK trial demonstrated a significant benefit of revascularization over medical therapy in patients with cardiogenic shock in whom revascularization could be performed within 18 hours of onset of shock.[14] Note that the benefit of such therapy did not extend to patients over 75 years of age in this randomized trial.

Free Wall Rupture
- Free wall rupture occurs most commonly 2 to 6 days after MI.
- It occurs most commonly in patients without prior angina or MI and with large infarcts by enzyme criteria.
- May present as hypotension, cardiac tamponade, or pulseless electrical activity. Mortality is very high, and management consists of volume resuscitation, inotropes, pericardiocentesis, and surgical repair.

Pseudoaneurysm
- A cardiac pseudoaneurysm consists of a contained rupture sealed by thrombus and pericardium.
- It is often found incidentally and may be associated with a to-and-fro murmur or a hemodynamically significant pericardial effusion.
- Diagnosis is by echocardiography.
- Treatment is surgical in nearly all cases.

VSD
- VSD typically occurs 2 to 5 days after AMI.
- It is more common in anterior MIs.
- It presents with a new harsh holosystolic murmur with or without hemodynamic compromise.

- Diagnosis by echocardiography with Doppler and pulmonary artery (PA) catheterization reveals oxygen step-up.
- Management involves an intraaortic balloon pump (IABP), inotropes, vasodilators, and surgical versus catheter-based closure.

Papillary Muscle Rupture

- Papillary muscle rupture usually occurs 2 to 7 days after AMI.
- It most frequently involves the posteromedial papillary muscle due to its single blood supply.
- Usually associated with inferior MI and presents with a new holosystolic murmur (heard only 50% of the time), cardiogenic shock, and pulmonary edema. Diagnosis can be made by echocardiography or PA catheter waveforms with prominent v waves.
- Treatment involves afterload reduction with IABP or vasodilators, revascularization, and surgical repair.

RV Infarct

- RV infarct occurs in the setting of inferior MI and presents with the triad of hypotension, elevated jugular venous pressure with Kussmaul sign, and clear lung fields.
- Diagnosed by right-sided ECG with STE in V3R and V4R or by witnessed RV wall motion abnormality on echocardiography.
- Treatment includes volume loading to PCWP of 18 to 20 mmHg, avoidance of nitrates, and low-dose dobutamine if needed to treat hypotension.

Arrhythmias

- Many arrhythmias are associated with STEMI.
- Accelerated idioventricular rhythm should not be treated unless there is hemodynamic disturbance.
- Prophylactic antiarrhythmic infusion after AMI to suppress ventricular tachycardia/ventricular fibrillation (VT/VF) does not improve mortality and is not indicated.
- Bradycardias may warrant a temporary transvenous pacer if associated with significant atrioventricular (AV) block.
  - AV block in association with an **inferior MI** usually portends a **good prognosis**, as the mechanism is ischemia of the AV node (the AV nodal branch derives from the RCA) and a compensatory Bezold–Jarisch reflex, which stimulates vagal tone. This may persist up to 1 to 2 weeks.
  - AV block in association with an **anterior MI** usually portends a **poor prognosis** (permanent pacer likely required), as the mechanism is infarction of part of the distal conduction system.

Post-MI Pericarditis

- Pericardial conditions are covered in detail in Chapter 17.
- Post-MI pericarditis typically occurs 1 to 4 days after MI.
- It may cause recurrent chest discomfort and widespread STE.
- PR depression may occur on ECGs but is uncommon; pericardial rub may be found on examination.
- Treatment consists of high-dose nonsteroidal antiinflammatory drugs (NSAIDs).
- Heparin should be avoided owing to the risk of hemorrhagic transformation.
- Glucocorticoids should be avoided because of the increased risk of rupture.

Dressler Syndrome

- Dressler syndrome presents 2 to 10 weeks after MI with fever, malaise, and pleuritic chest discomfort.

- Patients have an elevated erythrocyte sedimentation rate, and echocardiography may demonstrate pericardial effusion.
- Usually managed with high-dose NSAIDs.

LV Thrombus

- An LV thrombus may occur with large anteroapical MIs that produce akinetic or dyskinetic segments on echocardiogram or left ventriculogram.
- Treatment consists of anticoagulation with warfarin for 3 to 6 months.

Ventricular Aneurysm

- Persistent ST elevation more than 4 weeks after AMI is suggestive but not diagnostic of an aneurysm.
- Echocardiography establishes the diagnosis and provides information regarding LV function and the presence of thrombus.
- Patients may present with heart failure, ventricular arrhythmias, or an embolic event.
- Prevention involves timely reperfusion and afterload reduction, preferably with an angiotensin converting enzyme (ACE) inhibitor, to help reduce adverse LV remodeling and subsequent aneurysm formation.
- Once formed, additional treatment may include warfarin anticoagulation and potentially surgical resection in selected cases.

MONITORING/FOLLOW-UP

- Follow-up echocardiogram 3 months after an AMI is indicated in order to assess improvement in ventricular function and possible need for defibrillator therapy in patients with new LV dysfunction.
- Cardiac rehabilitation is indicated 2 weeks after AMI. Participation is these programs after an MI is associated with decreased mortality and recurrent MI as well as improvements in quality of life, functional capacity, and social support.

OUTCOME/PROGNOSIS

- Late risk stratification is primarily determined by ventricular function and residual ischemia. Patients with ejection fractions <30% are at particularly high risk.
- A number of other factors including age, the presence of renal insufficiency, and heart failure have been used in a variety of risk scores to further define prognosis.

REFERENCES

1. Thygesen K, Alpert JS, Jaffe AS, et al. Join ESC/ACCF/AHA/WHF Task Force for Universal Definition of Myocardial Infarction. Third universal definition of myocardial infarction. *J Am Coll Cardiol* 2012;60:1581-1598.
2. O'Gara PT, Kushner FG, Ascheim DD, et al. 2013 ACCF/AHA guideline for the management of ST-elevation myocardial infarction. *Circulation* 2013;127:e362-e425.
3. Killip T 3rd, Kimball JT. Treatment of myocardial infarction in a coronary care unit. A two-year experience with 250 patients. *Am J Cardiol* 1967;20:457-464.
4. Forrester JS, Diamond G, Chatterjee K, Swan HJ. Medical therapy of acute myocardial infarction by application of hemodynamic subsets (first of two parts). *N Engl J Med* 1976;295:1356-1362.
5. Morrow DA, Antman EM, Charlesworth A, et al. TIMI risk score for ST-elevation myocardial infarction: a convenient, bedside, clinical score for risk assessment at presentation. *Circulation* 2000;102:2031-2037.

6. Sgarbossa EB, Pinski SL, Barbagelata, et al. Electrocardiographic diagnosis of evolving acute myocardial infarction in the presence of left bundle-branch block. GUSTO-1 (Global Utilization of Streptokinase and Tissue Plasminogen Activator for Occluded Coronary Arteries) Investigators. *N Engl J Med* 1996;334:481-487.

7. The Assessment of the Safety and Efficacy of a New Thrombolytic Regimen (ASSENT)-3 Investigators. Efficacy and safety of tenecteplase in combination with enoxaparin, abciximab, or unfractionated heparin: the ASSENT-3 randomised trial in acute myocardial infarction. *Lancet* 2001;358:605-613.

8. Stone GW, Witzenbichler B, Guafliumi G, et al. Bivalirudin during primary PCI in acute myocardial Infarction. *N Engl J Med* 2008;358:2218-2230.

9. Brener SJ, Barr LA, Burchenal JE, et al. Randomized, placebo-controlled trial of platelet glycoprotein IIb/IIIa blockade with primary angioplasty for acute myocardial infarction. ReoPro and Primary PTCA Organization and Randomized Trial (RAPPORT) Investigators. *Circulation* 1998;98:734-741.

10. Levine GN, Bates ER, Blankenship JC, et al. 2011 ACCF/AHA/SCAI Guideline for Percutaneous Coronary Intervention: a report of the American College of Cardiology Foundation/American Heart Association Task Force on Practice Guidelines and the Society for Cardiovascular Angiography and Interventions. *Circulation* 2001;124:e574-e651.

11. Thrombolytic Therapy Trialists' (FTT) Collaborative Group. Indications for thrombolytic therapy in suspected acute myocardial infarction: collaborative overview of early mortality and major morbidity results from all randomised trials of more than 1000 patients. *Lancet* 1994;343:311-322.

12. Brass LM, Lichtman JH, Wang Y, et al. Intracranial hemorrhage associated with thrombolytic therapy for elderly patients with acute myocardial infarction: results from the Cooperative Cardiovascular Project. *Stroke* 2000;31:1802-1811.

13. Huynh T, Cox JL, Massel D, et al. Predictors of intracranial hemorrhage with fibrinolytic therapy in unselected community patients: a report from the FASTRAK II project. *Am Heart J* 2004;148:86-91.

14. Hochman JS, Sleeper LA, Webb JG, et al. Early revascularization in acute myocardial infarction complicated by cardiogenic shock. SHOCK Investigators. Should we emergently revascularize occluded coronaries for cardiogenic shock. *N Engl J Med* 1999;341:625-634.

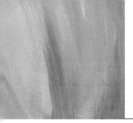

Primary and Secondary Prevention of Cardiovascular Disease

13

Kristen Scott-Tillery, Mohammad Ali
Kizilbash, and Andrew M. Kates

Primary Prevention

GENERAL PRINCIPLES

- Primary cardiovascular disease (CVD) prevention is prevention of disease in a person without prior symptoms of CVD by treating risk factors with lifestyle modifications or drugs.
- The main objective is to optimize or control risk factors directly responsible for atherosclerosis, left ventricular remodeling, and/or peripheral vascular disease.
- Prevention addressed at population-wide levels is highly effective at reducing risk factor levels in the community.
- Programs enacted to educate or effect policy change on the society as a whole from previous decades (e.g., government warnings on cigarette use [intial-1964], efforts to reduce dietary fat intake [the 1960s and 1970s], the National High Blood Pressure Education Program [the 1970s and 1980s], and the National Cholesterol Education Program [the 1980s and 1990s]) have produced dramatic declines in CVD death rates.
- Prevention efforts at the individual level are geared to identify patients at risk for CVD through risk stratification.
- The publication of guidelines on several areas of prevention occurred as the *3rd Edition* was going to press.

RISK ASSESSMENT

- Key to understanding who is at risk for CVD is in the identification of risk factors.
- Risk factors can be divided into nonmodifiable, modifiable (behavioral), and clinical (physiologic).[1]
- Routine risk-factor screening should begin at the age of 18 years.
- Blood pressure, body mass index (BMI), waist circumference, and pulse (to screen for atrial fibrillation) should be recorded at each visit and repeated every 2 years.
- Fasting serum lipoprotein profile (or total and high-density-lipoprotein [HDL] cholesterol if fasting is unavailable) and fasting blood glucose should be measured according to the patient's risk of hyperlipidemia and diabetes (every 5 years or every 2 years if risk factors are present).
- Please see ACC/AHA Guidelines on cardiovascular risk (http://circ.ahajournals.org/content/early/2013/11/11/01.cir.0000437741.48606.98).[2]

Risk Assessment in Asymptomatic Patients

- The goal of global risk assessment is to identify asymptomatic patients without established coronary heart disease (CHD) to both motivate lifestyle changes and identify those who may benefit from pharmacologic interventions.

- Global risk scores estimate the absolute risk of CVD over some time period, usually over the next 10 years.
- Risk scores combine individual traditional CVD risk factors into a single quantitative estimate.
- The Framingham risk score (FRS) has been commonly used to assess risk. This model, however, was derived in an exclusively white sample population and has limited applicability to others.
- A new pooled cohort atherosclerotic cardiovascular disease (ASCVD) risk equation has been developed to estimate the 10-year risk for ASCVD in African American and White men and women between 40 and 79 years of age (http://my.americanheart.org/professional/StatementsGuidelines/PreventionGuidelines/Prevention-Guidelines_UCM_457698_SubHomePage.jsp).
- Additional recommendations include:
  - Use of the sex-specific Pooled Cohort Equations for non-Hispanic whites may be considered when estimating risk in patients from populations other than African Americans and non-Hispanic whites.
  - If, after quantitative risk assessment, a risk-based treatment decision is uncertain, assessment of one or more of the following—family history, hs-CRP, CAC score, or ABI—may be considered to inform treatment decision making.
  - The contribution to risk assessment for a first ASCVD event using ApoB, CKD, albuminuria, or cardiorespiratory fitness is uncertain at present. N (no recommendation for or against).
  - CIMT is not recommended for routine measurement in clinical practice for risk assessment for a first ASCVD event.
  - It is reasonable to assess traditional ASCVD risk factors every 4 to 6 years in adults 20 to 79 years of age who are free from ASCVD and to estimate 10-year ASCVD risk every 4 to 6 years in adults 40 to 79 years of age without ASCVD.

Risk Groups and Management in Asymptomatic Patients

- For those individuals with ASCVD risk >7.5%, initiation of moderate-to-high intensity statin is recommended.
- Table 13-1 shows the thresholds for screening tests for those individuals in whom the initiation of pharmacologic therapy is uncertain.
- Note that CIMT is no longer recommended.

Lifetime Risk

- Lifetime risk is an emerging concept in primary prevention.
- Ten-year risk estimates greatly underestimate the risk of developing CHD in men <35 years and women <45 years.
- Stresses the importance of achieving and/or maintaining an ideal risk factor profile at early ages through lifestyle changes to promote healthy aging.[3]
- Assessing 30-year or lifetime ASCVD risk based on traditional risk factors may be considered in adults 20 to 59 years of age without ASCVD and who are not at high short-term risk.

BEHAVIORAL RISK FACTORS

- A healthy lifestyle is important in the prevention of cardiovascular disease. Recently published Guidelines on Lifestyle Management to Reduce CV Risk provide valuable assistance. http://circ.ahajournals.org/content/early/2013/11/11/01.cir.0000437740.48606.d1.[4]

Diet

- Healthy diet is a critical component in the prevention of CVD.
- It offers one of the greatest potentials for reducing the risk of CVD.

TABLE 13-1	EXPERT OPINION THRESHOLDS FOR USE OF OPTIONAL SCREENING TESTS WHEN RISK-BASED DECISIONS REGARDING INITIATION OF PHARMACOIOGICAL THERAPY ARE UNCERTAIN FOLLOWING QUANTITATIVE RISK ASSESSMENT	
Measure	Support revising risk assessment upward	Do not support revising risk assessment
Family history of premature CVD	Male <55 years of age Female <65 years of age (First degree relative)	Occurrences at older ages only (if any)
hs-CRP	≥2 mg/L	<2 mg/L
CAC score	≥300 Agatston units or ≥75th percentile for age, sex, and ethnicity	<300 Agatston units and <75th percentile for age, sex, and ethnicity
ABI	<0.9	≥0.9

- The American Heart Association (AHA) has published recommendations for a healthy diet applicable to patients both with and without CHD.
- Dietary advice to those who would benefit from LDL lowering include:
  - Consume a dietary pattern that emphasizes intake of vegetables, fruits, and whole grains; includes low-fat dairy products, poultry, fish, legumes, nontropical vegetable oils, and nuts; and limits intake of sweets, sugar-sweetened beverages, and red meats.
  - Adapt this dietary pattern to appropriate calorie requirements, personal and cultural food preferences, and nutrition therapy for other medical conditions (including diabetes mellitus).
  - Achieve this pattern by following plans such as the DASH dietary pattern, the USDA Food Pattern, or the AHA Diet.
  - Aim for a dietary pattern that achieves 5% to 6% of calories from saturated fat.
  - Reduce the percentage of calories from saturated fat and trans fat.
- Dietary advice to those who would benefit from BP lowering:
  - Consume a dietary pattern that emphasizes intake of vegetables, fruits, and whole grains; includes low-fat dairy products, poultry, fish, legumes, nontropical vegetable oils, and nuts; and limits intake of sweets, sugar-sweetened beverages, and red meats.
  - Adapt this dietary pattern to appropriate calorie requirements, personal and cultural food preferences, and nutrition therapy for other medical conditions (including diabetes mellitus).
  - Achieve this pattern by following plans such as the DASH dietary pattern, the USDA Food Pattern, or the AHA Diet.
  - Lower sodium intake.
  - Consume no more than 2,400 mg of sodium/day.
  - Further reduction of sodium intake to 1,500 mg/day is desirable since it is associated with even greater reduction in BP.
  - Reduce intake by at least 1,000 mg/day since that will lower BP.

Exercise

- In general, advise adults to engage in aerobic physical activity to reduce LDL-C and non-HDL-C and BP: three to four sessions a week, lasting on average 40 minutes per session, and involving moderate-to-vigorous intensity physical activity.
  - Lowering blood pressure
  - Improving insulin resistance and glucose tolerance
  - Lowering triglycerides
  - Raising HDL
  - Lowering fibrinogen levels and improving fibrinolytic capacity
- The AHA and the American College of Sports Medicine have published recommendations regarding exercise in healthy adults (Table 13-3).[5]
  - These guidelines stress the benefits of moderate-intensity exercise.
  - This point is important as it was once felt that only vigorous exercise had significant cardiovascular benefit.
  - Examples of moderate-intensity exercise include walking at 3 to 4 mph; leisurely sports such as bicycling on a flat surface at 10 to 12 mph, or golfing (without a cart).

Alcohol

- Moderate consumption has been shown to have beneficial effects on CVD.
  - 1 to 2 drinks/day for men and 1 drink/day for women.
  - One drink is a 4-oz glass of wine, a 12-oz beer, or 1.5 oz of 80-proof spirit.
  - Alcohol consumption at this level appears to reduce total and cardiovascular mortality.[6-8]

TABLE 13-2   DIET RECOMMENDATIONS

Eating pattern	DASH*	TLC†	Serving sizes
Grains‡	6 to 8 servings per day	7 servings§ per day	1 slice bread, 1 oz dry cereal,¶ ½ cup cooked rice, pasta, or cereal
Vegetables	4 to 5 servings per day	5 servings§ per day	1 cup raw leafy vegetable, ½ cup cutup raw or cooked vegetable, ½ cup vegetable juice
Fruits	4 to 5 servings per day	4 servings§ per day	1 medium fruit, ¼ cup dried fruit, ½ cup fresh, frozen, or canned fruit, ½ cup fruit juice
Fat-free or low-fat milk and milk products	2 to 3 servings per day	2 to 3 servings per day	1 cup milk, 1 cup yogurt, 1½ oz cheese
Lean‖ meats, poultry, and fish	<6 oz per day	≤5 oz per day	

TABLE 13-2 DIET RECOMMENDATIONS (*Continued*)

Eating pattern	DASH*	TLC†	Serving sizes
Nuts, seeds, and legumes	4 to 5 servings per week	Counted in vegetable servings	½ cup (1½ oz), 2 Tbsp peanut butter, 2 Tbsp or ½ oz seeds, ½ cup dry beans or peas
Fats and oils	2 to 3 servings# per day	Amount depends on daily calorie level	1 tsp soft margarine, 1 Tbsp mayonnaise, 2 Tbsp salad dressing, 1 tsp vegetable oil
Sweets and added sugars	5 or fewer servings per week	No recommendation	1 Tbsp sugar, 1 Tbsp jelly or jam, ½ cup sorbet and ices, 1 cup lemonade

*Dietary Approaches to stop Hypertension. For more information, please visit http://www.nhlbi.nih.gov/health/public/heart/hbp/dash.

†Therapeutic Lifestyle Changes. For more information, please visit http://www.nhlbi.nih.gov/cgi-bin/ chel/step2intro.cgi.TLC includes 2 therapeutic diet options: plant stanol/sterol (add 2 g per day) and soluble fiber (add 5 to 10 g per day).

‡Whole-grain foods are recommended for most grain servings to meet fiber recommendations.

§This number can be less or more depending on other food choices to meet 2,000 calories.

¶Equals ½ to 1¼ cups. Depending on cereal type. Check the product's Nutrition Facts Label.

‖Lean cuts include sirloin tip, round steak, and rump roast; extra lean hamburger; and cold cuts made with lean meat or soy protein. Lean cuts of pork are center-cut ham loin chops, and pork tenderloin.

#Fat content changes serving counts for fats and oils: For example, 1 Tbsp of regular salad dressing equals 1 serving: 1 Tbsp of low-fat dressing equals ½ serving: 1Tbsp of fat-free dressing equals 0 servings.

From Lichtenstein AH, Appel LJ, Brands M, et al. Diet and lifestyle recommendations revision 2006: a scientific statement from the American Heart Association Nutrition Committee. *Circulation* 2006;114:82-96, with permission.

- The effect of alcohol consumption and CVD is J-shaped curve such that, with moderation, there is a decrease in CVD death; but with increasing usage, there is increased death rates from all causes as well as from CVD.
- Increased alcohol consumption can have untoward medical and societal ramifications (i.e., hypertension, alcoholism, cirrhosis, accidents, suicide, and decreased economic productivity).

TABLE 13-3	PHYSICAL ACTIVITY RECOMMENDATIONS FOR HEALTHY ADULTS

- Maintain a physically active lifestyle to promote and maintain good health
- Perform moderate aerobic activity for ≥30 minutes/day on 5 days/week or vigorous aerobic activity for ≥20 minutes/day on 3 days/week
- Combinations of moderate and vigorous activities can be performed to meet the recommendations
- Recommended moderate and/or vigorous activities are in addition to the light intensity activities performed every day and very short activities
- Moderate aerobic activity should noticeably raise the heart rate and in roughly equivalent to brisk walking; it can be accumulated by shorter episode of activity that is ≥10 minutes, but <30 minutes
- Vigorous activity causes a substantial increase in heart rate (e.g., jogging)
- Additionally perform activities using the major muscle groups that maintain and/or increase strength and endurance
- Greater health benefits are achieved by exceeding the minimum recommendations

Modified from Haskell WL, Lee I-M, Pate RP, et al. Physical activity and public health: updated recommendation for adults from the American College of Sports Medicine and the American Heart Association. *Circulation* 2007;116:1081-1093.

- **Recommending alcohol consumption simply to improve cardiovascular risk profile does not outweigh the risks of alcohol use.**

Tobacco Abuse

- Smoking is the leading cause of preventable death among older adults.
- Recommendations include
  - **Ask** patients about their tobacco use at every visit.
  - In a clear, strong, and personalized manner, **advise** every tobacco user to quit.
  - **Assess** the tobacco user's willingness to quit.
  - **Assist** by counseling and developing a plan for quitting.
  - **Arrange** follow-up, referral to special programs, or pharmacotherapy.
  - Urge avoidance of exposure to secondhand smoke at work and at home.
  - Consider the use of pharmacotherapy.
- Nicotine patch, nicotine gum, nicotine spray, and nicotine inhalers have been shown to significantly increase the rate of cessation.[9]
- Bupropion, used alone or in combination with replacement therapy, has also been shown to increase cessation rates.[10]
  - The standard regimen is 150 mg by mouth (PO) daily for 3 days, followed by 150 mg PO twice daily for 8 to 12 weeks. The patient is instructed to avoid smoking on days 5 to 7.
  - Contraindicated in patients at risk for seizures.
- Varenicline, used for 12 to 24 weeks, has shown benefit in aiding in smoking cessation.[11]

CLINICAL/PHYSIOLOGIC RISK FACTORS

Cholesterol

- The ACC/AHA have recently published Recommendations for Lipid Management which focus on risk rather than target LDL: http://circ.ahajournals.org/content/early/2013/11/11/01.cir.0000437738.63853.7a
- These guidelines address treatment in four groups (Figure 13-1):[12]

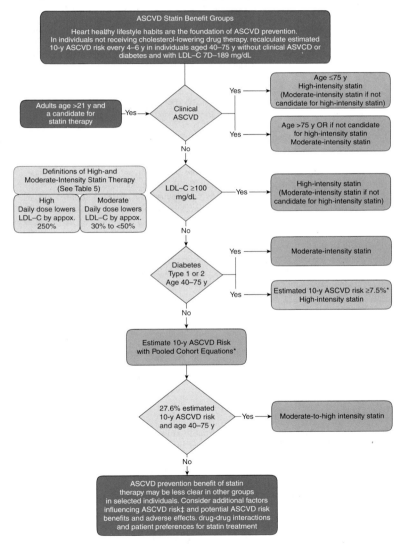

FIGURE 13-1. Major recommendations for statin therapy for ASCVD prevention.

| TABLE 13-4 | High- Moderate- and Low-Intensity Statin Therapy (Used in the RCTs reviewed by the Expert Panel)* |

High-Intensity Statin Therapy	Moderate-Intensity Statin Therapy	Low-Intensity Statin Therapy
Daily dose lowers LDL–C on average, by approximately ≥50%	Daily dose lowers LDL–C on average, by approximately 30% to <50%	Daily dose lowers LDL–C on average, by <30%
Atorvastatin (40†)–80 mg Rosuvastatin 20 (40) mg	Atorvastatin 10 (20) mg Rosuvastatin (5) 10 mg Simvastatin 20–40 mg‡ Pravastatin 40 (80) mg Lovastatin 40 mg *Fluvastatin XL 80 mg* Fluvastatin 40 mg bid *Pitavastatin 2–4 mg*	*Simvastatin 10 mg* Pravastatin 10–20 mg Lovastatin 20 mg *Fluvastatin 20–40 mg* *Pitavastatin 1 mg*

Specific statins and doses are noted in bold that were evaluated in RCTs included in CQ1, CQ2 and the CTT 2010 meta-analysis included in CQ3. All of these RCTs demonstrated a reduction in major cardiovascular events. Statins and doses that are approved by the U.S. FDA but were not tested in the RCTs reviewed are listed in *italics*.

*Individual responses to statin therapy varied in the RCTs and should be expected to vary in clinical practice. There might be a biologic basis for a less-than-average response.

†Evidence from 1 RCT only: down-titration if unable to tolerate atorvastatin 80 mg in IDEAL (47).

‡Although simvastatin 80 mg was evaluated in RCTs, initiation of simvastatin 80 mg or titration to 80 mg is not recommended by the FDA due to the increased risk of myopathy, including rhabdomyolysis.

bid indicates twice daily; FDA, Food and Drug Administration; IDEAL, Incremental Decrease through Aggressive Lipid Lowering Study; LDL–C, low-density lipoprotein cholesterol; and RCTs, randomized controlled trails.

- Recommendations now consider treatment in terms of moderate or high intensity statins.
- Recommendations for initiating statin therapy in patients with atherosclerotic cardiovascular disease are shown in Figure 13-2.

Hypertension
- Hypertension is the second leading modifiable cause of death.
- Detection of hypertension begins with proper blood pressure measurements.
- The 2014 Evidence-Based Guideline for the Management of High Blood Pressure in Adults (JNC 8) was recently published and can be found at http://jama.jamanetwork.com/article.aspx?articleid=1791497[13]
- Recommendations to achieve these goals are reviewed in Figure 13-4.

Diabetes Mellitus
- Moderate-to-high intensity statins are recommended for those with diabetes.
- A detailed discussion of this subject is found in Chapter 37.

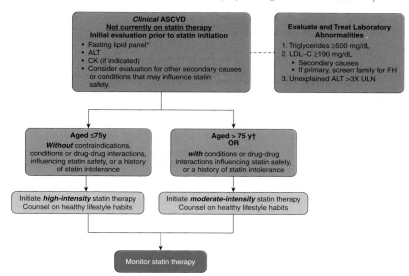

*Fasting lipid panel preferred. In a nonfasting individual, a nonfasting non-HDL–C >220 mg/dL may indicate genetic hypercholesterolemia that requires further evaluation or a secondary etiology. If nonfasting triglycerides are >500 mg/dL, a fasting lipid panel is required.

†It is reasonable to evaluate the potential for ASCVD benefits and for adverse effects, and to consider patient preferences, in initiating or continuing a moderate- or high-intensity statin, in individuals with ASCVD >75 years of age.

ALT indicates alanine transaminase; ASCVD indicates atherosclerotic cardiovascular disease; CK, creatine kinase; FH, familial hypercholesterolemia; LDL–C, low-density lipoprotein cholesterol; and ULN, upper limit of normal.

FIGURE 13-2. Initiating statin therapy in individuals with clinical ASCVD.

Obesity

- Obesity is associated with hyperlipidemia, hypertension, and insulin resistance.
- Both increased waist-to-hip ratios and BMI have been associated with CVD.
- Among obese individuals, those with central adiposity are at particularly high risk for CVD, especially in African-Americans.
- Although exercise is an important part of any weight loss program, dietary change is the mainstay of weight loss.
- Recommendations include
  - Initiation of a weight management program through caloric restriction and increased caloric expenditure as appropriate.
  - For overweight/obese persons, the goal is to reduce body weight by 10% in the first year of therapy.

Aspirin

- Aspirin as primary prevention is sometimes recommended for men with a 10-year risk of >10% and for women with risk of >20%, but this decision must be individualized and made on a case-by-case basis. Rates of serious vascular events are reduced, but cardiovascular mortality does not appear to be significantly lessened.[15,16]

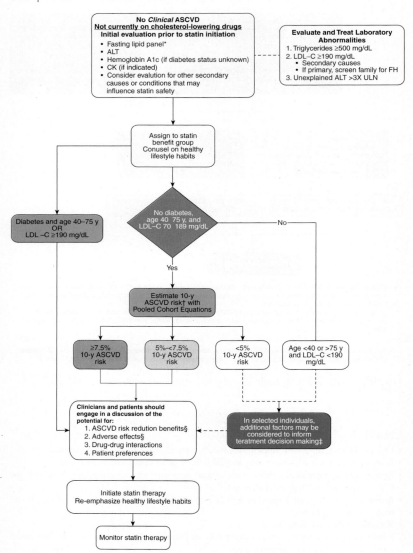

FIGURE 13-3. Initiating statin therapy in individuals *without clinical* ASCVD.

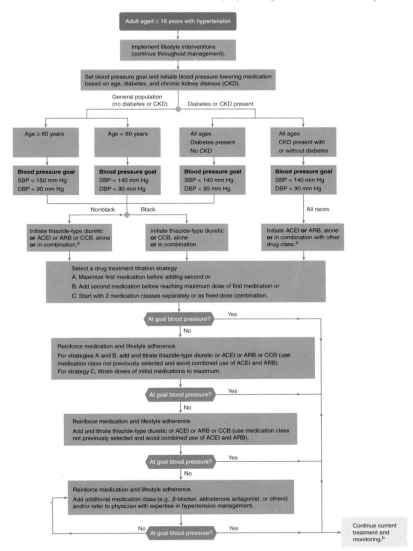

FIGURE 13-4. 2014 Hypertension Guideline Management AlgorithmSBP indicates systolic blood pressure; DBP, diastolic blood pressure; ACEI, angiotensin-converting enzyme; ARB, angiotensin receptor blocker; and CCB, calcium channel blocker. [a]ACEIs and ARBs should not be used in combination. [b]If blood pressure fails to be maintained at goal, reenter the algorithm where appropriate based on the current individual therapeutic plan.

- In the context of primary prevention, diabetes may not necessarily function as a CHD equivalent.[17]
- The higher the global risk score, the more beneficial aspirin is; however, the risk of aspirin use (gastrointestinal or intracranial bleeding) also increases with increasing global risk scores.

Metabolic Syndrome

- This syndrome is characterized by a group of metabolic risk factors that are associated with insulin resistance.
- The metabolic syndrome is identified by the presence of more than three of these components:
  - Central obesity as measured by waist circumference:
    - Men ≥40"
    - Women ≥35"
  - Fasting blood triglycerides ≥150 mg/dL
  - Blood HDL cholesterol:
    - Men <40 mg/dL
    - Women <50 mg/dL
  - Blood pressure ≥130/85 mmHg
  - Fasting glucose ≥100 mg/dL

Additional Risk Factors

- Testing the following risk factors could be considered for risk assessment in asymptomatic individuals:
  - Hemoglobin A1c levels in nondiabetics
  - Microalbuminuria in hypertensives and diabetics
  - Lipoprotein-associated phospholipase A2 levels >30 mg/dL are associated with increased risk of atherosclerosis.
  - Used to further risk stratify intermediate-risk individuals.
- The following are not currently recommended for routine risk assessment:
  - Lipoprotein and apolipoprotein assessment
  - Particle size and density
  - Homocysteine
  - Fibrinogen levels
  - Natriuretic peptides
  - Brachial/peripheral flow-mediated dilation

Secondary Prevention

GENERAL PRINCIPLES

- Secondary prevention is the prevention of death or progression/recurrence of disease in those patients who are symptomatic or have previously been diagnosed with CVD.
- Growing body of evidence confirms that aggressive comprehensive risk factor management improves survival, reduces recurrent events and the need for interventional procedures, and improves quality of life for these patients (Table 13-5).[14]

SPECIAL TOPICS IN SECONDARY PREVENTION

Lipid Management

- High-intensity statins are recommended for all individuals with ASCVD.

Cardiac Rehabilitation

- Comprehensive cardiac rehabilitation services include long-term programs involving medical evaluation, prescribed exercise, cardiac risk factor modification, education, and counseling.
- The simplest approach for clinicians prescribing exercise for patients with CHD is to refer them to an established cardiac rehabilitation program.
- Patients in such programs exercise three times a week for ≥30 minutes, including 5 minutes of warm-up and cooldown calisthenics and ≥20 minutes of exercise at 70% to 85% of the predetermined peak heart rate (about 60% to 75% of VO_2max).

TABLE 13-5	AHA/ACC CHD SECONDARY PREVENTION RECOMMENDATIONS
Risk	**Goal**
Smoking	Complete cessation No exposure or environmental tobacco smoke
Blood pressure	See HTN table
Cholesterol	High intensity statin therapy
Physical activity	At least 30 minutes 7 days/week (minimum 5 days/week)
Weight	BMI 18.5–24.9 Waist circumference men <40" Waist circumference women <35"
Diabetes	HbA1c ≤7%
Antiplatelet agents/ anticoagulants	Aspirin 75–162 mg daily If intolerant/allergic clopidogrel 75 mg daily Aspirin + P2Y12 receptor antagonist for those after ACS or PCI with stent
ACE inhibitors	Recommended for all who have heart failure or who have had an MI with LVEF ≤40% Also recommended in those with hypertension, diabetes, or chronic kidney disease ARBs recommended for those who are ACE inhibitor intolerant
Aldosterone blockers	Recommended for those post-MI patients without significant renal impairment or hyperkalemia who are already on therapeutic doses of ACE inhibitor and β-blocker, who have LVEF ≤40%, and who have either diabetes or heart failure
β-Blockers	Recommended in all patients who have had an MI/ACS and/or left ventricular dysfunction (with or without clinical heart failure) Consider chronic therapy for all patients with coronary or other vascular disease

(*Continued*)

TABLE 13-5	AHA/ACC CHD SECONDARY PREVENTION RECOMMENDATIONS (Continued)
Risk	**Goal**
Influenza vaccine	Recommended for all patients with CVD
Depression	Screen for depression in patients with recent CABG or MI
Cardiac rehabilitation	Recommended for all patients with ACS, CABG, PCI, chronic angina, and/or peripheral artery disease (either immediately post or within the past year) Can also be considered for those with clinical stable heart failure

AHA, American Heart Association; ACC, American College of Cardiology; CHD, coronary heart disease; LDL, low-density lipoprotein cholesterol; BMI, body mass index; HbA1c, hemoglobin A1c; ACS, acute coronary syndrome; PCI, percutaneous coronary intervention; ACE, angiotensin-converting enzyme; MI, myocardial infarction; LVEF, left ventricular ejection fraction; ARB, angiotensin receptor blocker; CVD, cardiovascular disease; CABG, coronary artery bypass grafting.

Data from Smith SC Jr, Benjamin EJ, Bonow RO, et al. AHA/ACCF secondary prevention and risk reduction therapy for patients with coronary and other atherosclerotic vascular disease: 2011 update: a guideline from the American Heart Association and American College of Cardiology Foundation. *Circulation* 2011;124:2458-2473.

- Most rehabilitation programs recommend other activities such as light yard work or brisk walking on other days.
- Enrollment in a cardiac rehabilitation program after discharge can enhance patient education and compliance with the medical regimen and assist with the implementation of a regular exercise program.
- Exercise training can generally begin within 1 to 2 weeks after unstable angina/non–ST-segment elevation myocardial infarction treated with percutaneous coronary intervention or coronary artery bypass grafting.
- Unsupervised exercise may target a heart rate range of 60% to 75% of maximal heart rate (maximal heart rate = 220 − age); supervised training may target a higher heart rate (70% to 85% of maximal heart rate). Additional restrictions apply when residual ischemia is present (see Table 13-6).[18]
- Patients with CHD should undergo symptom-limited exercise testing before referral to an exercise program to establish baseline exercise ability, determine maximal heart rate, and exclude ischemia, symptoms, or arrhythmias that would alter the therapeutic approach.
- The patient should take his or her cardiac medications to match the conditions likely to be encountered during the exercise sessions.
- Patients in medically supervised and unsupervised programs should include some resistance exercises in their training regimens. These exercises should be performed at least twice weekly with dumbbells light enough to permit 12 to 15 repetitions of each exercise.

Other Therapies

Hormone replacement therapy should not be used for primary or secondary prevention of CVD in women (see Chapter 38).

TABLE 13-6	EXERCISE RECOMMENDATIONS FOR PATIENTS WITH CHD		
Patients	**Intensity**	**Duration**	**Frequency**
Aerobic exercise			
General CHD	70–85% peak HR	≥20 minutes	≥3 times/week
With asymptomatic ischemia	70–85% ischemic HR	≥20 minutes	≥3 times/week
With angina	70–85% ischemic HR or angina onset	≥20 minutes	≥3 times/week
With PCI (± stent)	70–85% peak HR	≥20 minutes	≥3 times/week
With claudication	Walking to pain tolerance	≥30 minutes	≥3 times/week
With HF (NYHA class I–III)	70–85% peak HR	≥20 minutes	≥3 times/week
Resistance exercise			
For most CHD patients	30–50% 1-repetition maximal weight	12–15 repetitions	2–3 times/week

CHD, coronary heart disease; HR, heart rate; PCI, percutaneous coronary intervention; HF, heart failure; NYHA, New York Heart Association.

Data from Thompson PD. Exercise prescription and proscription for patients with coronary artery disease. *Circulation* 2005;112:2354-2363.

REFERENCES

1. Wilson MD, Pearsion TA. Primary Prevention. In: Wong ND, Black HR, Gardin JM, eds. *Preventive Cardiology: A Practical Approach*. New York: McGraw-Hill; 2005:493-514.
2. Goff Jr DC, Lloyd-Jones DM, Bennett G, O'Donnell CJ, Coady S, Robinson J, D'Agostino RB, Schwartz JS, Gibbons R, Shero ST, Greenland P, Smith SC, Lackland DT, Sorlie P, Levy D, Stone NJ, Wilson PWF, 2013 ACC/AHA Guideline on the Assessment of Cardiovascular Risk, Journal of the American College of Cardiology (2014), doi: 10.1016.
3. Lichtenstein AH, Appel LJ, Brands M, et al. Diet and lifestyle recommendations revision 2006: a scientific statement from the American Heart Association Nutrition Committee. *Circulation* 2006;114:82-96.
4. Eckel RH, Jakicic JM, Ard JD, Miller NH, Hubbard VS, Nonas CA, de Jesus JM, Sacks FM, Lee I-M, Smith Jr SC, Lichtenstein AH, Svetkey LP, Loria CM, Wadden TW, Millen BE, Yanovski SZ, 2013 AHA/ACC Guideline on Lifestyle Management to Reduce Cardiovascular Risk, Journal of the American College of Cardiology (2013), doi: 10.1016/j.jacc.2013.11.003.

5. Haskell WL, Lee I-M, Pate RP, et al. Physical activity and public health: updated recommendation for adults from the American College of Sports Medicine and the American Heart Association. *Circulation* 2007;116:1081-1093.

6. Thun MJ, Peto R, Lopez, et al. Alcohol consumption and mortality among middle-aged and elderly U.S. adults. *N Engl J Med* 1997;337:1705-1714.

7 Di Castelnuovo A, Costanzo S, Bagnardi V, et al. Alcohol dosing and total mortality in men and women: an updated meta-analysis of 34 prospective studies. *Arch Intern Med* 2006;166:2437-2445.

8. Ronksley PE, Brien SE, Turner BJ, et al. Association of alcohol consumption with selected cardiovascular disease outcomes: a systematic review and meta-analysis. *BMJ* 2011;342:d671.

9. Stead LF, Rerera R, Bullen C, et al. Nicotine replacement therapy for smoking cessation. *Cochrane Database Syst Rev* 2012;11:CD000146.

10. Hughes JR, Stead LF, Lancaster T. Antidepressants for smoking cessation. *Cochrane Database Syst Rev* 2007;1:CD000031.

11. Cahill K, Stead LF, Lancaster T. Nicotine receptor partial agonists for smoking cessation. *Cochrane Database Syst Rev* 2012;4:CD006103.

12. Stone NJ, Robinson J, Lichtenstein AH, Bairey Merz CN, Lloyd-Jones DM, Blum CB, McBride P, Eckel RH, Schwartz JS, Goldberg AC, Shero ST, Gordon D, Smith Jr SC, Levy D, Watson K, Wilson PWF, 2013 ACC/AHA Guideline on the Treatment of Blood Cholesterol to Reduce Atherosclerotic Cardiovascular Risk in Adults, Journal of the American College of Cardiology (2013), doi: 10.1016/j.jacc.2013.11.002.

13. James PA, Oparil S, Carter BL, Cushman WC, Dennison-Himmelfarb C, Handler J, Lackland DT, Lefevre ML, Mackenzie TD, Ogedegbe O, Smith SC Jr, Svetkey LP, Taler SJ, Townsend RR, Wright JT Jr, Narva AS, Ortiz E. 2014 Evidence-Based Guideline for the Management of High Blood Pressure in Adults: Report From the Panel Members Appointed to the Eighth Joint National Committee (JNC 8). JAMA. 2013 Dec 18. doi: 10.1001/jama.2013.284427. [Epub ahead of print] /j.jacc.2013.11.005.

14. Smith SC Jr, Benjamin EJ, Bonow RO, et al. AHA/ACCF secondary prevention and risk reduction therapy for patients with coronary and other atherosclerotic vascular disease: 2011 update: a guideline from the American Heart Association and American College of Cardiology Foundation. *Circulation* 2011;124:2458-2473.

15. Antithrombotic Trialists' (ATT) Collaboration. Aspirin in the primary and secondary prevention of vascular disease: collaborative meta-analysis of individual participant data from randomised trials. *Lancet* 2009;373:1849-1860.

16. Seshasai SR, Wijesuriva S, Sivakumaran R, et al. Effect of aspirin on vascular and nonvascular outcomes: meta-analysis of randomized controlled trials. *Arch Intern Med* 2012;172:209-216.

17. Pignone M, Alberts MJ, Colwell JA, et al. Aspirin for primary prevention of cardiovascular events in people with diabetes: a position statement of the American Diabetes Association, a scientific statement of the American Heart Association, and an expert consensus document of the American College of Cardiology Foundation. *Circulation* 2010;121:2694-2701.

18. Thompson PD. Exercise prescription and proscription for patients with coronary artery disease. *Circulation* 2005;112:2354-2363.

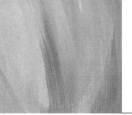

Evaluation and Management of Systolic Heart Failure

14

Shane J. LaRue and Susan M. Joseph

GENERAL PRINCIPLES

Definition

- Heart failure (HF) is a clinical syndrome characterized by dyspnea, exercise intolerance, and fluid retention in the setting of abnormal cardiac function.
- Cardiac dysfunction results from myocardial muscle dysfunction and is characterized by either left ventricular (LV) dilation or hypertrophy or both.
- The primary dysfunction may be systolic, diastolic, or mixed, though this chapter will focus on systolic HF.
- Most frequently, patients will present with either manifestations of poor cardiac output, such as **fatigue and exercise intolerance**, or volume overload/congestion, such as **pulmonary and peripheral edema**.
- Description of clinical presentation of acute decompensated HF is in Chapter 5.

Classification

- HF can be classified by several different characteristics, including mechanism, etiology, symptom severity, hemodynamic variables, and stage.
- Most simply, HF can first be divided by etiology as **ischemic** (a result of obstructive coronary artery disease [CAD]) and **nonischemic** (all other causes).
- Alternatively, HF can be characterized as a disorder of **systolic dysfunction** (LV ejection fraction [LVEF] ≤40%) versus **diastolic dysfunction**, which is known as HF with preserved systolic function (HF-PSF), described in Chapter 15.
- HF patients are frequently characterized by symptom severity on the New York Heart Association (NYHA) scale (Figure 14-1).[1]
- American Heart Association (AHA) staging system takes into account risk factors and cardiac function, ranging from those at risk for developing HF to those with the most severe consequences thereof.[2]
- Killip classification includes both hemodynamic and clinical data to stratify severity.[3]

Epidemiology

- As of 2008, approximately 5.7 million people in the United States had HF, with an estimated 670,000 new diagnoses each year.
- Despite significant advances in the management of HF, mortality remains high, especially after hospitalization, where rates of death are approximately 22% and 42% at 1 and 5 years, respectively.
- Notably almost half of all patients admitted to the hospital for HF have preserved systolic function, indicating the clinical importance of this disease entity.

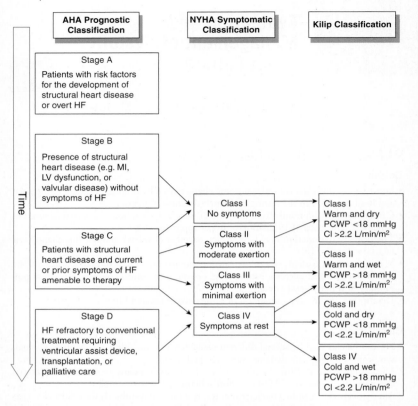

FIGURE 14-1. Classifications of heart failure. (From McBride BF, White CM. Acute decompensated heart failure: a contemporary approach to pharmacotherapeutic management. *Pharmacotherapy* 2003;23:997-1020, with permission.)

Etiology

• Among patients with abnormal systolic function, approximately two-thirds will have an ischemic cardiomyopathy (ICM), usually resulting from prior myocardial infarction (MI).
• The causes of nonischemic cardiomyopathy (NICM) in patients with systolic dysfunction are more varied and are shown in Table 14-1.

Pathophysiology

• Regardless of the initial insult leading to myocardial injury (e.g., ischemia, hypertension [HTN], and viral infection) a stereotypical pathologic remodeling response occurs.
• Over time, this **negative remodeling** leads to progressive cardiac enlargement and deterioration in cardiac function, largely due to activation of compensatory neurohormonal pathways such as the renin–angiotensin–aldosterone system (RAAS) and the sympathetic nervous system.

TABLE 14-1 CAUSE OF NONISCHEMIC CARDIOMYOPATHY

- Autoimmune/collagen-vascular:
  - Systemic lupus erythematosus
  - Dermatomyositis
  - Rheumatoid arthritis
  - Scleroderma
  - Polyarteritis nodosa
  - Churg–Strauss Syndrome
  - Cardiofacial
- Congenital heart disease:
  - Systemic right ventricular failure (TGA)
- Endocrine:
  - Diabetes mellitus
  - Hyperthyroidism
  - Hypothyroidism
  - Hyperparathyroidism
  - Pheochromocytoma
  - Acromegaly
- Endomyocardial
  - Endomyocardial fibrosis
  - Hypereosinophilic syndrome (Löeffler endocarditis)
- Genetic
  - Hypertrophic CM
  - ARVC/D
  - LVNC
  - Glycogen storage (PRKAG2, Danon)

- Conduction defects
- Mitochondrial myopathies
- Congenital heart diseases
- High-output states:
  - Arteriovenous malformation
  - Arteriovenous fistula
- Hypertensive heart disease
- Infiltrative:
  - Amyloidosis (primary, familial, senile, secondary forms)
  - Sarcoidosis
- Storage disorders:
  - Hemochromatosis
  - Fabry disease
  - Glycogen storage disease (type II, Pompe)
  - Gaucher disease
  - Hurler disease
  - Hunter disease
- Inflammatory (myocarditis)
- Neuromuscular/neurologic:
  - Friedreich ataxia
  - Duchenne, Becker, Emery–Dreifuss muscular dystrophy

- Myotonic dystrophy
- Neurofibromatosis
- Tuberous sclerosis
- Nutritional deficiencies:
  - Thiamine (beriberi/B1)
  - Pellagra (niacin/B3)
  - Scurvy (vit. C)
  - Keshan disease (selenium)
  - Carnitine
  - Kwashiorkor (protein)
- Pericardial constrict
- Peripartum
- Stress induced (takotsubo)
- Tachycardia induced
- Toxicity:
  - Chemotherapy (anthracyclines, cyclophosphamide)
  - Radiation
  - Alcohol
  - Cocaine
  - Amphetamines
  - Heavy metals
- Valvular

- The initial function of these responses is to maintain cardiac output by increasing ventricular filling pressures (preload) and myocardial contractility.
- However, over time, high levels of angiotensin II, aldosterone, and catecholamines lead to progressive myocardial fibrosis and apoptosis. This secondary injury promotes a further decline in cardiac function and contributes to the increased risk of arrhythmias.
- The neurohormonal model of HF is the basis for the most effective treatments used for HF management today.

Risk Factors

- There are many known factors that increase the chance of developing HF from many of the previously listed cardiomyopathies.
- The more common among these factors are **age, HTN, diabetes, CAD, and a strong family history of cardiomyopathy**.
- Additional risk factors have been attributed to specific cardiomyopathies. Examples include myocarditis or viral CM (recent viral illness or upper respiratory symptoms, rheumatologic disease history or symptoms), genetic CM (family history of HF or sudden cardiac death), toxic CM (alcohol or drug abuse, history of chemotherapy), and peripartum CM (recent pregnancy).

Prevention

- Early treatment and prevention of LV dysfunction are possible by identifying and treating high-risk individuals. **The critical modifiable risk factors are diabetes, HTN, and CAD; aggressive treatment of these diseases paramount**.
- HTN is present in about 75% of patients with HF and treatment significantly reduces the incidence of HF.
- Diabetes is associated with a two- to fivefold increased risk of developing HF independent of CAD. The term "**diabetic CM**" is used to describe the abnormal diastolic function (with or without systolic abnormalities) seen in diabetics. Up to 33% of patients hospitalized for HF have diabetes.

Associated Conditions

Other common associated conditions include sleep-disordered breathing, which is present in an estimated 30% to 40% of HF patients, and atrial fibrillation (AF), which affects approximately one-third of HF patients.

DIAGNOSIS

Clinical Presentation

- Full discussion can be found in Chapter 5.
- The presentation of systolic HF is essentially the same as that of diastolic HF and can be divided into three basic presentation phenotypes:
  - "Flash" or acute pulmonary edema with HTN.
  - Slowly progressive fluid accumulation.
  - Low-output state.

History

- Full discussion can be found in Chapter 5.
- Three main goals to elicit from the patient's history are:
  - Identify etiology and/or factors contributing to the decline in function.
  - Assess progression and severity of illness, particularly to classify the patient based on the NYHA class.
  - Assess volume status.

Physical Examination

- Full discussion can be found in Chapters 2 and 5.
- The primary function of the physical examination in patients with HF is to assess volume status.

Diagnostic Criteria

- HF is a clinical diagnosis based on history, physical examination findings, and chest radiography. Although there are no universally agreed-upon diagnostic criteria for HF, the Framingham criteria require two major or one major and two minor criteria.
  - **Major Criteria**: paroxysmal nocturnal dyspnea, jugular venous distention, crackles, cardiomegaly, pulmonary edema, S3, hepatojugular reflux, and weight loss with diuresis (>4.5 lb).
  - **Minor Criteria**: lower extremity edema, nocturnal cough, dyspnea on exertion, hepatomegaly, pleural effusions, tachycardia, and decrease in vital capacity.
- The diagnosis of HF is further supported by laboratory values (elevated brain natriuretic peptide [BNP]) and imaging studies (e.g., cardiac dysfunction on echocardiogram) as detailed below.

Diagnostic Testing

Laboratories

- Laboratory data play an important role in the early assessment of acute HF, but are also used for monitoring in the chronic setting.
- In the acute setting, laboratory data obtained should include **cardiac biomarkers, such as troponin**, to evaluate for myocardial ischemia, **metabolic panel** for renal function and electrolyte abnormalities, and **hemoglobin**.
- The presence of an elevated troponin may signify an acute coronary syndrome; however, mild troponin elevations can occur even in the absence of epicardial CAD. In either case, the presence of an elevated troponin signifies myocardial injury and identifies a high-risk subset of HF patients.
- **BNP** level may also be helpful, particularly if the dyspnea is of unclear etiology.
  - BNP is a small polypeptide released by myocytes in response to increased wall stress.
  - Systemic levels of BNP correlate with invasive intracardiac pressure measurements and are a reliable marker of volume status.
  - BNP specificity is reduced in patients with renal dysfunction, and the sensitivity is reduced in obese patients.
  - **A BNP level** >400 pg/L is consistent with HF. Levels ranging from 100 pg/mL to 400 pg/mL may represent underlying LV dysfunction; however, other diseases such as acute pulmonary embolism must be considered.
- In the absence of significant CAD, additional blood work should include an **iron panel and ferritin level**, a test for HIV, and **hepatitis C** testing (in at-risk individuals).
- Routine testing for viral infections is not recommended as the results do not alter therapy. However, if performed, the most common viruses associated with myocarditis include coxsackie B, adenovirus, cytomegalovirus (CMV), echovirus, HIV, hepatitis C, and parvovirus B19.
- In patients with physical findings consistent with a rheumatologic disease, additional testing such as an antinuclear antibody (ANA) and/or antineutrophil cytoplasmic antibody (ANCA) titer can be checked.
- Serum protein electrophoresis (SPEP) and urine protein electrophoresis (UPEP) should be checked if there is clinical suspicion for amyloidosis.
- If the patient has episodic HTN, tachycardia, and/or headaches, pheochromocytoma should be ruled out by testing catecholamine levels.
- Genetic testing and counseling can be considered if a strong family history of CM is present.

Electrocardiography

- In the acute setting, an ECG should be obtained rapidly to look for evidence of ischemia, infarct, or arrhythmia.
- ECG in a HF patient may also demonstrate prior infarct, left bundle branch block (LBBB), conduction disease, AF, left ventricular hypertrophy (LVH), and low voltage (infiltrative CM).

Imaging

- The **chest radiograph** (CXR) can assess for evidence of pulmonary edema or cardiomegaly and to rule other causes of dyspnea (pneumonia, pneumothorax). Up to 40% of chronic HF patients with significant elevations in pulmonary capillary wedge pressure will have no radiographic evidence of congestion.
- A **transthoracic echocardiogram** (TTE) provides information regarding systolic and diastolic function, valvular disease, LVH, asymmetric septal hypertrophy, and pericardial disease and provides an estimation of pulmonary artery (PA) systolic pressure.
- **Cardiac MRI** has been increasingly used in the assessment of new-onset cardiomyopathies, particularly for infiltrative disease.

Diagnostic Procedures

- In some cases, placement of a **pulmonary artery catheter** can help guide therapy.
  - A PA catheter should be considered for patients who present with hypotension and evidence of shock (see Chapter 8).
  - Invasive hemodynamic data can direct the use of inotropic and vasopressor agents and can help with volume assessment (Table 14-2).
  - However, the ESCAPE trial demonstrated that routine PA catheter placement does not alter mortality or length of hospital stay in acute decompensated HF. Therefore, placement of a **PA catheter should be reserved for hemodynamically unstable patients or for those not responding to empiric inotrope or diuretic therapy**.
- Patients with new systolic dysfunction should undergo an **ischemic evaluation**.
  - For patients with multiple cardiac risk factors, chest pain, and/or segmental wall motion abnormalities on echocardiography, coronary angiography is preferred.
  - Revascularization via percutaneous intervention or coronary artery bypass grafting is indicated in patients with reduced LVEF and viable myocardium.

TREATMENT

- The treatment goals during a hospitalization for acute decompensated HF (ADHF) are to **(1) improve patient symptoms, (2) correct hemodynamic and volume status, (3) minimize renal and cardiac injury, and (4) initiate lifesaving medical therapies**. Figure 14-2 provides a guideline for management of ADHF.
- The treatment goals for chronic HF are different than those for ADHF and include **(1) reduction of mortality, (2) improvement of symptoms, and (3) reduction of hospitalizations**.
- Being familiar with the large body of clinical trial data regarding medical therapy of chronic HF can guide decisions toward proper medical treatment.

Medications

First Line

Acute Pulmonary Edema and Hypertension

- **The immediate goal is to stabilize respiratory status by lowering blood pressure and removing fluid from the lungs**.

TABLE 14-2   INTERPRETING HEMODYNAMIC DATA IN THE HEART FAILURE PATIENT WITH A PA CATHETER

Cardiac index (2.5–4.5 L/min/m²)	CVP (5–8 mmHg)	Mean PAP (15–25 mmHg)	PCWP (5–10 mmHg)	SBP (100–120 mmHg)	SVR (800–1200 dynes/sec × cm⁻⁵)	Diagnosis and management
↓	↓	↓ or normal	↓	↓	↑	D: Hypovolemia M: IV fluids
↓	↑	↑	↑	↑ or normal	↑↑	D: HF with high vascular tone M: Vasodilators/afterload reduction
↓	↑	↑	↑	↓	↑↑	D: HF with poor systemic perfusion M: Inotropes, diuretics
↓	↑	↑	↑	↓↓	↑	D: HF with shock M: Inotrope, vasopressors, mechanical support
↓↑ or normal	↓ or normal	↓ or normal	↓ or normal	↓	→	D: Distributive shock (sepsis) M: IV fluids, vasopressors, antibiotics
↓	↑	↑	→ normal	↓	↑	D: Pulmonary HTN, Right heart failure M: Inotropes, pulmonary vasodilators

CVP, central venous pressure; HF, heart failure; HTN, hypertension; PAP, pulmonary artery pressure; PCWP, pulmonary capillary wedge pressure; SBP, systolic blood pressure; SVR, systemic vascular resistance. Normal values in parentheses.

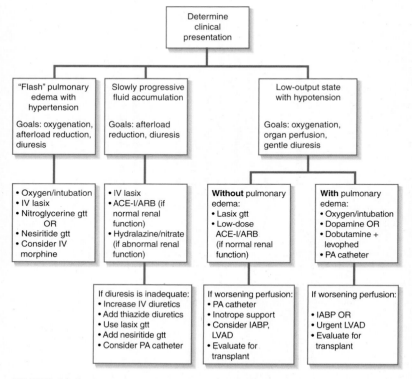

FIGURE 14-2. General approach to the management of acute decompensated heart failure (ADHF).

- These patients should receive oxygen, IV vasodilators, and IV diuretics.
- As high vascular tone (rather than marked volume overload) characterizes this presentation, vasodilators are more important than diuretics to rapidly lower cardiac filling pressures and improve patient symptoms.
  - The VMAC study is one of the few randomized controlled trials evaluating vasodilator therapy in patients with ADHF.[4]
  - In this study, both **nitroglycerin** and **nesiritide** infusions were effective at reducing patient symptoms and cardiac filling pressures compared to diuretics alone; however, nesiritide infusion led to a more rapid and sustained improvement in these parameters. Thirty-day mortality was not significantly different between the treatment arms. These short-term data and clinician experience have led to the recommendation **that one of these two vasodilator medications be used in the treatment of patients with acute pulmonary edema**.
- In addition to vasodilators, **diuretics** are useful for reducing preload and improving patient volume status and symptoms. An initial dose of **IV furosemide** should be administered. However, overaggressive diuresis can lead to renal dysfunction.
- **IV morphine** can also be considered in these patients, as it has venodilating properties and can reduce anxiety.

- If the respiratory status remains tenuous, noninvasive positive-pressure ventilation (BiPAP) or intubation may be necessary to improve oxygenation until the hemodynamic and volume status can be improved.

Slowly Progressive Volume Overload

- In patients with volume overload without respiratory distress, the primary goal is to **maximize afterload reduction and remove excess fluid without promoting kidney dysfunction**.
- Angiotensin converting enzyme (ACE)-inhibitor therapy should be initiated or continued if renal function is not significantly impaired (Cr < 2.0 to 2.5 mg/dL) and the potassium level is not elevated ($\geq$5.0 mEq/L).
  - If the patient is ACE inhibitor-naive, it is reasonable to start with a short-acting agent such as **captopril**.
  - Prior to discharge, patients should be transitioned to a long-acting ACE inhibitor.
  - In the setting of impaired renal function or hyperkalemia, a combination of **hydralazine** and **nitrates** can be used for afterload reduction.
- With diuretic therapy, the goal is to remove between 1.5 L per day and 3.0 L per day, depending on the degree of volume overload.
  - As an initial strategy, bolus **IV furosemide** is reasonable.
  - For patients on home oral furosemide, administer the same dose IV and assess response (for example, 40 mg PO twice daily can become 40 mg IV twice daily).
  - If the diuresis is inadequate, then the IV dose can be increased or a **thiazide** diuretic can be added. The addition of a thiazide diuretic can cause profound potassium and magnesium depletion, so aggressive monitoring and repletion are mandatory.
  - If the patient is still resistant to diuretic therapy, then a **furosemide or nesiritide infusion** can be considered.
- Poor diuresis with these measures and/or progressive renal dysfunction should lead to PA catheter placement and/or the use of **inotropes (dobutamine or milrinone)** or ultrafiltration.
  - Routine use of inotropes in ADHF was challenged by the OPTIME trial where milrinone infusion did not improve diuresis, but did lead to an increase in adverse events.[5]
  - In addition, the ADHERE database shows an association between inotrope use and worse clinical outcomes.[6] Therefore, **inotropes should be reserved for patients with reduced cardiac output, refractory edema, and evidence of end-organ hypoperfusion**.

Low-Output State $\pm$ Volume Overload

- Patients who present with ADHF and evidence of hypoperfusion represent <5% of hospital admissions for HF.
- These patients are generally the sickest and are often in overt cardiogenic shock. Acute renal failure, elevated liver enzymes, metabolic acidosis, and peripheral vasoconstriction are common.
- This situation is most frequently encountered in the setting of an acute MI, acute myocarditis, or at the end stage of a chronic CM.
- **Patients in early or overt cardiogenic shock require rapid triage and admission to an ICU for stabilization**. Urgent revascularization may be required if the underlying cause of the shock state is an acute MI.
  - If the systolic blood pressure (SBP) is between 80 and 100 mmHg, empiric treatment with **dobutamine or milrinone** can often help improve end-organ perfusion and facilitate diuresis. A **continuous furosemide infusion** is often the most effective means to remove fluid from such patients without promoting further hypotension. If the patients fail to respond to empiric therapy quickly, PA catheterization is warranted.

◦ In the situation where the SBP is <80 mmHg, patients are unlikely to tolerate the hypotension that dobutamine or milrinone can cause. Options include **dopamine** or the combination of **low-dose norepinephrine with dobutamine or milrinone**. These patients should receive a PA catheter to direct therapy (Chapter 8).

Second Line

- After stabilization of the acute patient, a number of medications have been shown to prevent the negative remodeling and prolong survival in chronic HF.
- **ACE inhibitors and angiotensin receptor blockers** (ARBs) have become the corner-stone of medical treatment for patients with systolic dysfunction.
  ◦ Much of the benefit of ACE inhibitors in HF comes from their action in blocking the effects of angiotensin II by inhibiting its formation.
    ▪ Angiotensin II is a potent vasoconstrictor that also stimulates pro-fibrotic and pro-inflammatory pathways and promotes adverse myocardial remodeling.
    ▪ V-HEFT 2 was the first clinical trial of ACE inhibitors in HF. In this study, enalapril therapy led to a 28% decrease in mortality as compared with hydralazine/nitrate therapy despite similar levels of blood pressure control.[7]
    ▪ Several subsequent randomized trials have established the benefit of ACE inhibitors in patients with chronic LV dysfunction (SOLVD, CONSENSUS) and with post-MI LV dysfunction (SAVE, TRACE, AIRE).[8-12] ACE inhibitors were consistently associated with a mortality reduction of approximately 20% to 25% at 1 to 5 years.
    ▪ When initiating an ACE inhibitor, low doses should be used at first and then gradually titrated upward. Plasma creatinine and potassium should be checked at 1 to 2 weeks after initiation or up titration of an ACE inhibitor. Small increases in creatinine (up to 30%) are common and should not prompt discontinuation of therapy.
    ▪ Side effects include cough (about 10%), hyperkalemia, hypotension, renal insufficiency, angioedema, and teratogenicity.
  ◦ ARBs act downstream of ACE inhibitors by inhibiting the type 1 angiotensin receptor, thereby attenuating the biologic effects of angiotensin II.
    ▪ The largest clinical trials of ARBs in patients with chronic HF are Val-HEFT and CHARM.[13,14] Both of these studies showed that **ARBs are equivalent to ACE inhibitors with regard to HF mortality reduction**. Similar findings were seen in VALIANT for patients with LV dysfunction post-MI.[15]
    ▪ Therefore, ARBs are an acceptable alternative for patients who are ACE inhibitor-intolerant (usually secondary to cough).
    ▪ ARBs should be initiated in a similar manner to ACE inhibitors. The expected side effects are the same as with ACE inhibitors with the exception of cough, which is not seen with ARB therapy.
- In addition to inhibitors of the RAAS, β-**blocker therapy is mandatory for all patients with LV dysfunction**. Once considered contraindicated in HF, β-blockers have become the most effective drugs for managing this condition.
  ◦ **Carvedilol** has been studied in patients with mild to moderate HF (US carvedilol studies) or severe HF (COPERNICUS) and in the post-MI setting (CAPRICORN).[16,17] All-cause and cardiovascular mortality was consistently reduced by 25% to 48%.
  ◦ Similar benefit was seen with **metoprolol** succinate in the MERIT-HF trial, where all-cause mortality was reduced by 34% at 1 year in class II to III HF patients.[18]
  ◦ The use of **bisoprolol** is also supported by clinical data from CIBIS I and II.[19,20]

- ○ β-Blockers should be started at low doses and titrated every 1 to 2 weeks until goal doses are achieved. **Patients should be stable, largely euvolemic, and already on an ACE inhibitor or ARB prior to the initiation of a β-blocker.**
- ○ Caution should be used in patients with underlying bradycardia or conduction system disease. Fatigue is also common with β-blocker treatment, but it generally improves after 1 to 2 weeks of treatment. If bronchospasm or low blood pressure is an issue, then β-1-selective agents (metoprolol succinate) are often better tolerated.
- **Aldosterone antagonists** are recommended in patients with severe HF (NYHA III to IV) and those with LV dysfunction post-MI.
  - ○ Aldosterone is an adrenal hormone whose production is stimulated through angiotensin II-dependent and -independent pathways. In the myocardium, aldosterone leads to fibrosis and progressive pathologic remodeling.
  - ○ The effects of inhibiting aldosterone in HF were first investigated in the RALES trial, where treatment with **spironolactone** led to a 30% mortality reduction and 36% decrease in hospitalizations in patients with NYHA class III to IV HF.[21]
  - ○ Subsequently, the EPHESUS trial demonstrated mortality benefit with the more selective aldosterone antagonist **eplerenone** in patients with post-MI LV dysfunction already taking an ACE inhibitor and β-blocker.[22]
  - ○ The major side effect is hyperkalemia, especially in the setting of reduced renal function or concomitant ACE inhibitor/ARB therapy; thus frequent monitoring is required. Aldosterone antagonists should be avoided in patients with a baseline potassium ≥ 5.0 mEq/L or with a baseline Cr >2.0 to 2.5 mg/dL. Gynecomastia can also be seen with spironolactone.
- **Hydralazine/nitrate combination can be used as an alternative to ACE inhibitor/ ARB therapy in patients intolerant of these medications.**
  - ○ The V-HEFT I study was the first trial to investigate hydralazine combined with nitrates (isosorbide dinitrate) in chronic HF.[23] This vasodilator combination improved patient symptoms and reduced mortality when compared to placebo and doxazosin.
  - ○ Further subgroup analysis of V-HEFT I and its counterpart V-HEFT II suggested that patients of African descent treated with this combination derived particular benefit.[7,23]
  - ○ These observations lead to the A-HEFT trial which demonstrated a 43% decrease in mortality and a 33% decrease in HF hospitalizations in African American patients with class III to IV HF already treated with ACE inhibitor and β-blocker.[24] Thus, the combination of hydralazine and nitrates is **recommended in African American patients with severe HF symptoms already on aggressive medical therapy.**
  - ○ The most common side effects are headache and hypotension. Patient compliance can also be an issue, given the number of pills required per day (TID to QID dosing).
- **Digoxin can be used for symptoms of HF, but it does not alter survival from HF.**
  - ○ Digoxin is a cardiac glycoside that inhibits the Na–K exchange ion channel, leading to increased intracellular calcium and enhanced contractility.
  - ○ The DIG trial demonstrated that digoxin therapy, **in addition to** ACE inhibitors and diuretics, decreased HF hospitalizations but did not alter mortality.[25] Of note, the best outcomes were seen in patients with digoxin levels <1 ng/mL. Based on these results and other studies demonstrating that digoxin can improve HF symptoms, this agent is **used for patients on optimal medical therapy who still have frequent hospitalizations for HF.**
  - ○ Caution must be used in patients with renal dysfunction as digoxin has a narrow therapeutic index and toxicity can occur. Adverse reactions with digoxin include cardiac arrhythmias (atrial tachycardia with atrioventricular block, bidirectional ventricular tachycardia, AF with regular ventricular response), gastrointestinal symptoms, and neurologic complaints (confusion, visual disturbances).

- ○ Digoxin toxicity usually manifests when serum levels exceed 2 ng/mL; however, hypokalemia and hypomagnesemia can lower this threshold.
- Despite the lack of randomized studies to guide the optimal approach to diuretic therapy, **diuretics are a mainstay of medical therapy for volume management in chronic HF.**
  - ○ The general consensus is to prescribe the **lowest dose of diuretic that is necessary to maintain euvolemia.**
  - ○ The loop diuretics **furosemide, torsemide, and bumetanide** are the primary options for volume control.
    - ▪ Torsemide or bumetanide should be considered in patients with significant right-sided HF and abdominal venous congestion, where the absorption of furosemide is frequently unpredictable.
    - ▪ The conversion from furosemide to torsemide to bumetanide is approximately 40:20:1.
  - ○ At times, loop diuretics may not be sufficient to maintain euvolemia. In these cases a **thiazide diuretic can be added to overcome distal tubular hypertrophy** and induce diuresis.
  - ○ Given the potency of combining a thiazide with a loop diuretic, it is recommended to use only short-term dosing or a 3 day per week dosing schedule. Electrolytes and renal function must be followed carefully as significant volume depletion can occur with any diuretic use.
- **Continuous inotrope infusion should only be considered for AHA stage D/NYHA class III to IV patients with refractory HF symptoms and evidence of end-organ hypoperfusion.**
  - ○ The two inotropes available in the United States are the nonselective β-agonist **dobutamine** and the phosphodiesterase inhibitor **milrinone.**
  - ○ Both of these medications increase cardiac output by increasing contractility and reducing afterload.
  - ○ The hemodynamic effects of these agents are similar; however, dobutamine is favored when renal function is impaired and/or the SBP is low (85 to 90 mmHg).
  - ○ Milrinone can be more effective for patients with elevated PA pressures, given its potent vasodilating action.
  - ○ Adverse events associated with inotrope infusion include hypotension (particularly when the patient is hypovolemic), atrial and ventricular arrhythmias, and acceleration in the decline of ventricular function. The risks and benefits must be considered very carefully before initiating inotrope therapy.
  - ○ Patients with severe HF symptoms may require continuous home inotrope infusion.
    - ▪ To qualify for continuous inotrope infusion, a patient's cardiac index must be <2 L/minute per square meter and must improve with inotropes.
    - ▪ Thus, initiation of inotropes for possible home infusion requires the placement of a PA catheter.

Other Nonpharmacologic Therapies

- Many patients in cardiogenic shock may require additional **mechanical support,** which includes an intra-aortic balloon pump (IABP) or a percutaneous LV assist device (LVAD) (Table 14-3).
  - ○ For critically ill patients who are poor surgical candidates, the Abiomed Impella (www.abiomed.com/, last accessed 6/7/13) and CardiacAssist, Inc. TandemHeart (www.cardiacassist.com/TandemHeart, last accessed 6/7/13) percutaneous LVADs are available for short-term mechanical circulatory support and have been shown to have superior hemodynamic effects compared to the IABP.

TABLE 14-3	PERCUTANEOUS CIRCULATORY SUPPORT OPTIONS			
Device	**Catheters**	**Support**	**Advantages**	**Limitations**
IABP	8-Fr Arterial	Counter-pulsation 0.5 L/minute	Ease of insertion Lower cost Increase coronary perfusion	Minimal increase in CO
Impella 2.5	13-Fr Arterial	Microaxial impeller 2.5 L/minute	Percutaneous insertion	Insufficient support for cardiogenic shock
Impella 5.0	21-Fr Arterial	Microaxial impeller 5 L/minute	Greater circulatory support	Large catheter size Requires surgical cutdown Vascular/bleeding complications
Tandem Heart	17-Fr Arterial 21-Fr Venous	Centrifugal pump (extracorporeal) 4 L/minute	Greater circulatory support	Large catheter size Trans-septal puncture Vascular/bleeding complications

IABP, intra-aortic balloon pump; CO, cardiac output.

- The Impella is an all-arterial system, which utilizes a contained micro-axial pump placed retrogradely across the aortic valve via the femoral artery. The catheter removes blood from the LV cavity and pumps it into the ascending aorta. Two different sizes are available, capable of providing 2.5 and 5 L/minute of cardiac output, respectively.
- The Tandem Heart is a left atrial to femoral artery bypass system capable of providing up to 4 L/minute of flow. It consists of an inflow cannula placed into the left atrium from femoral vein via trans-septal puncture, a continuous flow centrifugal (extracorporeal) pump, and an outflow cannula to the femoral artery.
- **Implantable cardiac defibrillators** (ICDs) are used to prevent sudden death from life-threatening ventricular arrhythmias.
  - MADIT-I and MADIT-2 trials established the survival benefit of ICDs in patients with ICM and an EF ≤30%.[26,27]
  - Subsequently, the SCD-HEFT trial demonstrated a similar benefit for ICDs in patients with ICM and NICM with EF ≤35%.[28]
  - In an appropriately selected population, 6 implanted CDs are needed to save one life over 8 years (number needed to treat NNT). Therefore **ICD implantation should be considered for all HF patients with EF ≤35%**. A full discussion of this subject can be found in Chapter 25.

- **Cardiac resynchronization therapy** (CRT) is designed to resynchronize ventricular contraction and improve cardiac function in patients with HF and dyssynchronous electromechanical activation of the left ventricle.
  - The three largest randomized trials in CRT are COMPANION and CARE-HF and MADIT-CRT.[29,30,31]
  - Biventricular pacing was associated with an improvement in symptoms and a reduction in hospitalizations compared to patients receiving medical therapy alone. The CARE-HF trial also demonstrated a marked decrease in mortality associated with biventricular pacing.
  - **CRT should be considered in patients with dyssynchrony (QRS >120 ms) who have NYHA class III to IV HF symptoms despite medical therapy**. More recent indications have endorsed the use of CRT in patients with less severe HF (NYHA class, I or II) and more dyssynchrony (QRS >150 ms).
- **Ultrafiltration** (UF) allows for fluid removal at a consistent rate without negative consequences associated with aggressive diuretic use, such as electrolyte depletion and renal injury.
  - The UNLOAD trial was a small study that compared UF to standard therapy in patients admitted with ADHF.[32]
  - Fluid removal was more effective and efficient using UF and the risk of future hospitalizations for HF was reduced. The downside of UF is that it requires specialized peripheral venous access and the machines/equipment can be costly.

Surgical Management

- **LVADs can be considered in select patients with acute or chronic end-organ hypoperfusion from cardiac dysfunction**.
- LVADs extract oxygenated blood from either the LA or LV, shuttle it through a palatial or continuous-flow pump, and then return it to the aorta.
- LVADs are designed for short- or long-term ventricular support.
  - The **short-term devices** include the percutaneously inserted TandemHeart and Impella and the surgically implanted Abiomed AB5000 (www.abiomed.com/products/ab5000/, lasted accessed 6/7/13) and Medtronic Bio-Medicus Bio-Pump (www.medtronic.com, last accessed 6/7/13). These devices can provide cardiac support for 1 to 2 weeks or 1 to 2 months, respectively.
- The **long-term LVADs** previously used in the United States were all pulsatile devices—Thoratec VAD and HeartMate IP, VE, and XVE (www.thoratec.com, last accessed 6/7/13) and WorldHeart Novacor (www.worldheart.com, last accessed 6/7/13).
  - In most situations, LVADs are used as a "bridge" to transplant. However, LVAD implantation can also be considered in select patients who are not transplant candidates. This is referred to as "destination" therapy.
  - Two randomized trials of destination therapy in end-stage HF patients are the REMATCH and INTrEPID studies, which compared LVAD to standard medical therapy in patients with advanced HF.[33,34]
    - Although mortality was significantly reduced in the LVAD arm of both trials, over half of the treated patients died within 1 year.
    - Device failure, sepsis, and embolic events are the primary causes of death in patients with LVADs.
  - The HeartMate II trial compared the continuous flow HeartMate II with the pulsatile HeartMate XVE and demonstrated superiority of the newer, continuous flow HeartMate II device.[35]
  - Totally implantable pulsatile devices and total artificial heart technologies continue to improve and are exclusively available in clinical trial settings.
- **Heart transplantation remains the definitive therapy for end-stage HF.**
  - Successful transplantation became possible in the 1980s, when the immunosuppressant cyclosporine was used to control rejection.

- Currently there are about 2,000 heart transplants in the United States each year.
- **Survival following heart transplantation is 85%, 70%, and 50% of patients alive at 1, 5, and 10 years, respectively.**
- Patients considered for transplantation have severe HF symptoms despite maximal medical therapy and have a limited life expectancy. A VO_2 max ≤ 14 mL/kg per minute on cardiopulmonary exercise testing portends a significantly reduced 1-year survival, and this criterion has been used to identify patients with the greatest need for transplant.
- Contraindications to transplant, some of which are relative, include severe, irreversible pulmonary HTN, active infection, severe chronic obstructive pulmonary disease, significant renal impairment (not related to poor cardiac output), severe peripheral vascular disease or carotid disease, severe psychiatric disease, primary liver disease with coagulopathy, advanced age (>70 to 75), diabetes with end-organ dysfunction, and active malignancy.

LIFESTYLE/RISK MODIFICATION

Diet

- Dietary instruction regarding sodium and fluid intake is critical in volume management in patients with HF.
- Sodium intake should generally be limited to 2 to 3 g per day in patients with HF, though more severe restriction to <2 g per day is necessary with moderate to severe HF.
- Fluid intake must also be limited, with 1.5 to 2 L per day recommended for those with hyponatremia or edema despite aggressive diuretic usage.

Activity

- Patients with HF should undergo exercise testing to evaluate for ischemia/arrhythmias prior to commencement of an exercise program.
- If appropriate, exercise training can then be started, preferably in a monitored setting to facilitate understanding of exercise expectations and to increase duration and intensity to a general exercise goal of 30 minutes of moderate activity/exercise, 5 days per week with warm up and cool down exercises.

SPECIAL CONSIDERATIONS

- For some patients, relieving symptoms and avoiding hospitalization may be the primary goals; therefore continuous inotrope infusion and/or hospice care may be reasonable.
- In patients who are not candidates for more aggressive HF therapy, discussions regarding end-of-life issues, including turning off ICD therapy, should be undertaken.
- The issue of what to do with β-blocker therapy during a HF exacerbation is a controversial and frequently discussed topic.
  - As the benefits of β-blocker are realized over the long term, it has been general practice to discontinue these medications during ADHF, given their negative inotropic effects.
  - However, HF exacerbations are associated with high levels of systemic catecholamines, and there are data to suggest that the withdrawal of β-blocker during ADHF can worsen outcomes.
  - In a β-blocker–naïve patient, it is reasonable to defer treatment until euvolemia has been achieved and the patient is on an afterload reduction regimen.
  - In patients already receiving β-blocker therapy, every attempt should be made to continue the medication at its current dose. If the patient is in a low-output state, the dose can be decreased.
  - In the event that the patient requires inotropic therapy it is appropriate to discontinue the β-blocker.

REFERRAL

Referral to HF/transplant specialists allows for evaluation for advanced mechanical therapy (e.g., left ventricular assist device support) or cardiac transplantation in appropriate situations.

PATIENT EDUCATION

- Key components to long-term success in HF management are patient education, optimal medical and device therapy, and adequate patient follow-up.
- The inpatient hospitalization provides an opportunity to ensure these issues are addressed. The **ABCs checklist for hospital discharge** is a useful device:
  - **A:** ACE inhibitor or ARB.
  - **B:** β–Blocker.
  - **C:** Counseling (smoking cessation, exercise).
  - **D:** Dietary education (low-sodium diet, fluid restriction), Device therapy (if appropriate).
  - **E:** Euvolemia achieved.
  - **F:** Follow-up appointment established.

MONITORING/FOLLOW-UP

- Hospital care:
  - It is critical to continually reassess the patient's volume status throughout the hospitalization, which is done by monitoring daily weights, fluid intake and urine output, and physical examination findings (jugular venous pulse, edema).
  - A basic metabolic panel should also be checked regularly to monitor electrolytes and renal function, with close attention to BUN and HCO_3 levels, as they often climb with intravascular volume contraction.
  - Prior to discharge, patients should be transitioned to a stable oral diuretic regimen. In general, the lowest dose of diuretic needed to maintain euvolemia should be used.
- Post-heart transplant:
  - During the first year after transplant, acute rejection and infection (from both common and opportunistic pathogens–CMV, *Nocardia*, and *Pneumocystis*) are the primary complications.
  - Patients receive three-drug immunosuppression, infection prophylaxis, and routine endomyocardial biopsies during this time period to reduce adverse events.
  - After the first year, coronary artery vasculopathy, renal insufficiency, and malignancy are the primary factors that limit survival.
  - Aggressive treatment of HTN, statin therapy, routine coronary angiography or intravascular ultrasound, lower doses of immunosuppression, and cancer screening are all important to maximize long-term survival.
- Remote monitoring and volume assessment:
  - In an effort to identify subclinical volume overload, when intervention can prevent hospitalization, several monitoring strategies have been developed.
  - Blood pressure, weight, and symptoms can be monitored wirelessly and remotely via the internet (Latitude Patient Management System, Boston Scientific, www.bostonscientific.com, last accessed 6/7/13), helping clinicians direct medical therapy.
  - Thoracic impedance levels recorded from an implantable defibrillator/CRT device can assess trends in fluid balance (OptiVol Fluid Status Monitoring, Medtronic, www.medtronic.com, last accessed 6/7/13).

OUTCOME/PROGNOSIS

- Up to 30% of patients admitted with HF will die within 1 year.
- However, there are many factors that alter prognosis in an individual patient.
- **The Seattle HF model** is a comprehensive risk-prediction tool for assessing survival probability in a given individual. A user-friendly calculator for the Seattle Heart Failure Model is available on the web at depts.washington.edu/shfm/index.php (last accessed 6/7/13).[36,37]
- The ability to risk-stratify patients with HF is useful to direct the aggressiveness of therapy and to guide discussions with patients and their families.

REFERENCES

1. McBride BF, White CM. Acute decompensated heart failure: a contemporary approach to pharmacotherapeutic management. *Pharmacotherapy* 2003;23:997-1020.
2. Hunt SA, Abraham WT, Chin MH, et al. 2009 Focused update incorporated into the ACC/AHA 2005 Guidelines for the Diagnosis and Management of Heart Failure in Adults A Report of the American College of Cardiology Foundation/American Heart Association Task Force on Practice Guidelines Developed. *J Am Coll Cardiol* 2009;119:e391-e479.
3. Killip T 3rd, Kimball JT. Treatment of myocardial infarction in a coronary care unit. A two-year experience with 250 patients. *Am J Cardiol* 1967;20:457-464.
4. Publication Committee for the VMAC Investigators. Intravenous nesiritide versus nitroglycerin for treatment of decompensated congestive heart failure: a randomized controlled trial. *JAMA* 2002;287(12):1531-1540.
5. Gheorghiade M, Shin DD, Thoms TO, et al. Congestion is an important diagnostic and therapeutic target in heart failure. *Rev Cardiovasc Med* 2006;7:S12-S24.
6. Abraham WT, Adams, KF, Fonarow GC, et al. In-hospital mortality in patients with acute decompensated heart failure requiring intravenous vasoactive medications: an analysis from the Acute Decompensated Heart Failure National Registry (ADHERE). *J Am Coll Cardiol* 2005;46:57-64.
7. Cohn JN, Johnson G, Ziesche S, et al. A comparison of enalapril with hydralazine–isosorbide dinitrate in the treatment of chronic congestive heart failure. *N Engl J Med* 1991;325(5):303-310.
8. The SOLVD Investigators. Effect of enalapril on survival in patients with reduced left ventricular ejection fractions and congestive heart failure. *N Engl J Med* 1991;325:293-302.
9. The CONSENSUS Trial Study Group. Effects of enalapril on mortality in severe congestive heart failure. Results of the Cooperative North Scandinavian Enalapril Survival Study (CONSENSUS). *N Engl J Med* 1987;316:1429-1435.
10. Pfeffer MA, Braunwald E, Moyé LA, et al. Effect of captopril on mortality and morbidity in patients with left ventricular dysfunction after myocardial infarction. Results of the survival and ventricular enlargement trial. The SAVE Investigators. *N Engl J Med* 1992;327:669-677.
11. Køber L, Torp-Pedersen C, Carlsen JE, et al. A clinical trial of the angiotensin-converting-enzyme inhibitor trandolapril in patients with left ventricular dysfunction after myocardial infarction. Trandolapril Cardiac Evaluation (TRACE) Study Group. *N Engl J Med* 1995;333:1670-1676.
12. The Acute Infarction Ramipril Efficacy (AIRE) Study Investigators. Effect of ramipril on mortality and morbidity of survivors of acute myocardial infarction with clinical evidence of heart failure. *Lancet* 1993;342:821-828.
13. Cohn JN, Tognoni G. A randomized trial of the angiotensin-receptor blocker valsartan in chronic heart failure. *N Engl J Med* 2001;345(23):1667-1675.
14. Pfeffer MA, Swedberg K, Granger CB, et al. Effects of candesartan on mortality and morbidity in patients with chronic heart failure: the CHARM-Overall programme. *Lancet* 2003;362(9386):759-766.
15. Pfeffer MA, McMurray JJ, Velazquez EJ, et al. Valsartan, captopril, or both in myocardial infarction complicated by heart failure, left ventricular dysfunction, or both. *N Engl J Med* 2003;349(20):1893-1906.
16. Packer M, Fowler MB, Roecker EB, et al. Effect of carvedilol on the morbidity of patients with severe chronic heart failure: results of the carvedilol prospective randomized cumulative survival (COPERNICUS) study. *Circulation* 2002;106(17):2194-2199.

17. Dargie HJ. Effect of carvedilol on outcome after myocardial infarction in patients with left-ventricular dysfunction: the CAPRICORN randomized trial. *Lancet* 2001;357:1385-1390.

18. Effect of metoprolol CR/XL in chronic heart failure: Metoprolol CR/XL Randomised Intervention Trial in Congestive Heart Failure (MERIT-HF). *Lancet* 1999;353:2001-2007.

19. A randomized trial of beta-blockade in heart failure. The Cardiac Insufficiency Bisoprolol Study (CIBIS). CIBIS Investigators and Committees. *Circulation* 1994;90:1765-1773.

20. The Cardiac Insufficiency Bisoprolol Study II (CIBIS-II): a randomised trial. *Lancet* 1999;353:9-13.

21. Pitt B, Zannad F, Remme WJ, et al. The effect of spironolactone on morbidity and mortality in patients with severe heart failure. Randomized Aldactone Evaluation Study Investigators. *N Engl J Med* 1999;341:709-717.

22. Pitt B, Remme W, Zannad F, et al. Eplerenone, a selective aldosterone blocker, in patients with left ventricular dysfunction after myocardial infarction. *N Engl J Med* 2003;348:1309-1321.

23. Cohn JN, Archibald DG, Ziesche S, et al. Effect of vasodilator therapy on mortality in chronic congestive heart failure. Results of a Veterans Administration Cooperative Study. *N Engl J Med* 1986;314:1547-1552.

24. Taylor AL, Ziesche S, Yancy C, et al. Combination of isosorbide dinitrate and hydralazine in blacks with heart failure. *N Engl J Med* 2004;351:2049-2057.

25. The Digitalis Investigation Group. The effect of digoxin on mortality and morbidity in patients with heart failure. *N Engl J Med* 1997;336(8):525-533.

26. Moss AJ, Hall WJ, Cannom DS, et al. Improved survival with an implanted defibrillator in patients with coronary disease at high risk for ventricular arrhythmia. Multicenter Automatic Defibrillator Implantation Trial Investigators. *N Engl J Med* 1996;335:1933-1940.

27. Moss AJ, Fadl Y, Zareba W, et al. Survival benefit with an implanted defibrillator in relation to mortality risk in chronic coronary heart disease. *Am J Cardiol* 2001;88:516-520.

28. Bardy GH, Lee KL, Mark DB, et al. Amiodarone or an implantable cardioverter-defibrillator for congestive heart failure. *N Engl J Med* 2005;352:225-237.

29. Bristow MR, Saxon LA, Boehmer J, et al. Cardiac-resynchronization therapy with or without an implantable defibrillator in advanced chronic heart failure. *N Engl J Med* 2004;350:2140-2150.

30. Cleland JG, Daubert JC, Erdmann N, et al. The effect of cardiac resynchronization on morbidity and mortality in heart failure. *N Engl J Med* 2005;352:1539-1549.

31. Moss AJ, Hall WJ, Cannom DS, et al. Cardiac-Resynchronization Therapy for the Prevention of Heart-Failure Events. *N Engl J Med* 2009;361(14):1329-1338.

32. Costanzo MR, Guglin ME, Saltzberg MT, et al. Ultrafiltration versus intravenous diuretics for patients hospitalized for acute decompensated heart failure. *J Am Coll Cardiol* 2007;49:675-683.

33. Rose EA, Gelijns AC, Moskowitz AJ, et al. Long-term mechanical left ventricular assistance for end-stage heart failure. *N Engl J Med* 2001;345:1435-1443.

34. Rogers JG, Butler J, Lansman SL, et al. Chronic mechanical circulatory support for inotrope-dependent heart failure patients who are not transplant candidates: results of the INTrEPID Trial. *J Am Coll Cardiol* 2007;50:741-747.

35. Slaughter MS, Rogers JG, Milano CA, et al. Advanced heart failure treated with continuous-flow left ventricular assist device. *N Engl J Med* 2009;361:2241-2251.

36. Levy WC, Mozaffarian D, Linker DT, et al. The Seattle Heart Failure Model: prediction of survival in heart failure. *Circulation* 2006;113:1424-1433.

37. Mozaffarian D, Anker SD, Anand I, et al. Prediction of mode of death in heart failure: the Seattle Heart Failure Model. *Circulation* 2007;116:392-398.

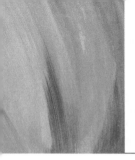

Evaluation and Management of Heart Failure with Preserved Ejection Fraction (Diastolic Heart Failure)

15

Ashwin Ravichandran and Gregory A. Ewald

GENERAL PRINCIPLES

- Heart failure (HF) is at epidemic levels in the United States. The societal and medical impact of this disorder is likely to continue to grow over the next several decades, given the increasing prevalence of diabetes and hypertension and the aging population.
- Early recognition and treatment of HF risk factors can curb the expected rise in HF incidence.
- A major contributor to the rise in HF hospitalizations has been HF with preserved left ventricular systolic function (HF-PSF), known as diastolic HF.

Definition

- Signs and symptoms of HF despite normal or near-normal ejection fraction, and evidence of diastolic dysfunction.
- Abnormal left ventricular (LV) filling and elevated filling pressures are the hallmark of this disease process.

Epidemiology

- More than 5 million people in the United States currently have HF, with an estimated 550,000 new diagnoses each year.
- Nearly 50% of patients with a diagnosis of HF, or hospitalized for acute HF, have preserved systolic function (PSF).
- Patients with HF-PSF are more likely to be elderly and/or female, and have hypertension or diabetes.
- Mean age of diagnosis is between 73 and 79 years.
- Patients with PSF were less likely to have a prior myocardial infarction (MI), and less likely to be on angiotensin-converting enzyme (ACE) inhibitor or angiotensin receptor blocker (ARB) therapy.
- Compared with patients with LV dysfunction, patients with PSF have nearly the same length of hospital stay, but a slightly lower hospital mortality (3% vs. 4%).[1]

Etiology

- The various etiologies of HF with PSF are depicted in Figure 15-1.[2]
- Hypertension: Over time, left ventricular hypertrophy (LVH) can develop and cause increased wall thickness and abnormal relaxation.
- Coronary artery disease (CAD): Akinetic myocardium causes decreased compliance during LV chamber filling. It also alters metabolic pathways necessary for myocyte relaxation.

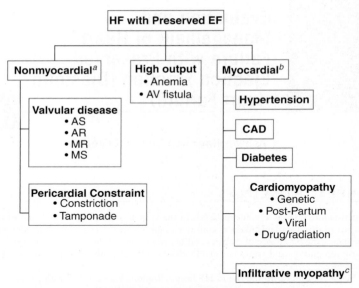

ᵃCause of HF or specific target for therapy
ᵇDisease process that may lead to HF
ᶜMay have stage in which EF is normal but often declines

FIGURE 15-1. Etiologies of heart failure with preserved EF. (From Lindenfeld J, Albert NM, Boehmer JP, et al. HFSA 2010 comprehensive heart failure practice guideline. Section II: evaluation and management of patients with heart failure and preserved left ventricular ejection fraction. *J Card Fail* 2010;16:e126-e133, with permission.)

- Diabetes mellitus: Causes microvascular disease leading to LV noncompliance during filling. It also leads to myocyte apoptosis and interstitial fibrosis.
- Restrictive/infiltrative cardiomyopathy (see the Special Considerations section).
- Hypertrophic cardiomyopathy (discussed in Chapter 16).
- Noncompaction cardiomyopathy.
- Pericardial disease: including tamponade and constriction (discussed in Chapter 17).
- Right HF due to pulmonary hypertension (discussed in Chapter 18).
- Congenital heart disease (discussed in Chapter 35).
- Valvular disease such as severe stenosis or regurgitation (discussed in Chapters 19 to 21).

Pathophysiology

- There is loss of normal relaxation patterns due to structural or functional abnormalities, causing increased filling pressures starting in the LV and eventually leading back to the left atrium (LA) and pulmonary vasculature.
- This is linked to abnormalities in myocyte relaxation, including calcium modulation, decreased availability of adenosine triphosphate (ATP), and increased intracellular glycolysis.
- There is upregulation of neurohormonal stimuli, including the renin–angiotensin–aldosterone system (RAAS) and the sympathetic nervous system.

- Relaxation is delayed or incomplete due to LVH or LV dyssynchrony, which will lead to early diastolic filling abnormalities.
- LV chamber dilation and restrictive/constrictive filling leading to late diastolic filling abnormalities.
- The LV chamber stiffness increased and there is decreased compliance from increased fibrosis/collagen deposition (from previous MI), infiltrative processes, LVH, and chamber dilation.
- This leads to a greater dependence on the late diastole since the initial LA-LV pressure gradient is less, and therefore a bigger reliance on atrial contraction.

Prevention

Prevention requires aggressive risk factor modification, including strict control of blood pressure, cholesterol levels, and glucose levels to prevent macrovascular and microvascular coronary disease.

Associated Conditions

- Because of increased atrial pressures, atrial arrhythmias are common. In advanced HF-PSF, the contribution of atrial systole is important, and atrial fibrillation can trigger HF symptoms quickly.
- With overlapping etiologies, renal insufficiency is common with HF-PSF.

DIAGNOSIS

Clinical Presentation

Clinical history and physical examination are described elsewhere (see Chapters 2, 5, and 14).

Diagnostic Criteria

- HF is a clinical diagnosis based on history, physical exam findings, and chest radiography. Although there are no universally agreed upon diagnostic criteria for HF, the Framingham criteria require two major or one major and two minor criteria:
  - **Major criteria**: paroxysmal nocturnal dyspnea (PND), jugular venous distention (JVD), crackles, cardiomegaly, pulmonary edema, S3, hepatojugular reflux (HJR), and weight loss with diuresis (>4.5 lb).
  - **Minor criteria**: lower extremity edema, nocturnal cough, dyspnea on exertion (DOE), hepatomegaly, pleural effusions, tachycardia, and decrease in vital capacity.
- The diagnosis of HF is further supported by laboratory values (elevated brain natriuretic factor [BNP]) and imaging studies (cardiac dysfunction on echocardiogram) as detailed in Figure 15-2.[2]
- A suggested diagnostic algorithm is presented in Figure 15-3.[2]

Differential Diagnosis

Other diseases that can mimic symptoms of HF: lung disease, thromboembolic disease, atrial arrhythmias, myocardial ischemia, obesity, pulmonary hypertension, valvular disorders, volume overload related to renal dysfunction, or increased afterload from hypertensive crisis (e.g., renovascular disease).[2,3]

Diagnostic Testing

Because macrovascular CAD is the most common etiology of all types of HF, an appropriate cardiac ischemia evaluation is an important first step in evaluating HF with PSF. This may include a combination of electrocardiogram, serum cardiac biomarkers, cardiac echocardiography (with and without stress), cardiac nuclear imaging (with and without stress), or cardiac catheterization.

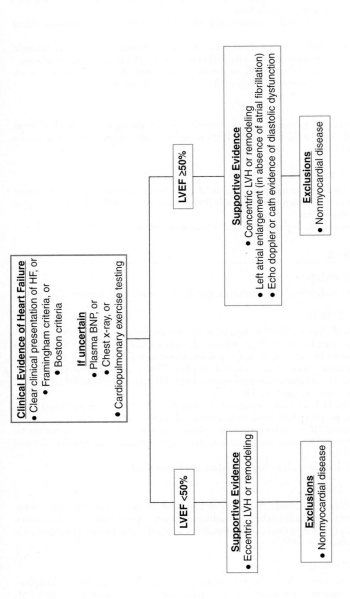

Clinical Evidence of Heart Failure
• Clear clinical presentation of HF, or
  • Framingham criteria, or
  • Boston criteria

If uncertain
  • Plasma BNP, or
  • Chest x-ray, or
• Cardiopulmonary exercise testing

LVEF <50%

Supportive Evidence
• Eccentric LVH or remodeling

Exclusions
• Nonmyocardial disease

LVEF ≥50%

Supportive Evidence
• Concentric LVH or remodeling
• Left atrial enlargement (in absence of atrial fibrillation)
• Echo doppler or cath evidence of diastolic dysfunction

Exclusions
• Nonmyocardial disease

Adapted from Yturralde FR et al. *Prog Cardiovasc Dis* 2005;47:314-319.

FIGURE 15-2. Diagnostic criteria for heart failure with preserved vs. decreased left ventricular ejection fraction. (From Lindenfeld J, Albert NM, Boehmer JP, et al. HFSA 2010 comprehensive heart failure practice guideline. Section II: evaluation and management of patients with heart failure and preserved left ventricular ejection fraction. *J Card Fail* 2010;16:e126-e133, with permission.)

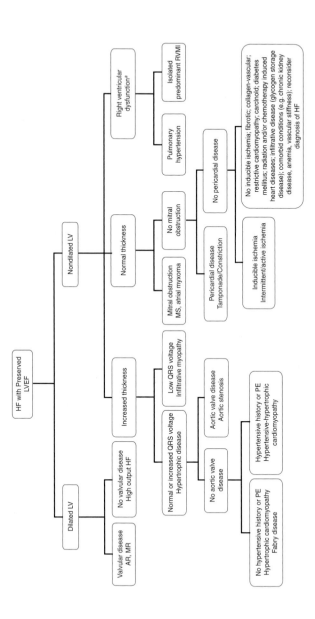

LVEF = left ventricular ejection fraction; HF = heart failure;
QRS = electrocardiographic ventricular depolarization; AR = aortic
Regurgitation; MR = mitral regurgitation; MS = mitral stenosis;
RVMI = right ventricular myocardial infarction; PE = pulmonary embolism.

aSome patients with right ventricular dysfunction
have LV dysfunction due to ventricular interaction

FIGURE 15-3. Diagnostic algorithm for heart failure with preserved systolic function. (From Lindenfeld J, Albert NM, Boehmer JP, et al. HFSA 2010 comprehensive heart failure practice guideline. Section II: evaluation and management of patients with heart failure and preserved left ventricular ejection fraction. *J Card Fail* 2010;16:e126-e133, with permission.)

Laboratories

- Brain natriuretic peptide:
  - BNP is usually elevated in HF with PSF, though not to the same degree as in systolic HF.
  - Can help distinguish from non-HF causes of symptoms.
  - BNP can falsely low in obese patients.[4,5]
- Other laboratory testing:
  - Blood glucose testing/HgbA1c for diabetes evaluation.
  - Iron studies: iron overload states including hemochromatosis, excessive transfusions.
  - Genetic testing is indicated if rare diseases such as storage disorders (see Restrictive Cardiomyopathy below).
  - Serum/urine protein electrophoresis: to evaluate for a protein gap that may indicate an overproduction and deposition process such as amyloidosis.
  - 5-Hydroxyindoleacetic acid (5-HIAA) testing if other features of carcinoid syndrome and tricuspid disease are present.

Electrocardiogram

- The ECG can provide clues to chamber enlargement and hypertrophy.
- It may provide evidence of ischemia and/or prior MI.
- Low voltage could indicate a restrictive process.

Imaging

- **Echocardiography**:
  - Assessment of systolic function, chamber sizes, and hypertrophy. Also, as mentioned previously, valvular dysfunction such as mitral regurgitation or aortic stenosis can lead to HF with PSF.
  - Regional wall motion abnormalities indicating ischemia and/or prior infarction can be identified.
  - LVH in the absence of a cause for pressure overload can indicate hypertrophic cardiomyopathy (see Chapter 16).
  - Infiltrative/restrictive processes can also be identified with features such as abnormal filling patterns and biatrial enlargement. LVH may be present.
  - Diastolic function is evaluated by using LV filling patterns through the mitral valve and tissue Doppler velocities at the mitral valve annulus (see Chapter 31).
- **Cardiac MRI** can be helpful in looking for infiltrative/restrictive, and constrictive processes (see Chapter 32).
- Other imaging such as renal ultrasound, MRA, or angiogram can be done if renal artery stenosis is under consideration. These may be especially helpful in patients with recurrent hypertensive crises.

Diagnostic Procedures

- **Cardiac catheterization**:
  - Left heart catheterization can be done as part of ischemic evaluation, as well as to measure LV end diastolic pressure (LVEDP).
  - Right heart catheterization to assess hemodynamics. Wedge pressure and/or LVEDP >15 mmHg indicates abnormally high filling pressures consistent with left heart disease/HF.
  - Simultaneous left and right heart catheterization can be done for hemodynamic evaluation as well as to assess for etiologies such as constrictive cardiomyopathy.
- **Endomyocardial biopsy** can identify pathologic changes, specifically for restrictive cardiomyopathies discussed below.

TREATMENT

- Unlike HF with decreased systolic function, there are very few clinical trials to direct optimal medical therapy in patients with HF with PSF.[3]
- No specific medications have been found to decrease morbidity and mortality from HF with PSF.
- Therapy is directed at symptom control, BP and dietary monitoring, and any possible underlying etiologies such as ischemia or restrictive/infiltrative processes. BP goal of <130/80 mmHg may be warranted.[3]

Medications

- **Loop diuretics** are used for volume control and maintenance of euvolemia.[2,3] Thiazide diuretics can help with volume, but is generally reserved more for treating hypertension.
- **ACE inhibitors and ARBs** are recommended in patients with history of CAD or those with coronary risk factors including diabetes.[3]
  - The HOPE study demonstrated that in a patient aged >55 years with documented vascular disease or multiple coronary risk factors, **ramipril** reduced the annual risk of developing HF by 23% and by 33% in those with systolic blood pressure (SBP) >139 mmHg.[6]
  - CHARM-Preserved trial demonstrated that **candesartan** therapy in patients with New York Heart Association (NYHA) class II to IV HF with LVEF >40% showed a trend toward the primary endpoint of reduced hospitalizations and cardiovascular death (adjusted hazard ratio of 0.86, with confidence interval 0.74 to 1.00, $p = 0.051$). This was driven largely by a reduction in hospitalization. Blood pressure was, not surprisingly, also improved in the candesartan group.[7]
  - The I-PRESERVE trial randomized over 4,000 patients older than 60 years with NYHA class II to IV symptoms and EF >45% to **irbesartan** or placebo. Overall rates of death and hospitalization were not different between the two groups, with hazard ratios of 0.95 to 1.00, not reaching statistical significance.[8]
- **β-Blockers are recommended in those with prior MI or atrial fibrillation.**[3]
  - No studies to date demonstrate clear mortality benefit in those without compelling indications.[9]
  - A small prospective cohort suggests a possible reduction in number of hospitalizations of patients with diastolic dysfunction and stable CAD who were using β-blockers.[10]
  - More rapid heart rates result in decreased contractile force, less diastolic filling time, and increased resting wall tension due to incomplete reuptake of calcium.
  - If rate control is necessary the goal resting rate is approximately 60.
- **Calcium channel blockers are recommended in those with symptom-limiting angina or atrial fibrillation requiring rate control and have intolerance to β-blockers.**[3] In addition to decreasing heart rate, can facilitate calcium signaling to decrease wall tension ("lusitropic effect").

Other Nonpharmacologic Therapies

- Restoration of sinus rhythm is of potential benefit.[2]
  - When loss of atrial contribution occurs, LV filling in an already noncompliant heart becomes even worse. Combined with the predisposition to tachycardia, sinus rhythm is theorized to be of benefit.
  - Consider in patients who are still symptomatic despite adequate rate control.
  - There are no randomized trials looking at symptomatic patients.
  - Amiodarone and dofetilide have been shown to increase conversion to and maintenance of sinus rhythm in HF patients.
  - Early experience with catheter ablation also suggests improvement in symptoms for HF patients.

Lifestyle Modifications

- Low sodium diet.
- Exercise as tolerated.
- Blood pressure monitoring.

SPECIAL CONSIDERATIONS

Restrictive Cardiomyopathy

- Restrictive cardiomyopathies are characterized by a rigid myocardium and poor ventricular filling.
- Pericardial disease can present similarly but have a considerably different prognosis and treatment (Chapter 17).
- MRI is a useful diagnostic imaging tool for diagnosis, with characteristic findings that can be specific for the disease state (Chapter 32).
- **Amyloidosis**:
  - Normal myocardial contractile elements are replaced by interstitial deposits, causing restriction.
  - There are many types of amyloidosis but cardiac involvement is seen most commonly in primary amyloidosis.
  - Amyloid deposits are seen histologically as insoluble amyloid fibrils in all chambers of the heart (Congo red stain).
  - Amyloid deposits found in the conduction system result in cardiac arrhythmias.
  - ECG classically shows low voltage with poor R-wave progression.
  - Echocardiographic findings characteristic of cardiac amyloidosis include a granular, sparkling appearance of thickened ventricular walls and significant biatrial enlargement.
  - The degree of wall thickness predicts survival; patients with normal wall thickness have a median survival of 2.4 years, and those with markedly increased wall thickness have an average survival of <6 months.[11]
- **Sarcoidosis**:
  - Cardiac involvement occurs in 5% of all sarcoid patients.
  - Myocardial restriction results from patchy scar formation around infiltrating, noncaseating granulomas.
  - Most common manifestation of cardiac sarcoid is conduction system disease, with the most dramatic presentations being sudden cardiac death due to ventricular tachyarrhythmias or high-degree heart block.
- **Hemochromatosis**:
  - Restriction is secondary to abnormal iron metabolism and myocardial iron deposition.
  - It may be primary, due to an autosomal recessive genetic abnormality, or secondary, due to iron overload.
  - Presents with diabetes, skin discoloration, and diastolic dysfunction.
  - Workup includes iron studies, with an elevated transferrin saturation being most suggestive, followed by biopsy of an accessible organ (often the liver).
  - Treatment of underlying disease is of utmost importance to prevent progression of disease, which includes phlebotomy and chelation therapy.
- **Hypereosinophilic syndrome** (Löffler endocarditis, parietalis fibroblastica):
  - This syndrome results in an obliterative, restrictive cardiomyopathy thought to result from toxic damage from the intracytoplasmic granular content of activated eosinophils.
  - It occurs in temperate climates and is associated with a hypereosinophilic syndrome.
  - Patients have endocardial thickening and obliteration of the cardiac apex.
  - It is usually an aggressive disease, more common in men than in women.
  - Corticosteroids and cytotoxic drugs in the early phase of disease may improve symptoms and survival.

- **Idiopathic restrictive cardiomyopathy**:
  - Idiopathic restrictive cardiomyopathy is characterized by a mild-to-moderate increase in cardiac weight.
  - Biatrial enlargement occurs commonly, with a 10% incidence of atrial appendage thrombi.
  - Patchy endocardial fibrosis is present and may extend into the conduction system, resulting in complete heart block.
- **Gaucher disease** is an autosomal recessive disease produced by mutations of the glucocerebrosidase gene that result in the accumulation of the lipid glucocerebroside in the heart.
- **Hurler syndrome** (a form of mucopolysaccharidosis type I) is an autosomal recessive genetic disorder caused by a mutation in the chromosome pair responsible for producing α-L-iduronidase, resulting in a mucopolysaccharide accumulation in the heart.
- **Carcinoid heart disease**:
  - Results from untreated carcinoid syndrome, where lesion formation correlates with the concentration of serotonin and 5-HIAA.
  - Lesions predominantly in the right ventricular (RV) endocardium, where tricuspid insufficiency is prominent. Tricuspid and pulmonic stenoses can also be seen.
  - Occasionally left-sided valvular lesions can be seen in patients with either pulmonary metastases or a patent foramen ovale (or other intracardiac shunt).

OUTCOME/PROGNOSIS

- HF with PSF has a fairly similar prognosis to systolic HF.[12,13] However, a recent individual patient data meta-analysis (including more than 10,000 with PSF) suggests that survival is better in those with PSF (3-year mortality about 25% vs. approximately 32% for those with reduced LVEF).[14]
- Many factors appear to alter prognosis in an individual patient, such as HF symptoms (NYHA class), laboratory tests (troponin, BNP, sodium, hemoglobin, creatinine), cardiac physiology (e.g., LVEF, diastolic function, pulmonary pressures, and wedge pressure), HF etiology (ischemic vs. nonischemic), associated conditions (e.g., atrial fibrillation, renal insufficiency), medication and device therapy, and age.[1]
- The Seattle HF model is a comprehensive risk-prediction tool for assessing survival probability in a given individual. A user-friendly calculator for the Seattle HF model is available on the web at http://depts.washington.edu/shfm/index.php (last accessed 6/11/13).
- Risk-stratification of patients with HF is useful to direct the aggressiveness of therapy and to guide discussions with patients and their families.

REFERENCES

1. Yancy CW, Lopatin M, Stevenson LW, et al. Clinical presentation, management, and in-hospital outcomes of patients admitted with acute decompensated heart failure with preserved systolic function: a report from the Acute Decompensated Heart Failure National Registry (ADHERE) Database. *J Am Coll Cardiol* 2006;47:76-84.
2. Hunt SA, Abraham WT, Chin MH, et al. 2009 Focused update incorporated into the ACC/AHA 2005 Guidelines for the Diagnosis and Management of Heart Failure in Adults A Report of the American College of Cardiology Foundation/American Heart Association Task Force on Practice Guidelines Developed. *J Am Coll Cardiol* 2009;119:e391-e479.
3. Lindenfeld J, Albert NM, Boehmer JP, et al. HFSA 2010 comprehensive heart failure practice guideline. Section II: evaluation and management of patients with heart failure and preserved left ventricular ejection fraction. *J Card Fail* 2010;16:e126-e133.
4. Anjan VY, Loftus TM, Burke MA, et al. Prevalence, clinical phenotype, and outcomes associated with normal B-type natriuretic peptide levels in heart failure with preserved ejection fraction. *Am J Cardiol* 2012;110:870-879.
5. Khan AM, Cheng S, Magnusson M, et al. Cardiac natriuretic peptides, obesity, and insulin resistance: evidence from two community-based studies. *J Clin Endocrinol Metab* 2011;96:3242-3249.

6. Arnold JM, Yusuf S, Young J, et al. Prevention of heart failure in patients in the Heart Outcomes Prevention Evaluation (HOPE) study. *Circulation* 2003;107:1284-1290.

7. Yusuf, Pfeffer MA, Swedber K, et al. Effects of candesartan in patients with chronic heart failure and preserved left-ventricular ejection fraction: the CHARM-Preserved Trial. *Lancet* 2003;362:777-781.

8. Massie BM, Carson PE, McMurray JJ, et al. Irbesartan in patients with heart failure and preserved ejection fraction. *N Engl J Med* 2008;359:2456-2467.

9. Clinical effectiveness of beta-blockers in heart failure: findings from the OPTIMIZE-HF (Organized Program to Initiate Lifesaving Treatment in Hospitalized Patients with Heart Failure) Registry. *J Am Coll Cardiol* 2009;53:184-192.

10. Smith DT, Farzaneh-Far R, Ali S, et al. Relation of beta-blocker use with frequency of hospitalization for heart failure in patients with left ventricular diastolic dysfunction (from the Heart and Soul Study). *Am J Cardiol* 2010;105:223-228.

11. Cueto-Garcia L, Reeder GS, Kyle RA, et al. Echocardiographic findings in systemic amyloidosis: spectrum of cardiac involvement and relation to survival. *J Am Coll Cardiol* 1985;6:737-743.

12. Bhatia RS, Tu JV, Lee DS, et al. Outcome of heart failure with preserved ejection fraction in a population-based study. *N Engl J Med* 2006;355:260-269.

13. Owan TE, Hodge DO, Herge RM, et al. Trends in prevalence and outcome of heart failure with preserved ejection fraction. *N Engl J Med* 2006;355:251-259.

14. Meta-analysis Global Group in Chronic Heart Failure (MAGGIC). The survival of patients with heart failure with preserved or reduced left ventricular ejection fraction: an individual patient data meta-analysis. *Eur Heart J* 2012;33:1750-1757.

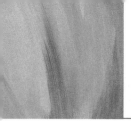

Hypertrophic Cardiomyopathy

16

Shimoli Shah and Keith Mankowitz

GENERAL PRINCIPLES

- Hypertrophic cardiomyopathy (HCM) is **the most common heritable cardiac disease** and is transmitted in an autosomal dominant fashion.
- The prevalence of HCM is approximately 1 in 500 and is caused by one of more than 400 **mutations in at least 13 genes** encoding proteins of the cardiac sarcomere.[1]
- Mutations of β-myosin heavy-chain, cardiac troponin T, and myosin-binding protein C are the most common. The various sarcomeric mutations result in **inappropriate myocardial hypertrophy, most commonly of the interventricular septum**.
- The clinical picture of HCM varies considerably and can be associated with chest pain, shortness of breath, syncope or no symptoms at all. It is the most common cause of **sudden death among young athletes in the United States**.[1]
- Summary of management of HCM:
  ○ Control symptoms.
  ○ Avoid strenuous exertion.
  ○ Screen for risk factors for sudden death and consider a prophylactic ICD in high-risk patients.
  ○ Screen first-degree relatives.

Definition

- A characteristic feature of HCM is **left ventricular (LV) wall thickening in the absence of a cardiac or systemic cause** (e.g., aortic stenosis or hypertension). The usual clinical diagnostic criterion for HCM is **maximal LV wall thickness >15 mm**.
- Dynamic obstruction of blood exiting the heart can occur, as the aortic outflow tract is geometrically narrowed due to the thick septum and an elongated mitral valve apparatus causing **systolic anterior motion (SAM)** and **mitral regurgitation**. This dynamic process of LV outflow tract (LVOT) obstruction is present in approximately one-third of patients at rest and another third with provocation.

Classification

- It is important to distinguish between the **obstructive or nonobstructive forms** of HCM via 2D echocardiography. A **subaortic gradient ≥30 mmHg** reflects a true mechanical impedance to outflow.
- Obstruction can be **subaortic** (caused by SAM) or **midcavity** (due to a hypertrophy of the basal portion of the septum and small outflow tract).
- In patients with no obstruction at rest, provocative maneuvers such as exercise or the Valsalva maneuver should be performed to identify latent obstruction.
- The pattern of hypertrophy in HCM is asymmetric and can involve any portion of the ventricular septum or LV free wall. Thickening confined to the most distal portion

of LV chamber (apical HCM) is a morphologic form often associated with a "spade" deformity of the left ventricle and marked T-wave negativity on the electrocardiogram and most commonly found in Japanese populations.

Epidemiology

- The prevalence of HCM in the adult general population is 1:500. It is the most common genetic cardiovascular disease.
- HCM is transmitted as an **autosomal dominant** trait and mutations in at least 13 different genes have been associated with the condition.
- Phenotypic expression of HCM is variable and **not all individuals with a genetic defect will manifest clinical signs of HCM**.

Etiology and Pathology

- HCM is a primary disorder of the sarcomere.
- Phenotypic expression of HCM is variable and depends on a complex interplay of genetic, environmental, and molecular factors. Myocytes of involved cardiac tissue in HCM show bizarre shapes and disorganized patterns. There is often replacement fibrosis in the interstitium of the myocardium.
- Coronary arteries in patients with HCM can have thickened walls with abnormal function.

Pathophysiology

- LVOT obstruction is produced by SAM of the mitral valve and/or midsystolic contact with the ventricular septum.
- SAM is felt to be a result of a combination of the Venturi phenomenon (high-velocity LV ejection jet pulls the mitral leaflet toward the septum), drag effect (a pushing force of flow directly on the leaflets), and intrinsic abnormalities of the mitral valve.
- **Obstruction can be dynamic** and reduced by maneuvers that decrease myocardial contractility and increase ventricular volume; and increased by maneuvers that reduce ventricular volume or increase myocardial contractility.

Prevention

All patients with a first-degree family member with HCM are at risk and should undergo surveillance screening (see below).

DIAGNOSIS

History

- The majority of patients with HCM are **asymptomatic**.
- The most commonly reported symptom is **dyspnea** secondary to elevated LV diastolic filling pressures and diastolic dysfunction.
- Other symptoms include **angina** (from myocardial oxygen mismatch due to increased myocardial mass, small-vessel disease, or wall stress), **syncope** (due to LVOT obstruction or arrhythmias), and **arrhythmia** (manifesting as palpitations, syncope, or sudden death).

Physical Examination

- A classic finding on auscultation is a **crescendo-decrescendo ejection systolic murmur** (ESM) audible in at least two-thirds of patients with HCM, best heard along the left sternal border but may be heard throughout the precordium.

- The **murmur intensifies** with maneuvers that decrease preload, like standing and the Valsalva maneuver. Exertion, such as having the patient squat 10 times or a brisk short walk, is useful to provoke the ESM.
- Conversely, the **murmur decreases** in intensity with squatting (which increases preload and afterload) and handgrip (which increases afterload). This type of dynamic murmur should not be attributed to a benign flow murmur and should be evaluated further with an echocardiogram.
- The carotid pulse typically rises briskly and then declines in midsystole as the gradient develops, followed by a secondary rise.
- The jugular venous pulse may demonstrate a prominent wave secondary to diminished ventricular compliance.
- Amyl nitrite decreases systemic vascular resistance and decreases LV volume, which increases the murmur of HCM.

Diagnostic Criteria

HCM can be diagnosed by a combination of physical examination, ECG, imaging techniques including echocardiography and magnetic resonance imaging (MRI), cardiac catheterization, and genetic testing.

Diagnostic Testing

Laboratories
- Genetic testing can be done to assess the proband and screen family members.
- Thirteen genes with multiple mutations have been discovered to date. Approximately 60% to 70% of HCM patients will be found to have mutations.
- Specific HCM phenotypes may be associated with higher prevalence of genetic mutations. Eight percent of the sigmoid morphology (with a prominent basal septal bulge) had a genetic mutation as opposed to 79% of the reverse curve (predominant mid septal thickening).[2]

Electrocardiography
- The ECG is usually abnormal in HCM patients; however, at least 10% of patients with HCM may have a normal ECG.
- **No particular ECG pattern is classic for HCM**. ST segment and T wave abnormalities are the most common, followed by evidence of LV hypertrophy.
- Prominent Q waves in the inferior leads, precordial leads, or both can occur in up to 50% of patients.
- Negative T waves in the mid-precordial leads are characteristic of apical HCM.

Imaging
- **Echocardiography is diagnostic for HCM**. Wall thickness, mitral valve abnormalities including elongated leaflets, mitral regurgitation, and LVOT obstruction can be accurately assessed.
- **MRI** has similar diagnostic capabilities as echocardiography and is particularly useful when echo images are suboptimal. It can also assess the presence of myocardial fibrosis (by gadolinium enhancement).

Diagnostic Procedures

- **Cardiac catheterization** is useful to quantify the LVOT obstruction and LV pressures.
- Most symptomatic patients with HCM complain of angina or chest pain. Left heart catheterization can rule out epicardial coronary artery disease as a cause for angina.

TREATMENT

The majority of patients with HCM have no or mild symptoms and do not require treatment. For symptomatic patients, the majority can be managed medically without the need for interventional procedures.

Medications

- **β-Blockers are usually the first-line drugs** and are useful to treat angina and palpitations. Shortness of breath due to dynamic LVOT gradients respond well to β-blockade.[1,3,4]
- **Calcium channel blockers** are useful for treating angina. They should be avoided in patients with evidence of elevated filling pressures and significant LVOT gradients.[1,3,5-7]
- **Disopyramide**, a class I antiarrhythmic drug, is a potent negative inotrope that reduces the LVOT gradient. Up to 70% of patients with symptomatic hypertrophic obstructive cardiomyopathy respond favorably to disopyramide. It should be initiated in hospital with telemetry monitoring. Disopyramide is usually combined with a β-blocker.[1,3,8]
- **Diuretics** are the best drugs to reduce high filling pressures and treat diastolic heart failure. They should be used cautiously because of a **potential to cause hypotension**.
- **Nitrates** are useful to relieve angina. They should be used cautiously because of the **potential to cause hypotension**. Transdermal nitrates, including nitro paste or a nitro patch, are probably the best route to deliver this class of drug.

Surgical Management

- **Myectomy** should be performed in patients with severely limiting symptoms refractory to medical therapy and a significant LVOT gradient (>50 mmHg) at rest or with physiologic provocation.[3,9-11]
- The procedure should be performed by an experienced surgeon.
- Myectomy is the gold standard for septal reduction treatment. There is over 45 years of experience, a low operative mortality (less than 1% to 2%), permanent reduction of LVOT obstruction, substantial reduction in heart failure symptoms, and possible evidence of decreased mortality over longer term follow up.
- **Alcohol septal ablation** is reserved for patients who have severe symptoms (New York Heart Association [NYHA] class III or IV) refractory to all medications and a LVOT gradient of 50 mmHg at rest or with provocation. Recovery time is less than surgical myectomy.[3,12]
- Alcohol ablation is associated with increased conduction abnormalities and a higher post-intervention LVOT gradient compared to surgical myectomy.
- The choice of treatment strategy should be made after a thorough discussion of the procedures with the individual patient.[3,13]

Lifestyle/Risk Modification

- Activity restriction is discussed below.
- Syncope in patients with HCM should be reported promptly, as it may represent aborted sudden cardiac arrest.
- The risk of transmitting the gene to children is approximately 50%.
- First-degree relatives should be screened with an echocardiogram and if possible genetic testing.

Activity

- HCM is the **most common cause of sudden death in athletes aged <35 years**.
- All patients with HCM should be advised to **avoid sports and activities involving burst exertion** such as basketball, football, hockey, and soccer. Exertion can trigger fatal arrhythmias in HCM patients.
- Patients can walk, jog, or ride a bike as long as they do so at a low workload, slow pace, and can speak in full sentences.

SPECIAL CONSIDERATIONS

- All patients with a first-degree family member with HCM should undergo a history and physical examination, 12-lead ECG, and 2D echo.
- Adolescents aged between 12 and 18 should have yearly evaluations as the phenotypic expression of HCM usually manifests some time during the teenage years.
- Adults (aged >18 years) with affected family members should undergo screening with echocardiography every 5 years due to the variable phenotypic expression of HCM which can be delayed for several decades.
- The utility of genetic testing in HCM is limited by the genetic heterogeneity, expense, and limited availability (see below).
- A genetic councilor can play an important role in helping patients and families cope with diognostic testing, family screening and other legal, ethical and social implications of having the diagnosis of HCM.

COMPLICATIONS

- Patients with HCM may be at **increased risk of sudden death** due to abnormal myocardial substrate (ischemia, fibrosis, necrosis, and abnormal myocytes). The risk of each individual patient should be assessed at every visit. One risk factor may be sufficient to recommend an internal cardiac defibrillator (ICD).
- **Risk factors for sudden death include**[1,14]:
  - Prior cardiac arrest.
  - Family history of sudden death.
  - Unexplained syncope particularly in young patients or when exertional and recurrent.
  - LV thickness >30 mm.
  - LVOT obstruction.[15]
  - Frequent runs of nonsustained ventricular tachycardia.
  - Abnormal blood pressure response during exercise.
- Approximately 5% of patients with HCM develop LV dilatation and LV systolic dysfunction. These patients have a poor prognosis and should be treated with drugs similar to other patients with dilated cardiomyopathy including angiotensin-converting enzyme (ACE) inhibitors.

REFERRAL

HCM patients should be managed by a cardiologist familiar with the disease.

PATIENT EDUCATION

- Time should be spent explaining HCM to patients and their families.
- The HCM associates can provide further education and advice; HCM is a useful resource for patients (www.4hcm.org, last accessed 6/21/13).

MONITORING/FOLLOW-UP

Patients should be seen at least every 6 months and a screening Holter should be done yearly. Periodic echocardiograms are appropriate as well. Family screening (1st degree relatives) is warranted.

OUTCOME/PROGNOSIS

There are some high-risk patients who have a mortality of 4% to 6% per year, but the prognosis of most HCM patients is excellent.[1] Studies done in communities demonstrate a similar mortality to age-matched population in low-risk HCM patients.

REFERENCES

1. Nishimura RA, Holmes DR Jr. Clinical practice. Hypertrophic obstructive cardiomyopathy. *N Engl J Med* 2004;350:1320-1327.
2. Binder J, Ommen SR, Gersh BJ, et al. Echocardiography-guided genetic testing in hypertrophic cardiomyopathy: septal morphological features predict the presence of myofilament mutations. *Mayo Clin Proc* 2006;81:459-467.
3. Maron BJ, McKenna WJ, Danielson GK, et al. American College of Cardiology/European Society of Cardiology clinical expert consensus document on hypertrophic cardiomyopathy. *J Am Coll Cardiol* 2003;42:1687-1713.
4. Nistri S, Olivotto I, Maron MS, et al. β Blockers for prevention of exercise-induced left ventricular outflow tract obstruction in patients with hypertrophic cardiomyopathy. *Am J Cardiol* 2012;110:715-719.
5. Bonow RO, Dilsizian V, Rosing DR, et al. Verapamil-induced improvement in left ventricular diastolic filling and increased exercise tolerance in patients with hypertrophic cardiomyopathy: short- and long-term effects. *Circulation* 1985;72:853-864.
6. Rosing DR, Idänpään-Heikkilä U, Maron BJ, et al. Use of calcium-channel blocking drugs in hypertrophic cardiomyopathy. *Am J Cardiol* 1985;55:185B-195B.
7. Gilligan DM, Chan WL, Joshi J, et al. A double-blind, placebo-controlled crossover trial of nadolol and verapamil in mild and moderately symptomatic hypertrophic cardiomyopathy. *J Am Coll Cardiol* 1993;21:1672-1679.
8. Sherrid MV, Barac I, McKenna WJ, et al. Multicenter study of the efficacy and safety of disopyramide in obstructive hypertrophic cardiomyopathy. *J Am Coll Cardiol* 2005;45:1251-1258.
9. Ommen SR, MAron BJ, Olivotto I, et al. Long-term effects of surgical septal myectomy on survival in patients with obstructive hypertrophic cardiomyopathy. *J Am Coll Cardiol* 2005;46:470-476.
10. Woo A, Williams WG, Choi R, et al. Clinical and echocardiographic determinants of long-term survival after surgical myectomy in obstructive hypertrophic cardiomyopathy. *Circulation* 2005;111:2033-2041.
11. Orme NM, Sarajja P, Dearani JA, et al. Comparison of surgical septal myectomy to medical therapy alone in patients with hypertrophic cardiomyopathy and syncope. *Am J Cardiol* 2013;111:388-392.
12. Nagueh SF, Groves BM, Schwartz L, et al. Alcohol septal ablation for the treatment of hypertrophic obstructive cardiomyopathy. A multicenter North American registry. *J Am Coll Cardiol* 2011;58:2322-2328.
13. Agarwal S, Tuzcu EM, Desai MY, et al. Updated meta-analysis of septal alcohol ablation versus myectomy for hypertrophic cardiomyopathy. *J Am Coll Cardiol* 2010;55:823-834.
14. Frenneaux MP. Assessing the risk of sudden cardiac death in a patient with hypertrophic cardiomyopathy. *Heart* 2004;90:570-575.
15. Maron MS, Olivotto I, Betocchi S, et al. Effect of left ventricular outflow tract obstruction on clinical outcome in hypertrophic cardiomyopathy. *N Engl J Med* 2003;348:295-303.

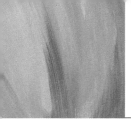

Diseases of the Pericardium

Jeremiah P. Depta and Craig K. Reiss

17

Introduction

- The pericardium is a fibrous sac surrounding the heart consisting of two layers:
  - Visceral pericardium which is a thin inner layer attached to the epicardium.
  - Parietal pericardium which is an outer layer of thicker connective tissue.
- The layers are separated by the pericardial space, which normally contains 15 to 50 mL of fluid.
- Pericardial fluid consists of an ultrafiltrate continuously produced from the mesothelial cells of the visceral pericardium and is resorbed via lymphatics and venules.
- Although it is not absolutely essential for cardiac performance, several functions have been attributed to the pericardium:
  - Tethering of the heart within the mediastinum.
  - Lubrication of the movements of the heart.
  - Augmentation of diastolic function.
  - Serving as a barrier to infection and inflammation.
  - Participation in autonomic reflexes and paracrine signaling.

Acute Pericarditis

GENERAL PRINCIPLES

- Acute pericarditis is the most common pericardial syndrome, caused by inflammation of the pericardium resulting in characteristic clinical features.
- Some clinicians prefer the term "myopericarditis," due to associated inflammation of the adjacent myocardium.[1]

Classification
- Pericarditis can be classified as acute or recurrent.
- Recurrent pericarditis can occur after the resolution of the inciting cause of an acute attack.

Epidemiology
- The exact incidence and prevalence are unknown.
- It is diagnosed in 1 out of every 1,000 hospital admissions.[1]

Etiology
- Table 17-1 lists the most common causes of acute pericarditis.
- **Idiopathic is the most common cause.**

TABLE 17-1	ETIOLOGIES OF ACUTE PERICARDITIS

- Infectious
  - Viral (coxsackie, echovirus, Epstein–Barr virus, HIV)
  - Tuberculosis
  - Lyme disease
  - Miscellaneous (other viral, bacterial, fungal, parasitic)
- Uremia
- Connective tissue disease
- Myocardial infarction, acute or subacute (Dressler syndrome)
- Post-cardiac surgery
- Trauma
- Cancer, chemotherapy, radiation
- Drugs (hydralazine, procainamide, isoniazid, phenytoin, penicillin)
- Hypothyroidism
- Idiopathic

- Diagnostic work-up for the cause of acute pericarditis rarely establishes a specific diagnosis.
- Some idiopathic causes may actually represent postviral causes.
- **Viral infections** represent the next most cause of acute pericarditis.
  - Patients typically will have upper respiratory tract symptoms prior to presentation.
  - Coxsackie and echoviruses are the most common viral agents.
- **Autoimmune** phenomena collectively represent a major cause of acute pericarditis, including connective tissue disease, drug-induced, postpericardiotomy, and Dressler syndrome.
- **Uremic** pericarditis occurs in one-third of patients with chronic uremia.
  - It is typically associated with a pericardial effusion.
  - It is associated with higher levels of azotemia (BUN > 60 mg/dL).
- **Tuberculous** or **HIV**-associated pericarditis should be suspected in high-risk patients (history of exposure, immunocompromised state).
- Pericarditis **after acute myocardial infarction** (AMI).
  - Post-MI pericarditis presents in the first few days up through 6 weeks after an infarct, often secondary to local pericardial irritation.
  - Dressler syndrome is a type of postinfarction pericarditis that occurs 1 to 8 weeks after the infarct. It occurs in 1% of patients after AMI and is thought to be immune-mediated.

DIAGNOSIS

Clinical Presentation

History
- Typically patients will present with recent-onset chest discomfort.
- The discomfort is described as:
  - Sharp pain.
  - Retrosternal or left-sided.

- ○ Radiation to the back, neck, and shoulders.
- ○ Pain along the trapezius ridge is classic for pericarditis and uncommon in ischemic disease.
- ○ Pleuritic in some cases, which can be associated with dyspnea.
- ○ May be worsened with swallowing.
- Classically, the pain will improve when the patient leans forward and worsen when the patient is supine.
- It is important to ask the patient about any fevers, chills, shaking, lethargy, myalgias, or upper respiratory symptoms which help to determine if an infectious etiology is suspected.
- In patients with suspected autoimmune disorders, it is key to also ask about arthralgias including morning stiffness, skin changes, Raynaud phenomenon, abdominal pain, and neuropathy.

Physical Examination

- Physical examination of patients with acute pericarditis is unimpressive unless a pathognomonic pericardial friction rub is present.
- A **pericardial friction rub** is:
  - ○ Caused by friction between the inflamed visceral and parietal pericardia.
  - ○ Described as high-pitched, grating, or scratching.
  - ○ Classically has three components per cardiac cycle (i.e., ventricular systole, early diastole, and atrial systole) but usually only one or two components are present.
  - ○ Often fleeting and dynamic.
  - ○ Best heard by placing the diaphragm of the stethoscope at the left lower sternal border while the patient is leaning forward.

Diagnostic Criteria

To diagnose acute pericarditis, at least two of the four symptoms should be present:
- Typical chest pain.
- Pericardial friction rub.
- Suggestive ECG changes.
- New or worsening pericardial effusion.

Differential Diagnosis

- Acute pericarditis-type chest discomfort can mimic several disease including:
  - ○ Acute coronary syndrome (ACS).
  - ○ Aortic dissection.
  - ○ Pulmonary embolism.
  - ○ Pneumonia.
  - ○ Pneumothorax.
- It can be difficult to differentiate pericarditis from ACS.

Diagnostic Testing

Laboratories

- Laboratory tests may reveal nonspecific markers of inflammation such as an elevated erythrocyte sedimentation rate (ESR), C-reactive protein (CRP), or leukocytosis.
- Serum cardiac enzymes (troponin or CK-MB) are often slightly elevated due to inflammation of the adjacent myocardium.
- More specific tests, such as antinuclear antibody (ANA), rheumatoid factor, thyroid function, tuberculin testing, blood or viral cultures, and cytology, should be ordered based on the clinical scenario.

Electrocardiography

- ECG changes are present in most cases, but its absence does not exclude pericarditis (Figure 17-1).
- Serial ECGs during the initial hours to days of acute pericarditis reveal a characteristic evolution present in about 60% of patients:
  - Stage 1: Diffuse concave ST-segment elevation and PR depression in all leads except aVR. Also, helpful is concomitant ST depression and PR elevation in lead aVR.
  - Stage 2: Normalized ST segments with decreasing or flattened T-waves.
  - Stage 3: T-wave inversion.
  - Stage 4: ECG normalization.
- Stage 1 is highly specific and diagnostic for acute pericarditis.

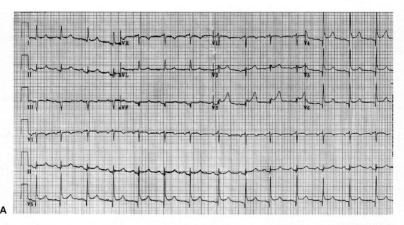

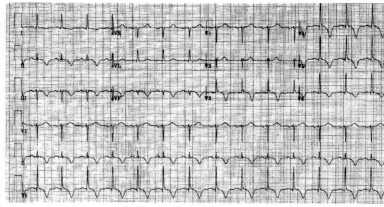

FIGURE 17-1. ECG in pericarditis. **A:** Stage 1 pericarditis, exhibiting diffuse concave ST-segment elevations and PR depression except in aVR, where the abnormalities are reversed. **B:** Stage 3 pericarditis, 1 day later in the same patient, showing diffuse T-wave inversion after ST segments had normalized.

- **The crucial distinction between stage 1 ECG changes in acute pericarditis and acute ST-segment elevation MI lies in the noncoronary distribution of the ST changes** (e.g., leads I, II, and III), as well as the presence of PR depression in acute pericarditis.
- An equally important distinction is that in acute pericarditis **T-wave inversion only occurs after the ST-segment elevation has resolved**, whereas in ST-segment elevation MI both T-wave inversion and ST-segment elevation are found concurrently.
- However, due to significant overlap in the ECG findings in these two entities, urgent echocardiography can be useful to rule out segmental wall motion abnormalities, which would be expected with ongoing myocardial ischemia.

Imaging

- Transthoracic echocardiography (TTE) is obtained at diagnosis and usually 1 to 2 weeks after initiation of treatment to rule out a significant pericardial effusion.
- Large effusions are not typical in uncomplicated viral or idiopathic pericarditis.
- The presence of larger ellusion alerts the physician to a broader differential diagnosis such as chronic inflammation, constriction, tamponade, or malignancy.

TREATMENT

- Typically, acute pericarditis is self-limited.
- Treatment typically consists of a short course of a nonsteroidal anti-inflammatory drug (NSAID) with or without the addition of colchicine.

Medications

- **NSAIDs**:
  - Typical NSAIDs that are used are aspirin, ibuprofen, naproxen, or indomethacin.
  - All patients should be treated for at least 2 weeks to minimize the risk for scarring.
    - Ibuprofen: 600 to 800 mg every 8 hours.
    - Aspirin (ASA): 650 mg every 4 to 6 hours for 2 to 4 weeks.
  - ASA is suggested in patients with post-MI pericarditis or Dressler syndrome as other NSAIDs are contraindicated in the setting of an acute MI. Glucocorticosteroids and NSAIDs are avoided after an MI due to a risk for impaired ventricular healing, which can increase the risk for ventricular rupture.
- **Colchicine**:
  - The COPE trial found that adding colchicine to an ASA regimen significantly reduced the recurrence of acute pericarditis compared with placebo with a number needed to treat of 5.[2]
    - Colchicine was given as 1 to 2 mg for 1 day then 0.5 to 1.0 mg per day for 3 months.
    - The ASA regimen for the study was 800 mg every 6 to 8 hours for 7 to 10 days with a gradual taper over 3 to 4 weeks.
  - Some patients may not be able to tolerate the gastrointestinal side effects.
  - Less frequent but important side effects include hepatoxicity, myotoxicity, and bone marrow suppression; thus, the patient's serum creatinine, creatine kinase, transaminases, and blood cell count should be followed.
  - To avoid toxicity, it must be used with caution in elderly patients and those with renal insufficiency.
- **Glucocorticoids**:
  - Corticosteroids are seldom used due to their substantial side effects but may be required in patients with:
    - Refractory symptoms despite NSAID therapy.
    - Autoimmune pericarditis (especially if secondary to connective tissue disease).
    - Uremic pericarditis.

- Prednisone dosing is highly variable but typically dosed as 1 mg/kg for 4 weeks followed by a slow taper.
- Some clinicians will add NSAIDs with or without colchicine during the steroid taper.
- The COPE trial found that the use of corticosteroids was an independent risk factor for predicting recurrent pericarditis.[2]

Other Nonpharmacologic Therapies

- Pericardiocentesis (diagnostic and/or therapeutic) may be considered in patients with moderate or large pericardial effusion in patients with:
  - Symptoms attributable to the effusion.
  - Cardiac tamponade (see below).
  - Concern for a purulent, tuberculous, or malignant effusion.
- Any patient with a high fever, bacteremia, or signs of sepsis should undergo urgent pericardiocentesis for diagnosis and the increased risk for development of tamponade, sepsis, and death in patients with purulent pericarditis.

Surgical Management

Pericardiectomy may be considered in patients with severe recurrent disease despite intensive medical therapy.

COMPLICATIONS

- Complications include:
  - Recurrent or chronic pericarditis.
  - Pericardial constriction (usually resulting from chronic pericarditis).
  - Pericardial effusion and tamponade (including hemopericardium). Large pericardial effusions are uncommon among patients with acute pericarditis, especially those with idiopathic or viral etiology.
  - Development of atrial fibrillation.
- **Anticoagulants should be avoided** to decrease the risk of hemopericardium, a rare complication.

MONITORING/FOLLOW-UP

- Patients should be seen with 2 to 4 weeks of initiating medical therapy for acute pericarditis.
- Patients with pericardial effusions should be followed with serial TTEs.
- Strenuous activity should be avoided for at least 4 weeks in case of concomitant myocardial involvement.

OUTCOMES/PROGNOSIS

- **The majority of cases are self-limited**.
- In idiopathic pericarditis, it is estimated that 15% to 30% of patients will develop recurrent pericarditis.

Pericardial Effusion

GENERAL PRINCIPLES

- A pericardial effusion represents an increased amount of fluid in the pericardial space.
- The significance of a pericardial effusion is determined by its size, rate of accumulation, and cause.
- Effusions become clinically detectable around 50 mL and can reach up to 2 L or more.

Classification
- Effusions are often classified based on their etiology.
- One distinction is based on the chronicity of the effusion.
  - Acute effusions may develop hemodynamic compromise (i.e., tamponade) with small amounts of fluid (<200 mL).
  - Chronic effusions can withstand large accumulations of fluid without cardiac tamponade due to pericardial stretching over time.

Etiology
- Typically a patient has an established underlying diagnosis prior to development of the pericardial effusion.
- Any cause of pericarditis (Table 17-1) can lead to a pericardial effusion.
- In one US study, malignancy was the most common cause (23%), followed by radiation (14%), viral (14%), collagen-vascular disease (14%), and uremia (12%).[3]

Pathophysiology
The etiology of an effusion can be categorized by the mechanisms leading to the effusion:
- Increased fluid production (e.g., chronic inflammation).
- Decreased resorption due to disruption of lymphatics and veins.
- Altered oncotic balance (e.g., congestive heart failure, renal failure, or hypoalbuminemia).
- Foreign substance (e.g., blood, pus, lymph, or tumor infiltration).

DIAGNOSIS

Clinical Presentation
Pericardial effusions have marked variability in their clinical presentation ranging from asymptomatic to life-threatening.

History
- Symptoms of pericardial effusion, when present, are often vague and nonspecific.
- Fatigue, decreased exercise capacity, and dyspnea are common.
- Patients may complain of a dull ache or chest pressure.
- Large effusions may compress extrinsic structures and lead to complaints of dysphagia, nausea, hiccups, hoarseness (due to recurrent laryngeal nerve impingement), or cough.

Physical Examination
- Physical examination often yields no unique findings.
- Large effusions may cause decreased heart sounds.
- Ewart sign may be present, which is dullness of the left lung base secondary to compression of the left lung.
- Despite a substantial effusion, a pericardial rub may still be present in the setting of pericarditis.
- Cardiac tamponade has unique physical examination findings and is discussed separately below.

Diagnostic Testing
Laboratories
If the clinical evaluation is suspicious for a certain etiology, lab studies may be indicated to support the clinical diagnosis.

Electrocardiography
- ECG may reveal low voltage of the QRS complex and/or electrical alternans.
- Amplitude of the entire QRS complex (R + S):
  - Limb leads <5 mm.
  - Precordial leads <10 mm.

Imaging
- **Transthoracic echocardiography**:
  - TTE is **the study of choice** for diagnosis and follow-up of pericardial effusions.
  - The size of an effusion can be estimated by evaluating the posterior echo-free space on the parasternal long-axis view during diastole (Table 17-2).
  - In addition to size and location of the effusion, TTE can detect other features, such as pericardial thickness, fibrinous stranding, and fluid loculations or masses.
  - When large effusions are present, findings of tamponade should be specifically excluded (see below).
  - It is important to differentiate a pericardial effusion from a left pleural effusion by the position of the aorta in the parasternal long axis view. A pericardial effusion will displace the aorta posteriorly, whereas the aorta will be located just posterior to the left atrium in a left pleural effusion.
  - TTE can also detect loculated effusions which occur more often in patients after recent cardiac surgery.
- **Ancillary imaging**:
  - Chest radiograpy (CXR) may reveal enlargement of the cardiac silhouette if the effusion is >250 mL.
  - A globular or water bottle-shaped heart may also be seen.
  - CT and MRI are capable of determining the size of an effusion, estimating pericardial thickness, and have the added advantage of imaging surrounding structures.

Diagnostic Procedures
- **Pericardiocentesis**:
  - Diagnostic pericardiocentesis should be considered if an effusion is large and readily accessible and if further diagnostic information would affect management decisions.
  - **The diagnostic yield of a diagnostic pericardiocentesis is but fairly low variable.**[1,3,4]
  - Pericardial effusion analysis should be considered in patients:
    - Undergoing drainage for tamponade.
    - With a high suspicion for neoplastic, purulent, or tuberculous pericarditis.
    - With a moderate-to-large effusion of unknown etiology.

TABLE 17-2	ESTIMATION OF PERICARDIAL EFFUSION BY ECHOCARDIOGRAPHY	
Effusion size	**Volume (mL)**	**Posterior effusion thickness**
Physiologic	<50	<10 mm, systole only
Small	50–100	<10 mm, seen in systole and diastole
Moderate	100–500	10–20 mm, seen anteriorly as well
Large	>500	>20 mm, seen anteriorly, posteriorly, and apically

- ○ Pericardial fluid is typically sent for:
  - ▪ Cell count and differential (though rarely helpful in establishing a cause).
  - ▪ Gram stain.
  - ▪ Culture.
  - ▪ Cytology.
  - ▪ Possibly polymerase chain reaction testing for certain organisms.
- ○ Further specific testing (e.g., adenosine deaminase in tuberculous) is based on the clinical scenario.
- ○ In patients with an established malignancy and a new pericardial effusion, it is important to perform a fluid analysis as up to 50% of patients will not have a malignant pericardial effusion (i.e., positive pathologic evidence of tumor).
- **Pericardial biopsy**:
  - ○ Pericardial biopsy can be performed percutaneously at experienced centers but is typically performed surgically.
  - ○ Biopsy is done in patients with an effusion of unknown etiology or in patients with recurrent effusions despite drainage.
  - ○ Patients with malignant effusions may undergo biopsy to help establish the primary cancer.

TREATMENT

- Therapy for pericardial effusion is directed at the underlying cause.
- Drainage is indicated for symptomatic or refractory cases or when an infectious cause is present.
- Drainage may be considered in large effusions with echocardiographic features of tamponade. Any patients with clinical signs of cardiac tamponade should be drained immediately (see below).
- Malignant effusions frequently recur and may require an indwelling catheter.
- Specific drainage procedures are discussed below and in Chapter 8.
- Anticoagulation is generally avoided until the effusion resolves to minimize the risk for hemopericardium.
- Pericardiectomy or "pericardial window" is warranted in patients with:
  - ○ Recurrent effusions.
  - ○ Loculated effusion, especially posterior effusions which cannot be approached percutaneously.
  - ○ In certain patients undergoing biopsy.

MONITORING/FOLLOW-UP

- Patients should be followed closely depending on the size of the pericardial effusions.
- All large pericardial effusions should be followed with serial TTE.

OUTCOMES/PROGNOSIS

Prognosis depends on the underlying cause for the pericardial effusion.

Cardiac Tamponade

GENERAL PRINCIPLES

- Cardiac tamponade is a complication of pericardial effusion which can be life-threatening.
- It is considered a medical emergency, as cardiogenic shock and death can rapidly ensue.

Definition

Cardiac tamponade is a condition that exists when the pericardial space contains fluid under sufficient pressure to interfere with cardiac filling resulting in decreased cardiac output.

Classification

Cardiac tamponade can be classified as:
- **Acute**: Typically occurs in the setting an acute cause of a small amount of pericardial fluid in a stiff pericardium resulting in profound hemodynamic compromise.
- **Subacute**: Occurs in patients with chronic effusions that slowly accumulate and tamponade will occur once the intrapericardial pressure overcomes the intracardiac pressure in the right atrium.
- **Low pressure**: Can occur in the setting of severe hypovolemia where smaller intrapericardial pressures can overcome the decreased intracardiac pressure leading to a decrease in cardiac output.

Etiology

- Any condition that can lead to a pericardial effusion can cause tamponade.
- The most common causes are idiopathic, malignancy, uremia, cardiac rupture, iatrogenic disease, bacterial infection, tuberculosis, radiation, myxedema, dissecting aortic aneurysm, postcardiotomy, and lupus.
- Tamponade is more common in pericardial effusions secondary to malignancy, bacterial infection, or tuberculosis.
- Purulent pericarditis should be suspected in any patient with high fevers or signs of sepsis.

Pathophysiology

- As fluid accumulates in the pericardial space, the parietal pericardium stretches (i.e., increase compliance) to minimize any change in intrapericardial pressure.
- When pericardial compliance reaches a maximum stretch, intrapericardial pressure begins to increase and impairs diastolic filling.
- During inspiration, venous return increases to the right side of the heart.
- In cardiac tamponade, the right side of the heart cannot expand the right ventricular (RV) free wall due to increased intrapericardial pressures; thus the right ventricle can only expand at the intraventricular septum.
- Distention (i.e., bowing) of the intraventricular septum during inspiration into the left ventricle (LV) decreases diastolic filling of the LV, thus reducing stroke volume.
- Decreased cardiac output results in adrenergic compensation to maintain organ perfusion (i.e., increased heart rate, contractility, and vasoconstriction).
- If the intrapericardial pressure continues to increase, the compensatory mechanisms eventually fail to augment cardiac output leading to shock.

DIAGNOSIS

Clinical Presentation

History
- Symptoms of tamponade include restlessness, dyspnea, cough, chest discomfort, extreme fatigue, presyncope, anxiety, or agitation.
- With progression, evidence of shock is found with decreased urine output, mental status changes, obtundation, and eventual cardiac arrest.

Physical Examination
- The three classic signs of cardiac tamponade are known as Beck triad which include **hypotension, jugular venous distention (JVD), and decreased heart sounds**.

- Physical examination findings of tamponade include the following:
  - JVD: The neck veins may also show a prominent x descent and lack of y descent (Figure 17-2), characteristic of tamponade.
  - Tachycardia.
  - Decreased heart sounds.
  - Hypotension.
  - Tachypnea.
  - Signs of cardiogenic shock.
  - Pulsus paradoxus:
    - **Pulsus paradoxus is an exaggerated drop in systolic pressure on inspiration**. It should be assessed in all patients with suspected cardiac tamponade.
    - With inspiration, RV filling increases causing a shift of the intraventricular septum into the LV leading to a decrease in LV filling, stroke volume, and lower systolic blood pressure.
    - In expiration, this process abates resulting in a higher systolic blood pressure.
    - This process is termed intraventricular dependence and is exaggerated in patients with cardiac tamponade.
    - Pulsus paradoxus can be checked by inflating the blood pressure cuff above the systolic pressure and deflating until Korotkoff sounds are heard only during expiration.
    - Then the cuff is further deflated until Korotkoff sounds are heard with both inspiration and expiration.
    - Pulsus paradoxus is the difference between these pressures.
    - The sensitivity is 98% if >10 mmHg and the specificity is 70% if >10 mmHg; and 83% if >12 mmHg.[5]
    - Other disorders that may be associated with an abnormal pulsus paradoxus include chronic obstructive pulmonary disease, constrictive pericarditis, and RV failure from infarction or pulmonary embolism.

Diagnostic Testing

Electrocardiography

- ECG findings are the same as with pericardial effusion and may show low voltage or electrical alternans.
- Neither finding is sensitive or specific for diagnosing cardiac tamponade.

Imaging

- **As soon as tamponade is suspected, TTE should be performed urgently to confirm the diagnosis**.

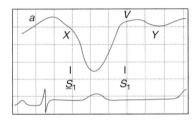

FIGURE 17-2. Right atrial pressure tracing in pericardial tamponade. Note the prominent x descent and absent y descent. (From Murphy JG. *Mayo Clinic Cardiology Review,* 2nd ed. Philadelphia, PA: Lippincott Williams & Wilkins; 2000:854, with permission.)

- TTE will typically reveal a large effusion and may show swinging of the heart within the effusion.
- The size of the effusion will depend on its chronicity.
- Some TTE findings that suggest cardiac tamponade are:
  - Right atrial notching in late diastole.
  - RV collapse in early diastole.
  - Abnormal ventricular septal motion.
  - Dilated, noncompressible inferior vena cava with blunted respiratory changes.
  - Respiratory variation of tricuspid valve inflow velocities of >40% or mitral valve inflow velocities of >25%.
- The absence of any chamber collapse is 90% sensitive for tamponade.[6]
- RV collapse (specifity = 90%) is more specific than RA collapse.[6]
- RV collapse may not be seen in patients with elevated pulmonary pressures.
- TTE reveals only a snapshot in time and, therefore, cannot assess the rate of progression or predict onset of fatal hemodynamic collapse.
- Tamponade is a clinical diagnosis, and echocardiography has a confirmatory role.
- The decision of how and when to best perform drainage is best determined by the patient's clinical status and not the specific echo findings.
- If tamponade is suspected in cases of postcardiotomy or cardiac trauma, TTE provides inadequate assessment because of the possibility of localized or loculated effusions and usually poor echocardiographic windows.
- The most common location of hemorrhage postcardiotomy is posterior to the left atrium, which is virtually invisible by TTE.
- Transesophageal echocardiography (TEE) should be used instead to confirm the diagnosis.

TREATMENT

- All patients with clinical tamponade need to be drained percutaneous or surgically expediently.
- Options for treatment include percutaneous needle pericardiocentesis or surgical drainage.
- Different drainage procedures should be selected on an individual basis determined by the clinical situation (degree of urgency, location of effusion, likelihood for recurrence).

Medication

- Before drainage, **patients must be resuscitated aggressively** with intravenous fluids to reduce chamber collapse.
- Pressor support (e.g., norepinephrine) may be added for blood pressure support if necessary.
- Additionally, endotracheal intubation must be undertaken with caution owing to the decrease in preload both with sedative agents and with positive-pressure ventilation, which could precipitate complete circulatory collapse.

Other Nonpharmacologic Therapies

- Percutaneous needle **pericardiocentesis** is a rapid method for draining pericardial fluid and is appropriate for all emergent and most urgent cases involving hemodynamic compromise (see Chapter 8).
- It can be performed at the bedside or in a cardiac catheterization lab.
- Most operators use echocardiographic guidance and agitated saline injected through the pericardiocentesis needle to visually confirm entry into the pericardial space.
- There is a low but significant risk of complications, including cardiac puncture or coronary laceration.

- A pericardial drain is usually left in place for several days postprocedure until drain output tapers off to prevent short-term reaccumulation.
- For patients who have persistent elevated right atrial pressures following pericardiocentesis, effusive constrictive pericarditis should be considered (see below).

Surgical Management

- If the patient is not experiencing imminent hemodynamic collapse, **subxiphoid pericardiotomy** is a minimally invasive surgical procedure that can provide a more definitive treatment and reduced risk of recurrence.
- Additionally, a pericardiotomy allows for visualization, thorascopic inspection, and tissue biopsy.
- A pericardial window may also be created which allows for direct drainage of fluid into the peritoneal cavity.
- More definitive surgical management of malignant pericardial disease may require partial or complete **pericardiectomy**.
- General anesthesia is required for an anterior thoracotomy or sternotomy and is associated with significant morbidity and mortality.
- Less invasive treatments are usually preferred, but pericardiectomy can be considered in those with a relatively good prognosis in whom more definitive therapy is desired.

Constrictive Pericarditis

GENERAL PRINCIPLES

- Constrictive pericarditis occurs when chronic inflammation renders the pericardium thickened and scarred.
- The pericardial space is obliterated resulting in a **loss of normal pericardial compliance**.
- This exerts an **external volume constraint** on the heart, thus interfering with normal cardiac filling.

Etiology

- Any chronic insult to the pericardium, including host immune response, can result in constriction.
- The **most common causes** include:
  - Idiopathic or viral pericarditis account for roughly half of the cases.
  - Post-cardiac surgery constrictive pericarditis occurs as a late complication and more is common in surgeries complicated by postoperative pericarditis or hemorrhage into the pericardial space.
  - Constrictive pericarditis post-chest radiation is a late complication, occurring years after radiation therapy.
  - Connective tissues disorders.
  - Postinfectious, with tuberculosis being the most common cause in developing countries.
  - End-stage renal disease.
  - Malignancy, typical associated cancers include breast, lung, and lymphoma.
- **Effusive constrictive pericarditis** is a unique and rare variant of constrictive pericarditis caused by **constriction of the visceral layer of pericardium**.
  - Its hallmark feature is constrictive physiology (see below) in the presence of a pericardial effusion.

- ○ Typically patients will present with suspected tamponade and undergo pericardiocentesis. However, right atrial pressures will remain elevated after drainage.
- ○ Specifically, the diagnosis should be suspected in patients who fail to reduce right atrial pressure by >50% or <10 mmHg following adequate drainage (i.e., intrapericardial pressure = 0 mmHg),[7] though this can also occur in patients with RV failure or severe tricuspid regurgitation.
- ○ Treatment and clinical course depend on the cause for pericarditis, though some patients may require pericardiectomy.

Pathophysiology

- Thickening and fibrosis of the pericardium decrease pericardial compliance.
- The pericardium often becomes calcified and adherent to the epicardium of the heart.
- This results in **decreased ventricular compliance** as the ventricle cannot expand during diastolic filling.
- As the ventricle fills, **diastolic pressures rapidly increase and filling ceases** due to the elevated pressures in both ventricles.
  - ○ Rapid ventricular filling occurs in early diastole only.
  - ○ Atrial systole does not contribute to ventricular filling due to the elevated ventricular pressures.
- The increased end-diastolic pressures become equal in all four chambers of the heart.
- The elevated pressures in both ventricles lead to **elevated systemic and pulmonary venous pressures**.

DIAGNOSIS

Clinical Presentation

History

- The signs and symptoms of constrictive pericarditis are due to elevated filling pressures causing left- and right-sided heart failure.
- In early stages, patients may complain of fatigue, weakness, and decreased exercise tolerance.
- As filling pressures continue to rise, patients complain of right-sided symptoms, such as lower extremity edema, increased abdominal girth and ascites, and eventually left-sided symptoms, such as dyspnea on exertion, orthopnea, and paroxysmal nocturnal dyspnea.

Physical Examination

- Physical examination in constriction typically reveals impressive **findings of right-sided heart failure**, including markedly elevated jugular venous pulse (JVP), hepatomegaly, ascites, and lower extremity edema.
- Findings of left-sided heart failure, such as frank pulmonary edema, are less common.
- Physical examination findings that are more specific for constriction include:
  - ○ Increased JVP with prominent *y* descent due to rapid early diastolic filling (Figure 17-3).
  - ○ **Kussmaul sign**: Lack of expected decrease or obvious increase of JVP on inspiration.
  - ○ **Pericardial knock**: Early, loud, high-pitched S3 derived from rapid pressure equalization after initial ventricular filling.

Diagnostic Testing

No single study provides definitive evidence of constrictive pericarditis; thus it is often necessary to obtain several different studies to support any clinical suspicion.

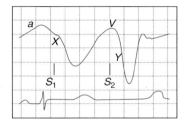

FIGURE 17-3. Right atrial pressure tracing in constrictive pericarditis. Note the prominent *y* descent. (From Murphy JG. *Mayo Clinic Cardiology Review*, 2nd ed. Philadelphia, PA: Lippincott Williams & Wilkins; 2000, with permission.)

Electrocardiography

- ECG findings commonly include low QRS voltage, generalized T-wave flattening, or left atrial enlargement.
- Atrial fibrillation is fairly common in patients with constrictive pericarditis.

Imaging

- CXR may reveal:
  - Calcified pericardium (best seen in the lateral views).
  - Pleural effusions.
  - Evidence of biatrial enlargement.
- TTE can reveal several indirect features suggestive of constriction:
  - Thickened, echogenic pericardium.
  - Tram-tracking: Adherence to and movement of the pericardium with the myocardium during contraction.
  - Dilated, noncompressible inferior vena cava.
  - Septal bounce due to rapid early diastolic filling.
  - Posterior LV wall flattening in diastole (equalization of pressures, equivalent to the "square root" sign).
  - **Ventricular interdependence** on Doppler examination. No findings are particularly pathognomonic, although ventricular interdependence is the closest physiologic correlate. Because of the external volume constraint, RV and LV fill at the expense of each other. Mitral inflow velocities decrease with inspiration and increase with expiration, and tricuspid velocities conversely increase with inspiration and decrease with expiration.
- CT and MRI are useful for detecting pericardial thickening, dilated hepatic veins, dilated right atrium, and other findings that support constrictive pericarditis. These studies are not diagnostic and should be used only to support a diagnosis of pericardial constriction.

Diagnostic Procedures

- **Right- and left-heart catheterizations** are done simultaneously to assess right- and left-sided pressures, determine cardiac output, and help differentiate constrictive from restrictive physiology.
- Hemodynamic measurements reveal **elevated and equal pressure in all four chambers in diastole** before the wave.
- Right atrial measurements reveal a preserved *x* descent and a **steep *y* descent** from the increased flow during early diastole (Figure 17-3) and Kussmaul sign.

- Ventricular hemodynamic measurements reveal the **dip-and-plateau ("square root" sign) during diastole** due to rapid early diastolic filling, which is abruptly halted once the constricted volume is reached (Figure 17-4).
- A common diagnostic dilemma is the **distinction between pericardial constriction and restrictive cardiomyopathy.**
  - Decreased compliance of either the pericardium or myocardium leads to similar defects in ventricular filling, and substantial overlap exists in signs, symptoms, and hemodynamic measurements.
  - The distinction is critical, however, as patients with restrictive cardiomyopathy carry an exceptionally high mortality risk with cardiac surgery.
  - Restrictive cardiomyopathy and constriction can be present in the same patient (e.g., after chest radiation).
  - The most sensitive (97%) and specific (100%) catheterization criterion for constrictive pericarditis is a **systolic area index** >1.1 (the ratio of RV to LV systolic pressure-time area in inspiration versus expiration).[8]
  - Endomyocardial biopsy may occasionally be required to rule out a myocardial process prior to surgery.
  - Table 17-3 highlights some the major differences between these entities.

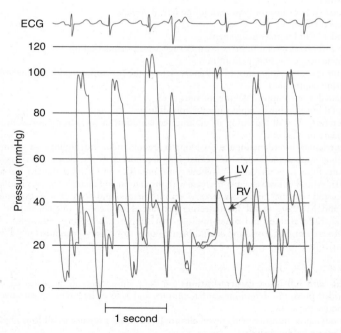

FIGURE 17-4. Simultaneous RV and LV pressure tracings in constrictive pericarditis. Note the prominent dip and plateau (square root sign), particularly post-PVC. (From Marso SP, Griffin BP, Topol EJ, eds. *Manual of Cardiovascular Medicine.* Philadelphia, PA: Lippincott Williams & Wilkins; 2000, with permission.)

TABLE 17-3	DISTINGUISHING PERICARDIAL CONSTRICTION AND RESTRICTIVE CARDIOMYOPATHY	
Constriction		**Restriction**
Ventricular interdependence present		Absent
Abnormal pericardial features (thick, echogenic, adherent, calcified)		Abnormal myocardial features (infiltration, abnormal biopsy, conduction system disease)
Preserved tissue Doppler velocities		Restrictive diastolic filling pattern
Pulmonary hypertension mild or absent		Significant pulmonary hypertension
Septal bounce		Normal septal motion
LVEDP–RVEDP <5 mmHg (equalization)		LVEDP-RVEDP >5 mmHg
RVEDP/RVSP >1/3		RVEDP/RVSP <1/3
Systolic area index >1.1		Systolic area index ≤1.1
BNP low or mildly elevated (<200)		BNP elevated (>200)

BNP, B-type natriuretic peptide; LVEDP, left ventricular end-diastolic pressure; RVEDP, right ventricular end-diastolic pressure; RSVP, right ventricular systolic pressure.

TREATMENT

- Constrictive pericarditis is a difficult disease to manage medically.
- If possible, it is desirable to treat underlying cause.
- A small subset of patients will have spontaneous resolution or respond to medical therapy.

Medication

- Medical therapy is dictated by the underlying cause for constriction.
- For patients with heart failure symptoms, diuretics, angiotensin-converting enzyme (ACE) inhibitors, and a low-salt diet form the cornerstone of therapy but often meet with limited success.

Surgical Management

- **Surgical pericardiectomy (stripping) is the definitive therapy of choice**.
- The operative mortality rate can be as high as 20%.
- The majority of patients report symptomatic improvement with pericardiectomy.
- Surgery should be performed early, as constrictive pericarditis is a progressive disease, and patients with poor functional class are at higher risk of perioperative death.

Pericardial Tumors

GENERAL PRINCIPLES

- It is not infrequent for a patient to present with a mass (or multiple masses) within the pericardium.

- Tumors can be categorized as primary (i.e., derived initially from pericardial tissue) or metastatic.

Etiology

- **Primary pericardial tumors are very rare.** Five entities make up the bulk of tumors in this category.
  - Pericardial cyst:
    - Pericardial cysts are fluid-filled fibrous sacs lined with mesothelial cells and represent **the most common primary pericardial tumor.**
    - They are usually <3 cm in size and are often located at the right heart border.
    - Surgery is curative but is often not necessary, as there is no malignant potential.
  - Teratoma:
    - Teratomas occur more often in young women.
    - **Although benign, they are quite aggressive** and are likely to cause compressive symptoms.
  - Mesothelioma:
    - Mesotheliomas are malignant, with features similar to the better-known pleural mesothelioma.
    - Association with asbestos exposure is still controversial.
  - Angiosarcoma: Angiosarcomas are aggressive malignancies that can be derived from pericardial or myocardial tissue.
  - Lipoma: Pericardial lipomas are similar to lipomas in other locations.
- **Pericardial metastases are 100- to 1,000-fold more common than primary tumors.**
  - They typically represent a late-stage process; thus, identification of the primary tumor is usually well established at the time of presentation.
  - The most common malignancies (accounting for two-thirds of cases) found to metastasize to the pericardium include:
    - Lung cancer (most common).
    - Breast cancer.
    - Hematologic malignancies.
  - Although less common overall, **melanoma has the highest propensity to spread to the pericardium.**
  - There are three routes of metastasis to the pericardium:
    - Lymphatic spread (lung and breast cancer), associated with significant pericardial effusion.
    - Hematogenous spread (leukemia, lymphoma, melanoma), which tend to result in hemorrhagic effusion.
    - Direct extension (lung and esophageal cancer).

DIAGNOSIS

Clinical Presentation

Common presentations include:
- Symptoms from compression of the cardiac chambers (usually dyspnea or syncope).
- Pericarditis.
- Effusion/tamponade.
- Arrhythmias.

Diagnostic Testing

Diagnosis typically involves:
- Imaging with multiple modalities (CXR, TTE, CT, or MRI).
- Pericardial fluid analysis.
- Tissue biopsy (if needed).

TREATMENT

In addition to systemic chemotherapy, treatment includes local control with drainage procedures, radiation, and occasionally instillation of chemotherapeutic drugs into the pericardial space.

REFERENCES

1. Imazio M, Trinchero R. Triage and management of acute pericarditis. *Int J Cardiol* 2007;118:286-294.
2. Imazio M, Bobbio M, Cecchi E, et al. Colchicine in addition to conventional therapy for acute pericarditis: results of the COlchicine for acute PEricarditis (COPE) trial. *Circulation* 2005;112:2012-2016.
3. Corey GR, Campbell PT, Van Trigt P, et al. Etiology of large pericardial effusions. *Am J Med* 1993;95:209-213.
4. Permanyer-Miralda G, Sagristá-Sauleda J, Soler-Soler J. Primary acute pericardial disease: a prospective series of 231 consecutive patients. *Am J Cardiol* 1985;56:623-630.
5. Roy CL, Minor MA, Brookhart MA, et al. Does this patient with a pericardial effusion have cardiac tamponade? *JAMA* 2007;297:1810-1818.
6. Mercé J, Sagristá-Sauleda, J, Permanyer-Miralda G, et al. Correlation between clinical and Doppler echocardiographic findings in patients with moderate and large pericardial effusion: implications for the diagnosis of cardiac tamponade. *Am Heart J* 1999;138:759-764.
7. Sagristá-Sauleda J, Angel J, Sánchez A, et al. Effusive-constrictive pericarditis. *N Engl J Med* 2004;350:469-475.
8. Talreja DR, Nishimura RA, Oh JK, et al. Constrictive pericarditis in the modern era: novel criteria for diagnosis in the cardiac catheterization laboratory. *J Am Coll Cardiol* 2008;51:315-319.

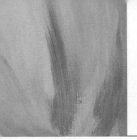

Pulmonary Hypertension: Pulmonary Arterial Hypertension and Right Heart Failure

18

Mohammed Hadi and Murali M. Chakinala

GENERAL PRINCIPLES

Definition

- Pulmonary hypertension (PH) is a general term that denotes an increase in blood pressure within the pulmonary vasculature.
- The ACCF/AHA consensus statement defines pulmonary arterial hypertension (PAH) as **mean pulmonary artery pressure (PAP) ≥25 mmHg with normal pulmonary artery capillary wedge pressure (PCWP), i.e., ≤15 mmHg and pulmonary vascular resistance (PVR) of >3 Wood units with the following** relationship between pressure, flow, and resistance:[1]

$$PVR = (mean~PAP - mean~PAOP)/cardiac~output$$
$$PVR = pulmonary~vascular~resistance$$
$$PAP = pulmonary~artery~pressure$$
$$PAOP = pulmonary~artery~occlusion~pressure$$

Classification

Five major categories of PH are based upon the driving etiology for the pathophysiology (Table 18-1).[1,2]

Epidemiology

- **Group 1 PAH** has a prevalence of approximately 25 cases/million.[1]
  - Idiopathic PAH (IPAH) is a sporadic disease with prevalence of five cases/million.
  - There are well-established links between PAH and exposure to potent anorexigens (e.g., fenfluramine, dexfenfluramine), toxic rapeseed oil, and methamphetamines.
  - PAH associated with systemic sclerosis is most common form of PAH associated with collagen vascular disease with about 12% prevalence in the systemic sclerosis population.
  - Other forms of associated PAH (APAH) are rare (e.g., 0.5% of HIV-positive individuals and 5% to 7% of cirrhotics with portal hypertension referred for liver transplantation).
- The highest prevalence PH in the developed world is overwhelmingly **Group 2** (PH secondary to left heart disease), followed by Group 3 (PH secondary to lung disease).
  - The presence of diastolic dysfunction and elevated left ventricular (LV) filling pressures appears to be instrumental for the development of PH in the setting of heart failure with preserved ejection fraction (HFpEF), LV systolic heart failure, or aortic valve stenosis.

TABLE 18-1	**UPDATED CLINICAL CLASSIFICATION OF PULMONARY HYPERTENSION**

Group 1: Pulmonary arterial hypertension (PAH)

Idiopathic PAH (IPAH)

Heritable PAH (HPAH)

  Bone morphogenetic protein receptor II mutation (BMPR-II)

  Activin-like kinase receptor 1 (ALK-1)/endoglin (with or without hereditary hemorrhagic telangiectasia)

  Unknown

Drug- and toxin-induced

Associated with (APAH)

  Collagen vascular disease/connective tissue disorder

  HIV infection

  Portal hypertension

  Congenital heart disease

  Schistosomiasis

  Chronic hemolytic anemia

Persistent pulmonary hypertension of the newborn

Group 1′: Pulmonary veno-occlusive disease and/or pulmonary capillary hemangiomatosis

Group 2: Pulmonary hypertension owing to left heart disease

Systolic dysfunction

Diastolic dysfunction

Valvular disease

Group 3: Pulmonary hypertension due to lung diseases and/or hypoxia

Chronic obstructive pulmonary disease

Interstitial lung disease

Other pulmonary diseases with mixed restrictive and obstructive pattern

Sleep-disordered breathing

Alveolar hypoventilation disorders

Chronic exposure to high altitude

Developmental abnormalities

Group 4: Pulmonary hypertension due to chronic thromboembolic pulmonary hypertension (CTEPH)

Group 5: Pulmonary hypertension with unclear multifactorial mechanisms

Hematologic disorders/splenectomy

Systemic disorders: sarcoid, pulmonary Langerhans cell histiocytosis, lymphangioleiomyomatosis, neurofibromatosis

(Continued)

TABLE 18-1	UPDATED CLINICAL CLASSIFICATION OF PULMONARY HYPERTENSION (*Continued*)

Metabolic disorders: glycogen storage diseases, Gaucher disease

Other: tumor-related obstruction, fibrosing mediastinitis, chronic renal failure on dialysis

Modified from Simonneau G, Robbins I, Beghetti M, et al. Updated clinical classification of pulmonary hypertension. *J Am Coll Cardiol* 2009;54:S43-S54.

- Cases of **Group 3** PH (PH due to lung diseases and/or hypoxia) generally tend to be mild and correlate with the degree of severity of underlying lung disease and/or hypoxemia.
  - PH can be severe in idiopathic pulmonary fibrosis, hypoventilation syndromes, chronic obstructive pulmonary disease, or a combination of these entities.
  - Disproportionately high pressures in Group 3 PH (i.e., mean PAP >40) should prompt workup for additional contributory factors (e.g., obstructive sleep apnea [OSA], chronic thromboembolic disease, and HFpEF).
- **Group 4** PH or chronic thromboembolic pulmonary hypertension (CTEPH) occurs in 1% to 2% of pulmonary emboli (PE) survivors.
  - Approximately 40% do not have acutely defined venothrombotic events prior to detection of PH.
  - The cumulative burden of emboli appears to be a risk factor.
  - About 10% of CTEPH cases are linked to antiphospholipid syndrome.
  - Association of CTEPH has been made with postsplenectomy, chronic osteomyelitis, inflammatory bowel disease, chronic endovascular devices (e.g., pacemaker leads, ventriculoatrial shunts).
- **Group 5** encompasses a broad category of disorders that can develop PH from multiple mechanisms.
  - Sarcoid-associated PH can result from interstitial lung disease, LV cardiomyopathy, mediastinal compression of central pulmonary vessels, or granulomatous involvement of small pulmonary arteries/veins.
  - Some Group 5 cases behave like Group 1 conditions and may be treated similarly, only after thorough evaluation of the underlying mechanisms for PH (e.g., sarcoid, Langerhans cell histiocytosis).

Pathophysiology

- Complex origins of PAH include infectious/environmental insults in the setting of predisposing comorbidities and/or underlying genetic predisposition, for example, gene mutation of bone morphogenetic protein receptor II (BMPR II) or activin-like kinase receptor 1 (ALK 1).
- BMPR II mutations found in 70% of familial PAH and 25% of IPAH, while ALK 1 mutations causative for hereditary hemorrhagic telangiectasia rarely presents with PAH.[1,3]
- The pathogenesis of PAH may vary with the different etiologies but converges to a **common pathway of endothelial and smooth muscle cell proliferation and dysfunction** that results in the complex interplay of the following factors:

○ Vasoconstriction caused by overproduction of vasoconstrictor compounds such as endothelin and insufficient production of vasodilators such as prostacyclin and nitric oxide/cyclic GMP.[4]

○ Endothelial and smooth muscle proliferation due to mitogenic properties of endothelin and thromboxane A2 in the setting of low levels of inhibitory molecules, such as prostacyclin and nitric oxide.

○ In situ thrombosis of small- and medium-sized pulmonary arteries resulting from platelet activation and aggregation due to increased thromboxane A2 and low levels of platelet inhibitors, such as prostacyclin and nitric oxide.

○ The physiologic consequences of this proliferative vasculopathy are an increase in PAP and right ventricle (RV) afterload for any given flow through the pulmonary circuit with resultant elevated PVR.

Associated Conditions

• **Right heart failure (RHF) is the late consequence and most common cause of death in PAH**.

• Factors that portend a poor prognosis in PAH and are linked to RV compensation include:

  ○ Modified World Health Organization functional class III or IV (Table 18-2)

  ○ Elevated mean right atrial pressure (RAP) (>20 mmHg)

  ○ Low cardiac index (<2.0 L/minute/m^2)

  ○ Exertional syncope

• Pathophysiology of RHF associated with PH:

  ○ Increased PVR is initially compensated by RV hypertrophy with maintenance of cardiac output, but chronically this results in RV dilation and dysfunction, and ultimately a decrease in cardiac output.

  ○ In advanced cases, RV function and cardiac output decline with a concomitant decline in PAP due to the RV's inability to generate pressure (Figure 18-1).[5]

• Other causes of RHF:

  ○ **RHF is most commonly caused by PH due to left heart failure**.

  ○ RHF can exist without PH: RV infarction, arrhythmogenic right ventricular dysplasia, Uhl anomaly (also known as "parchment heart," congenital absence of RV myocardium), and massive acute PE.

TABLE 18-2	MODIFIED WORLD HEALTH ORGANIZATION (WHO) FUNCTIONAL CLASSIFICATION SCHEME

Class I: No limitation of physical activity. Ordinary physical activity does not cause undue dyspnea or fatigue, chest pain, or near syncope.

Class II: Slight limitation of physical activity. Comfortable at rest. Ordinary physical activity causes undue dyspnea or fatigue, chest pain, or near syncope.

Class III: Marked limitation of physical activity. Comfortable at rest. Less than ordinary activity causes undue dyspnea or fatigue, chest pain, or near syncope.

Class IV: Unable to carry out any physical activity without symptoms. Dyspnea and/or fatigue may be present at rest. Discomfort is increased by any physical activity. Signs of right heart failure are present.

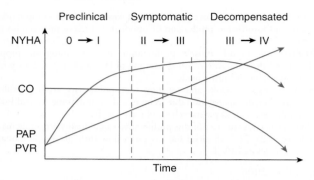

FIGURE 18-1. Schematic progression of pulmonary arterial hypertension. NYHA, New York Heart Association; CO, cardiac output; PAP, pulmonary artery pressure; PVR, pulmonary vascular resistance. (From Galiè N, Manes A, Palazzini M, et al. Pharmacological impact on right ventricular remodeling in pulmonary arterial hypertension. *Eur Heart J Suppl* 2007;9(H):H68-H74, with permission.)

DIAGNOSIS

Clinical Presentation

- High level of suspicion is needed to diagnose PAH.
- Symptoms of PAH are quite nonspecific and include exertional dyspnea, fatigue, palpitations, and chest pain.
- The average delay to diagnosis remains very high (about 2.5 years).

History

- The history should explore for underlying risk factors and comorbid conditions (Table 18-1).[2]
- In addition to nonspecific symptoms, exertional chest pain and syncope are important clues for advanced right heart dysfunction.

Physical Examination

- Lower extremity edema and increasing abdominal girth suggest RHF.
- Cardiac auscultation reveals accentuated S2 with a loud P2 component.
- Development of RV dysfunction results in a systolic tricuspid regurgitant murmur (early), diastolic pulmonary insufficiency murmur (late), and a right ventricular S3.
- Peripheral manifestations of RHF include distended jugular venous pulsation, hepatojugular reflux, hepatomegaly, pulsatile liver, ascites, and lower extremity edema.
- Findings of underlying conditions linked to PH should be sought out (e.g., skin changes of scleroderma, stigmata of liver disease, clubbing in congenital heart disease, abnormal breath sounds in parenchymal lung disease).

Diagnostic Testing

- A multistep strategy is necessary to distill the finding of PH ultimately to one of the diagnostic categories in Table 18-1.[2]
- Findings on basic investigations such as chest radiography (CXR, pulmonary arteries, and right atrial prominence) and ECG (RV hypertrophy: dominant R wave of >7 mm

or R/S ratio >1 with strain and possible right axis deviation) are helpful when present, but insensitive, especially in milder cases.

- A series of investigations (Figure 18-2) is employed to[6]:
  ○ Confirm the diagnosis.
  ○ Clarify the clinical group of PH and the specific etiology within the PAH group (Table 18-1).[2]
  ○ Evaluate the severity of functional and hemodynamic impairment in PAH.

Laboratory Tests

- Lab test can be used to evaluate for causative conditions (hepatic function panel, HIV antinuclear antibody [ANA], extractable nuclear antigens [ENA], antitopoisomerase antibody, hemoglobin, thyroid function tests) and gauge degree of cardiac impairment (B-type natriuretic peptide [BNP]).
- Additional testing is based on the initial evaluation and may include hepatitis B and C serologies, hemoglobin electrophoresis, antiphospholipid antibody, and lupus antico-agulant.
- **Arterial blood gas assessment** is an important for identifying a hypoventilation syndrome.

Imaging

- **Transthoracic echocardiography** (TTE) with Doppler and agitated saline injection is preferred initial test to identify presence of PH.
  ○ If tricuspid regurgitation is present, Doppler interrogation allows for the most common method for estimating pulmonary artery systolic pressure (PASP).

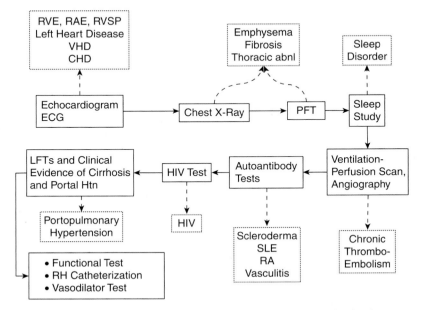

FIGURE 18-2. Diagnostic flowchart for the evaluation of unexplained pulmonary hypertension. (From McLaughlin VV, McGoon MD. Pulmonary arterial hypertension. *Circulation* 2006;114:1417-1431, with permission.)

- Sensitivity for PH is 80% to 100% and the correlation coefficient with invasive measurement 0.6 to 0.9.
  - The ACCF/AHA consensus statement encourages further evaluation if PASP >40 mmHg.[1]
- ○ TTE can identify possible left-sided cardiac causes of PH, including aortic valve disease or LV dysfunction. Clues for diastolic heart disease and HFpEF include left atrial enlargement, grade II or III diastolic dysfunction based on typical Doppler mitral inflow patterns (i.e., pseudonormalization or restrictive filling), and decreased tissue Doppler velocities.
- ○ TTE provides important functional and morphologic information about the RV, including degree of hypertrophy and/or dilatation, tricuspid annular plane systolic excursion (TAPSE <1.8 portends poorer prognosis), and the Tei index.[1]
- ○ Agitated saline or a "bubble study" is useful to identify congenital shunts (e.g., atrial septal defects [ASD], ventricular septal defects [VSD]) or the acquired patent foramen ovale.
- **Transesophageal echocardiography** (TEE) can be performed contingent upon the TTE findings to better evaluate atrial septal anatomy (for ASD) and mitral valve disease.
- **Cardiac MRI** can also define cardiac anomalies, especially if TEE is contraindicated, and may also provide pertinent functional information of the RV.
- **Ventilation-perfusion (V/Q) lung scan** is the screening test of choice to exclude chronic thromboembolic disease but can also be abnormal in pulmonary veno-occlusive disease and fibrosing mediastinitis.
- **Chest CT** can reveal relevant parenchymal and mediastinal findings when suspected.
- **CT angiography** may miss subtle findings of chronic thromboembolic disease, particularly when read by inexperienced radiologists.
- **Pulmonary angiography** can be performed safely in the setting of severe PH to confirm chronic thromboembolic disease and determine surgical accessibility of organized thrombotic material.

Diagnostic Procedures

- **Pulmonary function testing** (PFT) includes spirometry and lung volumes to assess for obstructive (e.g., COPD) or restrictive (e.g., interstitial lung diseases) ventilatory abnormalities.
- **Polysomnography** should be done if symptoms of sleep-disordered breathing are uncovered (e.g., daytime hypersomnolence, snoring, apneas, early morning headaches).
- **Nocturnal oximetry** can disclose nocturnal desaturations, which are fairly common in PH even when daytime hypoxemia is not documented and should be treated with supplemental oxygen.
- **Six-minute walk** is a critical test in the evaluation of PH, for both establishing severity of impairment and predicting short and intermediate term survivals:
  - ○ Baseline distance walked of <330 m is a predictor of worse outcome in PAH.
  - ○ Ability to walk ≥380 m (while on treatment) is considered a favorable predictor in PAH. Distance covered also correlates with modified WHO functional classification, Table 18-2.
- **Right heart catheterization** (RHC) remains the gold standard for diagnosis and allows concomitant vasoreactivity testing.
  - ○ Inability to reliably assess trans-pulmonary blood flow and pulmonary venous pressure represents the most relevant limitations of echocardiography. **Therefore RHC should be performed on all patients suspected with PAH prior to initiation of therapy**, unless in the rare circumstance that cardiac anatomy precludes catheterization.
  - ○ Some initially suspected of PAH will not require catheterization, if an alternative diagnosis established by noninvasive testing. **RHC should be reserved for those who after noninvasive screening are still considered probable PAH patients**.

○ RHC measurements should include PAP, RAP, pulmonary capillary wedge pressure (PCWP), mixed venous saturation, cardiac output (thermodilution or Fick methods), and PVR.
  ▪ If a reliable PCWP is not determined, direct LV end-diastolic pressure (LVEDP) should be checked.
  ▪ If PCWP or LVEDP ≥15, LV dysfunction is confirmed and may account for the elevated PAP, depending on the remainder of the evaluation.
• **Acute vasodilator testing** is recommended in PAH is confirmed by RHC.[1]
  ○ Short-acting vasodilators, such as intravenous adenosine, epoprostenol, or inhaled nitric oxide, should be used.
  ○ Rationale for vasodilator testing is based on two factors:
    ▪ Acute vasoresponsiveness identifies patients with better prognosis.
    ▪ Responders are more likely to have a sustained response to oral calcium channel blockers (CCBs).
  ○ Vasodilator testing should not be done if severe RHF exists (i.e., RAP >20 mmHg or cardiac index <1.5 L/minute/m²).
  ○ **Definition of a vasoresponder is decline in mean PAP ≥10 mmHg and concluding mean PAP <40 mmHg while at least maintaining cardiac output.**
  ○ Vasoresponders should undergo CCB trial with nifedipine or diltiazem while a pulmonary artery catheter in place in order to recapitulate the response to short-acting vasodilators.

TREATMENT

• Management of PH entirely depends on the specific category isolated from a comprehensive evaluation.
• PH secondary to left heart disease (Group 2) should receive appropriate therapy for underlying causative left heart condition with a hemodynamic goal of lowering the PCWP (and LVEDP) as much as possible.
  ○ **Patients with HFpEF** often develop secondary PH and exertional dyspnea and require **afterload-reducing agents** (to minimize LV afterload), **diuretics** (to avoid excess volume), and **negative chronotropes**. Severe anemia and chronic use of nonsteroid anti-inflammatory drugs (NSAIDs) can aggravate the situation and should be avoided.
  ○ The subset of patients of **LV systolic heart failure and associated PH** appear to benefit from **sildenafil** (a phosphodiesterase-5 inhibitors [PDE5-I]), in terms of exertional capacity, hemodynamics during exercise, and quality of life. Sildenafil should only be used if PH is persistent and relevant after careful hemodynamic assessment, which should document an elevated PVR, after optimization of LV filling pressures (i.e., near normal PCWP or LVEDP) and optimization of LV systolic function.
• **PH caused by parenchymal lung diseases** (Group 3) should be treated with appropriate **therapies for their underlying pulmonary condition**: bronchodilators, pulmonary rehabilitation (obstructive lung disease), immunomodulators (interstitial lung diseases), noninvasive ventilation (OSA and/or hypoventilation syndrome). It is critical to ensure adequate saturations (SpO₂ ≥ 0%), as much as possible throughout the day and night in order to avoid hypoxic vasoconstriction and cor pulmonale.
• Group 4, **chronic thromboembolic PH**, can be cured by **pulmonary thromboendarterectomy** at specialized centers and requires careful screening to determine resectability and expected hemodynamic response. When the disease is considered nonsurgical due to distal predominance of the culprit lesions, medical therapy as for PAH can be attempted.
• **Treatment of acute decompensated right ventricular failure** involves a complex interaction between volume status, hypoxemia, and hypotension. Figure 18-3 demonstrates an organized treatment algorithm.[7-9]

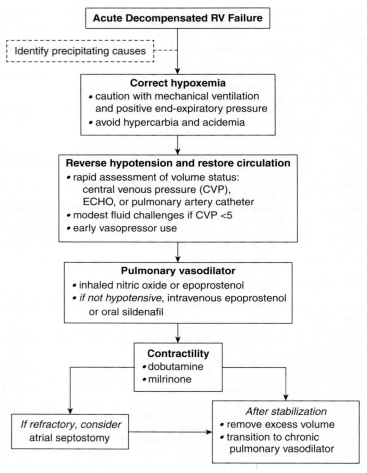

FIGURE 18-3. Treatment algorithm for management of acute decompensated right ventricular failure.

○ **Identify and correct precipitating factors**:
  ■ Possibilities included interruption of chronic PAH therapy, dietary/fluid indiscretion, infection (particularly blood-stream infection in patients with indwelling central venous catheters), PE, atrial tachyarrhythmias, thyrotoxicosis, pregnancy, induction for general anesthesia, and RV infarction.
  ■ Sepsis in particular is poorly tolerated due to systemic vasodilation and an inability to augment cardiac output due to poor RV function; fluid resuscitation has to be balanced with overdistention of a dilated hypokinetic RV that can impair LV filling due to acute encroachment.
○ **Correct hypoxemia**
○ **Reverse hypotension and restore circulation**:

- Factors governing RV stroke volume are similar to those of LV (i.e., preload, afterload, and myocardial contractility). Pulmonary artery catheter may assist management in selected patients.
- **Preload**: Cautious volume challenge of crystalloid until CVP is 10 to 12 mmHg. Measures of system perfusion should be monitored.
- **Systemic hypotension**: Low systemic diastolic pressure coupled with elevated RV end-diastolic pressure narrows the myocardial perfusion gradient and promotes RV ischemia. Vasopressors are critical to restoring systemic blood pressure and maintain organ perfusion and minimize RV ischemia. While no agent is superior, norepinephrine or dopamine can be used at the lowest needed doses to minimize tachycardia, dysrhythmias, myocardial oxygen consumption, and pulmonary vasoconstriction.
- **Afterload reduction**: Selective pulmonary arterial dilation is critical to breaking the spiral of RV decompensation and hypotension. Inhaled agents preferentially lower PVR with minimal decreases in systemic vascular resistance and minimize ventilation-perfusion mismatching and hypoxemia. Two available agents are inhaled nitric oxide (up to 40 parts per million) and inhaled epoprostenol (5,000 to 20,000 ng/mL) as a continuous nebulization. Nonselective vasodilators (e.g., nitroprusside, nitrates, hydralazine, and calcium channel antagonists) must be avoided.
- **Contractility**: In normotensive patients with persistently unmet peripheral metabolic needs, inotropic support is indicated. Options include dobutamine or milrinone—guard against hypotension and tachyarrhythmias.
  - ○ **Treat volume overload and RV encroachment**.

Medications

First Line

- **Vasomodulator/vasodilator therapy**. At present, the following medications are only approved for treatment of Group 1 conditions. Approved PAH therapies have generally been shown in the short term to improve exercise capacity, functional classification, reduce hospitalizations, and "time to clinical worsening." Long-term outcome of prolonging survival is being inferred based on observational data and large-scale contemporary registries.[10]
  - ○ **CCBs should only be used for treating PAH after confirming acute vasoresponsiveness with a short-acting vasodilator and safety with acute CCB challenge** (as above).[1,11]
    - Indiscriminate CCB use can lead to hemodynamic collapse and syncope in patients with advanced RHF who are not acute vasoresponders.
    - Chronic CCB therapy (e.g., amlodipine, nifedipine, or diltiazem) can be prescribed, at an initial low dose and titrated over several weeks, while monitoring systemic pressures and guarding against the aggravation of RHF. Patients that do not have near normalization of PA pressures with long-term CCB usage should be considered for additional vasodilator/vasomodulator therapy (see below).
  - ○ **Endothelin receptor antagonists** block binding of endothelin-1 to A or B receptors on pulmonary artery smooth muscle cells and endothelial cells, which mitigates the signal to vasoconstrict and for cellular hypertrophy/growth.[1]
    - Two available agents are **bosentan** and **ambrisentan**, which are approved for functional class II or greater patients.[12,13]
    - Both drugs are teratogenic, and bosentan requires monthly laboratory monitoring for hepatotoxicity.
  - ○ **PDE5-I** block the phosphodiesterase, which degrades intracellular cGMP necessary for vasodilatory and cellular inhibition effects of nitric oxide.[1,4]

- Two available agents are **sildenafil** and **tadalafil**, which are approved for functional class II or greater patients.[14,15]
- No specific laboratory monitoring is needed but potent drug interaction with organic nitrates must be avoided.
  - **Prostanoids** are generally considered the most potent, but also the most potentially toxic, class of therapies due to their complex delivery system and wider therapeutic window. Prostanoids induce vasodilation, inhibit cellular growth, and inhibit platelet aggregation.[1]
    - Commercially available prostanoids include **epoprostenol** (intravenous), room-temperature stable epoprostenol (intravenous), **treprostinil** (intravenous, subcutaneous, or inhaled), and **iloprost** (inhaled).[16-18]
    - Approved for functional class III or greater (subcutaneous treprostinil is also approved in class II).
    - Choice of therapy is variable across experts and **dosing of parenteral agents is highly individualized to the patient and requires great expertise and impeccable nursing**.
    - Prostanoids are used in treatment-naïve patients who present in advanced RHF, but are mostly used as add-on therapies when oral agents provide ineffective or inadequate treatment response. Several randomized controlled trials of combination therapy have confirmed the benefits of combining prostanoids with an oral agent.
    - Adverse effects include drug-related side effects (e.g., jaw pain, nonpruritic rash, flushing, headache, gastrointestinal side effects, and extremity pain) and delivery-system complications (e.g., blood-stream infections, catheter-related thrombosis, inadvertent interruptions of drug administration with very short-acting continuous infusions).

Second Line

- **Warfarin to target an INR between 1.5 and 2.5 is recommended for PAH patients that have a favorable risk benefit profile for anticoagulation**, based on scant data favoring survival in IPAH patients.[1]
  - Anticoagulant therapy is not urgent and can be stopped for invasive procedures or active bleeding.
  - Caution with anticoagulation in patients with portopulmonary patients, complex congenital heart disease, systemic sclerosis, or prior history of significant hemoptysis.
- **Diuretic therapy** alleviates improves right heart function and improves symptoms.[1]
  - Often requires some combination of a loop diuretic, aldosterone antagonist, and thiazide.
  - **Too rapid of a diuresis can be poorly tolerated due to preload dependency** of the RV and limited ability of the cardiac output to compensate for systemic hypotension.
  - Avoid aggravating chronic renal dysfunction, particularly in an individual with long-standing RHF or intrinsic renal disease.
- **Digoxin** offers weak inotropic support and maybe particularly helpful if concomitant atrial tachyarrhythmias are present.[1]
- **Inotropic agents** (i.e., dobutamine, dopamine, milrinone, digoxin) modestly improve right heart function, cardiac output, and symptoms. Dobutamine, dopamine, and milrinone are best suited for short-term use in acutely decompensated states especially when overt organ hypoperfusion is evident.

Other Nonpharmacologic Therapies

- **Supplemental oxygen** should be used to maintain normoxemia and avoid hypoxic vasoconstriction as much as possible.
  - Normoxemia may be impossible to achieve if significant intracardiac right-to-left shunting is occurring.

○ Also consider supplemental oxygen during airline travel.
- **In-line intravenous filters** may prevent paradoxical air emboli in patients with significant intracardiac right-to-left shunts.
- **Fluid and sodium restriction** is appropriate for individuals with RHF.
- **Pulmonary rehabilitation** and exercise training is desirable for select individuals to overcome deconditioning.

Surgical Management

- **Lung or heart-lung transplantation** is reserved for suitable PAH patients that remain in advanced functional classes (III to IV) with ominous hemodynamics (RAP >15 and cardiac index <2.0 L/minute/m^2) despite maximal medical therapy, including a parenteral prostanoids.[1]
  ○ RV recovery after isolated lung transplantation allows for reserving heart-lung transplantation primarily in cases of irreparable complex congenital defects.
  ○ Median survival after lung transplantation is approximately 6 years while survival for IPAH patients at 5 years is 50%.
- **Atrial septostomy** percutaneously creates a right-to-left shunt across the interatrial septum and increases delivery of blood to the arterial circulation and oxygen to peripheral tissues—indicated in cases of refractory RHF (e.g., recurrent syncope, severe ascites, or poor systemic end-organ perfusion).[1]
- Septal defect closure is feasible in carefully selected cases of intracardiac defects in order to prevent development or minimize progression of PAH.
  ○ Requirements for closure include significant net left-to-right shunting (pulmonary/systemic flow ratio ≥2.0) and low pulmonary vascular resistance (PVR <5 Wood units and pulmonary/systemic resistance ratio ≤0.3).
  ○ Ostium secundum defects can be closed percutaneously while other defects require surgery.

SPECIAL CONSIDERATIONS

- The initial choice of PAH-specific therapy should be individualized based on risk factor stratification of an individual, with reliance on several clinical variables[19]:
  ○ Functional class (II or III vs. IV)
  ○ Clinical evidence of RHF (no vs. yes)
  ○ Rate of progression (gradual or months vs. rapid or weeks)
  ○ Degree of exercise impairment (6-minute walk distance of >400 m vs. <300 m)
  ○ Degree of hemodynamic derangement (RAP <10 mmHg vs. >20 mmHg or cardiac index >2.5 L/minute/m^2 vs. <2.0 L/minute/m^2)
- If most of the variables are in the concerning end of the spectrum, the aggregate impression should be that an individual is at high risk for serious event, including death in the near term, and should be started on a parenteral prostanoid.
- Other potentially worrisome findings are underlying PAH diagnosis (collagen vascular disease, portopulmonary hypertension, and HPAH), presence of pericardial effusion, degree of BNP elevation, degree of concomitant renal dysfunction, male gender, age >60, resting systolic blood pressure (<110 mmHg), pulse rate (92 beats), and diffusing capacity (<32%).
- The REVEAL registry has identified 19 clinical variables that may provide a simple risk calculator for any individual patient and awaits further validation.[18]
- Comorbid conditions, social support, and the patient's overall level of health-care sophistication are also critical, as delivery systems for PAH-specific therapies differ widely.
- ***Streptococcus pneumonia* and influenza vaccinations** should be used to avoid respiratory tract infections.
- Patients should **avoid high-risk behaviors** that can acutely decrease RV preload and/or increase RV afterload in advanced RHF:

○ Deep **Valsalva maneuvers** (e.g., severe coughing paroxysm, straining during defecation or micturition, vigorous exercise including resistance training, or lifting heavy items) should be avoided.

○ **High altitudes** (>5,000 feet) may be dangerous due to low inspired concentration of oxygen.

• **Avoid pregnancy** due to the marked hemodynamic alterations that can further strain a compromised RV. Contraception choice is highly variable but caution against thromboembolic events.

• **Systemic sympathomimetic agents** have vasoactive properties and should be avoided (e.g., over-the-counter decongestants, nicotine, and cocaine).

• **NSAIDs** also have multiple counterproductive effects in RHF.

MONITORING/FOLLOW-UP

• PAH remains incurable and current treatments are still largely palliative.

• Patients require close monitoring to detect deteriorating RV function and clinical progression.

• While no consensus exists for monitoring PAH patients, most centers use composite clinical variables (modified WHO functional class), exercise measures (6-minute walk time), and an objective RV assessment (e.g., echocardiogram, catheterization, BNP, cardiac MRI).

• If patients are declining, therapeutic classes are switched or, more likely, a second or third drug from a different therapeutic class is added.

REFERENCES

1. McLaughlin V, Archer S, Badesch D, et al. ACCF/AHA 2009 expert consensus document on pulmonary hypertension. *J Am Coll Cardiol* 2009;53:1573-1619.
2. Simonneau G, Robbins I, Beghetti M, et al. Updated clinical classification of pulmonary hypertension. *J Am Coll Cardiol* 2009;54:S43-S54.
3. Elliot CG. Genetics of pulmonary arterial hypertension: current and future implications. *Semin Respir Crit Care Med* 2005;26:365-371.
4. Lindman BR, Chakinala MM. Modulating the NO–cGMP pathway in the pressure-overloaded left ventricle and group II pulmonary hypertension. *Intl J Clin Pract Suppl* 2010;168:15-22.
5. Galiè N, Manes A, Palazzini M, et al. Pharmacological impact on right ventricular remodeling in pulmonary arterial hypertension. *Eur Heart J Suppl* 2007;9(H):H68-H74.
6. McLaughlin VV, McGoon MD. Pulmonary arterial hypertension. *Circulation* 2006;114:1417-1431.
7. DeMarco T, McGlothin D. Managing right ventricular failure in PAH. *Adv Pulm Hypertens* 2005;14:1626.
8. Lahm T, McCaslin C, Wozniak T, et al. Medical and surgical treatment of acute right ventricular failure. *J Am Coll Cardiol* 2010;56:1435-1446.
9. Piazza G, Goldhaber S. The acutely decompensated right ventricle: pathways for diagnosis and management. *Chest* 2005;128:1836-1852.
10. Galiè N, Manes A, Negro L. A meta-analysis of randomized controlled trials in pulmonary artery hypertension. *Eur Heart J* 2009;30:394-403.
11. Rich S, Kaufmann E, Levy PS. The effect of high doses of calcium-channel blockers on survival in primary pulmonary hypertension. *N Engl J Med* 1992;327:76-81.
12. Rubin LJ, Dadesch DB, Barst RJ, et al. Bosentan therapy for pulmonary arterial hypertension. *N Engl J Med* 2002;346:896-903.
13. Oudiz RJ, Galiè N, Olschewski H, et al. Long-term ambrisentan therapy for the treatment of pulmonary arterial hypertension. *J Am Coll Cardiol* 2009;54:1971-1981.
14. Galiè N, Ghofrani HA, Torbicki A, et al. Sildenafil citrate therapy for pulmonary arterial hypertension. *N Engl J Med* 2005;353:2148-2157.
15. Galiè N, Brundage BH, Ghofrani HA, et al. Tadalafil therapy for pulmonary hypertension. *Circulation* 2009;119:2894-2903.

16. Barst RJ, Rubin LJ, Long WA, et al. A comparison of continuous intravenous epoprostenol (prostacyclin) with conventional therapy for primary pulmonary hypertension. *N Engl J Med* 1996;334:296-301.

17. Simonneau G, Barst RJ, Galie N, et al. Continuous subcutaneous infusion of treprostinil, a prostacyclin analogue, in patients with pulmonary arterial hypertension: a double-blind, randomized, placebo-controlled trial. *Am J Respir Crit Care Med* 2002;165:800-804.

18. Olschewski H, Simonneau G, Galie N, et al. Inhaled iloprost for severe pulmonary hypertension. *N Engl J Med* 2002;347:322-329.

19. Benza R, Miller DP, Gomberg-Maitland M, et al. Predicting survival in pulmonary arterial hypertension: insights from the Registry to Evaluate Early and Long-term Pulmonary Arterial Hypertension Disease Management (REVEAL). *Circulation* 2010;122:164-172.

Aortic Valve Disease

19

Suzanne V. Arnold and Brian R. Lindman

- Aortic valve disease, particularly aortic stenosis (AS), is common and, as the population ages, increasing in prevalence.
- AS is present in 2% of people aged >65 years and in 4% of those aged >85 years.
- Rheumatic valve disease is quite common worldwide, and due to antibiotic usage and the aging of the population, degenerative/calcific AS is more common in the developed world.
- Inadequate understanding of the pathophysiology of aortic valve disease has limited efforts at medical therapy. Both AS and regurgitation remain "surgical diseases." However, emerging data on valvular and ventricular biology may pave the way for more effective medical therapy.
- Transcatheter techniques for valve implantation will likely play an increasingly important role in the treatment of patients with aortic valve disease.
- An aortic valve is a trileaflet valve that permits unidirectional flow from the left ventricle (LV) into the aorta.
- AS is characterized by incomplete opening of the valve during systole, which limits antegrade flow, yielding a systolic pressure gradient between the LV and ascending aorta.
- Aortic regurgitation (AR) is caused by incompetence of the valve, allowing backward flow of blood from the aorta into the LV during diastole.

Aortic Stenosis

GENERAL PRINCIPLES

Background

- Lesions of the aortic valve are the most common cause for obstruction of flow from the LV into the aorta.
- Other causes of obstruction and the consequent pressure gradient between the LV and aorta include obstruction above the valve (supravalvular) and below the valve (subvalvular), both fixed (i.e., subaortic membrane) and dynamic (i.e., hypertrophic cardiomyopathy with obstruction).
- Aortic sclerosis is thickening of the aortic valve leaflets, which causes turbulent flow through the valve and a murmur but no gradient and therefore no stenosis. Aortic sclerosis is considered a risk factor for progression to stenosis.

Epidemiology

- AS is a progressive disease typically characterized by an asymptomatic phase until the valve area reaches a minimum threshold, generally <1 cm^2.
- In the absence of symptoms, patients with AS generally have a good prognosis with a risk of sudden death estimated to be <1% per year.
- Predictors of decreased event-free survival (free of aortic valve replacement [AVR] or death) include higher peak aortic jet velocity, extent of valve calcification, elevated B-type natriuretic peptide (BNP), and coexistent coronary artery disease (CAD).[1,2]

- Once patients experience symptoms, their average survival is 2 to 3 years, with an increased risk of sudden death.

Etiology

- **Calcific/degenerative:**
  - Common cause in the United States.[3]
  - Trileaflet calcific AS usually presents in the seventh through ninth decades of life (mean age mid-70s).
  - Risk factors are similar to CAD including age, male gender, smoking, and hypertension and exacerbated by abnormal calcium metabolism.[4]
  - Active biological process with bone formation in the valve.
  - Calcification leading to stenosis affects both trileaflet and bicuspid valves.
- **Bicuspid:**
  - Occurs in 1% to 2% of population (congenital lesion).
  - Usually presents in the sixth through seventh decades (mean age mid- to late-60s).
  - Approximately 50% of patients needing AVR for AS have a bicuspid valve.[5]
  - More prone to endocarditis than trileaflet valves.
  - Associated with aortopathies (i.e., dissection, aneurysm) in a significant proportion of patients.
- **Rheumatic:**
  - Most common cause worldwide and usually presents in the third through fifth decades.
  - Almost always accompanied by mitral valve (MV) disease.

Pathophysiology

The pathophysiology for calcific AS involves both the valve and the ventricular adaptation to the stenosis. There is growing evidence for an active biological process within the valve that begins much like the formation of an atherosclerotic plaque and eventually leads to the formation of calcified bone (Figure 19-1).

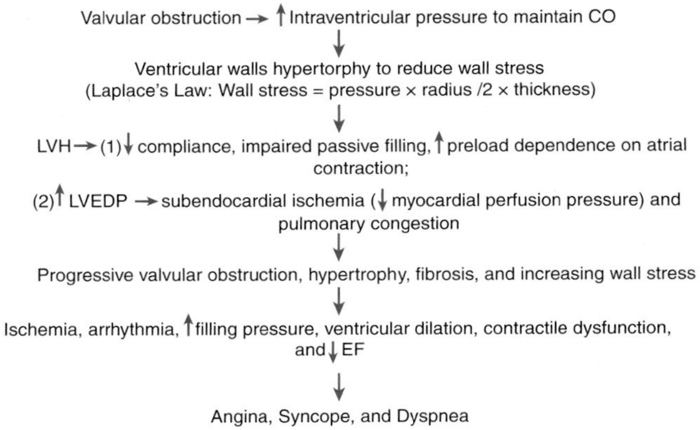

Valvular obstruction → ↑Intraventricular pressure to maintain CO
↓
Ventricular walls hypertorphy to reduce wall stress
(Laplace's Law: Wall stress = pressure × radius /2 × thickness)
↓
LVH → (1)↓compliance, impaired passive filling, ↑preload dependence on atrial contraction;
(2)↑LVEDP → subendocardial ischemia (↓myocardial perfusion pressure) and pulmonary congestion
↓
Progressive valvular obstruction, hypertrophy, fibrosis, and increasing wall stress
↓
Ischemia, arrhythmia, ↑filling pressure, ventricular dilation, contractile dysfunction, and↓EF
↓
Angina, Syncope, and Dyspnea

FIGURE 19-1. Pathophysiology of aortic stenosis.

DIAGNOSIS

Clinical Presentation

History

- Classic symptoms include:
  - Angina
  - Syncope
  - Heart failure
- Not infrequently, patients may limit their activity in ways that mask the presence of symptoms but indicate a progressive and premature decline in functional capacity. In the setting of severe AS, these patients should be viewed as symptomatic.

Physical Examination

- Harsh systolic crescendo–decrescendo murmur heard best at the right upper sternal border and radiating to both carotids; time to peak intensity correlates with severity (later peak = more severe).
- Diminished or absent A2 (soft S2) suggests severe AS.
- An opening snap suggests bicuspid AV.
- S4 reflects atrial contraction on a poorly compliant ventricle.
- Point of maximum impact (PMI) is sustained and diffuse and not displaced (unless the ventricle has dilated).
- Pulsus parvus et tardus: late-peaking and diminished carotid upstroke in severe AS.
- Gallavardin phenomenon is an AS murmur in which the musical element of the murmur is heard best at the apex (easily confused with Mitral regurgitation (MR)).
- Between extremes, it is often difficult to assess AS severity on examination.

Diagnostic Criteria

The diagnostic criteria for severe AS are presented in Table 19-1.

Diagnostic Testing

- The standard evaluation of AS is presented in Table 19-2.
- Further evaluation in selected patients is presented in Table 19-3.

TREATMENT

Medications

- Severe symptomatic AS is a surgical disease. **There are currently no medical treatments proven to decrease mortality or delay surgery**.
- Nevertheless, there are some guidelines for medical therapy in nonsurgical candidates, asymptomatic patients, or those with less severe stenosis.

TABLE 19-1	SEVERE AORTIC STENOSIS
Jet velocity (m/second)	>4.0
Mean gradient (mmHg)	>40
Valve area (cm²)	<1.0

Modified from Bonow RO, Carabello BA, Chatterjee K, et al. ACC/AHA 2006 guidelines for the management of patients with valvular heart disease. *J Am Coll Cardiol* 2006;48:e1-e148.

TABLE 19-2   STANDARD EVALUATION OF AORTIC STENOSIS

ECG	• LAE and LVH
CXR	• LVH, cardiomegaly, and calcification of the aorta, AV, or coronaries
	• Rib notching suggests coarctation and BAV.
TTE	• Leaflet number, morphology, and calcification
	• Calculate valve area using continuity equation [Area$_{AV}$ × Velocity$_{AV}$ = Area$_{LVOT}$ × Velocity$_{LVOT}$]. The continuity equation is based on the principle that flow (velocity × area) is equal both proximal to and at the level of the obstruction.
	• Transvalvular mean and peak gradients

LAE, left atrial enlargement; LVH, left ventricular hypertrophy; AV, aortic valve; BAV, bicuspid aortic valve; LVOT, left ventricular outflow tract.

TABLE 19-3   FURTHER EVALUATION IN SELECTED PATIENTS WITH AORTIC STENOSIS

TEE	• Clarify whether there is a bicuspid valve if unclear on TTE.
	• Occasionally needed to evaluate for other or additional causes of LVOT obstruction.
Exercise testing	• Evaluate for exercise capacity, abnormal blood pressure response (<20 mmHg increase with exercise), or exercise-induced symptoms.
Dobutamine stress echo	• Useful to assess the patient with LV dysfunction with a small valve area (suggesting severe AS) but a low (<30–40 mmHg) mean transvalvular gradient (suggesting less severe AS)
	• Can help distinguish truly severe AS from pseudosevere AS
	• Assess for the presence of contractile reserve.
Cath	• In patients undergoing AVR who are at risk for CAD
	• Evaluate for CAD in patients with moderate AS and symptoms of angina.
	• Hemodynamic assessment of the severity of AS in patients in whom noninvasive tests are inconclusive or when there is a discrepancy between noninvasive tests and clinical findings regarding AS severity (utilizes the Gorlin formula).
CTA	• CTA may be an alternative to cath to evaluate coronary anatomy prior to valve surgery (the role and accuracy of CTA is still being investigated).

TEE, transesophageal echocardiogram; TTE, transthoracic echocardiogram; LVOT, left ventricular outflow tract; LV, left ventricle; AS, aoritic stenosis; AVR, aortic valve replacement; CAD, coronary artery disease; CTA, computed tomographic angiography.

- **Hypertension:**
  - Hypertension is very common in patients with AS.
  - Inadequate treatment of hypertension adds an additional load on the LV and contributes to the progression of disease.
  - **Angiotensin-converting enzyme (ACE) inhibitors**: some data suggest that ACE inhibition may interfere with the valvular biology that leads to valve calcification.
  - **Statins**: some early data suggested that statins may slow progression of AS, but several subsequent clinical trials of patients with mild-to-severe AS failed to show any benefit with statins.[6–9] It is unknown if earlier intervention with statins (i.e., when the valve is sclerotic) would slow progression of the disease.
  - **Use vasodilators, particularly nitroglycerin, cautiously so as to avoid hypotension.**
- **Severe AS with decompensated heart failure:**
  - Patients with severe AS and LV dysfunction may experience decompensated heart failure.
  - Depending on the clinical scenario, several options may help bridge the patient to definitive surgical management (i.e., AVR):
    - Intra-aortic balloon pump (IABP) (contraindicated in patients with moderate to severe AR)
    - Sodium nitroprusside
    - Percutaneous aortic valvuloplasty
  - Each of the above measures provides some degree of afterload reduction, either at the level of the valve (valvuloplasty) or by reduction in systemic vascular resistance (IABP, nipride); this afterload reduction can facilitate forward flow.
  - Operative mortality may decrease as heart failure improves and transient end-organ damage is reversed.

Surgical Management
- Therapeutic decisions are primarily based on the presence or absence of symptoms (Figure 19-2).[3,10]
- The treatment of severe AS is almost exclusively surgical AVR.
- **Symptomatic severe AS is a deadly disease and deserves prompt surgical intervention.**
- Certain associated high-risk features or the need for another cardiac surgical intervention may lead to the recommendation for an AVR even when the patient is asymptomatic or has less than severe stenosis.
- Operative mortality varies significantly depending on age, comorbidities, and concurrent surgical procedures to be performed.

Transcatheter Aortic Valve Replacement
- In high-risk or inoperable patients, **transcatheter aortic valve replacement (TAVR)** is rapidly becoming a promising treatment option.
- TAVR can be performed via transfemoral, transapical, or transaortic approaches.
- As demonstrated in the randomized Placement of AoRtic TraNscathetER Valves (PARTNER) Trial, TAVR can substantially reduce mortality and improve quality of life as compared to medical therapy in patients deemed "inoperable."[11]
- In patients who are not inoperable but high risk, TAVR is a reasonable option. The risk of stroke is higher in TAVR in the periprocedural period but similar at three years. Paravalvular leak associated with TAVR is associated with worse outcomes. Ongoing trials will help further identify additional groups who may benefit from TAVR.
- TAVR may become a good option for an aging population with numerous comorbidities accompanying severe AS.

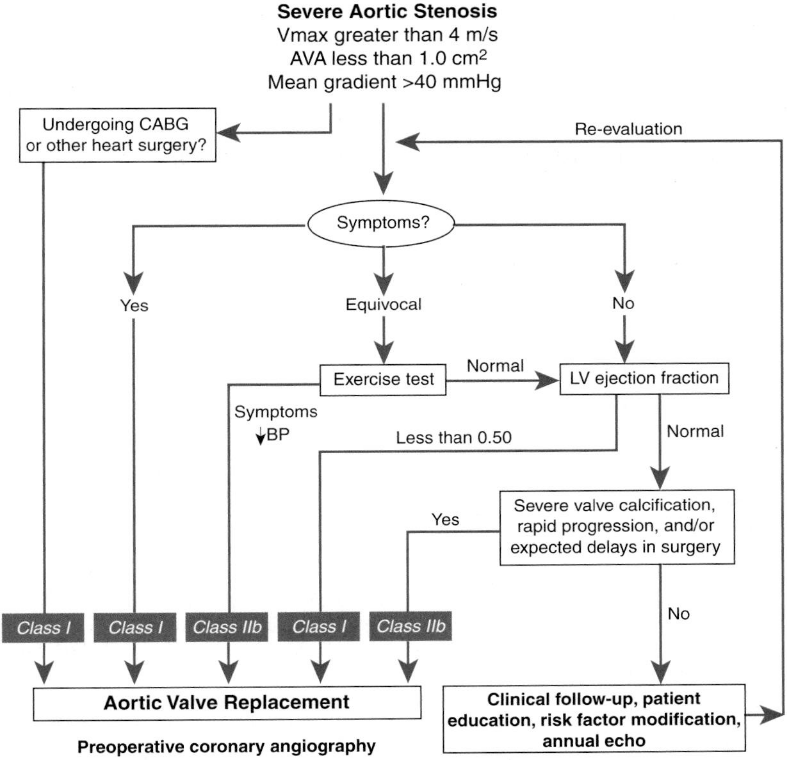

FIGURE 19-2. Evaluation and treatment of severe aortic stenosis. (From Bonow RO, Carabello BA, Chatterjee K, et al. ACC/AHA 2006 guidelines for the management of patients with valvular heart disease. *J Am Coll Cardiol* 2006;48(3): e1-e148, with permission.)

Percutaneous Aortic Valvuloplasty

Valvuloplasty has a limited role in the management of AS; aortic valve area increases very modestly and restenosis occurs in weeks to months. It may be used:

- As a bridge to AVR in patients with decompensated heart failure.
- As a palliative measure in patients not undergoing valve replacement.
- **If urgent noncardiac surgery is needed in patients with severe symptomatic AS.**
- To clarify optimal management in high-risk operative candidates who have concomitant severe lung disease in whom it is not clear whether shortness of breath is primarily due to lung versus valve disease. If there is a clinical response (improvement in shortness of breath) with valvuloplasty, there is greater confidence that the clinical benefit of AVR may outweigh the risk.

Challenging Clinical Scenarios

- Asymptomatic severe AS—**is the patient really asymptomatic?**
  - Determine whether the patient is really asymptomatic with an exercise stress test.
  - An elevated BNP may predict earlier symptom onset or worse outcome if surgery is delayed.
  - A CT scan to assess the extent of valve calcification can predict earlier symptom onset.
- Concomitant CAD and moderate AS in a patient with angina—**what is causing the angina?**
  - Incorporate all the data (including Doppler assessment of the coronary lesion in the cath lab, perfusion imaging, and severity of AS) to guide management.
  - If AS is moderate and the coronary lesion appears obstructive, consider percutaneous coronary intervention to relieve angina; if there is no relief, then consider AVR.
- Combined AS/AR—**what if symptoms develop when the lesion(s) are only moderate?**
  - Generally, surgical timing is still determined by the guidelines for isolated AS or AR.
  - However, patients with combined moderate AS and AR may develop symptoms and/or LV dysfunction before either lesion is severe.
  - It is reasonable to pursue AVR in combined moderate AS/AR when symptoms are present, LV function is reduced, or at the time of other cardiac surgery.
- Aortic root disease—**how does aortic root dilation influence the timing and extent of surgery?**
  - Almost 50% of patients with severe AS have a bicuspid aortic valve (BAV).[5]
  - This is associated with aortic pathology that may predispose these patients to aortic dilation and dissection.
  - It is critical to evaluate the aortic dimensions in patients with BAV, as significant enlargement may indicate a need for surgery even before valve stenosis is severe. Regardless of which drives the timing of surgery (aortic dimension or AV disease), both may need to be repaired or replaced at the time of surgery.
  - All patients identified with a BAV should have imaging—computed tomography (CT) or magnetic resonance imaging (MRI)—to evaluate for thoracic aortic pathology.
- LV dysfunction—**should surgery be done when the valve area suggests severe AS but the gradient is low?**
  - Dobutamine stress echo can be used to distinguish truly severe AS from pseudosevere AS as well as to evaluate for the presence of contractile reserve.
  - Lack of contractile reserve predicts an increased operative mortality.
  - Long-term survival is better with AVR than medical management in those with or without contractile reserve.
  - Recovery of LV function after AVR cannot be predicted based on the absence/presence of contractile reserve.

Aortic Regurgitation

GENERAL PRINCIPLES

- For the natural history of AR, see Table 19-4.[3]
- AR results from pathology of the aortic valve with or without involvement of the aortic root.
- Several potential causes for AR variably affect the valve and aortic root. AR usually develops insidiously, but may be acute.
- **More common causes** include BAV, rheumatic disease, calcific degeneration, infective endocarditis, idiopathic dilatation of the aorta, myxomatous degeneration, systemic hypertension, dissection of the ascending aorta, and Marfan syndrome (MFS).

TABLE 19-4	NATURAL HISTORY OF AORTIC REGURGITATION
Asymptomatic patients with normal LV systolic function	
Progression to symptoms and/or LV dysfunction	<6% per year
Progression to asymptomatic LV dysfunction	<3.5% per year
Sudden death	<0.2% per year
Asymptomatic patients with LV dysfunction	
Progression to cardiac symptoms	>25% per year
Symptomatic patients	
Mortality rate	>10% per year

From Bonow RO, Carabello BA, Chatterjee K, et al. ACC/AHA 2006 guidelines for the management of patients with valvular heart disease. *JACC* 2006;48(3):e1-e148, with permission.

- **Less common causes** include traumatic injury to the aortic valve, collagen vascular diseases (e.g., ankylosing spondylitis, rheumatoid arthritis, Reiter's syndrome, giant-cell aortitis, and Whipple disease), syphilitic aortitis, osteogenesis imperfect, Ehlers–Danlos syndrome (EDS), discrete subaortic stenosis, ventricular septal defect (VSD) with prolapse of an aortic cusp, and anorectic drugs.
- **Acute causes** are infective endocarditis, dissection of the ascending aorta, and trauma.
- The pathophysiologies of acute and chronic AR are presented in Figures 19-3 and 19-4, respectively.

DIAGNOSIS

Clinical Presentation

History

- Acute: Patients with acute AR typically present with **pulmonary edema manifested by severe dyspnea**. Other presenting symptoms may be related to the causes of acute AR listed above.
- Chronic: **Symptoms depend on the presence of LV dysfunction and whether the patient is in the compensated versus decompensated stage.** Compensated patients are typically asymptomatic, whereas those in the decompensated stage may note decreased exercise tolerance, dyspnea, fatigue, and/or angina.

Physical Examination

- **Acute AR:**
  - Tachycardia
  - Wide pulse pressure may be present but often is not because forward stroke volume (and therefore systolic blood pressure) is reduced.
  - A brief soft diastolic murmur heard best at the third left intercostal space (often not heard)
  - Systolic flow murmur (due to volume overload and hyperdynamic LV)

Pathophsiology of Acute Aortic Regurgitation

Sudden large regurgitant volume imposed on LV of
normal (or small) size with normal (or decreased) compliance

↓

Rapid ↑LVEDP and ↑LAP
LV attempts to maintain CO with ↑HR and ↑contractility

↓

Attempts to maintain forward SV/CO may be inadequate

↙   ↓   ↘

Pulmonary edema ischemia   Cardiogenic shock   Myocardial
(↑LVEDP and ↑LAP pressure)   (↓forward SV/CO)   (↓coronary perfusion
                                                                ↑demand myocardial O$_2$)

LV, left ventricle; LVEDP, left ventricular end diastolic pressure; LAP, left atrial pressure; CO,
cardiac output; HR, heart rate; SV, stroke volume.

FIGURE 19-3. Pathophysiology of acute aortic regurgitation.

Pathophysiology of Chronic Aortic Regurgitation

Regurgitant volume load

↓

Compensatory mechanisms:
(1)↑LV dilation → ↑LVED volume and ↑chamber compliance
(2)↑LV hypertrophy (eccentric and concentric) stimulated by ↑LV afterload

↓

These compensatory mechanisms maintain a relatively low LVEDP,
adequate forward SV/CO, and sufficient coronary perfusion pressure

↓

Decompensation

↓

Steadily increasing regurgitant volume load
Further ventricular dilation → ↑ wall stress
Inability to continue further hypertrophy to ↓afterload
Contractile dysfunction → ↓EF/SV/CO
↓LVEDP

↙   ↘

CHF symptoms   Angina
(due both to congestion   (↓coronary perfusion pressure
and ↓CO)   and marked LVH)

LV, left ventricle; LVED, left ventricular end diastolic; LVEDP, left ventricular end diastolic
pressure; EF, ejection fraction; SV, stroke volume; CO, cardiac output; CHF, congestive
heart failure.

FIGURE 19-4. Pathophysiology of chronic aortic regurgitation.

- Diminished S1 due to increased LV end-diastolic pressure (LVEDP) and premature MV closure
- LV heave
- Pulsus paradoxus (may suggest cardiac tamponade secondary to aortic dissection)
- Measure blood pressure in both arms (a significant difference suggests aortic dissection).
- Look for evidence of infective endocarditis.
- Look for Marfanoid characteristics.

- **Chronic AR:**
  - LV heave
  - PMI is laterally displaced.
  - Diastolic decrescendo murmur heard best at lower sternal border (LSB) leaning forward at end-expiration (severity of AR correlates with duration, not intensity, of the murmur).
  - Systolic flow murmur (due mostly to volume overload; concomitant AS may also be present)
  - Austin Flint murmur—low-pitched diastolic murmur, heard best at the apex, caused by antegrade flow through a mitral orifice narrowed by severe AR, which restricts the motion of the anterior MV leaflet.
  - S3 is often heard as a manifestation of the volume overload and is not necessarily a sign of congestive heart failure (CHF).
  - Widened pulse pressure (often >100 mmHg) with a low diastolic pressure.
  - Characteristic signs related to wide pulse pressure:
    - Musset sign: head bobbing with each cardiac cycle
    - Corrigan pulse: rapid carotid upstroke followed by arterial collapse
    - Müller sign: pulsation of the uvula
    - Traube sign: pistol-shot murmur heard on the femoral artery
    - Duroziez sign: to-and-fro murmur over the femoral artery when partially compressed
    - Quincke pulse: visible capillary pulsation in the nail bed after holding the tip of the nail

Diagnostic Criteria

The diagnostic criteria for severe AR are presented in Table 19-5.[12]

Diagnostic Testing

The diagnostic evaluation will depend somewhat on the acuity of the presentation.

Electrocardiography

ECG findings include tachycardia, LV hypertrophy (LVH), and left atrial enlargement (LAE) (more common in chronic AR). New heart block may suggest an aortic root abscess.

Imaging

- **Chest radiograph (CXR):** look for pulmonary edema, widened mediastinum, and cardiomegaly.
- **Transthoracic echocardiography (TTE):**
  - LV systolic function
  - LV dimensions at end systole and end diastole
  - Leaflet number and morphology
  - Assessment of the severity of AR (see Table 19-5)[12]
  - Look for evidence of endocarditis or aortic dissection.
  - Dimension of aortic root
- **Transesophageal echocardiogrpahy (TEE):**
  - Clarify whether there is a bicuspid valve if unclear on transthoracic echo.
  - Better sensitivity and specificity for aortic dissection than transthoracic echo
  - Clarify whether there is endocarditis ± root abscess if unclear on transthoracic echo.
  - Better visualization of aortic valve in patients with a prosthetic aortic valve

TABLE 19-5 SEVERE AORTIC REGURGITATION

Qualitative

Angiographic grade	3–4+
Color Doppler jet width	>65% of LVOT
Doppler vena contracta width (cm)	>0.6
PHT of AR jet (ms)	<200
Quantitative (cath or echo)	
Regurgitant volume (mL/beat)	≥60
Regurgitant fraction (%)	≥50
Regurgitant orifice area (cm²) (ERO)	≥0.30
Additional essential criteria	
LV size	Increased[a]

[a]Except in acute AR in which the ventricle has not had time to dilate.

LVOT, left ventricular outflow tract; PHT, pressure half-time; AR, aortic regurgitation; ERO, effective regurgitant orifice; LV, left ventricular.

Modified from Zoghbi WA, Enriquez-Sarano M, Foster E, et al. Recommendations for evaluation of the severity of native valvular regurgitation with two-dimensional and Doppler echocardiography. *J Am Soc Echocardiogr* 2003;16:777-802.

- **MRI/CT:**
  - Depending on the institution, either of these may be the imaging modality of choice for evaluating aortic dimensions and/or aortic dissection.
  - If echo assessment of the severity of AR is inadequate, MRI is useful for assessing the severity of AR.
  - CT angiography (CTA) may be an alternative to cath to evaluate coronary anatomy prior to valve surgery (the role and accuracy of CTA are still being investigated).

Diagnostic Procedures

- **Coronary angiography** is performed in patients undergoing AVR who are at risk for CAD.
- Assessment of LV pressure, LV function, and severity of AR (via aortic root angiography) is indicated in symptomatic patients in whom the severity of AR is unclear on noninvasive imaging or discordant with clinical findings.

TREATMENT

Medications

- The role of medical therapy in patients with AR is limited. No randomized, placebo-controlled data show that vasodilator therapy delays the development of symptoms or LV dysfunction warranting surgery.[13]
- **Vasodilator therapy** (i.e., nifedipine, ACE inhibitor, hydralazine) has a potential role in three situations:

○ Chronic therapy in patients with severe AR who have symptoms or LV dysfunction but are not surgical candidates.

○ Short-term therapy to improve hemodynamics in patients with severe heart failure and severe LV dysfunction prior to surgery.

○ Long-term therapy in asymptomatic patients with severe AR who have some degree of LV dilatation but normal systolic function is indicated to reduce systolic blood pressure in hypertensive patients with AR.

○ In the absence of hypertension, it is not indicated for those who are asymptomatic, with mild or moderate AR, normal LV function, and normal LV cavity size.

• **β-Blockers** may be considered in the medical therapy of chronic severe AR.

○ It was previously believed that prolonging the diastolic filling time by slowing the heart rate would worsen the regurgitation; thus β-blockers were contraindicated in severe AR.

○ While this is likely true in the case of acute severe AR, a recent observational study of patients with chronic severe AR showed a marked reduction in 1- and 5-year mortality in the patients treated with β-blockers.[14] Randomized trials will need to confirm this finding.

Surgical Management

• **Surgery is indicated for any symptomatic patient with severe AR** regardless of LV systolic function (see Figure 19-5 and Table 19-6).[15]

• Acute, severe AR is almost always symptomatic.

• Valve repair may be feasible in a small subset of patients, usually those in whom aortic dissection is the cause of the AR.

• If the aortic root is dilated, it may be repaired or replaced at the time of AVR.

• AVR is usually a better alternative than medical therapy in improving overall mortality and morbidity although worse New York Heart Association (NYHA) functional class, LV dysfunction, and the chronicity of these abnormalities are predictors of higher operative and postoperative mortality.

• Short-term treatment with vasodilator therapy (i.e., nitroprusside) is reasonable to improve hemodynamics prior to surgery in the patient with decompensated heart failure.

TABLE 19-6	ACC/AHA GUIDELINES—CLASS I INDICATIONS FOR AORTIC VALVE REPLACEMENT FOR AORTIC REGURGITATION

• Symptomatic with severe AR irrespective of LV systolic function

• Asymptomatic with chronic severe AR and LV systolic dysfunction (EF ≤50%)

• Chronic severe AR while undergoing CABG, surgery on the aorta, or other valve surgery

AR, aortic regurgitation; LV, left ventricular; EF, ejection fraction; CABG, coronary artery bypass grafting.

Modified from Bonow RO, Carabello BA, Chatterjee K, et al. ACC/AHA 2006 guidelines for the management of patients with valvular heart disease. *J Am Coll Cardiol* 2006;48(3):e1-e148.

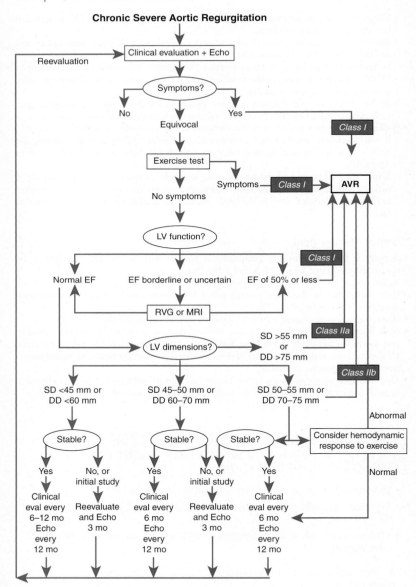

FIGURE 19-5. Evaluation and treatment of chronic severe aortic regurgitation. (From Bonow RO, Carabello BA, Chatterjee K, et al. ACC/AHA 2006 guidelines for the management of patients with valvular heart disease. *J Am Coll Cardiol* 2006;48(3):e1-e148, with permission.)

REFERENCES

1. Rosenhek R, Klaar U, Schemper M, et al. Mild and moderate aortic stenosis—natural history and risk stratification by echocardiography. *Eur Heart J* 2004;25:199-205.
2. Rosenhek R, Binder T, Parenta G, et al. Predictors or outcome in severe, asymptomatic aortic stenosis. *N Engl J Med* 2000;343:611-617.
3. Bonow RO, Carabello BA, Chatterjee K, et al. 2008 focused update incorporated into the ACC/AHA 2006 guidelines for the Management of Patients with Valvular Heart Disease. *J Am Coll Cardiol* 2008;52:e1-e142.
4. Stewart BF, Siscovick DS, Lind BK, et al. Clinical factors associated with calcific aortic valve disease. *J Am Coll Cardiol* 1997;29:630-644.
5. Roberts WC, Ko JM. Frequency by decades of unicuspid, bicuspid, and tricuspid aortic valves in adults having isolated aortic valve replacement for aortic stenosis, with or without associated aortic regurgitation. *Circulation* 2005;111:920-925.
6. Chan KL, Teo K, Dumesnil JG, et al. Effect of lipid lowering with rosuvastatin on progression of aortic stenosis. *Circulation* 2010;121:306-314.
7. Cowell SJ, Newby DE, Prescott RJ, et al. A randomized trial of intensive lipid lowering therapy in calcific aortic stenosis. *N Engl J Med* 2005;352:2389-2397.
8. Moura LM, Ramos SF, Zamorano JL, et al. Rosuvastatin Affecting Aortic Valve Endothelium to slow the progression of aortic stenosis (RAAVE). *J Am Coll Cardiol* 2007;49:554-561.
9. Rossebo AB, Pedersen TR, Boman K, et al. Intensive lipid lowering with simvastatin and ezetimibe in aortic stenosis. *N Engl J Med* 2008;359:1343-1356.
10. Otto CM. Valvular aortic stenosis: disease severity and timing of intervention. *J Am Coll Cardiol* 2006;47:2141-2151.
11. Leon MB, Smith CR, Mack M, et al. Transcatheter aortic-valve implantation for aortic stenosis in patients who cannot undergo surgery. *N Engl J Med* 2010;363(17):1597-1607.
12. Zoghbi WA, Enriquez-Sarano M, Foster E, et al. Recommendations for evaluation of the severity of native valvular regurgitation with two-dimensional and Doppler echocardiography. *J Am Soc Echocardiogr* 2003;16:777-802.
13. Evangelista A, Tornos P, Sambola A, et al. Long-term vasodilator therapy in patients with severe aortic regurgitation. *N Engl J Med* 2005;353:1342-1349.
14. Sampat U, Varadarajan P, Turk R, et al. Effect of beta-blocker therapy on survival in patients with severe aortic regurgitation. *J Am Coll Cardiol* 2009;54:452-457.
15. Bonow RO, Carabello BA, et al. American College of Cardiology/American Heart Association Task Force on Practice Guidelines; Society of Cardiovascular Anesthesiologists; Society for Cardiovascular Angiography and Interventions; Society of Thoracic Surgeons.HYPERLINK "http://www.ncbi.nlm.nih.gov/pubmed/16880336"ACC/AHA 2006 guidelines for the management of patients with valvular heart disease: a report of the American College of Cardiology/American Heart Association Task Force on Practice Guidelines (writing committee to revise the 1998 Guidelines for the Management of Patients With Valvular Heart Disease): developed in collaboration with the Society of Cardiovascular Anesthesiologists: endorsed by the Society for Cardiovascular Angiography and Interventions and the Society of Thoracic Surgeons. *Circulation* 20061;114(5):e84-231.

Mitral Valve Disease

20

William J. Nienaber and Jose A. Madrazo

- The mitral valve permits unidirectional flow from the left atrium (LA) to the left ventricle (LV).
- The mitral apparatus is composed of an annulus, two leaflets, posteromedial and anterolateral papillary muscles, and chordae tendineae. The latter two are considered part of the mitral subvalvular apparatus.
- Together with the LV, the proper interaction between these various parts is necessary for the adequate function of the mitral valve.

Mitral Stenosis

GENERAL PRINCIPLES

Etiology

- Mitral stenosis (MS) is characterized by incomplete opening of the mitral valve during diastole, which limits anterograde flow and yields a sustained diastolic pressure gradient between the LA and LV.
- MS is classified based on its etiology.
- **Rheumatic heart disease is the predominant cause of MS.** Rheumatic fever can cause fibrosis, thickening, and calcification, leading to fusion of the commissures, cusps, chordae, or some combination.
- Other causes are less common and include mitral annular calcification (MAC), congenital heart disease, carcinoid (in setting of right to left shunt or pulmonary involvement), systemic lupus erythematosus, rheumatoid arthritis, and mucopolysaccharidoses. Patients with end-stage renal disease are predisposed to MAC and calcific MS.
- "Functional MS" may occur with obstruction of left atrial outflow due to any number of causes including myxoma, LA thrombus, endocarditis with a large vegetation, congenital membrane of the LA (i.e., cor triatriatum), MV prosthesis dysfunction, or an oversewn mitral annuloplasty ring.

Pathophysiology

- Physiologic states that either increase the transvalvular flow (enhance cardiac output) or decrease diastolic filling time (via tachycardia) can lead to elevation in LA pressure and increase symptoms at any given valve area.
- Pregnancy, exercise, hyperthyroidism, atrial fibrillation (AF) with rapid ventricular response, and fever are examples in which either or both of these conditions occur. Symptoms are often first noticed at these times (Figure 20-1).

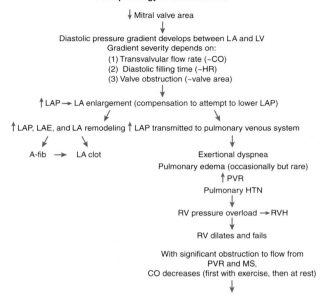

Pathophsiology of Mitral Stenosis

↓ Mitral valve area

Diastolic pressure gradient develops between LA and LV
Gradient severity depends on:
(1) Transvalvular flow rate (~CO)
(2) Diastolic filling time (~HR)
(3) Valve obstruction (~valve area)

↑LAP → LA enlargement (compensation to attempt to lower LAP)

↑LAP, LAE, and LA remodeling ↑LAP transmitted to pulmonary venous system

A-fib → LA clot

Exertional dyspnea
Pulmonary edema (occasionally but rare)
↑PVR
Pulmonary HTN

RV pressure overload → RVH

RV dilates and fails

With significant obstruction to flow from
PVR and MS,
CO decreases (first with exercise, then at rest)

Fatigue, dyspnea, ↓ functional capacity

FIGURE 20-1. Pathophysiology of mitral stenosis.

DIAGNOSIS

Clinical Presentation

- MS usually progresses slowly, with a long latent period (several decades) between rheumatic fever and the development of stenosis severe enough to cause symptoms (usually <2 to 2.5 cm^2 with exercise or <1.5 cm^2 at rest).
- Ten-year survival of untreated patients with MS depends on the severity of symptoms at presentation: asymptomatic or minimally symptomatic patients have an 80% survival of 10 years, whereas those with significant limiting symptoms have a 10-year survival of 0% to 15%.[1]
- Once severe pulmonary hypertension develops, mean survival is 3 years. Mortality in untreated patients is due (in order of frequency) to progressive pulmonary and systemic congestion, systemic embolism, pulmonary embolism, and infection.[1]

History

After a prolonged asymptomatic period, patients may present with any of the following symptoms: dyspnea, reduced functional capacity, orthopnea and/or paroxysmal nocturnal dyspnea, fatigue, palpitations (often due to AF), systemic embolism, hemoptysis, chest pain, or signs and symptoms of infective endocarditis.

Physical Examination

- Findings on physical examination will depend on the severity of valve obstruction and the associated adaptations that have had time to develop in response to it.
- Accentuation of S1 may occur when the leaflets are flexible.
- Opening snap (OS)—caused by sudden tensing of the valve leaflets after they have completed their opening excursion; the A2–OS interval varies inversely with the severity of stenosis (shorter interval = more severe stenosis).
- Middiastolic rumble—low-pitched murmur heard best at the apex with the bell of the stethoscope; the severity of stenosis is related to the duration of the murmur, not intensity (more severe = longer duration).
- Irregularly irregular pulse due to AF.
- MR murmur may be present.
- Loud P2, tricuspid regurgitation (TR) murmur, pulmonary artery (PA) tap, and/or right ventricular (RV) heave can indicate pulmonary hypertension.
- Increased jugular venous pressure (JVP), hepatic congestion, and peripheral edema can indicate varying degrees of right heart failure (HF).

Diagnostic Criteria

The criteria for severe MS are presented in Table 20-1.[1]

Diagnostic Testing

- The standard evaluation of MS is presented in Table 20-2.
- ECG: The presence of P mitrale (P-wave duration in lead II ≥0.12 seconds, indicating left atrial enlargement [LAE]) is an important clue to presence of MS. ECG signs of right ventricular hypertrophy (RVH) and AF often coexist.
- Chest X-ray (CXR): Imaging with chest radiography will often reveal signs of LAE, enlargement of RA/RV and/or pulmonary arteries, and calcification of the MV and/or annulus.
- Transthoracic echo (TTE): Provides an opportunity to assess etiology of MS and assess the severity of MS.
  - Leaflet mobility, leaflet thickening, subvalvular thickening, and leaflet calcification are determinants of the echocardiographic mitral valve score (Wilkins score), which ranges from 0 to 16, and is important in determining candidacy for percutaneous mitral balloon valvotomy (PMBV).[2]
  - Echocardiography remains the primary modality for determining mean **transmitral gradient**.
  - **Valve area** can also be assessed by several methods (pressure half-time, continuity equation, direct planimetry by 2D or 3D visualization).
  - Measurement of **pulmonary artery systolic pressure** (PASP) (using the TR jet velocity) is a crucial component of the echocardiographic examination of the patient with MS.
  - Measurement of **RV size and function** remains important for prognostic purposes.

TABLE 20-1	SEVERE MITRAL STENOSIS
Mean gradient (mmHg)	>10
Pulmonary artery systolic pressure (mmHg)	>50
Valve area (cm^2)	<1.0

Modified from Bonow RO, Carabello BA, Chatterjee K, et al. ACC/AHA 2006 guidelines for the management of patients with valvular heart disease. *J Am Coll Cardiol* 2006;48:e1-e148.

TABLE 20-2	STANDARD EVALUATION OF MITRAL STENOSIS
ECG	• LAE and LVH
CXR	• LVH, cardiomegaly, and calcification of the aorta, AV, or coronaries
	• Rib notching suggests coarctation and BAV
TTE	• Leaflet number, morphology, and calcification
	• Calculate valve area using continuity equation $[Area_{AV} \times Velocity_{AV} = Area_{LVOT} \times Velocity_{LVOT}]$
	○ The continuity equation is based on the principle that flow (velocity × area) is equal both proximal to and at the level of the obstruction.
	○ Transvalvular mean and peak gradients

LAE, left atrial enlargement; LVH, left ventricular hypertrophy; AV, aortic valve; BAV, bicuspid aortic valve; TTE, transthoracic echocardiogram; LVOT, left ventricular outflow tract.

- ○ Exercise testing with echo is helpful in clarifying functional capacity of those with an unclear history. It allows assessment of the transmittal gradient and PASP with exercise when there is a discrepancy between resting Doppler findings, clinical findings, and signs/symptoms.
- Transesophageal echocardiography (TEE): Provides valuable adjunct information in the assessment of MS.
  - ○ The presence of absence of clot and severity of MR in patients being considered for PMBV is most accurately assessed.
  - ○ More careful examination of the MV morphology and hemodynamics in patients with MS for whom TTE was suboptimal.
- 3D echocardiography: Imaging the MV with real-time 3D TTE or TEE allows for orienting the image in such a way that the **most accurate** plannimetry of the narrowest portion of the MV can be performed.
- Cardiac catheterization (CC) is often indicated:
  - ○ To determine the severity of MS when clinical and echo assessment are discordant (see Figure 20-2).[3]
  - ○ Reasonable to assess hemodynamic response of PA and LA pressures to exercise.
  - ○ Can provide clues to the etiology of severe pulmonary hypertension when out of proportion of the severity of MS as determined by noninvasive testing. Typically performed in patients going for mitral valve replacement (MVR) with risk factors for CAD.

TREATMENT

Treatment of MS depends on the patient's symptoms, the severity of stenosis, the presence and severity of associated pulmonary hypertension, presence of an associated arrhythmia, and the risk of thromboembolism (Table 20-3).[1]

Medications

- Medical therapy is aimed at **slowing progression of pulmonary hypertension, preventing endocarditis, reducing the risk of thromboembolism**, and **reducing HF symptoms**.

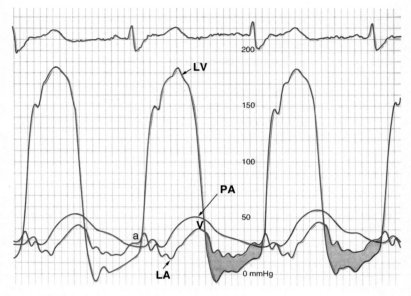

FIGURE 20-2. Hemodynamics observed in mitral stenosis. (From Murphy JG. *Mayo Clinic Cardiology Review*, 2nd ed. Philadelphia, PA: Lippincott Williams & Wilkins; 2000, with permission.)

TABLE 20-3	ACC/AHA GUIDELINES—CLASS I INDICATIONS FOR PREVENTION OF SYSTEMIC EMBOLIZATION IN PATIENTS WITH MITRAL STENOSIS

- Anticoagulation is indicated in patients with MS and AF (paroxysmal, persistent, or permanent).
- Anticoagulation is indicated in patients with MS and a prior embolic event, even in sinus rhythm.
- Anticoagulation is indicated in patients with MS with left atrial thrombus.

AF, atrial fibrillation; MS, mitral stenosis.

Modified from Bonow RO, Carabello BA, Chatterjee K, et al. ACC/AHA 2006 guidelines for the management of patients with valvular heart disease. *J Am Coll Cardiol* 2006;48:e1-e148.

- For HF, intermittent diuretics and a low-salt diet are often adequate if there is evidence of pulmonary congestion.
- For patients who develop symptoms only with exercise (likely associated with tachycardia), negative chronotropic agents such as β-blockers or nondihydropyridine calcium channel blockers may be of benefit.
- Since almost all MS is rheumatic in origin, prophylaxis against rheumatic fever may be appropriate.

Other Nonpharmacologic Therapies

- **PMBV** is generally performed via a transseptal approach. Class I indications are listed in Table 20-4.[1]
- After transseptal puncture of the interatrial septum, a catheter with a balloon is passed across the interatrial septum and the balloon is positioned across the mitral valve. Balloon inflation separates the commissures and fractures some of the nodular calcium in the leaflets, yielding an increased valve area.
- Usually, the transmitral pressure gradient decreases by 50% to 60%, cardiac output increases 10% to 20%, and valve area increases from 1.0 to 2.0 cm^2.[1]
- Contraindications to PMBV include LA thrombus, moderate-to-severe MR ($>2+$), and an echo score >8 (the latter is a relative contraindication).
- Complications include death (approximately 1%), stroke, cardiac perforation, severe MR requiring surgical correction, and residual atrial septal defect requiring closure.
- When done in those with favorable MV morphology, event-free survival (freedom from death, repeat valvotomy, or MV replacement) is 80% to 90% at 3 to 7 years.[1,4] This approach compares favorably with surgical mitral commissurotomy (open or closed) and is the procedure of choice in experienced centers for patients without contraindications.

Surgical Management

- Class I indication for surgery in MS are presented in Table 20-5.[1]
- Surgical treatment is usually reserved for those who are not candidates for PMBV because of the presence of one or more contraindications to PMBV or because the percutaneous option is unavailable.
- Surgical valvotomy can be done either closed (bypass unnecessary) or open (done under direct visualization on bypass). An open valvotomy yields a better outcome and is the preferred approach in developed countries; closed valvotomy continues to be used in some developing countries without access to open-heart surgery or percutaneous approaches.
- When the valve cannot be repaired, valve replacement is required.

TABLE 20-4	ACC/AHA GUIDELINES—CLASS I INDICATIONS FOR PERCUTANEOUS MITRAL BALLOON VALVOTOMY

- Symptomatic (NYHA functional class II, III, or IV) with moderate or severe MS and valve morphology favorable for PMBV in the absence of LA thrombus or moderate–severe MR
- Asymptomatic with moderate or severe MS and valve morphology favorable for PMBV who have pulmonary hypertension (PASP >50 mmHg at rest or >60 mmHg with exercise) in the absence of LA thrombus or moderate–severe MR

NYHA, New York Heart Association; MS, mitral stenosis; MR, mitral regurgitation; PMBV, percutaneous mitral balloon valvotomy; LA, left atrial; PASP, pulmonary artery systolic pressure.

Modified from Bonow RO, Carabello BA, Chatterjee K, et al. ACC/AHA 2006 guidelines for the management of patients with valvular heart disease. *J Am Coll Cardiol* 2006;48:e1-e148.

TABLE 20-5	ACC/AHA GUIDELINES—CLASS I INDICATIONS FOR SURGERY FOR MITRAL STENOSIS

- MV surgery (repair if possible) is indicated in symptomatic patients (NYHA functional class III or IV) with moderate-to-severe MS in a patient with acceptable operative risk when:
- PMBV is unavailable.
- PMBV is contraindicated because:
  - ○ Presence of LA thrombus despite anticoagulation or
  - ○ Concomitant moderate to severe MR is present, or
  - ○ Valve morphology not favorable for PMBV
- Symptomatic moderate-to-severe MS and also have moderate-to-severe MR should receive MV replacement unless valve repair is possible at the time of surgery.

MV, mitral valve; NYHA, New York Heart Association; MS, mitral stenosis; PMBV, percutaneous mitral balloon valvotomy; LA, left atrium; MR, mitral regurgitation.

Modified from Bonow RO, Carabello BA, Chatterjee K, et al. ACC/AHA 2006 guidelines for the management of patients with valvular heart disease. *J Am Coll Cardiol* 2006;48:e1-e148.

Mitral Regurgitation

GENERAL PRINCIPLES

Classification

- Mitral regurgitation (MR) is caused by inadequate coaptation of the valve leaflets, allowing blood to flow backward from the LV into the LA during systole.
- Prevention of MR is dependent on the integrated and proper function of the mitral valve (annulus and leaflets), subvalvular apparatus (chordae tendineae and papillary muscles), LA, and the ventricle. Abnormal function of any one of these components can lead to MR.
- Given the complexity of the interaction, the terminology to describe MR (the final common pathway of all abnormalities of the valve apparatus or ventricle that lead to MR) is often confusing.
- **Organic MR** is MR caused **primarily** by abnormalities of the valve leaflets and/or chordae tendinae (e.g., myxomatous degeneration, endocarditis, and rheumatic).
- **Functional MR** refers to MR caused **primarily** by ventricular dysfunction usually with accompanying annular dilatation (e.g., cardiomyopathy and ischemic MR).

Etiology

- **Degenerative** (essentially analogous to mitral valve prolapse syndrome):
  - ○ Usually occurs as a primary condition (Barlow disease or fibroelastic deficiency) but has also been associated with heritable diseases affecting the connective tissue, including Marfan syndrome (MFS), Ehlers–Danlos syndrome (EDS), osteogenesis imperfecta, etc.

- Myxomatous proliferation and cartilage formation can occur in the leaflets, chordae tendineae, and/or annulus.
- May be familial or nonfamilial.
- Occurs in 1% to 2.5% of the population (based on stricter echo criteria).
- Female-to-male ratio is 2:1.
- Either or both leaflets may prolapse.
- Most common reason for MV surgery.
- **Dilated cardiomyopathy (DCM):**
  - Mechanism of MR due to both:
    - Annular dilatation from ventricular enlargement.
    - Papillary muscle displacement due to ventricular enlargement and remodeling, which prevents adequate leaflet coaptation.
  - May occur in the setting ischemic DCM (where there is often an overlap of mechanism for MR in the setting of previous infarction) or nonischemic DCM.
- **Ischemic MR:**
  - Ischemic MR is a misnomer, as this is primarily postinfarction MR, not MR caused by active ischemia.
  - The MR is due primarily to ventricular dysfunction, not papillary muscle dysfunction. The mechanism of MR usually involves one or both of the following:
    - Annular dilatation from ventricular enlargement.
    - Local LV remodeling with papillary muscle displacement (both the dilatation of the ventricle and the akinesis/dyskinesis of the wall to which the papillary muscle is attached can prevent adequate leaflet coaptation).
- **Rheumatic MR:**
  - May be pure MR or combined MR/MS.
  - Caused by thickening and/or calcification of the leaflets and chords.
- **Infective endocarditis:** Usually caused by destruction of the leaflet tissue (i.e., perforation).
- **Other causes:**
  - Congenital (cleft, parachute, or fenestrated mitral valves)
  - Infiltrative diseases (i.e., amyloid)
  - Systemic lupus erythematosus (Libman–Sacks lesion)
  - Hypertrophic cardiomyopathy with obstruction
  - MAC
  - Paravalvular prosthetic leak
  - Drug toxicity (e.g., fenfluramine/phentermine)
- **Acute causes:**
  - Ruptured papillary muscle
  - Ruptured chordae tendineae
  - Infective endocarditis

Pathophysiology

The pathophysiology of acute MR is presented in Figure 20-3 and that of chronic MR in Figure 20-4.

DIAGNOSIS

Clinical Presentation

- The natural history and progression of MR depend on etiology, associated LV dysfunction, and severity of MR at the time of diagnosis.
- **MVP with little or no MR is most often associated with a benign prognosis and normal life expectancy;** a minority of these patients (10% to 15%) will go on to develop severe MR.

A. Acute Mitral Regurgitation

Sudden large volume load imposed on LA and LV of normal size and compliance

↓

Rapid ↑LVEDP, ↑LAP

↑LV preload (from volume load) facilitates the attempt of LV to maintain forward SV/CO with ↑HR and ↑contractility via Frank-Starling mechanisms and catecholamines

↓

Attempts to maintain forward SV/CO may be inadequate despite a supra-normal EF because a large portion is ejected backwards due to the lower resistance of the LA

↙   ↘

Pulmonary edema (↑LAP)   Hypotension (or shock) (↓forward SV/CO)

FIGURE 20-3. Pathophysiology of acute mitral regurgitation.

B. Chronic Mitral Regurgitation

Volume load imposed on LA and LV (usually it gradually increases over time)

↓

↑LVEDP and ↑LAP

↓

Compensatory dilatation of the LA and LV to accommodate volume load at lower pressures; this helps relieve pulmonary congestion
LV hypertrophy (eccentric) stimulated by LV dilatation (increased wall stress–LaPlace 's Law)

↓

↑Preload, LV hypertrophy, and reduced or normal afterload (low resistance LA provides unloading of LV) → large total SV (supra-normal EF) and normal forward SV

↓

"MR begets more MR" (vicious cycle in which further LV/annular dilatation ↑MR)

↓

Contractile dysfunction→ ↓EF, ↑end-systolic volume → ↑LVEDP/volume, ↑LAP

↙   ↘

Pulmonary congestion and pHTN   Reduced forward SV/CO

LA, left atrium; LV, left ventricle; LVEDP, left ventricular end diastolic pressure; LAP, left atrial pressure; SV, stroke volume; CO, cardiac output; EF, ejection fraction; pHTN, pulmonary hypertension.

FIGURE 20-4. Pathophysiology of chronic mitral regurgitation.

- The compensated asymptomatic phase of patients with severe organic MR (mostly degenerative but also due to rheumatic fever and endocarditis) with normal LV function is variable but may last several years.
- Two studies involving patients with severe asymptomatic MR showed an event-free survival (free of death or an indication for surgery) of 10% at 10 years and 55% at 8 years. Factors independently associated with increased mortality after surgery include preoperative ejection fraction (EF) <60%, New York Heart Association (NYHA) functional class III to IV symptoms, age, associated CAD, AF, and effective regurgitant orifice (ERO) >40 mm[2,5,6] Several of these factors and others are also associated with postoperative LV dysfunction and HF.
- The natural history of ischemic MR and MR due to DCM (these populations overlap) is generally worse than for degenerative MR because of the associated comorbidities in these patients, namely CAD and LV dysfunction with or without HF. Ischemic MR is independently associated with increased mortality after myocardial infarction (MI), in chronic HF, and after revascularization. Its impact on mortality increases with the severity of regurgitation.[7] The presence of MR in the setting of DCM is common (up to 60% of patients) and independently associated with increased mortality.[8]
- In both ischemic MR and MR due to DCM, because "MR begets MR," the ventricles of these patients dilate further and their HF symptoms worsen.

History

- Acute MR:
  - The most prominent symptom is relatively rapid onset of significant dyspnea, which may progress quickly to respiratory failure.
  - Symptoms of reduced forward flow may also be present, depending on the patient's ability to compensate for the regurgitant volume.
- Chronic MR:
  - The etiology of the MR and the time at which the patient presents will influence symptoms.
  - In degenerative MR that has progressed gradually, the patient may be asymptomatic even when the MR is severe.
  - As compensatory mechanisms begin to fail, patients may develop dyspnea on exertion (which may be due to pulmonary hypertension and/or pulmonary edema exacerbated by increased regurgitant volume during exercise), palpitations (from AF), fatigue, volume overload, and other symptoms of HF.
  - Patients with ischemic MR and MR due to DCM may report similar symptoms. In general, these patients will tend to be more symptomatic because of associated LV dysfunction.

Physical Examination

- Acute MR:
  - Tachypnea with respiratory distress
  - Tachycardia
  - Systolic murmur, usually at the apex—may not be holosystolic and may be absent.
  - S3 and/or early diastolic flow rumble may be present due to rapid early filling of LV during diastole because of large regurgitant volume load in the LA.
  - Apical impulse may be hyperdynamic.
  - Crackles on lung examination
  - Relative hypotension (even shock)
- Chronic MR:
  - Apical holosystolic murmur that radiates to the axilla.

- Murmur may radiate to the anterior chest wall if the posterior leaflet is prolapsed or toward the back if the anterior leaflet is prolapsed.
- In mitral valve prolapse, a midsystolic click is heard before the murmur.
- The LV apical impulse is displaced laterally.
- S3 and/or early diastolic flow rumble may be present due to significant early antegrade flow over the MV during diastole; this does not necessarily indicate LV dysfunction.
- Irregularly irregular rhythm of AF.
- Loud P2 indicates pulmonary hypertension.
- S2 may be widely split due to an early A2.
- Other signs of HF (i.e., lower extremity edema, elevated central venous pressure, crackles, etc.)

Diagnostic Criteria

The qualitative and quantitative measures of MR severity are presented in Table 20-6.[9]

Diagnostic Testing

Electrocardiography

ECG may sometimes show the following:

- LAE, left ventricular enlargement (LVE), and LVH
- AF
- Pathologic Q waves from previous MI in ischemic MR

TABLE 20-6	SEVERE MITRAL REGURGITATION
Qualitative	
Angiographic grade	3–4+
Color Doppler jet area	>40% LA area[a]
Doppler vena contracta width (cm)	≥0.7
Quantitative (cath or echo)	
Regurgitant volume (mL/beat)	≥60
Regurgitant fraction (%)	≥50
Regurgitant orifice area (cm²) (ERO)	≥0.40[b]
Additional essential criteria	
LA size	Enlarged[c]
LV size	Enlarged[c]

LA, left atrium; ERO, effective regurgitant orifice; LV, left ventricular.

[a]Or with a wall-impinging jet of any size swirling in the LA.

[b]Severe ischemic MR is defined by ERO ≥0.20.

[c]Enlargement should be present with chronic severe MR but often is not present with acute severe MR.

Modified from Zoghbi WA, Enriquez-Sarano M, Foster E, et al. Recommendations for evaluation of the severity of native valvular regurgitation with two-dimensional and Doppler echocardiography. *J Am Soc Echocardiogr* 2003;16:777-802.

Imaging

- CXR may reveal the following abnormalities:
  - LAE
  - Pulmonary edema
  - Enlarged pulmonary arteries
  - Cardiomegaly
- TTE:
  - Used to assess the etiology of MR.
  - MVP is defined by valve prolapse of 2 mm or more above the mitral annulus in certain echo views.
  - LA size (should be increased in chronic, severe MR)
  - LV dimensions at end-systole and end-diastole (should be dilated in chronic, severe MR of any etiology)
  - EF (LV dysfunction is present if EF $\leq$60%)
- TEE:
  - Provides better visualization of the valve to help define prolapsing leaflet(s)/scallop(s), presence of endocarditis, and feasibility of repair.
  - May help determine severity of MR when TTE is nondiagnostic, particularly in the setting of an eccentric jet.
  - Intraoperative TEE is indicated to guide repair and assess success.
- 3D echocardiography may provide additional and more accurate anatomic insights that can guide repair.
- Exercise testing with echocardiography:
  - Helpful in clarifying functional capacity of those with an unclear history.
  - Assess severity of MR with exercise in patients with exertional symptoms that seem discordant with the assessment of MR severity at rest.
  - Assess PASP with exercise.
  - Assess contractile reserve (change in EF with exercise); may indicate onset of contractile dysfunction.
- MRI:
  - Assess EF in patients with severe MR but with an inadequate assessment of EF by echocardiography.
  - Assess quantitative measures of MR severity when echo is nondiagnostic.
  - Viability assessment may play a role in considering therapeutic strategy in ischemic MR.
- Nuclear:
  - Assess EF in patients with severe MR but with an inadequate assessment of EF by echocardiography.
  - Viability assessment may play a role in considering therapeutic strategy in ischemic MR.
- Coronary CT angiography may be an alternative to left heart catheterization to evaluate coronary anatomy prior to valve surgery.

Diagnostic Procedures

- PA catheter:
  - To assess pulmonary hypertension in patients with chronic severe MR.
  - LA filling pressure in patients with unclear symptoms.
  - Giant v waves on pulmonary capillary wedge pressure (PCWP) tracing suggest severe MR.
- Coronary angiography:
  - May influence therapeutic strategy in ischemic MR.
  - Evaluation of CAD in patients with risk factors undergoing MV surgery.
  - Left ventriculogram can evaluate LV function and severity of MR.

TREATMENT

An outline of the treatment of chronic MR is presented in Figure 20-5.[1]

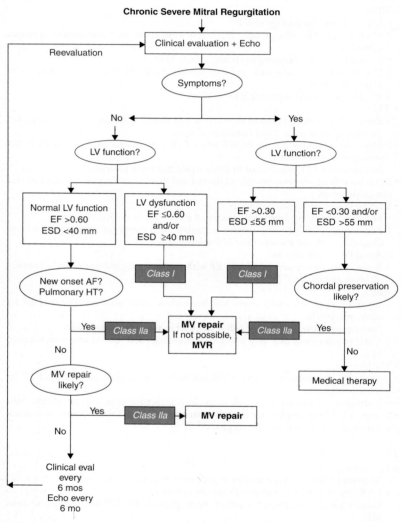

FIGURE 20-5. Treatment of chronic severe mitral regurgitation. (From Bonow RO, Carabello BA, Chatterjee K, et al. ACC/AHA 2006 guidelines for the management of patients with valvular heart disease. *J Am Coll Cardiol* 2006;48:e1-e148, with permission.)

Medication

- Acute MR:
  - In the setting of severe acute MR, surgical treatment is indicated, often urgently or emergently.
  - **Aggressive afterload reduction** with IV nitroprusside or intra-aortic balloon pump (IABP) can diminish the amount of MR and stabilize the patient by promoting forward flow and reducing pulmonary edema.
  - These patients are usually tachycardic but attempts to slow their heart rate should be avoided, as cardiac output is heart rate dependent in these patients with reduced stroke volume.
- Chronic MR:
  - The role of medical therapy may differ with different etiologies.
  - In the asymptomatic patient with normal LV function and chronic severe MR due to leaflet prolapse, there is no generally accepted medical therapy. In the absence of systemic hypertension, there is no known indication for vasodilating drugs. Whether angiotensin-converting enzyme (ACE) inhibitors or β-blockers delay ventricular remodeling and the need for surgery is being investigated in prospective studies.
  - Patients with functional MR (ischemic MR and MR due to DCM) should be treated as other patients with LV dysfunction. ACE inhibitors and β-blockers are indicated and have been shown to reduce mortality and the severity of MR.[10-18] Some patients may also qualify for cardiac resynchronization therapy, which has also been shown to reduce the severity of MR.[19-22]

Other Nonpharmacologic Therapies

- An ever-expanding number of percutaneous approaches are being considered for the treatment of MR, some of which are quite complex.
- Various approaches target each of the interrelated components that can contribute to MR: annular dilatation, lack of leaflet coaptation, and ventricular remodeling causing papillary muscle displacement.
- A. Many patients who could benefit from mitral valve repair are denied surgery owing to high surgical risk, advanced age, or other comorbidities. A catheter-based device is used that repairs the mitral valve by delivering a clip percutaneously to approximate the valve leaflet edges and improve leaflet coaptation. The device is approved for patients with significant symptomatic degenerative or functional mitral regurgitation who are at a prohibitive risk for mitral valve surgery.

Surgical Management

- Class I indication for surgery in MR are presented in Table 20-7.[1]
- Surgery for MR is most commonly performed in patients with degenerative mitral valve disease.
- Operative mortality is about 2%, even <1% in some centers for the best operative candidates.
- With advances in surgical technique (including more frequent and better repairs instead of replacements) and lower operative mortality, there is a push in some centers to operate earlier on patients with severe MR, even when they are still asymptomatic.[23,24] A move toward earlier surgery, however, particularly in asymptomatic patients, requires that all efforts be made to repair the valve and that the surgery be done by surgeons experienced in valve repair. Watchful waiting is an option in those with asymptomatic severe mitral MR.[6]
- Preoperative factors that increase operative and/or postoperative mortality include worse NYHA functional class, LV dysfunction (EF <60%), age, associated CAD, and AF.[1]
- Compared with valve replacement, valve repair yields improved operative survival, long-term survival, and improved postoperative LV function.[23,25]

TABLE 20-7	ACC/AHA GUIDELINES—CLASS I INDICATIONS FOR SURGERY IN MITRAL REGURGITATION

- Symptomatic acute severe MR
- Chronic severe MR and NYHA functional class II, III, or IV symptoms in the absence of severe LV dysfunction (EF <30%) and/or ESD >55 mm
- Asymptomatic chronic severe MR and mild-to-moderate LV dysfunction (EF 30–60%), and/or ESD ≥40 mm
- MV repair rather than MV replacement is recommended in the majority of patients with chronic severe MR who require surgery; patients should be referred to surgical centers experienced in MV repair.

MR, mitral regurgitation; NYHA, New York Heart Association; LV, left ventricle; EF, ejection fraction; ESD, end-systolic dimension; MV, mitral valve.

Modified from Bonow RO, Carabello BA, Chatterjee K, et al. ACC/AHA 2006 guidelines for the management of patients with valvular heart disease. *J Am Coll Cardiol* 2006;48:e1-e148.

- **Surgery for organic mitral disease:**
  - This generally involves repair of the valve (with triangular or quadrangular resection) and ring annuloplasty.
  - Long-term results at high-volume centers are excellent, with reoperation rates of 5% to 10% at 10 years and about 20% at 20 years.
  - If repair cannot be performed, replacement should be performed with preservation of the subvalvular chordal structures.
- **Surgery for ischemic MR and MR due to DCM:**
  - These procedures are more controversial and more complex.
  - Isolated annuloplasty likely inadequate.
  - Revascularization alone (coronary artery bypass grafting [CABG] or percutaneous intervention [PCI]) for chronic ischemic MR can decrease the severity of MR.
  - Annuloplasty and CABG can help reduce the presence and severity of postoperative MR but the rate of persistent and recurrent significant MR is high, often >30%, even in experienced centers. Surgery in these situations does not improve postoperative mortality or decrease HF symptoms.[26,27]
- **Severe LV dysfunction and moderate-to-severe MR:**
  - Surgery in this context is not associated with improved long-term survival.[28,29]
  - Annuloplasty has been shown to improve HF symptoms, EF, and ventricular size.
  - Optimal surgical solution will likely incorporate more than just an annuloplasty ring that addresses the dilated annulus.
  - The contribution of the dysfunctional ventricle (dilated, spherical, and with poor contractile function) will need to be therapeutically targeted as well.
- **Certain patients with AF** should be considered for a concomitant surgical maze procedure to restore sinus rhythm.[1,30-32] This may prevent future thromboembolic events, eliminate the need for anticoagulation, and prevent future HF.

REFERENCES

1. Bonow RO, Carabello BA, Chatterjee K, et al. ACC/AHA 2006 guidelines for the management of patients with valvular heart disease. *J Am Coll Cardiol* 2006;48:e1-e148.
2. Wilkins GT, Weyman AE, Abascal VM, et al. Percutaneous balloon dilation of the mitral valve: an analysis of echocardiographic variables related to outcome and the mechanism of dilation. *Br Heart J* 1988;60:299-308.

3. Murphy JG. *Mayo Clinic Cardiology Review*, 2nd ed. Philadelphia, PA: Lippincott Williams & Wilkins; 2000.

4. The National Heart, Lung, and Blood Institute Balloon Valvuloplasty Registry Participants. Multicenter experience with balloon mitral commissurotomy: NHLBI Balloon Valvuloplasty Registry Report on immediate and 30-day follow-up results. *Circulation* 1992;85:448-461.

5. Enriquez-Sarano M, Avierinos J-F, Messika-Zeitoun D, et al. Quantitative determinants of the outcome of asymptomatic mitral regurgitation. *N Engl J Med* 2005;352:875-883.

6. Rosenhek R, Rader F, Klaar U, et al. Outcome of watchful waiting in asymptomatic severe mitral regurgitation. *Circulation* 2006;113:2238-2244.

7. Grigioni F, Enriquez-Sarano M, Zehr KJ, et al. Ischemic mitral regurgitation: long-term outcome and prognostic implications with quantitative Doppler assessment. *Circulation* 2001;103:1759-1764.

8. Trichon BH, Felker M, Shaw LK, et al. Relation of frequency and severity of mitral regurgitation to survival among patients with left ventricular systolic dysfunction and heart failure. *Am J Cardiol* 2003;91:538-543.

9. Zoghbi WA, Enriquez-Sarano M, Foster E, et al. Recommendations for evaluation of the severity of native valvular regurgitation with two-dimensional and Doppler echocardiography. *J Am Soc Echocardiogr* 2003;16:777-802.

10. Schön HR, Schröter G, Barthel P, Schömig A. Quinapril therapy in patients with chronic mitral regurgitation. *J Heart Valve Dis* 1994;3:303-312.

11. Seneviratne B, Moore GA, West PD. Effect of captopril on functional mitral regurgitation in dilated heart failure: a randomised double blind placebo controlled trial. *Br Heart J* 1994;72:63-68.

12. Wisenbaugh T, Sinovich V, Dullabh A, Sareli P. Six month pilot study of captopril for mildly symptomatic, severe isolated mitral and isolated aortic regurgitation. *J Heart Valve Dis* 1994;3:197-204.

13. Høst U, Kelbaek H, Hildebrandt P, et al. Effect of ramipril on mitral regurgitation secondary to mitral valve prolapse. *Am J Cardiol* 1997;80:655-658.

14. Marcotte F, Honos GN, Walling AD, et al. Effect of angiotensin-converting enzyme inhibitor therapy in mitral regurgitation with normal left ventricular function. *Can J Cardiol* 1997; 13:479-485.

15. Levine AB, Muller C, Levine TB. Effects of high-dose lisinopril-isosorbide dinitrate on severe mitral regurgitation and heart failure remodeling. *Am J Cardiol* 1998;82:1299-1301.

16. Lowes BD, Gill, EA, Abraham WT, et al. Effects of carvedilol on left ventricular mass, chamber geometry, and mitral regurgitation in chronic heart failure. *Am J Cardiol* 1999;83:1201-1205.

17. Campomolla S, Febo O, Gnemmi M, et al. Beta-blockade therapy in chronic heart failure: diastolic function and mitral regurgitation improvement by carvedilol. *Am Heart J* 2000;139:596-608.

18. Ahmed MI, Aban I, Lloyd SG, et al. A randomized controlled phase IIb trial of beta(1)-receptor blockade for chronic degenerative mitral regurgitation. *J Am Coll Cardiol* 2012;60:833-838.

19. Abraham WT, Fisher WG, Smith AL, et al. Multicenter InSync Randomized Clinical Evaluation (MIRACLE) Study Group. Cardiac resynchronization in chronic heart failure. *N Engl J Med* 2002;346:1845-1853.

20. St John Sutton MG, Plappert T, Abraham WT, et al. Multicenter InSync Randomized Clinical Evaluation (MIRACLE) Study Group. Effect of cardiac resynchronization therapy on left ventricular size and function in chronic heart failure. *Circulation* 2003;107:1985-1990.

21. Cleland JG, Daubebert JC, Erdmann E, et al. Cardiac Resynchronization-Heart Failure (CARE-HF) study investigators. *N Engl J Med* 2005;352:1539-1549.

22. van Bommel RJ, Marsan NA, Delgado V, et al. Cardiac resynchronization therapy as a therapeutic option in patients with moderate–severe functional mitral regurgitation and high operative risk. *Circulation* 2011;124:912-919.

23. Enriquez-Sarano M, Schaff HV, Orszulak TA, Tajik AJ, Bailey KR, Frye RL. Valve repair improves the outcome of surgery for mitral regurgitation: a multivariate analysis. *Circulation* 1995;91:1022-1028.

24. Enriquez-Sarano M. Timing of mitral valve surgery. *Heart* 2002;87:79-85.

25. Mohty D, Orszulak TA, Schaff HV, et al. Very long-term survival and durability of mitral valve repair for mitral valve prolapse. *Circulation* 2001;104(Suppl I):I1-I7.

26. Diodato MD, Moon MR, Pasque MK, et al. Repair of ischemic mitral regurgitation does not increase mortality or improve long-term survival in patients undergoing coronary artery revascularization: a propensity analysis. *Ann Thorac Surg* 2004;78:794-799.

27. Mihaljevic T, Lam B-K, Rajeswaran J, et al. Impact of mitral valve annuloplasty combined with revascularization in patients with functional ischemic mitral regurgitation. *J Am Coll Cardiol* 2007;49:2191-2201.

28. Bolling SF, Pagani FD, Deeb GM, et al. Intermediate-term outcome of mitral reconstruction in cardiomyopathy. *J Thorac Cardiovasc Surg* 1998;115:381-386.

29. Wu AH, Aaronson KD, Bolling SF, et al. Impact of mitral valve annuloplasty on mortality risk in patients with mitral regurgitation and left ventricular systolic dysfunction. *J Am Coll Cardiol* 2005;45:381-387.

30. Handa N, Schaff HV, Morris JJ, et al. Outcome of valve repair and the Cox maze procedure for mitral regurgitation and associated atrial fibrillation. *J Thorac Cardiovasc Surg* 1999;118:628-635.

31. Raanani E, Albage A, David TE, et al. The efficacy of the Cox/maze procedure combined with mitral valve surgery: a matched control study. *Eur J Cardiothorac Surg* 2001;19:438-442.

32. Kobayashi J, Sasako Y, Bando K, et al. Eight-year experience of combined valve repair for mitral regurgitation and maze procedure. *J Heart Valve Dis* 2002;11:165-171.

Tricuspid Valve Disease　21

William J. Nienaber and Jose A. Madrazo

- The tricuspid valve (TV) lies between the right atrium (RA) and right ventricle (RV).
- It has three leaflets: anterior, posterior, and septal. Primary TV disease is relatively uncommon.

Tricuspid Stenosis

GENERAL PRINCIPLES

Definition

Tricuspid stenosis (TS) is characterized by incomplete opening of the TV during diastole, which limits anterograde flow and yields a sustained diastolic pressure gradient between the RA and RV.

Etiology

- **Rheumatic heart disease** (most common cause)
- Carcinoid syndrome
- Congenital abnormalities (see Chapter 35)
- Infective endocarditis (with bulky vegetations)
- Endocardial fibroelastosis
- Fabry disease
- Methysergide toxicity
- Löeffler syndrome
- RA mass may cause functional obstruction of the valve

DIAGNOSIS

Clinical Presentation

History

Patients typically note symptoms consistent with right heart failure, including peripheral edema, increased abdominal girth, fatigue, and palpitations (if there are associated arrhythmias).

Physical Examination

- Elevated jugular venous pulsations (JVP) with a giant *a* wave and diminished rate of *y* descent
- Hepatomegaly with a pulsatile liver
- Mid-diastolic murmur (low-pitched) that increases with inspiration
- Opening snap
- Edema in lower extremities, often anasarca

Diagnostic Testing

- **ECG:** May show right atrial enlargement (RAE) and/or atrial fibrillation (AF).
- **CXR:** May reveal an enlarged right heart border.
- **Transthoracic echocardiography (TTE):**
  - Evaluate morphology of valve.
  - RAE
  - Associated congenital abnormalities
  - TV gradient
  - Calculate valve area (<1.0 cm^2 is severe).
- **Transesophageal echocardiography (TEE):** Provides better visualization of valve leaflets, RA, and subvalvular apparatus.
- **Cardiac catheterization:** May be indicated to evaluate diastolic gradient between RA and RV.

TREATMENT

Medications

Medical treatment consists mostly of **diuretic therapy** for volume overload. Further medical management depends on other comorbidities.

Surgical Management

- The most common cause of TS is rheumatic valve disease, which inevitably will involve the mitral and/or artic valves as well.
- Timing of surgical intervention is usually driven by the severity of the left-sided valvular lesions.
- Tricuspid valvuloplasty or TV replacement (preferably bioprosthetic) may be indicated for severe TS but can result in TR.[1,2]
- For congenital TS, there may be other associated abnormalities that influence management and therapeutic decisions.

Tricuspid Regurgitation

GENERAL PRINCIPLES

Definition

- Tricuspid regurgitation (TR) is caused by inadequate coaptation of the valve leaflets, allowing blood to flow backward from the RV into the RA during systole.
- **Mild TR is found in up to 70% of normal patients**. It is clinically unremarkable in the majority of patients.

Etiology

- Secondary TR is caused by RV and annular dilatation and RV failure, most commonly secondary to left ventricular (LV) failure with or without valvular disease which causes pulmonary hypertension or pulmonary hypertension independent of left-sided cardiac disease.
- Abnormalities of the TV itself leading to TR can be caused by:
  - **Infective endocarditis is the most common etiology** and frequently associated with IV drug abuse.

- Carcinoid heart disease, commonly presenting as TR but also associated with TS.
- Right-sided myocardial infarction (MI), causing papillary muscle dysfunction
- Trauma (e.g., from pacemaker/implanted cardiac defibrillator [ICD] lead or repeated RV biopsy after transplant)
- Rheumatoid arthritis
- Rheumatic heart disease, indicating severe aortic or mitral valve disease
- Marfan syndrome (MFS)
- Radiation-induced valvulitis

Pathophysiology

- Severe TR leads to volume overload of the RV and RV dilatation.
- In the absence of pulmonary hypertension, severe TR may be well tolerated for many years.
- Patients with severe TR and pulmonary hypertension typically develop right-sided congestion due to elevated RA and central venous pressure (CVP), resulting in peripheral edema or anasarca, and may develop cardiac cirrhosis.

DIAGNOSIS

Clinical Presentation

History

- **Generally, TR is clinically insignificant and well tolerated**.
- Patients may complain of fatigue, lower extremity edema, increased abdominal girth, early satiety, or loss of appetite, depending on the degree of hepatic congestion, bowel wall edema, and ascites.

Physical Examination

- Examination of the JVP may reveal prominent v waves.
- A systolic murmur (usually holosystolic) may be heard best at the left lower sternal border that increases with inspiration (Carvallo sign).
- Right-sided S3 or increased P2 intensity may be present.
- Pulsatile liver, hepatomegaly, lower extremity edema, and ascites may be present.

Diagnostic Criteria

Severe TR is diagnosed when:
- Vena contracta width >0.7 cm, and
- Systolic flow reversal in hepatic veins

Diagnostic Testing

- **ECG:** May show RAE, AF, incomplete or complete right bundle branch block (RBBB), and right ventricular hypertrophy (RVH).
- **CXR:** May reveal an enlarged right heart border.
- **TTE:**
  - Evaluate morphology and motion of valve leaflets.
  - RAE, RV function, annular dilatation
  - Signs of RV volume overload (paradoxical septal motion)
  - Signs of RV pressure overload (flattened septum, D-shaped LV)
  - Pulmonary artery systolic pressure (PASP) is calculated using the Bernoulli equation (assuming no pulmonary stenosis):

$$PASP = 4V^2 + RAP$$

where V is the TR jet velocity and RAP (RA pressure) is estimated by inferior vena cava (IVC) size and collapsibility.
- **TEE:** Better visualizes the valve leaflets, RA, and subvalvular apparatus.
- Pulmonary artery catheterization:
  - Prominent v waves in the RA
  - Direct measurement of RA, RV, and PA pressures which may help in diagnosing etiology of TR.

TREATMENT

Medications
- Medical therapy is limited to **diuretics and afterload reduction** to decrease the severity of right-sided heart failure.
- Usually TR is secondary to some other process—pulmonary hypertension, left-sided heart failure, or other valvular abnormality—that is the primary focus of treatment.

Surgical Management
- **Repair with annuloplasty ring** is preferred to replacement when surgery is indicated (severe TR with symptoms).[1-7]
- TR may recur after repair.
- **If replacement is necessary, bioprosthetic valves are preferred** to mechanical valves owing to the risk of thrombosis (lower pressure on the right side of the heart predisposes to thrombosis of mechanical valves).[1-3]
- Increasing evidence suggests the value of a TV annuloplasty for secondary TR (particularly with a dilated annulus) at the time of mitral valve surgery, even if the TR is not severe.[1,2,8-10]

REFERENCES

1. Bonow RO, Carabello BA, Chatterjee K, et al. ACC/AHA 2006 guidelines for the management of patients with valvular heart disease. *J Am Coll Cardiol* 2006;48(3):e1-e148.
2. Bonow RO, Carabellow BA, Chatterjee K, et al. 2008 focused update incorporated into the ACC/AHA 2006 guidelines for the management of patients with valvular heart disease. *J Am Coll Cardiol* 2008;52:e1-e142.
3. Vahanian A, Baumgartner H, Bax J, et al. Task Force on the Management of Valvular Heart Disease of the European Society of Cardiology; ESC Committee for Practice Guidelines. *Eur Hear J* 2007;28:230-268.
4. Carrier M, Pellerin M, Guertin MC, et al. Twenty-five years' clinical experience with repair of tricuspid insufficiency. *J Heart Valve Disease* 2004;13:952-956.
5. McCarthy PM, Bhudia SK, Rajeswaran J, et al. Tricuspid valve repair: durability and risk factors for failure. *J Thorac Cardiovasc Surg* 2004;127:674-685.
6. Singh SK, Tang GH, Maganti MD, et al. Midterm outcomes of tricuspid valve repair versus replacement for organic tricuspid disease. *Ann Thorac Surg* 2006;82:1735-1741.
7. Guenther T, Noebauer C, Mazzitelli D, et al. Tricuspid valve surgery: a thirty-year assessment of early and late outcome. *Eur J Cardiothorac Surg* 2008;34:402-409.
8. Dreyfus GD, Corbi PJ, Chan KM, et al. Secondary tricuspid regurgitation or dilatation: which should be the criteria for surgical repair? *Ann Thorac Surg* 2005;79:127-132.
9. Chan V, Burwash IG, Lam BK, et al. Clinical and echocardiographic impact of functional tricuspid regurgitation repair at the time of mitral valve replacement. *Ann Thorac Surg* 2009;88: 1209-1215.
10. Kim JB, Yoo DG, Kim GS, et al. Mild-to-moderate functional tricuspid regurgitation in patients undergoing valve replacement for rheumatic mitral disease: the influence of tricuspid valve repair on clinical and echocardiographic outcomes. *Heart* 2012;98:24-30.

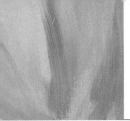

Infective Endocarditis and Cardiac Devices

<mark>22</mark>

Risa M. Cohen and Pablo F. Soto

Infective Endocarditis

GENERAL PRINCIPLES

Definition

- Infective endocarditis (IE) is a microbial infection involving the endothelial surface of the heart.
- It is predominantly characterized by the presence of vegetations consisting of microorganisms, inflammatory cells, and platelet–fibrin deposits.
- Valves are the most common location, although IE can also occur at ventricular septal defect (VSD) and atrial septal defect (ASD), chordae tendineae, or damaged mural endocardium.
- Multiple organisms can also cause IE (Table 22-1).[1]

Classification

IE may be categorized according to the following (see Table 22-2):
- Type of presentation
- Underlying valve characteristics
- Predisposing factors

Epidemiology

- In a multinational review of 15 studies, incidence of IE was found to be 1.4 to 6.2 cases per 100,000 patient-years, with mortality ranging from 14% to 46%.[2]
- In developed countries, the proportion of IE cases in patients with underlying rheumatic heart disease has markedly decreased. There has been a shift toward an older population (with degenerative valve disease) with a median age in the 5th to 7th decades.
- A higher incidence of IE is seen in the setting of IV drug use, cardiac and vascular prostheses, and nosocomial infections.

Pathophysiology

The pathophysiology of IE is outlined in Figure 22-1.

Risk Factors

- The major risk factor for the development of IE is a structural abnormality of a heart valve, often causing a stenotic or regurgitant lesion (e.g., bicuspid aortic valve, myxomatous mitral disease).
- Predisposing risk factors for native valve endocarditis (NVE) include **degenerative valve disease**, **age**, **IV drug use**, **poor dental hygiene**, **long-term hemodialysis**, and **diabetes mellitus**.

TABLE 22-1	FREQUENCY OF VARIOUS ORGANISMS CAUSING INFECTIVE ENDOCARDITIS			
Organism	NVE (%)	IV Drug abusers (%)	Early PVE (%)	Late PVE (%)
Streptococci	60	15–25	5	35
Viridans	35	5–10	<5	25
Bovis	10	<5	<5	<5
Enterococcus faecalis	10	10	<5	<5
Staphylococci	25	50	50	30
Coagulase-positive	23	50	20	10
Coagulase-negative	<5	<5	30	20
Gram-negative aerobic bacilli	<5	5	20	10
Fungi	<5	<5	10	5
Culture-negative endocarditis	5–10	<5	<5	<5

NVE, native valve endocarditis; PVE, prosthetic valve endocarditis.

From O'Rourke RA, Fuster V, Alexander RW, eds. *Hurst's the Heart*, 10th ed. New York, NY: McGraw-Hill; 2000:596, with permission.

TABLE 22-2	CLASSIFICATION OF ENDOCARDITIS
ABE	• Highly infective and particularly toxic • Develops within 1–2 days • Can cause significant valvular destruction and embolic infections • Most commonly caused by *Staphylococcus aureus*
SBE	• More indolent course than ABE • Develops within weeks to months • More often associated with immunologic phenomena • Often caused by streptococcal organisms, particularly *Streptococcus viridans*; also HACEK organisms and other gram-negative bacilli • *Streptococcus bovis* is often associated with colon cancer and polyps.
NVE	• Often predisposed by an abnormal native heart valve (e.g., mitral valve prolapse, bicuspid aortic valve)

TABLE 22-2	CLASSIFICATION OF ENDOCARDITIS (*Continued*)
	• Common organisms: *Streptococcus viridans*, *Staphylococcus aureus*, *Streptococcus bovis*, and *Enterococcus*
PVE	• Increased incidence in recent decades accounting for 10–30% of all IE
	• *Early* if it occurs within 2 months of valve replacement
	◦ Early PVE often involves coagulase-negative staphylococci
	• *Late* if it occurs after 2 months
	◦ Late PVE involves the usual NVE pathogens such as *Streptococcus viridans*, *Staphylococcus aureus*, and *Enterococcus*
	• Fungal endocarditis (*Candida* and *Aspergillus*) is more common in PVE than in NVE.
	• Greatest risk of IE within 6 months of valve replacement
	• Rates of infection appear to be similar between mechanical and bioprosthetic valves
Right-sided endocarditis	• Often seen in IV drug users; almost always involves the *tricuspid valve*
	• Most common pathogen is *Staphylococcus aureus* (60%).
NBTE	• Requires endothelial injury and a hypercoagulable state:
	◦ *Marantic endocarditis*, when associated with cancer
	◦ Libman–Sacks endocarditis, often with lupus
	◦ Antiphospholipid antibody syndrome
Culture-negative endocarditis	◦ Often related to prior antibiotic treatment
	• Incidence may be as high as 5–10%
	• Caused by fastidious or slow-growing organisms such as *HACEK*, fungi, anaerobes, *Legionella*, *Chlamydia psittaci*, *Coxiella*, *Brucella*, and *Bartonella*
Pacemaker/ defibrillator endocarditis	• Increased incidence due to increased indications for implantation
	• Often caused by *Staphylococcus aureus* or coagulase-negative staphylococci
Fungal endocarditis	• Often involves *Candida* or *Aspergillus*
	• Due to prosthetic valves, indwelling intravascular devices, immunosuppression, or IV drug use

(*Continued*)

TABLE 22-2	CLASSIFICATION OF ENDOCARDITIS (*Continued*)
HIV-related endocarditis	• *Staphylococcus aureus* is the most common pathogen. • Usually related to IV drug use or indwelling IV catheters

ABE, acute bacterial endocarditis; SBE, subacute bacterial endocarditis; NVE, native valve endocarditis; PVE, prosthetic valve endocarditis; NBTE, nonbacterial thrombotic endocarditis; HACEK, *Haemophilus aphrophilus*, *H. parainfluenzae*, and *h. paraphrophilus*; *Actinobacillus actinomycetemcomitans*; *Cardiobacterium hominis*; *Eikenella corrodens*; and *Kingella kingae*; IE, infective endocarditis.

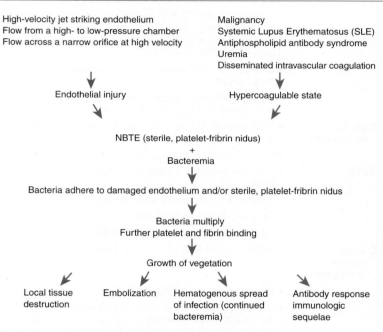

FIGURE 22-1. Pathophysiology of infective endocarditis.

DIAGNOSIS

Clinical Presentation

• The clinical spectrum can range from subtle, indolent manifestations of subacute infection presenting as a fever of undetermined origin (FUO) to extensive valve destruction and fulminant heart failure (HF).

• The most common clinical features of IE are **fever and a new heart murmur**.

• Fever may not be present in the elderly, the immunocompromised, patients with HF, or those with chronic renal disease.

History

A thorough history should take into account a detailed assessment of conditions that may predispose a patient to IE as noted above.

Physical Examination

- The physical examination is an important component of the evaluation of a patient with IE, and several organ systems may be involved (Table 22-3).
- Particular emphasis should be placed on searching for immunologic and embolic findings that may support the diagnosis of IE.

Diagnostic Criteria

There are several proposed criteria for the diagnosis of IE. The Duke criteria are shown in Tables 22-4 and 22-5.[3-5]

TABLE 22-3	PHYSICAL EXAMINATION FINDINGS IN ENDOCARDITIS
Organ system	**Findings**
Neurologic	• Any neurologic finding is associated with increased mortality • Range of clinical presentations (e.g., confusion, decreased alertness, focal deficit) • Due to embolic stroke, hemorrhagic stroke (transformed embolic stroke or mycotic aneurysm rupture), cerebritis from microabscesses, and meningitis
Cardiac	• Assess for new or worsening murmur due to valvular destruction, ruptured chordae tendineae, or obstruction due to large vegetation • Congestive heart failure • Irregular and/or bradycardic rhythm may indicate the presence of heart block
Abdominal	• Abdominal pain due to emboli and subsequent intestinal, splenic, and/or renal ischemia/infarcts • Splenomegaly may be present, more commonly in subacute IE
Skin and extremities	• Assess for signs of IV drug use • Noteworthy peripheral manifestations are • **Petechiae:** usually found on conjunctiva, buccal and palatal mucosa, and behind ears • **Osler nodes:** tender subcutaneous nodules often found at the pulp of the fingers • **Janeway lesions:** painless, blanchable, macular red spots at the palms and soles • **Splinter hemorrhages:** dark linear streaks seen at the nail bed
Ophthalmologic	• **Roth spots:** round retinal hemorrhages with a pale center

TABLE 22-4	**DEFINITION OF TERMS USED IN THE PROPOSED MODIFIED DUKE CRITERIA FOR THE DIAGNOSIS OF IE**

Major criteria

Blood culture positive for IE

Typical microorganisms consistent with IE from two separate blood cultures;
  Viridans streptococci, *Streptococcus bovis*, HACEK group. *Staphylococcus aureus*; or

Community-acquired enterococci, in the absence of a primary focus; or

Microorganisms consistent with IE from persistently positive blood cultures, defined as follows:

  At least two positive cultures of blood samples drawn >12 hours apart; or

  All of three or a majority of four or more separate cultures of blood (with first and last sample drawn at least 1 hour apart)

Single positive blood culture for *Coxiella burnetii* or antiphase I IgG antibody titer >1:800

Evidence of endocardial involvement

Echocardiogram positive for IE (TEE recommended for patients with prosthetic valves, rated at least "possible IE" by clinical criteria, or complicated IE [paravalvular abscess]: TTE as first test in other patients) defined as follows:

  Oscillating intracardiac mass on valve or supporting structures, in the path of regurgitant jets, or on implanted material in the absence of an alternative anatomic explanation; or

  Abscess; or

  New partial dehiscence of prosthetic valve

New valvular regurgitation (worsening or changing of preexisting murmur not sufficient)

Minor criteria

Predisposition, predisposing heart condition, or injection drug use

Fever, temperature >38°C

Vascular phenomena, major arterial emboli, septic pulmonary infarcts, mycotic aneurysm, intracranial hemorrhage, conjunctival hemorrhages, and Janeway lesions

Immunologic phenomena: glomerulonephritis, Osler nodes, Roth spots, and rheumatoid factor

Microbiological evidence: positive blood culture but does not meet a major criterion as noted above or serologic evidence of active infection with organism consistent with IE

Echocardiographic minor criteria eliminated

IE, infective endocarditis; HACEK, *Haemophilus aphrophilus, H. parainfluenzae, and H. paraphrophilus; Actinobacillus actinomycetemcomitans; Cardiobacterium hominis; Eikenella corrodens;* and *Kingella kingae*; TEE, transesophageal echocardiogram; TTE, transthoracic echocardiogram.

From Li JS, Sexton DJ, Mick N, et al. Proposed modifications to the Duke criteria for the diagnosis of infective endocarditis. *Clin Infect Dis* 2000;30:633-638, with permission.

TABLE 22-5	DEFINITION OF IE ACCORDING TO THE PROPOSED MODIFIED DUKE CRITERIA

Definite IE

Pathologic criteria:

- Microorganisms demonstrated by culture or histologic examination of a vegetation, a vegetation that has embolized, or an intracardiac abscess specimen; or
- Pathologic lesions: Vegetation or intracardiac abscess confirmed by histologic examination showing active endocarditis

Clinical criteria[a]:

- Two major criteria; or
- One major criterion and three minor criteria; or
- Five minor criteria

Possible IE

- One major criterion and one minor criterion; or
- Three minor criteria

Rejected

- Firm alternate diagnosis explaining evidence of IE; or
- Resolution of IE syndrome with antibiotic therapy for ≤4 days; or
- No pathologic evidence of IE at surgery or autopsy, with antibiotic therapy for ≤4 days; or
- Does not meet criteria for possible IE, as above

---

[a]Excludes single positive cultures for coagulase-negative staphylococci and organisms that do not cause endocarditis.

IE, infective endocarditis; HACEK, *Haemophilus aphrophilus*, *H. parainfluenzae*, and *H. paraphrophilus*; *Actinobacillus actinomycetemcomitans*; *Cardiobacterium hominis*; *Eikenella corrodens*; and *Kingella kingae*; TEE, transesophageal echocardiography; TTE, transthoracic echocardiography.

From Li JS, Sexton DJ, Mick N, et al. Proposed modifications to the Duke criteria for the diagnosis of infective endocarditis. *Clin Infect Dis* 2000;30:633-638, with permission.

Diagnostic Testing

Laboratories

- **Blood cultures**: Draw at least two sets from different sites and over a period of time (i.e., at least 1 hour between the first and last sets, ideally at least 24 hours) before administering antibiotics; obtain fungal cultures if fungal endocarditis is suspected.
- **Complete blood count** (CBC): Evaluate for leukocytosis, thrombocytosis (acute-phase reactant), thrombocytopenia (sepsis), and anemia (subacute bacterial endocarditis [SBE] can lead to anemia of chronic disease).
- **Blood urea nitrogen** (BUN)/**creatinine** and urinalysis to evaluate for evidence of immune complex glomerulonephritis.
- **Erythrocyte sedimentation rate** (ESR), **C-reactive protein** (CRP), and **rheumatoid factor** (RF) are usually elevated.

- Serologic testing for *Brucella, Legionella, Bartonella, Coxiella burnetii, Mycoplasma,* and *Chlamydia* species as indicated for culture-negative endocarditis.
- Occasionally, polymerase chain reaction (PCR) testing of explanted valve tissue is needed to confirm the microbe.

Electrocardiography

- An electrocardiogram should be obtained to assess for conduction abnormalities (such as varying and progressive degrees of atrioventricular [AV] block) suggestive of abscess formation, which are particularly associated with aortic valve endocarditis.
- Ischemic/infarct changes suggestive of coronary emboli.

Imaging

- CXR:
  - Evidence of HF (pulmonary edema).
  - Septic emboli, particularly in IV drug users with suspected right-sided endocarditis.
- **Transthoracic echocardiography** (TTE)[4,5]:
  - TTE may detect valvular vegetations with or without positive blood cultures.
  - It is used to characterize the hemodynamic severity of valvular lesions in known IE.
  - It can also assess for complications of IE (e.g., abscesses, perforation, and shunts).
  - TTE can be used to reassess high-risk patients (e.g., those with a virulent organism, clinical deterioration, persistent or recurrent fever, new murmur, or persistent bacteremia).
  - TTE can be considered a reasonable option:
    - To diagnose IE of a prosthetic valve in the presence of persistent fever without bacteremia or a new murmur.
    - For the re-evaluation of prosthetic valve endocarditis (PVE) during antibiotic therapy in the absence of clinical deterioration.
  - High-risk features on transthoracic echo that should be further evaluated by transesophageal echocardiography (TEE):
    - Large vegetation(s)
    - Moderate-to-severe valvular regurgitation or stenosis
    - Suggestion of perivalvular extension (i.e., abscess, pseudoaneurysm, fistula)
    - Evidence of ventricular dysfunction
  - TTE is generally not recommended to re-evaluate uncomplicated (including no regurgitation on baseline echocardiogram) NVE during antibiotic treatment in the absence of clinical deterioration, new physical findings, or persistent fever.
- **TEE**[4,5]:
  - Assess the severity of valvular lesions in symptomatic patients with IE if TTE is nondiagnostic.
  - Diagnose IE in patients with valvular heart disease and positive blood cultures if TTE is nondiagnostic.
  - Diagnose complications of IE with potential impact on prognosis and management (e.g., abscesses, perforation, and shunts).
  - First-line diagnostic study to diagnose PVE and to assess for complications.
  - Preoperative evaluation in patients with known IE:
    - Unless the need for surgery is evident on transthoracic imaging or
    - Preoperative imaging will delay surgery in urgent cases.
  - Intraoperative TEE is recommended to patients undergoing valve surgery for IE.
  - TEE can be considered reasonable to
    - Diagnose possible IE in patients with persistent staphylococcal bacteremia without a known source.
    - Detect IE in patients with nosocomial staphylococcal bacteremia.

- Coronary computed tomography angiography (CCTA) is a useful alternative to left heart catheterization to evaluate coronary anatomy, particularly in less stable patients and those with complicated AV endocarditis.
- Brain CT/MRI:
  - Assess any new neurologic symptoms.
  - MRI may be needed to assess the severity of damage and the presence of hemorrhage caused by emboli to the brain.
  - MR angiography (MRA) may be needed to evaluate for cerebral mycotic aneurysms.

Diagnostic Procedures

Cardiac catheterization may be done to evaluate coronary anatomy in patients with risk factors for CAD needing valve surgery.

TREATMENT

Medications

- Effective treatment involves a coordinated multidisciplinary approach including cardiology, infectious diseases, and cardiac surgery. See Table 22-6 for recommended antibiotic regimens.[4]

TABLE 22-6	RECOMMENDED ANTIBIOTIC REGIMENS FOR IE
Microbe	**Regimen (options listed for each microbe)**
Streptococcus viridans and *Streptococcus bovis*	• IV PCN G or ceftriaxone
Highly PCN-susceptible	• IV PCN G or ceftriaxone + gentamicin
	• Vancomycin
Streptococcus viridans and *Streptococcus bovis*	• IV PCN G or ceftriaxone + gentamicin
Relatively PCN-resistant	• Vancomycin
Enterococcus	• Ampicillin or IV PCN G + gentamicin
Susceptible to PCN, gentamycin, vancomycin	• Vancomycin + gentamicin
Staphylococcus (native)	MSSA:
	• Nafcillin or oxacillin + gentamicin (optional)
	• Cefazolin + gentamicin (optional)
	MRSA:
	• Vancomycin

(Continued)

TABLE 22-6	RECOMMENDED ANTIBIOTIC REGIMENS FOR IE (*Continued*)
Microbe	Regimen (options listed for each microbe)
Staphylococcus (prosthetic)	MSSA: • Nafcillin or oxacillin + rifampin + gentamicin MRSA: • Vancomycin + rifampin + gentamicin
HACEK	• Ceftriaxone or ampicillin-sulbactam or ciprofloxacin
Culture-negative (native)	• Ampicillin + gentamicin • Vancomycin + gentamicin + ciprofloxacin
Culture-negative (prosthetic) <1 year	• Vancomycin + gentamicin + cefepime + rifampin
Culture-negative (prosthetic) >1 year	• Ampicillin + gentamicin • Vancomycin + gentamicin + ciprofloxacin
Culture-negative	• Ceftriaxone + gentamicin ± doxycycline
Bartonella suspected	• Doxycycline + gentamicin
Bartonella documented	• Amphotericin B ± long-term suppressive therapy with an oral azole
Fungal IE	

IE, infective endocarditis; HACEK, *Haemophilus aphrophilus, H. parainfluenzae and H. paraphrophilus, Actinobacillus actinomycetemcomitans, Cardiobacterium hominis, Eikenella corrodens, Kingella kingae;* PCN, penicillin; MSSA, methicillin-sensitive *Staphylococcus aureus;* MRSA, methicillin-resistant *S. aureus.*

Modified from Baddour LM, Wilson WR, Bayer AS, et al. AHA guidelines–infective endocarditis: diagnosis, antimicrobial therapy, and management of complications. *Circulation* 2005;111:394-434.

- **Empiric antibiotic coverage** for the most likely organisms (*Staphylococcus aureus*, gram-negative bacilli, and streptococci, including *Enterococcus*) is appropriate once adequate samples for blood cultures have been drawn.[4,5]
  - Vancomycin is often recommended by infectious diseases consultants as initial empiric therapy for *S. aureus* while awaiting culture results due to the high prevalence of methicillin-resistant *S. aureus* (MRSA).
  - Dosed for weight and renal function with a goal trough level of 15 to 25 µg/mL.
  - Oxacillin or nafcillin 2 g IV every 4 hours (if MRSA not suspected).
  - Ampicillin 2 g IV every 4 hours (if MRSA not suspected).
  - Gentamicin 1 to 1.5 mg/kg IV every 8 hours.
  - Rifampin can be added to nafcillin or vancomycin plus gentamicin for prosthetic valves.

- Anticoagulation[4,6]:
  - There is no clear role for antiplatelet or anticoagulant agents in preventing thromboemboli.
  - Warfarin should be changed over to unfractionated heparin in anticipation of possible surgery and/or for easy reversal if neurologic symptoms develop in patients with an indication for anticoagulation (e.g., mechanical valve).

Surgical Management

- Advances in surgical technique and a growing understanding that surgery may improve the natural history of the disease have made early surgical involvement crucial.
- In general, surgery is performed in any patient with hemodynamic instability, HF, complicated IE, or IE caused by a highly resistant organism (see Table 22-7).[5,7]
- Prompt surgical intervention should be initiated for hemodynamic instability and/ or HF.
- There should be no delays for "sterilization" of the surgical field with several days of preoperative antibiotic therapy.

TABLE 22-7	**ACC/AHA GUIDELINES—INDICATIONS FOR SURGERY FOR ENDOCARDITIS**

Surgery for NVE

Class I

1. Surgery of the native valve is indicated in patients with acute IE who present with valve stenosis or regurgitation resulting in heart failure. (Level of Evidence: B)

2. Surgery of the native valve is indicated in patients with acute IE who present with AR or MR with hemodynamic evidence of elevated LV end-diastolic or left atrial pressures (e.g., premature closure of MV with AR, rapid decelerating MR signal by continuous-wave Doppler (v-wave cutoff sign), or moderate or severe pulmonary hypertension). (Level of Evidence: B)

3. Surgery of the native valve is indicated in patients with IE caused by fungal or other highly resistant organisms. (Level of Evidence: B)

4. Surgery of the native valve is indicated in patients with IE complicated by heart block, annular or aortic abscess, or destructive penetrating lesions (e.g., sinus of Valsalva to right atrium, right ventricle, or left atrium fistula; mitral leaflet perforation with aortic valve endocarditis; or infection in annulus fibrosa). (Level of Evidence: B)

Class IIa

1. Surgery of the native valve is reasonable in patients with IE who present with recurrent emboli and persistent vegetations despite appropriate antibiotic therapy. (Level of Evidence: C)

Class IIb

1. Surgery of the native valve may be considered in patients with IE who present with mobile vegetations in excess of 10 mm with or without emboli. (Level of Evidence: C)

(Continued)

TABLE 22-7	ACC/AHA GUIDELINES—INDICATIONS FOR SURGERY FOR ENDOCARDITIS *(Continued)*

Surgery for PVE

Class I

1. Consultation with a cardiac surgeon is indicated for patients with IE of a prosthetic valve. (Level of Evidence: C)

2. Surgery is indicated for patients with IE of prosthetic valve who present with heart failure. (Level of Evidence: B)

3. Surgery is indicated for patients with IE of a prosthetic valve who present with dehiscence evidenced by cine fluoroscopy or echocardiography. (Level of Evidence: B)

4. Surgery is indicated for patients with IE of a prosthetic valve who present with evidence of increasing obstruction or worsening regurgitation. (Level of Evidence: C)

5. Surgery is indicated for patients with IE of a prosthetic valve who present with complications (e.g., abscess formation). (Level of Evidence: C)

Class IIa

1. Surgery is reasonable for patients with IE of a prosthetic valve who present with evidence of persistent bacteremia or recurrent emboli despite appropriate antibiotic treatment. (Level of Evidence: C)

2. Surgery is reasonable for patients with IE of a prosthetic valve who present with relapsing infection. (Level of Evidence: C)

Class III

1. Routine surgery is not indicated for patients with uncomplicated IE of a prosthetic valve caused by first infection with a sensitive organism. (Level of Evidence: C)

ACC, American College of Cardiology; AHA, American Heart Association; AR, aortic regurgitation; IE, infective endocarditis; LA, left atrium; LV, left ventricle; MR, mitral regurgitation.

From Bonow RO, Carabello BA, Chatterjee K, et al. American College of Cardiology/American Heart Association Task Force on Practice Guidelines. 2008 focused update incorporated into the ACC/AHA 2006 guidelines for the management of patients with valvular heart disease. *J Am Coll Cardiol* 2008;52:e1-142, with permission.

- When an acute neurologic event occurs, timing of surgery is more difficult, as early surgery can worsen neurologic function and increase mortality. Consider delaying surgery for 2 to 3 weeks after a significant embolic infarct or for at least 1 month after intracerebral hemorrhage.
- **Native valve surgery**[4,5]:
  - Acute IE that presents with valve stenosis or regurgitation resulting in HF.
  - Acute IE that presents with aortic regurgitation (AR) or mitral regurgitation (MR) with hemodynamic evidence of elevated left ventricle (LV) end-diastolic or left atrial pressures (e.g., premature closure of Mitral valve (MV) with AR, rapid decelerating MR signal by continuous-wave Doppler, or moderate-to-severe pulmonary hypertension).
  - IE caused by fungal or other highly resistant organisms.
  - IE is considered complicated if heart block, annular or aortic abscesses, or destructive penetrating lesions are present.
  - Recurrent emboli and persistent vegetations despite appropriate antibiotic therapy.

- **Surgery for PVE**[4,5]:
  - Indications include
    - HF
    - Valve dehiscence evidenced by cine fluoroscopy or echocardiography
    - Increasing obstruction or worsening regurgitation
    - Abscess
  - Reasonable to consider redo valve surgery for
    - Persistent bacteremia or recurrent emboli despite appropriate antibiotic treatment
    - Relapsing infection
    - The Early Surgery versus Conventional Treatment in Infective Endocarditis (EASE) trial indicated that early surgery (within 48 hours after randomization) in patients with infective endocarditis and large vegetations (>10 mm) significantly reduced the composite end point of death from any cause and embolic events by effectively decreasing the risk of systemic embolism.[8]
  - Routine surgery is not indicated for patients with uncomplicated IE of a prosthetic valve caused by the first infection with a sensitive organism.

SPECIAL CONSIDERATIONS

In 2008, the recommendations for **endocarditis prophylaxis** were revised (Tables 22-8, 22-9, and 22-10).[9]

OUTCOME/PROGNOSIS

- Several factors have been shown to independently predict increased mortality, including advanced age, presence of CHF, prosthetic valve, type of organism (*S. aureus*), diabetes mellitus type 2, renal insufficiency, and larger vegetation size, among others. A risk classification of mortality has been developed for patients with complicated left-sided NVE (see Table 22-11).[10-12]

TABLE 22-8	AHA GUIDELINES—CARDIAC CONDITIONS FOR WHICH INFECTIVE ENDOCARDITIS PROPHYLAXIS IS RECOMMENDED

- Patients with prosthetic cardiac valve or prosthetic material used for cardiac valve repair
- Previous IE
- CHD
  - Unrepaired cyanotic CHD, including palliative shunts and conduits
  - Completely repaired congenital heart defect with prosthetic material or device, whether placed by surgery or by catheter intervention, during the first 6 months after the procedure
  - Repaired CHD with residual defects at the site of or adjacent to the site of a prosthetic patch or prosthetic device (which inhibits endothelialization)
- Cardiac transplantation recipients with valve regurgitation due to a structurally abnormal valve

AHA, American Heart Association; IE, infective endocarditis; CHD, congenital heart disease.
From Wilson W, Taubert KA, Gewitz M, et al. Prevention of infective endocarditis guidelines from the American Heart Association. *Circulation* 2007;116:1736-1754, with permission.

TABLE 22-9	AHA GUIDELINES—SCENARIOS IN WHICH INFECTIVE ENDOCARDITIS PROPHYLAXIS IS RECOMMENDED

- The recommendations below only apply to patients with the cardiac conditions listed in Table 22-8.
- All dental procedures that involve manipulation of gingival tissues or periapical region of teeth or perforation of oral mucosa.
- Prophylaxis against infective endocarditis is **not recommended for nondental procedures** (such as transesophageal echocardiogram, esophagogastroduodenoscopy, or colonoscopy) in the absence of active infection.

AHA, American Heart Association; IE, infective endocarditis.

Modified from Wilson W, Taubert KA, Gewitz M, et al. Prevention of infective endocarditis guidelines from the American Heart Association. *Circulation* 2007;116:1736-1754.

- Complications significantly contribute to the morbidity and mortality of IE and can include valvular dysfunction and HF, abscess formation (which can lead to heart block or fistulas between various chambers of the heart), emboli, and uncontrolled infection.

Infections of Implantable Cardiac Devices

GENERAL PRINCIPLES

- Implanted cardiac devices can become infected, similar to any other foreign body.
- Examples of these devices include permanent pacemakers (PPMs), implantable cardioverter-defibrillators (ICDs), cardiac stents, left ventricular assist devices (LVADs), and intra-aortic balloon pumps (IABPs).
- Most device infections are associated with cardiac implantable electrophysiologic devices (CIEDs), such as PPMs and ICDs.
- The use of CIED therapy is increasing with the improvement in technology. As a result, CIED-related infections are also increasing and have become a significant clinical problem.
- Symptoms and signs, presentation, consequences, and treatment vary according to the device type, the location of the infected part(s) of the device, the extent of infection, and the clinical characteristics of the patient.

Epidemiology

- The incidence of cardiac device infection is difficult to determine due to the lack of a comprehensive registry or mandatory reporting. Reported rates have varied between 0.2% and 5.8%.[13-16]
- Infection in CIED is associated with a twofold increase in mortality.[14]

Pathophysiology

- CIED contamination and secondary infection happen at the time of implant or during subsequent manipulation of the device.

TABLE 22-10	AHA GUIDELINES—REGIMENS FOR A DENTAL PROCEDURE		
		Regimen: Single dose 30–60 minutes before the procedure	
Situation	Agent	Adults	Children
Oral	Amoxicillin	2 g	50 mg/kg
Unable to take oral medication	Ampicillin OR	2 g IM or IV	50 mg/kg IM or IV
	Cefazolin or ceftriaxone	1 g IM or IV	50 mg/kg IM or IV
Allergic to penicillins or ampicillin, oral	Cephalexin[a,b] OR	2 g	50 mg/kg
	Clindamycin OR	600 mg	20 mg/kg
	Azithromycin or clarithro-mycin	500 mg	15 mg/kg
Allergic to penicillins or ampicillin and unable to take oral medication	Cefazolin or ceftriaxone[b] OR	1 g IM or IV	50 mg/kg IM or IV
	Clindamycin	600 mg IM or IV	20 mg/kg IM or IV

[a]Or other first- or second-generation oral cephalosporin in equivalent adult or pediatric dosage.
[b]Cephalosporins should not be used in an individual with a history of anaphylaxis, angioedema, or urticaria with penicillins or ampicillin.
From Wilson W, Taubert KA, Gewitz M, et al. Prevention of infective endocarditis guidelines from the American Heart Association. *Circulation* 2007;116:1736-1754, with permission.

- The surgical pocket can also become infected from seeding from the bloodstream in the setting of bacteremia or fungemia.
- Staphylococcal species account for 60% to 80% of infections, particularly coagulase-negative *Staphylococcus* and *S. aureus*.[17]
- Gram-negative bacilli, *Propionibacteroi acnes*, *Corynebacterium*, and *Candida* spp. account for the rest of CIED-related infections.

Risk Factors[17]

- Diabetes mellitus
- HF
- Renal failure
- Previous generator replacement
- Underlying malignancy

TABLE 22-11	PROGNOSIS WITH COMPLICATED LEFT-SIDED ENDOCARDITIS			
Parameter	Points			
Mental status				
Alert	0			
Lethargy or disorientation	4			
Charlson comorbidity scale score				
0–1	0			
≥2	3			
Congestive heart failure[a]				
None or mild	0			
Moderate or severe	3			
Microbiology				
Viridans streptococci	0			
Staphylococcus aureus	6			
Other[b]	8			
Treatment				
Surgery	0			
Medical	5			
Points	≤6	7–11	12–15	>15
6-month mortality	9%	25%	39%	63%

[a]None or mild: Absence of rales, no shortness of breath at rest, and no pulmonary edema; moderate or severe: presence of at least one.

[b]Includes other streptococci, *Enterococcus*, coagulase-negative staphylococci, Enterobacteriaceae, other gram-negative bacilli, HACEK, fungi, and culture negative endocarditis.

Data from Hasbun R, Vikram HR, Barakat LA, et al. Complicated left-sided native valve endocarditis in adults–risk classification for mortality. *JAMA* 2003;289:1933-1940.

- Dermatologic disorders
- Urgent placement of device
- Fever within 24 hours
- Use of periprocedural temporary pacing[18]
- Low procedural volume

Prevention

- Strict aseptic technique
- Prophylactic antibiotics:
  - Administered 60 minutes prior to starting the procedure.
  - 1 to 2 g of cefazolin IV.
  - Vancomycin if the patient has had MRSA or is allergic to penicillin.
- Avoiding implantation in patients with signs of clinical infection.

DIAGNOSIS

Clinical Presentation

- Symptoms and signs are dependent on the organism, the presence of bacteremia, and the degree and specific site of infection.
- **Generator pocket infection:**
  - Superficial wound infections may or may not have surgical pocket involvement. They typically involve pain, swelling, erythema, and possible wound discharge and dehiscence.
  - Surgical pocket infection or subcutaneous lead infection typically involves pain, swelling, erythema over the area of infection, pocket erosion, and wound discharge.
  - Occasionally, deep-seated pocket infections can present with pain in the pocket and no other systemic signs or symptoms.
  - Pocket erosion can also occur without major systemic signs or symptoms and must be treated as a pocket infection.
- **Infection of PPM or ICD leads** (CIED-related endocarditis)[19]:
  - Systemic signs are more common with associated fevers, rigors, malaise, anorexia, and even hemodynamic compromise.
  - Signs and symptoms of endocarditis are often seen, such as infective and thrombotic embolization, mostly affecting the right-sided valves, and can also present with tricuspid regurgitation (TR), tricuspid stenosis (TS), pulmonary emboli, and pneumonia.
  - The clinical presentation can be acute or subacute and seldom involves signs of left-sided endocarditis.

Diagnostic Testing

- A high index of clinical suspicion is necessary, and the diagnosis should be considered in patients with devices and underlying fever.
- No single test is specific or sensitive enough to make the diagnosis.
- At least two sets of blood cultures should be collected before antimicrobial therapy is intitated (Table 22-12).[17]
- Positive blood cultures often confirm the diagnosis, particularly in *Staphylococcus* spp.
- Other findings that may aid in the diagnosis of CIED-related infections include leukocytosis, elevated CRP, and ESR.
- **TEE is the test of choice to exclude endocarditis**, especially in patients with *Staphylococcus aureus* bacteremia, because the rate of endocarditis is high.
- Chest X-ray, CT pulmonary angiography, and ventilation–perfusion pulmonary scintigraphy may also be helpful.
- Gallium and radiolabled leukocyte scintigraphy are neither sensitive nor specific for device infection.
- Cultures of the generator, surgical pocket, and lead tips at the time of device removal can be potentially helpful to determine the causative microorganism.
- **Percutaneous aspiration of the CIED pocket should not be performed** because of poor diagnostic yield and the potential to introduce pathogens into the surgical pocket.[17]

TREATMENT

Medications

- **Superficial or incisional infections** that do not involve the surgical pocket or the device itself do not require removal of the device.[17]
  - Managed with **antibiotics that cover *Staphylococcus* spp.**, such as oral cephalexin or cloxacillin for 7 to 14 days.
  - Can be very difficult to distinguish from early deep infection.

TABLE 22-12	AHA GUIDELINES FOR DIAGNOSIS OF CIED INFECTION AND ASSOCIATED COMPLICATIONS

Class I

1. All patients should have at least two sets of blood cultures drawn at the initial evaluation before prompt initiation of antimicrobial therapy for CIED infection. (*Level of Evidence: C*)

2. Generator-pocket tissue gram stain and culture and lead-tip culture should be obtained when the CIED is explanted. (*Level of Evidence: C*)

3. Patients with suspected CIED infection who either have positive blood cultures or have negative blood cultures but have had recent antimicrobial therapy before blood cultures were obtained should undergo TEE for CIED infection or valvular endocarditis. (*Level of Evidence: C*)

4. All adults suspected of having CIED-related endocarditis should undergo TEE to evaluate the left-sided heart valves, even if transthoracic views have demonstrated lead-adherent masses. In pediatric patients with good views, TTE may be sufficient. (*Level of Evidence: B*)

Class IIa

1. Patients should seek evaluation for CIED infection by cardiologists or infectious disease specialists if they develop fever or bloodstream infection for which there is no initial explanation. (*Level of Evidence: C*)

Class III

1. Percutaneous aspiration of the generator pocket should not be performed as part of the diagnostic evaluation of CIED infection. (*Level of Evidence: C*)

AHA, American Heart Association; CIED, cardiac implantable electrophysiologic device; TTE, transthoracic echocardiography.

Data from Baddour LM, Epstein AE, Erickson CC, et al. Update on cardiovascular implantable electronic device infections and their management: a scientific statement from the American Heart Association. *Circulation* 2010;121:458-477, with permission.

- ○ A wound swab and culture should be performed to help direct antimicrobial treatment.
- ○ Patients should be closely monitored and management escalated if needed, including alternative more broad-spectrum antibiotics or prolonged duration of treatment, and consideration of device removal if the infection does not resolve.
- **Otherwise, antimicrobial therapy is largely adjunctive to CIED removal.**[17,20]
  - ○ Antibiotics should be chosen based on in vitro antibiotic sensitivity.
  - ○ There are no definitive data on the optimal duration of treatment.
  - ○ Blood cultures should be obtained after extraction and, if positive, at least 2 weeks of parenteral antibiotic therapy should be considered prior to reimplantation.
  - ○ For persistently positive blood cultures greater than 24 hours after extraction, clinicians should consider 4 weeks of antibiotic therapy.
- CIED infections limited to the surgical pocket without erosion may be adequately treated within 7 to 10 days of oral antibiotics, which can be extended to 14 days if erosion is present.[17]
- **Generator pocket infections** require the removal of the device but removal of leads may be avoided. **Intravenous anti-staphylococcal antibiotic therapy**, usually with vancomycin, is recommended.

- **CIED-related endocarditis should be treated with a full course of antibiotics as for NVE.**
  - Complete removal of the entire CIED including generator, suture sleeves, sutures, and leads in cases where infection is strongly suspected or established is the goal in most cases.
  - This applies to all CIED infections other than superficial or incisional wound infections.
  - Recurrence of infection is high if any components are retained.
  - Erosion of any part of the CIED components implies contamination of the entire system and necessitates extraction of the entire system.
  - American Heart Association (AHA) guidelines for the diagnosis of CIED-related endocarditis are listed in Table 22-12.[17]
- **Patients with positive blood cultures but no evidence of local infection in the CIED** pose difficult management questions.[17]
  - The clinical parameters that are indicative of the above scenario are relapsing bacteremia after an appropriate period of antibiotic treatment and
    - no other source for bacteremia identified
    - bacteremia >24 hours
    - ICD
    - presence of a prosthetic valve
    - bacteremia within 3 months of device implantation
  - Strong consideration should be given to device extraction when blood cultures remain positive.

Other Non-Pharmacologic Therapy

- **Percutaneous CIED lead extraction** has become the preferred method to remove leads due to improved technologies, including excimer laser, cautery, and rotational dissection systems.[17,20]
- The procedure has significant risks, including tamponade, hemothorax, pulmonary embolism, lead migration, pneumonia, and death.
- In institutions with a high volume of cases, percutaneous lead removal can be performed relatively safely with a high success rate (95% to 97.5%), a low rate of complication (0% to 0.4%), and a high eradication rate of infection.[21]
- Surgical management should be considered when percutaneous management has failed or when hardware is retained.
- Larger vegetations (>2 cm) can be done safely percutaneously.
- Should not be postponed due to timing of antimicrobial therapy.

SPECIAL CONSIDERATIONS

- **CIED reimplantation after extraction:**
  - Every patient should be evaluated for the need for CIED reimplantation after extraction of an infected device.
  - It should be performed on the contralateral side when necessary. If this is not possible, then the leads should be tunneled to a device placed subcutaneously elsewhere, such as in the abdomen.
  - Reimplantation should be delayed until infection has fully resolved.
  - There are no prospective data that have examined the optimal timing of reimplantation; however, a minimum period of 24 to 48 hours is recommended and 2 weeks is preferred.[17,20]
- **LVAD Infections:**
  - Infection is a frequent complication of LVAD placement and is a significant source of morbidity and mortality.[22]

- The risk of infection increases with the duration of use, most commonly occurring after 2 weeks. Incidence of infection has been highly variable among different surveys, reported to range between 13% and 80%.
- Newer generation continuous-flow (CF) LVADs are associated with smaller pump pockets and drive-line exit sites versus pulsatile-flow (PF) devices.
- LVAD patients have also benefitted from increased provider awareness and experience of infectious complications.
- Sepsis is the most common cause of death, accounting for 41% of deaths in PF LVAD patients and 20% of deaths in CF LVAD patients.[22,23]
- Studies have shown a reduction in the incidence of sepsis in CF LVAD patients vs. PF LVAD patients.[24,25]
- **Types of infection**[26]:
  - **Drive-line infection is the most common** type of infection and usually presents with local inflammation and drainage at the exit site.
  - **Pocket infection** can also occur which causes local inflammatory changes.
  - Rarely, **endocarditis** can also occur due to infection involving the valve and/or the internal (blood-contacting) lining of the device.
  - Patients can have more than one type of infection simultaneously.
- **Organisms:**
  - The organisms involve depend on the type of infection and on whether there is an associate bloodstream infection.
  - Staphylococci are the most common, followed by gram-negative bacilli (including *Pseudomonas aeruginosa* and *Escherichia coli*), *Enterococcus, Corynebacterium,* and *Candida* spp.
  - Catheter-related blood stream infections (CRBSIs) tend to involve staphylococci or *Candida* spp.
  - Device-related infections usually involve gram-positive cocci (*Staphylococcus* or *Enterococcus* spp.), although gram-negative infections also occur which involve *P. aeruginosa, Enterobacter,* or *Klebsiella.*[26]
- **Risk factors** are usually related to patient comorbidities including diabetes and obesity.[26] They are also related to perioperative events such as bleeding, blood product transfusion, thrombosis, and surgical reexploration.
- **The clinical presentation** may include fever, leukocytosis, and/or local signs of infection. LVAD-related endocarditis can present with fever, bacteremia, embolic events, and valvular incompetence.
- Not considered to be a contraindication to cardiac transplantation.
- **Treatment** should be targeted against causative organism and an unresolved infection may require device removal.
- **Coronary artery stent infections:**
  - Infections of intracoronary stents are rare but are often fatal due to severe damage to the arterial wall.[27-29]
  - They occur secondary to contamination of stent at the time of implantation or due to subsequent bacteriemia. Infection can occur within 4 weeks of placement.
  - Fever, phlebitis, local infection, and bacteremia occur in <1% of all procedures.[30]
  - *Staphylococcus aureus* and *P. aeruginosa* are most common pathogens.
  - There may also be findings of associated abscess, suppurative pancreatitis, and pericardial empyema.
  - Brachial artery access has been associated with a 10-fold higher incidence of infectious complications, due to a cutdown approach. Repeated puncture of ipsilateral femoral artery or indwelling sheaths post procedure is associated with an increased incidence of infection.[30]
  - Prevention strategies should involve sterile technique, avoidance of access through endovascular grafts, avoidance of access ipsilateral to a prosthetic hip, and minimization of indwelling catheters after the procedure.

- ○ Treatment should involve empiric antibiotics effective against multidrug resistant gram-positive cocci and gram-negative bacilli.
- **IABP infections**
  - ○ Infections of IABPs are uncommon, and the rate of infection is related to the duration of therapy.
  - ○ Local wound infections are the most common, and usually bacteremia is secondary to contamination from a colonized or infected insertion site.[30]
  - ○ Risk factors for infection include contamination of the femoral site, especially in obese patients, and emergent placement is not done in the operating room or catherization laboratory.[30]
  - ○ Treatment should be with appropriate antimicrobial therapy, local wound care, and removal of the IABP whenever possible.

REFERENCES

1. O'Rourke RA, Fuster V, Alexander RW, eds. *Hurst's the Heart*, 10th ed. New York, NY: McGraw-Hill; 2000:596.
2. Tleyjeh IM, Abdel-Latif A, Rahbi H, et al. A systematic review of population-based studies of infective endocarditis. *Chest* 2007;132:1025-1035.
3. Li JS. Proposed modifications to the Duke criteria for the diagnosis of infective endocarditis. *Clin Infect Dis* 2000;30:633-638.
4. Baddour LM, Wilson WR, Bayer AS, et al. AHA guidelines—infective endocarditis: diagnosis, antimicrobial therapy, and management of complications. *Circulation* 2005;111:e394-e434.
5. Bonow RO, Carabello BA, Chatterjee K, et al. American College of Cardiology/American Heart Association Task Force on Practice Guidelines. 2008 focused update incorporated into the ACC/AHA 2006 guidelines for the management of patients with valvular heart disease. *J Am Coll Cardiol* 2008;52:e1-e142.
6. Whitlock RP, Sun JC, Fremes SE, et al. Antithrombotic and thrombolytic therapy for valvular disease: Antithrombotic Therapy and Prevention of Thrombosis, 9th ed: American College of Chest Physicians Evidence-Based Clinical Practice Guidelines. *Chest* 2012;141:e576S-e600S.
7. Vikram HR, Buenconsejo J, Hasbun R, et al. Impact of valve surgery on 6-month mortality in adults with complicated, left-sided native valve endocarditis. *JAMA* 2003;290:3207-3214.
8. Kang DH, Kim YJ, Kim SH, et al. Early surgery versus conventional treatment for infective endocarditis. *N Engl J Med* 2012;366(26):2466-2473. doi: 10.1056/NEJMoa1112843.
9. Wilson W, Taubert KA, Gewitz M, et al. Prevention of infective endocarditis guidelines from the American Heart Association. *Circulation* 2007;116:1736-1754.
10. Hasbun R, Vikram HR, Barakat LA, et al. Complicated left-sided native valve endocarditis in adults–risk classification for mortality. *JAMA* 2003;289:1933-1940.
11. Chu VH, Cabell CH, Benjamin DK, et al. Early predictors of in-hospital death in infective endocarditis. *Circulation* 2004;109:1745-1749.
12. Thuny F, Disalvo G, Belliard O, et al. Risk of embolism and death in infective endocarditis: prognostic value of echocardiography—a prospective multicenter study. *Circulation* 2005;112:69-75.
13. Gold MR, Peters RW, Johnson JW, Shorofsky SR. Complications associated with pectoral cardioverter-defibrillator implantation: comparison of subcutaneous and submuscular approaches. Worldwide Jewel Investigators. *J Am Coll Cardiol* 1996;28:1278-1282.
14. Voigt A, Shalaby A, Saba S. Rising rates of cardiac rhythm management device infections in the United States: 1996 through 2003. *J Am Coll Cardiol* 2006;48:590-591.
15. Gandhi T, Crawford T, Riddell J IV. Cardiovascular implantable electronic device associated infections. *Infect Dis Clin North Am* 2012;26:57-76.
16. Uslan DZ, Sohail MR, St Sauver JL, et al. Permanent pacemaker and implantable cardioverter defibrillator infection: a population-based study. *Arch Intern Med* 2007;167:669-675.
17. Baddour LM, Epstein AE, Erickson CC, et al. Update on cardiovascular implantable electronic device infections and their management: a scientific statement from the American Heart Association. *Circulation* 2010;121:458-477.
18. Klug D, Balde M, Pavin D, et al. Risk factors related to infections of implanted pacemakers and cardioverter–defibrillators: results of a large prospective study. *Circulation* 2007;116:1349-1355.
19. Le KY, Sohail MR, Friedman PA, et al. Clinical predictors of cardiovascular implantable electronic device-related infective endocarditis. *Pacing Clin Electrophysiol* 2011;34:450-459.

20. Gould P, Gula LJ, Yee R, et al. Cardiovascular implantable electrophysiological device-related infections: a review. *Curr Opin Cardiol* 2011;26:6-11.
21. Jones SO IV, Eckart RE, Albert CM, Epstein LM. Large, single-center, single-operator experience with transvenous lead extraction: outcomes and changing indications. *Heart Rhythm* 2008;5:520-525.
22. Holman WL, Park SJ, Long JW, et al. Infection in permanent circulatory support: experience from the REMATCH trial. *J Heart Lung Transplant* 2004;23:1359-1365.
23. Miller LW, Pagani FD, Russell SD, et al. Use of a continuous-flow device in patients awaiting heart transplantation. *N Engl J Med* 2007;357:885-896.
24. Slaughter MS, Rogers JG, Milano CA, et al. Advanced heart failure treated with continuous-flow left ventricular assist device. *N Engl J Med* 2009;361:2241-2251.
25. Schaffer JM, Allen JG, Weiss ES, et al. Infectious complications after pulsatile-flow and continuous-flow left ventricular assist device implantation. *J Heart Lung Transplant* 2011;30:164-174.
26. Califano S, Pagani FD, Malani PN. Left ventricular assist device-associated infections. *Infect Dis Clin North Am* 2012;26:77-87.
27. Liu JC, Cziperle DJ, Kleinman B, et al. Coronary abscess: a complication of stenting. *Catheter Cardiovasc Interv* 2003;58:69-71.
28. Alfonso F, Moreno R, Vergas J. Fatal infection after rapamycin eluting coronary stent implantation. *Heart* 2005;91:e51.
29. Elieson M, Mixon, Carpenter J. Coronary stent infections: a case report and literature review. *Tex Heart Inst J* 2012;39:884-889.
30. Baddour LM, Bettman MA, Bolger AF, et al. Nonvalvular cardiovascular device-related infections. *Circulation* 2003;108:2015-2031.

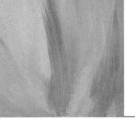

Advanced Electrocardiography: ECG 201

23

Shivak Sharma and Timothy W. Smith

GENERAL PRINCIPLES

Building on the overriding principles of Chapter 3 (read the electrocardiogram [ECG] the same way every time to avoid mistakes; practice, practice, practice; keep a file of interesting ECGs), this chapter highlights some of the common clinical situations where more subtle ECG findings help clinch the diagnosis.

DIAGNOSIS

Myocardial Infarction

- ST-segment elevations found in anatomically adjacent ECG leads are the classic finding for myocardial infarction (MI). The diagnosis is further confirmed with **reciprocal changes**, or sinus tachycardia (ST) depressions, in the area of the heart opposite the infarct.[1]
  - Inferior MI is usually caused by an occlusion of the right coronary artery (RCA). The RCA supplies the atrioventricular (AV) node in most people, so **PR prolongation or AV block** is often found with inferior MI.
  - Additionally, the RCA supplies the right ventricle (RV) through RV marginal arteries. Occlusion of the RCA proximal to these branch arteries can cause an **RV infarct**.
    - Clinically, this is important, because the RV systolic function is dependent on pre-load, and in the setting of an RV infarct, nitrates can cause precipitous drops in blood pressure due to decrease in venous return.
    - An RV infarct is suspected when **ST elevations are greater in lead III than in lead II or lead aVF**.
    - Diagnosis can be made using right-sided ECG leads (Figure 23-1), looking for **any ST elevation in right-sided V_4 (V_4R)**.
  - In most people, the posterior aspect of the heart is supplied by the distal left circumflex artery. Unfortunately, the standard 12-lead ECG does not have leads near this area of the heart, so posterior MIs may be invisible. The diagnosis of a posterior MI can be suspected by finding the reciprocal changes of a posterior ST elevation (i.e., **anterior ST depression**), particularly in lead V_1. Diagnosis can be made by finding ST elevations on additional leads V_7 to V_9 (Figure 23-1).
- The diagnosis of MI can also be made with a new or suspect new left-bundle-branch block (LBBB) pattern **in the correct clinical setting**.
  - It is important to know that the left bundle is richly supplied, primarily by the left anterior descending (LAD) artery and several septal and diagonal branches. Thus, a new LBBB pattern would suggest a large anterior infarct from a proximal LAD occlusion.
  - Many patients with a proximal LAD occlusion will present dramatically, with signs and symptoms of chest pain, hypotension, and/or new heart failure.
  - In contrast, an LBBB pattern is often found on a screening ECG in an asymptomatic patient. It is unlikely that a clinically stable and asymptomatic patient is having an acute, large anterior MI to cause this LBBB pattern, so good clinical judgment is essential.

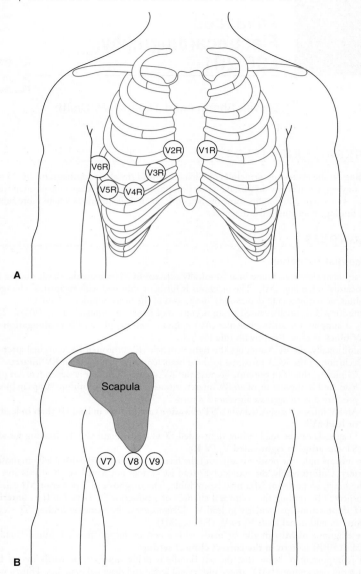

FIGURE 23-1. Alternate positions for ECG leads. **(A)** Right-sided leads (V$_1$R to V$_6$R) for diagnosing an RV infarct. **(B)** Posterior leads (V$_7$ to V$_9$) for diagnosing a posterior infarct.

- Patients presenting with chest pain and a known preexisting LBBB pattern can pose a diagnostic challenge. It is often incorrectly said that the diagnosis of acute MI cannot be made with an underlying LBBB pattern on the ECG. In fact, several ECG findings in this situation can be virtually diagnostic of an acute MI. Commonly cited criteria include[2]:
  - ST elevation $\geq$1 mm and concordant with QRS
  - ST depression $\geq$1 mm in V_1, V_2, or V_3
  - ST elevation $\geq$5 mm and discordant with QRS
- There are many causes of ST elevations on the ECG that are not due to infarcting myocardium.[3] **There is more to the ST segment than just elevation.** These causes range from benign to life-threatening.
  - Many young adult men have an especially **rapid ventricular repolarization**, which causes concave ST elevations, usually largest in lead V_2.
  - An **early repolarization pattern** has been described with a notched J point (immediately after the QRS complex) and tall, upright T waves, most pronounced in lead V_4.
  - The LBBB pattern causes ST-segment deviation in the direction opposite the major QRS deflection.
  - Hyperkalemia, pulmonary embolism (PE), and left ventricular hypertrophy (LVH) can cause ST elevations in distinct ways.
  - Brugada syndrome can manifest with distinctive downsloping ST elevations in leads V_1 and V_2.
  - Cardiac contusions and cardioversions can cause striking transient ST elevations as well.
  - A common mimic of MI is **pericarditis**. Patients with either disease can present with significant chest pain and have ST elevations on the ECG. Several important clinical and ECG distinctions are outlined in Table 23-1.

Tachycardias

- The interpretation of an ECG during a tachycardia can be invaluable for correctly diagnosing and treating the arrhythmia. Management of patients with various tachycardias is outlined in Chapter 7.
- A diagnostic approach to tachyarrhythmias as summarized in Figure 23-2 is a clinically useful classification to approach these patients.
- Tachycardias can be classified as either **narrow complex or wide complex**, based on QRS duration of less than or greater than 120 milliseconds, respectively.

Wide-Complex Tachycardias

- Wide-complex tachycardias have some degree of aberrant conduction through the ventricles and can be found in one of three scenarios: **ventricular tachycardia (VT)**, **supraventricular tachycardia (SVT) with aberrancy**, or **pre-excited tachycardia** (discussed in detail in Chapters 7 and 25).
- Determining the rhythm of an ECG with a wide-complex tachycardia has important prognostic and treatment implications, as each of the three situations on the differential diagnosis list is treated very differently.
- Clinical clues that favor VT or SVT with aberrancy are outlined in Table 23-2.
- In general, VT does not use the rapidly conducting His-Purkinje system, so the ventricular activation is more bizarre, with notching and extremely wide QRS complexes.
- Often, the atria and ventricles are dissociated, and sinus P waves can be seen marching through the VT.
- Further tools, such as the Brugada criteria, are often needed to discriminate VT from SVT with aberrancy (Figure 23-3).

TABLE 23-1	FEATURES TO HELP DISTINGUISH PERICARDITIS FROM MYOCARDIAL INFARCTION	
	MI	**Pericarditis**
History	Risk factors of prior CAD, advanced age, diabetes, hypertension, hypercholesterolemia, tobacco use, early family history of CAD	Recent viral illness History of chest radiation History of cancer
Chest pain characteristics	Variable, but classically "constant, severe squeezing" in the substernal area, with or without radiation to the left jaw and arm.	Variable, but worse with respiration and lying down. Improved with sitting forward.
Physical examination	Variable, but dyspnea, diaphoresis, rales more specific for MI	Variable, but friction rub is specific for pericarditis.
ECG characteristics	ST elevations in an "anatomic" distribution. Reciprocal ST-segment depressions	Diffuse ST elevations. PR depression.
Cardiac-specific biomarkers (troponin)	With large MI, markedly elevated biomarkers	Mild to absent elevation of biomarkers
Echocardiogram	Wall motion abnormalities in the distribution of the infarcting artery	No wall motion abnormalities

MI, myocardial infarction; CAD, coronary artery disease; ECG, electrocardiogram.

- Patients with Wolff-Parkinson-White (WPW) syndrome, a form of ventricular pre-excitation, can develop life-threatening atrial fibrillation (AF) with rapid ventricular conduction. This should be suspected if the tachycardia is irregular or especially fast (ventricular rates 150 to 250 beats per minute [bpm]).

Narrow-Complex Tachycardias

- **Narrow-complex tachycardias** use the His-Purkinje system to activate the ventricles, and most of these arrhythmias are supraventricular in origin.
- **AF:** The most common sustained tachyarrhythmia is discussed as a separate topic in Chapter 26.
- **Atrial flutter (AFL):**
  ○ The second most common atrial arrhythmia with a reported incidence of about 1% per year.

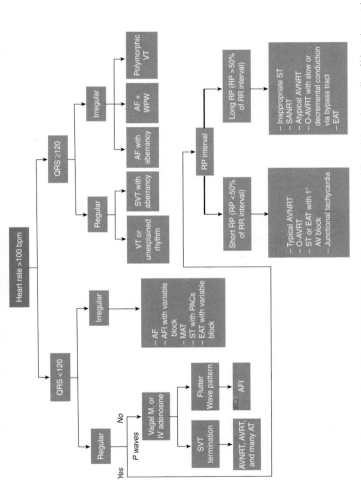

FIGURE 23-2. Approach to tachycardias. AF, atrial fibrillation; AFL, atrial flutter; AT, atrial tachycardia; AVNRT, atrioventricular nodal reentrant tachycardia; AVRT, atrioventricular reentrant tachycardia; AV, atrioventricular; EAT, ectopic atrial tachycardia; MAT, multifocal atrial tachycardia; O-AVRT, orthodromic atrioventricular reentrant tachycardia; PACs, premature atrial contraction; SANRT, sinoatrial nodal reentrant tachycardia; ST, sinus tachycardia; SVT, supraventricular tachycardia; VT, ventricular tachycardia; WPW, Wolff–Parkinson–White. (From Sharma S, Cooper DH, Faddis MN. Cardiac arrhythmias. In: Foster C, Mistry NF, Peddi PF, Sharma S, eds. *The Washington Manual of Medical Therapeutics*, 33rd ed. Philadelphia, PA: Lippincott Williams & Wilkins; 2010:201-248, with permission.)

TABLE 23-2	CLINICAL CLUES TO DISTINGUISH BETWEEN VENTRICULAR AND SUPRAVENTRICULAR TACHYCARDIAS FOR A WIDE-COMPLEX TACHYCARDIA	

Clinical clue	Ventricular tachycardia	Supraventricular tachy-cardia with aberrancy
History	Structural heart disease present	No structural heart disease
Initiation	VPD initiates	APD initiates "Long–short" sequence prior to initiation
P-wave timing	AV dissociation	AV relationship
QRS morphology	Tachycardia QRS morphology similar to prior VPDs	Characteristic QRS morphology for aberrant conduction (V_1, V_6)
	Fusion beats or capture beats	
	Positive QRS concordance (positive QRS $V_1 - V_6$)	
	QRS duration >140 ms if RBBB	
	QRS duration >160 ms if LBBB	
	Extreme axis (−90 to 180 degrees)	
Response to vagal maneuvers	No change	Can slow or terminate with vagal maneuvers

VPD, ventricular premature depolarization; APD, atrial premature depolarization; AV, atrioventricular; RBBB, right-bundle-branch block; LBBB, left-bundle-branch block.

- ○ It is associated with increasing age and underlying heart disease and is more common in men.
- ○ AFL usually presents as a **regular rhythm** but can be **irregularly irregular** when associated with variable AV block (2:1 to 4:1 to 3:1, etc.).
- ○ **Mechanism:** Reentrant circuit around functional or structural conduction barriers within the atria. Atrial rate is 250 to 350 bpm with conduction to ventricle that is usually not 1:1; most often 2:1. **SVT with regular ventricular rate of 150 bpm should raise suspicion for AFL.**
- ○ Like AF, commonly associated with patients post-cardiac surgery, pulmonary disease, thyrotoxicosis, and atrial enlargement.
- ○ **ECG:** In typical AFL, "sawtooth" pattern best visualized in leads II, III, and aVF with positive deflections in lead V_1.
- **Multifocal atrial tachycardia (MAT):**
  - ○ **Irregularly irregular.**
  - ○ SVT seen generally in elderly hospitalized patients with multiple comorbidities.

- ○ MAT is most often associated with chronic obstructive pulmonary disease (COPD) and heart failure but is also associated with glucose intolerance, hypokalemia, hypomagnesemia, drugs (e.g., theophylline), and chronic renal failure.
  - ○ **ECG:** SVT with at least **three distinct P-wave morphologies**, generally best visualized in leads II, III, and V_1.
- • **Sinus tachycardia (ST):**
  - ○ The most common mechanism of long RP tachycardia.
  - ○ Most often, ST is a normal physiologic response to hyperadrenergic states (e.g., fever, pain, hypovolemia, anemia, and hypoxia) but can also be induced by illicit drugs

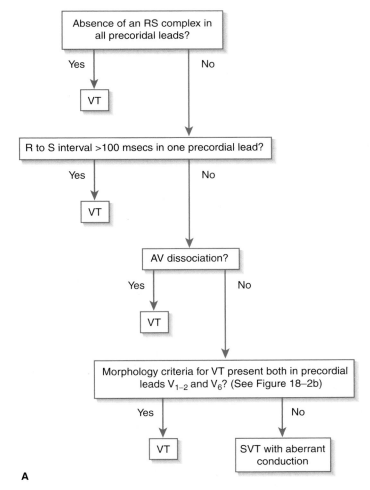

A

FIGURE 23-3. A and **B:** Brugada criteria for distinguishing ventricular tachycardia from supraventricular tachycardia with aberrancy in wide-complex tachycardias.

	LBBB		RBBB	
	VT	**SVT**	**VT**	**SVT**
Lead V1	In V1, V2 any of: (a) r ≥0.04 sec (b) Notched S downstroke (c) Delayed S nadir >0.06 sec	In V1, V2 absence of: (a) r ≥0.04 sec (b) Notched S downstroke (c) Delayed S nadir >0.06 sec	Taller left peak Biphasic RS or QR	Triphasic rsR' or rR'
Lead V6	Monophasic QS 		Biphasic rS 	Triphasic qRs

B

FIGURE 23-3. (*Continued*)

(e.g., cocaine, amphetamines, and methamphetamine) and prescription drugs (e.g., theophylline, atropine, and β-adrenergic agonists).

- ○ **Inappropriate ST** refers to persistently elevated sinus rate in the absence of an identifiable physical, pathologic, or pharmacologic influence.
- **Ectopic atrial tachycardia (EAT):**
  - ○ EAT with variable block can present as an **irregularly irregular** rhythm and can be distinguished from AFL by an **atrial rate of 150 to 200 bpm.**
  - ○ EAT with variable block is associated with **digoxin toxicity**.
  - ○ EAT is characterized by a regular atrial activation pattern with a P-wave morphology originating outside of the sinus node complex resulting in a **long RP tachycardia**.
  - ○ **Mechanism:** Enhanced automaticity, triggered activity, and possibly micro-reentry.
- **Atrioventricular nodal reentrant tachycardia (AVNRT):**
  - ○ This reentrant rhythm occurs in patients who have functional dissociation of their AV node into "slow" and "fast" pathways. It can occur at any age, but predilection for middle age and female gender. Structural heart disease is not a prerequisite.
  - ○ **"Typical" AVNRT** is the more common variety.
    - ▪ Conduction proceeds antegrade down the slow pathway and retrograde up the fast pathway, leading to **short RP tachycardia**.

- **ECG:** P waves hidden in QRS complexes or buried at the end of QRS complexes creating a pseudo-r' (V$_1$) or a pseudo-s' (II). Compare QRS in tachycardia and sinus rhythm to find retrograde P waves.
  - "**Atypical**" **AVNRT:** Antegrade conduction proceeds over the fast AV nodal pathway with retrograde conduction over the slow AV nodal pathway, leading to **long RP tachycardia**.
- **Atrioventricular reentrant tachycardia (AVRT):**
  - **Orthodromic atrioventricular reentrant tachycardia (O-AVRT)** is the most common reentrant tachycardia accounting for about 95% of all AVRT and is discussed further below.
  - Accessory pathway-mediated reentrant rhythm that occurs when antegrade conduction to the ventricle takes place through the AV node and retrograde conduction to the atrium occurs through the accessory or "bypass" tract. **Short RP tachycardia**.
  - **ECG:** Retrograde P waves are frequently seen after the QRS complex and are usually distinguishable from the QRS.
  - O-AVRT is the most common mechanism of SVT in patients with pre-excitation syndromes, like WPW syndrome (defined by short PR and a delta wave on upstroke of QRS) present on sinus rhythm ECG.
  - O-AVRT can occur without pre-excitation in which conduction through the bypass tract occurs only during tachycardia in a retrograde fashion ("concealed pathway").
  - Less commonly, retrograde conduction over the accessory pathway to the atrium proceeds slowly enough for atrial activation to occur in the second half of the RR interval, leading to a **long RP tachycardia**. Associated incessant tachycardia can cause tachycardia-induced cardiomyopathy.
- **Junctional tachycardia:**
  - Arises from automaticity within the AV junction as the electrical impulses conduct to the ventricle and atrium simultaneously, similar to typical AVNRT, so that the retrograde P waves are frequently buried in the QRS complex.
  - Common in young children but rare in adults.
- **Sinoatrial nodal reentrant tachycardia:**
  - Reentrant circuit is localized at least partially within the sinoatrial (SA) node.
  - Abrupt onset and termination, triggered by a premature atrial contraction.
  - **ECG:** P-wave morphology and axis are identical to the native sinus P wave during normal sinus rhythm.
- Two keys to determine the underlying rhythm in narrow-complex tachycardias are the analysis of the **P wave** and the administration of **adenosine** or the use of **vagal maneuvers** (Figure 23-4).[4]
  - **Analysis of the P wave:**
    - P waves are absent or very irregular in AF.
    - Flutter waves, which are regular, sawtooth atrial activations at about 300 bpm, can be seen in AFL.
    - **Short RP tachycardia:** P waves can be "buried" near the end of the QRS complex during typical AVNRT (activating the ventricle through the slow pathway and activating the atrium through the fast pathway of the AV node) or O-AVRT (activating the ventricle through the AV node [slow] and activating the atrium through the accessory pathway [fast]).
    - **Long RP tachycardia:** P waves are more visible; they are closer to following QRS complex than preceding QRS complex. Causes include EAT and atypical AVNRT (activating the ventricle through the fast pathway and activating the atrium through the slow pathway of the AV node).

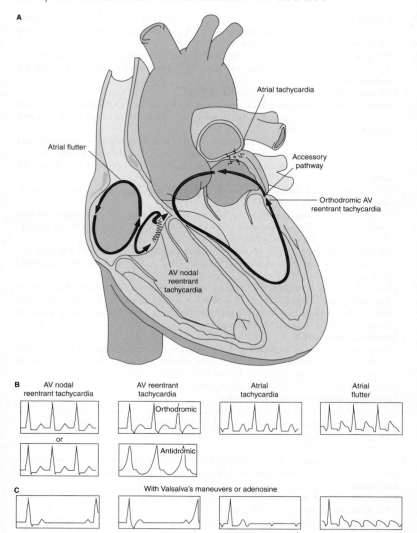

FIGURE 23-4. Main mechanisms and typical ECG recordings of supraventricular tachycardia. **(A)** Schematic of mechanisms for regular tachycardias, **(B)** ECG tracings for specific mechanisms of tachycardia and **(C)** ECG tracings for specific mechanisms of tachycardia after iv adenosine or valsalva maneuver to temporarily stop conduction through the AV node. (Modified from Delacretaz E. Supraventricular tachycardia. *N Engl J Med* 2006;354:1039-1051, with permission.)

- Vagal maneuvers and adenosine temporarily slow conduction through the AV node, which accomplishes two important functions:
  - It **reduces the ventricular rate** that allows the physician to see purely atrial tracings (AF, AFL, EAT, and MAT).
  - It **terminates an arrhythmia that uses the AV node** as part of the circuit (AVNRT and AVRT).
  - **Caveat:** Some EATs will be terminated with adenosine.

SPECIAL CONSIDERATIONS

- **Common ECG patterns**: If you approach the ECG in the same way every time with a reasonable method of interpretation (see Chapter 3), it is unlikely that you will miss the following diagnoses.
- Nevertheless, these are common ECG patterns and buzzwords associated with some classic clinical situations:
  - **Hyperkalemia:** Multiple ECG findings are seen as potassium levels rise, and include peaked T waves, wide QRS, PR prolongation, loss of P wave, and finally a sine wave pattern.
  - **Digitalis effect:** Downsloping, curved ST segments are seen with a characteristic "uptick" T wave.
  - **Digitalis toxicity:** Because digitalis increases the automaticity of the atrial and ventricular tissues while slowing the SA and AV nodes, two common ECG findings with digitalis toxicity are atrial tachycardia with AV block and bidirectional VT.
  - **Wellens waves:** Described as deep, symmetric T-wave inversions in the precordial leads. Wellens waves can indicate a critical proximal LAD occlusion, a central nervous system catastrophe (subarachnoid hemorrhage, where they are known as Birch waves), or an apical variant of hypertrophic cardiomyopathy.
  - **Osborne waves:** Also called J waves, these are seen as additional notching at the end of the QRS complex and are associated with profound hypothermia.
  - **LVH:** Many criteria have been studied to determine the presence of LVH by ECG (Table 23-3). These criteria have proven to be quite specific ($>$90%) but not very sensitive ($<$50%).[5]
  - **Ventricular pre-excitation:** Known as WPW syndrome, this disease is characterized by an accessory connection between the atrium and the ventricle, which bypasses the AV node to activate the ventricle. ECG findings include a short PR interval ($<$120 milliseconds), a slurring of the QRS complex (known as a delta wave), and ST-T-wave changes in the opposite direction of the QRS vector.
  - **Pulmonary disease pattern:** Because of hyperinflated lungs, a more vertical heart, and elevated pulmonary artery pressures, patients with COPD may have smaller QRS size, right axis deviation, incomplete right-bundle-branch block (RBBB) in V_1 (rSR' pattern), right atrial enlargement, and delayed R-wave transition in the precordial leads (QRS becomes more positive than negative in V_5 or V_6).
  - **PE:** Acute elevation of pulmonary pressures, as seen with acute PE, can cause ST or atrial arrhythmias, incomplete RBBB pattern, and the classic S1Q3T3 pattern (S wave in lead I, Q wave in lead III, and inverted T wave in lead III).
- This chapter concludes with several unknown ECG tracings (with interpretations, Figures 23-5 through 23-9) to exercise your ECG analysis skills.

TABLE 23-3	VARIOUS ELECTROGRAPHIC CRITERIA FOR DETERMINING THE PRESENCE OF LEFT VENTRICULAR HYPERTROPHY	
Criteria	Measurement	Points
Cornell voltage	S in V_3 + R in aVL >28 mm (men) S in V_3 + R in aVL >20 mm (women)	
Framingham	R in aVL >11 mm, R in V_4 to V_6 >25 mm S in V_1 to V_3 >25 mm S in V_1 or V_2 + R in 5 or V_6 >35 mm R in I + S in III >25 mm	
Sokolow-Lyon-index	S in V_1 + R in V_5 or V_6 >35 mm	
Romhilt-Estes point score	Any limb lead R wave or S wave ≥20 mm or S in V_1/ V_2 ≥30 mm or R in V_5/ V_6 ≥30 mm	3
	ST-T-wave abnormality (with or without digitalis)	1 or 3
	Left atrial abnormality	3
	Left axis deviation	2
	QRS duration ≥90 ms	1
	Intrinsicoid deflection in V_5/ V_6 ≥50 ms	1
	Definite LVH = 5 or more points; probable LVH = 4 points	

aVL, lead augmented vector left; LVH, left ventricular hypertrophy.

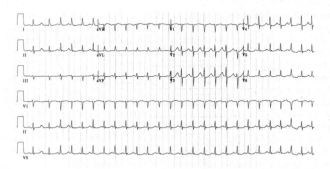

FIGURE 23-5. ECG tracing for interpretation. **Rate:** 160 bpm. **Rhythm:** Regular rhythm with a narrow QRS and **no P obvious waves**. This is a narrow-complex tachycardia. Differential diagnosis includes AV nodal reentry tachycardia (AVNRT), atrioventricular reentrant tachycardia, or (AVRT), automatic atrial tachycardia, atrial flutter, and atrial fibrillation. **Axis:** Up in lead I and up in lead II, so normal axis. **Intervals:** Without a P wave there is no PR interval. QRS is narrow, and there is no LVH. QT interval is <400 milliseconds. **Injury:** No significant ST-segment elevation no depression. No significant Q waves. **Putting it all together:** Narrow-complex tachycardia, likely due to **AVNRT**. Note that the retrograde P waves are likely buried within the QRS complex.

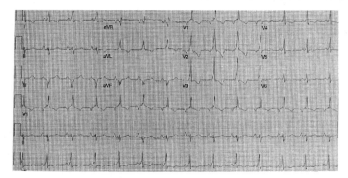

FIGURE 23-6. ECG tracing for interpretation. **Rate:** 80 bpm. **Rhythm:** Sinus rhythm. **Axis:** Up in lead I and down in lead II, so left axis deviation. **Intervals:** P waves are markedly negative in lead V_1 Left Atrial Enlargement (LAE) and markedly positive in lead II Right Atrial Enlargement (RAE). **PR interval is <120** milliseconds, seen best in the precordial leads. QRS is wide, but only at the initial upstroke **(delta wave)**. No LVH. QT intervals are normal. **Injury:** Neither significant ST-segment deviations nor Q waves, but **marked T-wave inversions V_2 to V_3. Putting it all together:** With a short PR interval, a delta wave, and localized T-wave inversions, this patient has ventricular pre excitation through an accessory pathway.

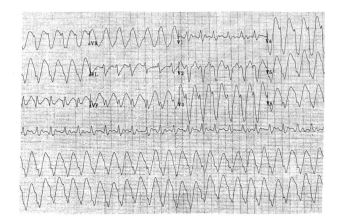

FIGURE 23-7. ECG tracing for interpretation. **Rate:** 150 bpm. **Rhythm:** No obvious P waves. Wide, regular QRS complex. This is a wide-complex tachycardia. Differential diagnosis includes ventricular tachycardia, SVT with aberrancy, ventricular pre-excitation. **Axis:** Down in lead I and down in lead II. This is **extreme left axis deviation**. **Intervals:** No P waves, so no PR interval. **QRS is markedly wide (200** milliseconds**)**. It is neither an LBBB nor RBBB morphology, so it is termed **idioventricular conduction delay (IVCD)**. LVH and QT intervals cannot be assessed in this wide-complex tachycardia. **Injury:** Difficult to assess in this wide-complex rhythm. **Putting it all together:** Using the various tools available, including Brugada criteria, this is a ventricular tachycardia. Because the QRS is extremely wide and of IVCD morphology (neither a true RBBB nor LBBB), suspect **hyperkalemia** as well.

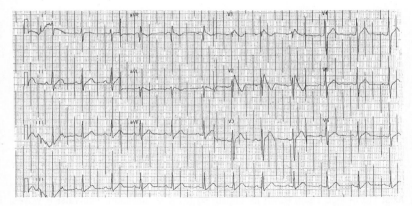

FIGURE 23-8. ECG tracing for interpretation. **Rate:** 70 bpm. **Rhythm:** Sinus. **Axis:** Down in lead I and up in lead II. Right axis deviation. **Intervals:** P-wave and PR intervals are normal. QRS is narrow without LVH. **QT interval is short** (QTc = 340 milliseconds). **Injury: Large, rapidly downsloping ST-segment elevations in leads V_1 and V_2.** No reciprocal changes or Q waves. **Putting it all together:** This is a classic ECG of a patient with **Brugada syndrome**, with coved ST elevations in leads V_1 to V_2 and an incomplete RBBB pattern.

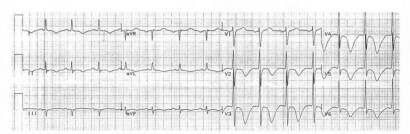

FIGURE 23-9. ECG tracing for interpretation. **Rate:** 90 bpm. **Rhythm:** Sinus. **Axis:** Up in lead I and up in lead II. Normal axis. **Intervals:** P wave and PR intervals are normal. QRS is narrow. LVH by Sokolow-Lyon criteria (S in lead I + R in lead V_5 is >35 mm). **QT interval is long** (QTc >600 milliseconds). Differential diagnosis includes hypo's, anti's, congenital, cerebral or impending infarction (Wellens waves). **Injury:** No significant ST-segment deviations. Isolated Q wave in lead III is generally normal. **Large, deep, symmetric T-wave inversions, primarily in the precordial leads. Putting it all together:** This is a classic ECG of a patient with **Wellens waves** due to a critical proximal left anterior descending (LAD) artery lesion.

REFERENCES

1. Zimetbaum PJ, Josephson ME. Use of the electrocardiogram in acute myocardial infarction. *N Engl J Med* 2003;348:933-940.
2. Sgarbossa EB, Pinski SL, Barbagelata A, et al. Electrocardiographic diagnosis of evolving acute myocardial infarction in the presence of left-bundle branch block. *N Engl J Med* 1996;334:481-487.
3. Wang K, Asinger RW, Marriott HJL. ST-segment elevation in conditions other than acute myocardial infarction. *N Engl J Med* 2003;349:2128-2135.
4. Delacretaz E. Supraventricular tachycardia. *N Engl J Med* 2006;354:1039-1051.
5. Hancock EW, Deal BJ, Mirvis DM, et al. AHA/ACCF/HRS recommendations for the standardization and interpretation of the electrocardiogram: part V: electrocardiogram changes associated with cardiac chamber hypertrophy. *J Am Coll Cardiol* 2009;53:992-1002.

Bradyarrhythmias and Permanent Pacemakers

24

Derrick R. Fansler and Jane Chen

GENERAL PRINCIPLES

Definition

- Bradycardia is a common cardiac rhythm defined as a ventricular rate less than 60 beats per minute (bpm).
- Bradycardias can be attributed to dysfunction somewhere within the native conduction system. Therefore, a review of normal propagation of the wave of depolarization, the respective vascular supply to each section, and the intrinsic and extrinsic influences (Table 24-1) on the conduction system is useful.
- The **sinus node** is a collection of specialized pacemaker cells located in the high right atrium. Under normal conditions, it initiates a wave of depolarization that spreads inferiorly and leftward via atrial myocardium and intranodal tracts, producing atrial systole.
  - The typical resting rate of the sinus node, between 50 and 90 bpm, is determined by the relative balance of the sympathetic and parasympathetic inputs.
  - Arterial blood is supplied to the sinus node via the sinus node artery, which has variable anatomic origins: Right coronary artery (RCA), 65%; circumflex, 25%; or dual (RCA and circumflex), 10%.[1]
- The wave of depolarization then reaches another grouping of specialized cells, **the atrioventricular (AV) node**, located in the right atrial side of the intra-atrial septum. Normally, the AV node should serve as the lone electrical connection between the atria and ventricles.
  - Conduction through the AV node is decremental, producing a delay typically in the range of 55 to 110 milliseconds; this accounts for the majority of the PR interval measured on electrocardiogram (ECG).
  - The AV node consists of slow-response fibers that, like the sinus node, possess inherent pacemaking properties and produce rates of 40 to 50 bpm. Because of its slower rate of depolarization, this becomes clinically relevant only in the setting of sinus node dysfunction.
  - The ventricular response to atrial depolarization is modulated by the effects of the autonomic nervous system on the AV node.
  - Blood supply to the AV node is primarily via the AV nodal artery, which typically originates from the proximal posterior descending artery (PDA) (80%), but can also come off the circumflex (10%), or both (10%). In addition, it receives collateral flow from the left anterior descending (LAD) artery.[1]
- From the AV node, the wave of depolarization travels down the **His bundle**, located in the membranous septum, and into the **right and left bundle branches** before reaching the Purkinje fibers, which depolarize the rest of the ventricular myocardium.
  - The His and right bundle receive blood via the AV nodal artery and from septal perforators off the LAD.

TABLE 24-1	CAUSES OF BRADYCARDIA

Intrinsic

Congenital disease (may present later in life)

Idiopathic degeneration (aging)

Infarction or ischemia

Cardiomyopathy

Infiltrative disease: sarcoidosis, amyloidosis, and hemochromatosis

Collagen vascular diseases: systemic lupus erythematosus, rheumatoid arthritis, and scleroderma

Surgical trauma: valve surgery and transplantation

Infectious disease: endocarditis, Lyme disease, and Chagas disease

Extrinsic

Autonomically mediated

Neurocardiogenic syncope

Carotid sinus hypersensitivity

Increased vagal tone: coughing, vomiting, micturition, defecation, and intubation

Drugs: β-blockers, calcium channel blockers, digoxin, and antiarrhythmic agents

Hypothyroidism

Hypothermia

Neurologic disorders: increased intracranial pressure

Electrolyte imbalances: hyperkalemia and hypermagnesemia

Hypercarbia/obstructive sleep apnea

Sepsis

- ○ The left bundle divides further into an anterior fascicle, supplied by septal perforators, and a posterior fascicle, which runs posterior and inferior to the anterior fascicle and is supplied by branches off the PDA and septal perforators off the LAD.

Classification

- With a basic understanding of the cardiac conduction system, it is possible to classify bradycardias based on their location of dysfunction, which determines prognosis and guides therapy.
- **Sinus node dysfunction:**
  - ○ Sinus node dysfunction, or **sick sinus syndrome**, is the most common reason for pacemaker implantation in the United States. It can be manifested in several ways:
  - ○ **Sinus bradycardia** is defined as a regular rhythm with QRS complexes preceded by "sinus" P waves (upright in II, III, aVF) at a rate of <60 bpm. Young patients and athletes often have resting sinus bradycardia that is well tolerated. Nocturnal heart rates are lower in all patients.

- Sinus arrest and sinus pauses refer to failure of the sinus node to depolarize, which manifest as periods of atrial asystole (no P waves). This may be accompanied by ventricular asystole or escape beats from junctional tissue or ventricular myocardium. Pauses of 2 to 3 seconds can be found in healthy, asymptomatic people, especially during sleep. Pauses >3 seconds, particularly during daytime hours, raise concern for sinus node dysfunction.
- Sinus exit block represents the appropriate firing of the sinus node but the wave of depolarization fails to traverse past the perinodal tissue. It is nearly indistinguishable from sinus arrest on surface ECGs except that the P-P interval will be a multiple of the P-P preceding the bradycardia.
- Tachy–brady syndrome occurs when tachyarrhythmias alternate with bradyarrhythmias. A classic example can be seen in the termination of atrial fibrillation (tachy), where a long pause may occur before the sinus node recovers (brady).
- Chronotropic incompetence is the inability to increase the heart rate appropriately in response to metabolic need.
- AV conduction disturbances:
  - AV conduction can be delayed (first-degree AV block), occasionally interrupted (second-degree AV block), frequently but not always interrupted (advanced or high-degree AV block), or completely absent (third-degree AV block).
  - First-degree AV block describes a conduction delay, usually localized to the AV node, that results in a PR interval >200 milliseconds on the surface ECG. "Block" is a misnomer because, by definition, there are no dropped beats (i.e., there is a P wave for every QRS complex).
  - Second-degree AV block is present when there are periodic interruptions (i.e., "dropped beats") in AV conduction. Distinction between Mobitz I and Mobitz II is important because each has a different natural history of progression to higher degrees of heart block.
    - Mobitz type I block (Wenckebach) is represented by a progressive delay in AV conduction with successive atrial impulses until an impulse fails to conduct, followed by reiterations of the sequence. Type I block is usually within the AV node and portends a more benign natural history, with progression to complete heart block unlikely. On surface ECG, classic Wenckebach block manifests as
      □ Progressive prolongation of the PR interval before a nonconducted P wave. Another hallmark of AV Wenckebach is that the first PR interval after the non-conducted P wave is shorter than the last PR interval before the nonconducted P wave.
      □ Shortening of each subsequent RR interval before the dropped beat. Therefore, the RR interval of the dropped beat will equal less than twice the shortest RR on the tracing.
      □ A regularly irregular grouping of QRS complexes (group beating).
    - Mobitz type II block carries a less favorable prognosis and is characterized by an abrupt AV conduction block without evidence of progressive conduction delay. On ECG, the PR intervals remained unchanged preceding the nonconducted P wave. The presence of type II block is associated with high incidence of progression to complete heart block.
  - Third-degree (complete) AV block is present when all atrial impulses fail to conduct to the ventricles. There is complete dissociation between the atria and ventricles. The ventricular depolarizations (escape rhythm) will be regular.
  - Advanced or high-degree AV block is present when the third-degree heart block is predominantly present, but occasionally, a P wave will conduct to the ventricle with a stable PR interval. Unlike the complete third-degree AV block, the ventricular depolarizations will have some irregularities due to intermittent conduction.

DIAGNOSIS

Clinical Presentation

- The clinical manifestations of bradyarrhythmias are variable, ranging from asymptomatic to nonspecific (e.g., light-headedness, fatigue, weakness, and exercise intolerance) to overt (i.e., syncope). Tolerance for bradyarrhythmias is largely dictated by the patient's ability to augment cardiac output in response to the decreased heart rate. Emphasis should be placed on delineating whether the presenting symptoms have a direct temporal relationship to underlying bradycardia. Other historical points of emphasis include the following:
  - Ischemic heart disease, particularly involving the right-sided circulation, can precipitate a number of bradyarrhythmias. Therefore, **symptoms of acute coronary syndrome** should always be sought.
  - **Precipitating circumstances** (e.g., micturition, coughing, defecation, and noxious smells) surrounding episodes may help to identify a neurocardiogenic etiology.
  - Tachyarrhythmias, in patients with underlying sinus node dysfunction, can be followed by long pauses due to sinus node suppression during tachycardia. Therefore, symptoms of palpitations may reveal the presence of an underlying **tachy–brady syndrome**. Given that the agents used to treat tachyarrhythmias are designed to promote decreased heart rates, this syndrome leads to management dilemmas.
  - History of structural heart disease, hypothyroidism, obstructive sleep apnea, collagen vascular disease, infections (e.g., bacteremia, endocarditis, Lyme disease, and Chagas disease), infiltrative diseases (e.g., amyloid, hemochromatosis, and sarcoid), neuromuscular diseases, and prior cardiac surgery (e.g., valve replacement and congenital repair) should be sought.
  - **Medications** should be reviewed, with particular emphasis on those that affect the sinus and AV nodes (i.e., calcium channel blockers [CCBs], β-blockers, and digoxin).
- If the bradycardia is ongoing, the initial history and physical examination should be truncated, focusing on assessing the hemodynamic stability of the arrhythmia. If the patient is demonstrating signs of poor perfusion (e.g., hypotension, confusion, decreased consciousness, cyanosis, etc.), **immediate management per the acute cardiac life support (ACLS) protocol** should be initiated. If the patient is stable, a more thorough examination can be obtained, with particular emphasis on the cardiovascular examination and any findings consistent with the aforementioned comorbidities (Figure 24-1).

Diagnostic Testing

- The **12-lead ECG** is the cornerstone diagnostic tool in any workup where arrhythmia is suspected. Rhythm strips from leads that provide the best view of atrial activity (II, III, aVF, or V1) should be examined.
- Emphasis should be placed on identifying evidence of **sinus node dysfunction** (P-wave intervals) or **AV conduction abnormalities** (PR interval, presence of bundle branch block). Evidence of both old and acute manifestations of ischemic heart disease should be sought as well.

Laboratories

- Laboratory studies should include electrolytes and thyroid function tests in most patients.
- Digoxin levels and cardiac troponins should be checked when clinically appropriate.

Electrocardiography

- The analysis of ECGs in the setting of bradycardia should focus on localizing the likely site of dysfunction along the conduction system.
- Along with correlating symptoms to the arrhythmia, localization of the block will help determine whether pacemaker implantation is necessary. See Figures 24-2 and 24-3 for some representative ECG strips of the rhythms described under **Classification** section.

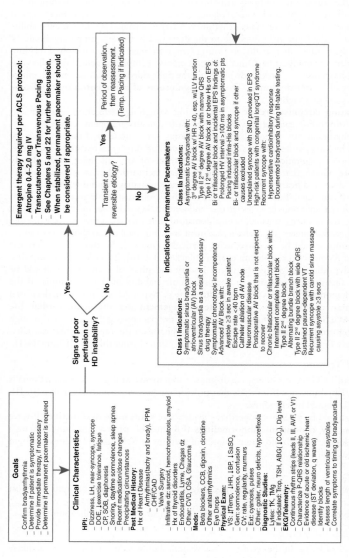

FIGURE 24-1. Approach to bradyarrhythmias. LH, light-headedness; DOE, dyspnea on exertion; CP, chest pain; SOB, shortness of breath; PPM, permanent pacemaker; CHF, congestive heart failure; CAD, coronary artery disease; CVD, cerebrovascular disease; OSA, obstructive sleep apnea; CCB, calcium channel blocker; ↓HR, bradycardia; ↓BP, hypotension; ↓SaO$_2$, hypoxia; ↑K, hyperkalemia; ↑Mg, hypermagnesemia; AF, atrial fibrillation; HD, hemodynamic; VT, ventricular tachycardia; EPS, electrophysiologic study; SND, sinus node dysfunction.

Goals
- Confirm bradyarrhythmia
- Determine if patient is symptomatic
- Provide immediate therapy, if necessary
- Determine if permanent pacemaker is required

Clinical Characteristics

HPI:
- Dizziness, LH, near-syncope, syncope
- DOE, ↓exercise tolerance, fatigue
- CP, SOB, diaphoresis
- Snoring, daytime somnolence, sleep apnea
- Recent medication/dose changes
- Precipitating circumstances

Past Medical History:
- Hx of Heart Disease
    – Arrhythmias(tachy and brady), PPM
    – CHF/CAD
    – Valve Surgery
- Infiltrative dz: sarcoid, hemochromatosis, amyloid
- Hx of thyroid disorders
- Endocarditis, Lyme, Chagas dz
- Other: CVD, OSA, Glaucoma

Meds:
- Beta blockers, CCB, digoxin, clonidine
- Other antiarrhythmics
- Eye Drops

Physical Exam:
- VS:↑Temp, ↓HR, ↓BP, ↓SaO$_2$
- Gen: somnolence, confusion
- CV: rate, regularity, murmurs
- Ext: cyanosis, pulses
- Other: goiter, neuro deficits, hyporeflexia

Diagnostic Studies:
- Lytes: ↑K, ↑Mg
- If indicated: Trop, TSH, ABG(↓CO$_2$), Dig level

EKG/Telemetry:
- Continuous rhythm strips (leads II, III, AVF, or V1)
- Characterize P-QRS relationship
- Evidence of acute or old ischemic heart disease (ST deviation, q waves)
- Identify blocks
- Assess length of ventricular asystoles
- Correlate symptoms to timing of bradycardia

Signs of poor perfusion or HD instability?

Yes →

Emergent therapy required per ACLS protocol:
- Atropine 0.4–2.0 mg IV
- Transcutaneous or Transvenous Pacing
- See Chapters 5 and 22 for further discussion.
- When stabilized, permanent pacemaker should be considered if appropriate.

No ↓

Transient or reversible etiology?

Yes → Period of observation, then reassessment. (Temp. Pacing if indicated)

No ↓

Indications for Permanent Pacemakers

Class I Indications:
- Symptomatic sinus bradycardia or atrioventricular (AV) block
- Sinus bradycardia as a result of necessary drug therapy
- Symptomatic chronotropic incompetence
- Advanced AV Block with:
    - Asystole ≥3 sec in awake patient
    - Escape rate <40 bpm
    - Catheter ablation of AV node
    - Neuromuscular disease
    - Postoperative AV block that is not expected to recover
- Chronic bifascicular or trifascicular block with:
    - Intermittent complete heart block
    - Type II 2nd degree block
    - Alternating bundle branch block
- Type II 2nd degree block with wide QRS
- Sustained pause-dependent VT
- Recurrent syncope with carotid sinus massage causing asystole ≥3 secs

Class IIa Indications:
- Asymptomatic bradycardia with:
    - 3rd degree AV block w/ HR >40, esp. w/LV function
    - Type II 2nd degree AV block with narrow QRS
    - Type II 2nd degree AV block at or below His on EPS
- Bi or trifascicular block and incidental EPS findings of:
    - Prolonged HV interval >100 ms in asymptomatic pts
    - Pacing induced infra-His block
- Bi- or trifascicular block and syncope if other causes excluded
- Unexplained syncope with SND provoked in EPS
- High-risk patients with congenital long-QT syndrome
- Recurrent syncope with:
    - Hypersensitive cardioinhibitory response
    - Documented bradycardia during tilt-table testing.

Sinus Bradycardia

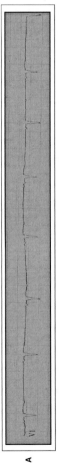

A

Sinoatrial Node Exit Block

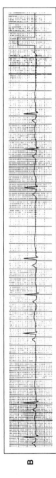

B

Sinus Rhythm with Blocked Premature Atrial Complexes

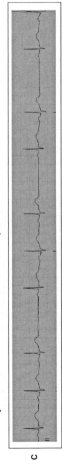

C

Tachy–Brady Syndrome with Prolonged Sinus Pause

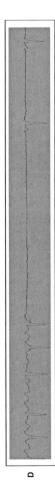

D

FIGURE 24-2. Examples of sinus node dysfunction. **(A)** Sinus bradycardia. The sinus rate is approximately 45 bpm. **(B)** Sinoatrial node exit block. Note that the P-P interval in which the pause occurs is exactly twice that of the nonpaused P-P interval. **(C)** Blocked premature atrial complexes. This rhythm is often taken for sinus node dysfunction or AV block. Note the premature, nonconducted P waves inscribed in the T wave that resets the sinus node leading to the observed pauses. **(D)** Tachy–brady syndrome. Note the termination of the irregular tachyarrhythmia followed by a prolonged 4.5-second pause prior to the first sinus beat.

First Degree AV Block

A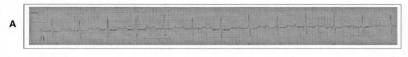

Second Degree AV Block- Mobitz type I (Wenckebach Block)

B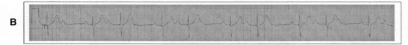

Second Degree AV Block- Mobitz type II

C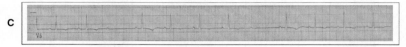

2:1 Second Degree AV Block

D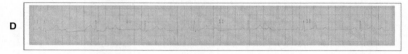

Third Degree (Complete) AV Block

E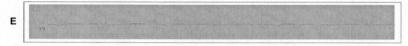

FIGURE 24-3. Examples of atrioventricular block. **(A)** First-degree AVB. There are no dropped beats and the PR interval is >200 milliseconds. **(B)** 3:2 second-degree AVB–Mobitz I. Note the "group beating" and the prolonging PR interval prior to the dropped beat. The third P wave in the sequence is subtly inscribed in the T wave of the preceding beat. **(C)** Second-degree AVB–Mobitz II. Note the abrupt AV conduction block without evidence of progressive conduction delay. **(D)** 2:1 AVB. This pattern makes it difficult to distinguish between a Mobitz I and a Mobitz II–type mechanisms of block. Note the narrow QRS complex, which supports a more proximal origin of block (type I mechanism). A wider QRS (concomitant bundle-branch or fascicular block) would suggest a type II mechanism. **(E)** Complete heart block. Note the independent regularity of both the atrial and ventricular rhythms (junctional escape), which have no clear association with each other throughout the rhythm strip.

Diagnostic Procedures

- ECG may not be sufficient if the arrhythmia is episodic and transient. In these circumstances, some form of continuous monitoring is indicated. In the inpatient setting, **continuous central telemetry monitoring** can be utilized.
- To evaluate the sinus node's response to exertion (chronotropic competence), walking the patient in the hallway or up a flight of stairs is easy and inexpensive. A formal **exercise ECG** can be useful to elicit Mobitz type II AV block in patients with symptoms of dyspnea with exertion, due to a drop in ventricular rate with increasing sinus rate.
- If the workup is continued on an outpatient basis, **24- to 72-hour Holter monitoring** can be used if the episodes occur daily.

- If symptoms are less frequent, an **event recorder** or **implantable loop recorder** should be considered. Patients should be encouraged to maintain accurate symptom diaries.

TREATMENT

- Bradyarrhythmias that lead to significant symptoms and hemodynamic instability are considered cardiovascular emergencies and should be managed as outlined in ACLS guidelines.
- See Chapters 7 and 8 for a more in-depth discussion of temporary pacing and management of severe, hemodynamically unstable bradycardia.

Medications

- **Atropine**, an anticholinergic agent given in doses of 0.5 to 2.0 mg intravenously, is the cornerstone pharmacologic agent for the emergent treatment of bradycardia.
- Intravenous (IV) **dopamine** infusion (5 to 10 µg/kg/minute) or IV **epinephrine** infusion (2 to 10 µg/minute) may be used for symptomatic bradycardia unresponsive to atropine and is considered equally effective to external pacing as a temporizing measure. IV **isoproterenol** infusion is a reasonable alternative.

Other Non-pharmacologic Therapies

- For bradyarrhythmias that are unresponsive to pharmacologic interventions or that have irreversible etiologies, pacemaker therapy should be considered.
- **Temporary pacing** is indicated for symptomatic second-degree or third-degree heart block caused by transient drug intoxication or electrolyte imbalance and complete heart block or Mobitz II second-degree AV block in the setting of an acute myocardial infarction (MI).
- Sinus bradycardia, atrial fibrillation (AF) with a slow ventricular response, or Mobitz I second-degree AV block should be treated with temporary pacing only if significant symptoms or hemodynamic instability is present.
- Temporary pacing is achieved preferably via insertion of a transvenous pacemaker. Transcutaneous external pacing can be used, although the lack of reliability of capture and patient discomfort clearly makes this a second-line modality.
- Transcutaneous pacing is contraindicated for patients with hypothermia and is not recommended for asystole.

Surgical Management

- Once hemodynamic stability has been confirmed or re-established as above, the focus turns to determining whether the patient's condition warrants placement of a permanent pacemaker (PPM).
- In symptomatic patients, key determinants include potential **reversibility of causative factors** and **temporal correlation of symptoms** to the arrhythmia.
- In asymptomatic patients, the key determinant is based on whether the discovered conduction abnormality has a **natural history of progression to higher degrees of heart block**.

Permanent Pacing

- Permanent pacing involves the placement of anchored, intracardiac pacing leads for the purpose of maintaining a heart rate sufficient to avoid symptoms and hemodynamic consequences of bradyarrhythmias.
- Advances in pacemaker technology allow contemporary pacers, through maintenance of AV synchrony and rate adaptive programming, to more closely mimic normal physiologic pacing.
- Class I (general agreement/evidence for benefit) and IIa (weight of conflicting opinion/evidence in favor of benefit) indications for permanent pacing are listed in Figure 24-1.[2,3]

- Pacemakers are designed to provide an electrical stimulus to the heart whenever the rate drops below a preprogrammed **lower rate limit**. Therefore, the ECG appearance of a PPM varies with the pacer's programming relative to the individual's heart rate.
- Pacing spikes immediately precede the generated P wave or QRS complex, indicating capture of the chamber. Atrial leads are typically placed in the right atrial appendage and therefore generate P waves of normal (sinus) morphology. Right ventricular (RV) pacing leads are usually placed at the RV apex, and therefore the QRS complexes typically assume a left bundle branch block (LBBB) like morphology. The axis may be negative in the inferior leads (II, III, and aVF). Figure 24-4 illustrates some common ECG appearances of normally and abnormally functioning pacemakers.

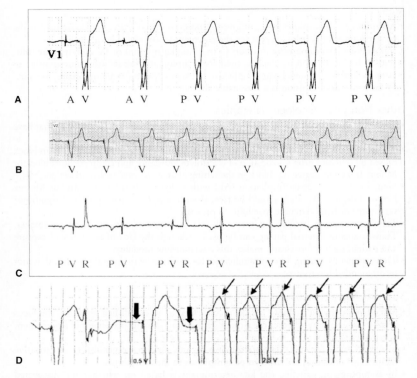

FIGURE 24-4. Pacemaker rhythms. **(A)** Normal dual-chamber (DDD) pacing. First two complexes are atrioventricular (AV) sequential pacing, followed by sinus with atrial sensing and ventricular pacing. **(B)** Normal single-chamber (VVI) pacing. The underlying rhythm is atrial fibrillation (no distinct P waves), with ventricular pacing at 60 bpm. **(C)** Pacemaker malfunction. The underlying rhythm is sinus (P) at 80 bpm with 2:1 heart block and first-degree AV block (long PR). Ventricular pacing spikes are seen (V) after each P wave, demonstrating appropriate sensing and tracking of the P waves; however, there is failure to capture. **(D)** Pacemaker-mediated tachycardia. Two ventricular paced events (vertical arrows) lead to atrial sensed events (angled arrows). Each atrial sensed event is followed by ventricular pacing, which causes another atrial sensed event, and the cycle continues. (A to C from Cooper DH, Faddis MN. Cardiac Arrhythmias. In: Cooper DH, et al., eds. *The Washington Manual of Medical Therapeutics*, 32nd ed. Philadelphia, PA: Lippincott Williams & Wilkins; 2007, with permission.)

- The pacemaker generator is commonly placed subcutaneously in the pectoral region. The electronic lead(s) are placed in their cardiac chamber(s) via central veins. Complications of placement include **pneumothorax, device infection, bleeding, and, rarely, cardiac perforation with tamponade.**
- Before implantation, the patient must be free of any active infections, and any anticoagulation issues must be considered. Hematomas in the pacemaker pocket develop most commonly in patients who are receiving IV heparin or subcutaneous low-molecular-weight heparin. In severe cases, surgical evacuation is required.

Pacing Modes
- Pacing modes are classified by a sequence of three or four letters.[4]
  ○ **Position I** denotes the chamber that is paced: A for atria, V for ventricle, D for dual (A + V), or O for none.
  ○ **Position II** refers to the chamber that is sensed: A for atria, V for ventricle, D for dual (A + V), or O for none.
  ○ **Position III** denotes the type of response that the pacemaker will have to a sensed signal: I for inhibition, T for triggering, D for dual (I + T), or O for none.
  ○ **Position IV** is used to signify the presence of rate-adaptive pacing (R) in response to increased metabolic need. Almost all contemporary pacers implanted have rate-modulating capabilities.
- There are several variables to consider in choosing the most appropriate pacing system for your patient: The primary indication for placement, the responsiveness of the SA node, the state of AV conduction, the presence of comorbid tachyarrhythmias, and the patient's activity level.
  ○ **The most common pacing systems used today include VVIR, DDDR, or AAIR devices.**[5]
  ○ In general, AAI systems should be used only for sinus node dysfunction in the absence of any AV conduction abnormalities.
  ○ The presence of AV nodal or His-Purkinje disease makes a dual-chamber device (DDD) more appropriate than AAI.
  ○ Patients with chronic AF warrant a single ventricular lead with VVI programming.
  ○ Modern-day pacemakers also have the capability of **mode switching.** This is useful in patients with DDD pacers who have paroxysmal tachyarrhythmias. When such a patient develops tachycardia, the pacer switches to a non-tracking mode (DDI) to avoid tracking the atrial arrhythmia. It will return to DDD when the tachyarrhythmia resolves.

Pacemaker Malfunction
- Pacemaker malfunction is a potentially life-threatening situation, particularly for patients who are pacemaker dependent. The workup of suspected malfunction should begin with a 12-lead ECG (Figure 24-4).
- If no pacing activity is seen, one can place a magnet over the pacemaker to assess for output failure and ability to capture. **Application of the magnet switches the pacemaker to an asynchronous pacing mode.** For example, VVI mode becomes VOO (ventricular asynchronous pacing) and DDD mode becomes DOO (asynchronous AV pacing).
- All implantable defibrillators also have pacing functions and the pacing functions are not affected by a magnet.
- If malfunction is obvious or if the ECG is unrevealing and malfunction is still suspected, then a formal interrogation of the device should be done. **Patients are given a card to carry upon implantation that will identify the make and model of the device.**
- A chest radiograph (two views) should also be obtained to assess for evidence of overt lead abnormalities (dislodgement, fracture, migration, etc.).

- General categories of pacemaker malfunction include oversensing, failure to capture, failure to sense (undersensing), and pacemaker-mediated tachycardia.
  - **Oversensing** refers to situations where a pacemaker does not deliver a stimulus when it should. It generally occurs when the pacemaker senses an external signal as cardiac in origin. An example of oversensing is seen during surgery when electrocautery can be inappropriately sensed as cardiac activity, leading to inappropriate inhibition of pacing. In patients who are pacemaker dependent, programming the pacemaker temporarily in asynchronous mode is recommended. Noise from lead fracture can also be a cause of oversensing. Pure output failure from battery or generator failure is rare.
  - **"Failure to capture"** refers to those situations where the pacing stimulus is delivered but fails to generate evidence of myocardial depolarization (i.e., P or QRS complex). Elevation in the threshold voltage required to initiate a wave of depolarization, due to changes in the tissue surrounding the electrode (i.e., new MI) or antiarrhythmic drugs, is often at fault. Lead fractures or microdislodgement should also be considered.
  - **Undersensing** occurs when the preprogrammed amplitude and/or frequency thresholds for sensing are no longer sufficient to identify native cardiac activity. This may lead to pacing spikes being identified on top of native P, QRS, or T complexes.
  - **Pacemaker-mediated tachycardia is** an "endless loop tachycardia" created by tracking of retrograde atrial impulses created by the previous ventricular paced beat. The ECG typically shows a ventricular paced rhythm at the programmed upper rate limit (URL) of the pacemaker (See Figure 24-4).

SPECIAL CONSIDERATIONS

- **Acute MI and conduction abnormalities:**
  - Bradyarrhythmias and conduction abnormalities in the setting of MI are common. Careful consideration must be given to the artery involved, the extent of infarct, prior conduction disease, and success of reperfusion to best determine if the arrhythmia will be self-limiting or irreversible.
  - During **inferior MI**, the site of block is typically at the level of the AV node. These dysrhythmias are often due to **heightened vagal tone (Bezold–Jarisch reflex) during the first 24 hours post-MI** and are typically responsive to atropine. After 24 hours, persistent or worsening block may occur, which is less responsive to atropine. These later blocks may respond to a methylxanthine, such as theophylline or aminophylline. In most cases, conduction abnormalities resolve within 1 to 2 weeks and permanent pacing is not needed.
  - **Anterior MI**, on the other hand, is more likely to cause conduction abnormalities due to ischemia and tissue necrosis. **The site of block is typically infranodal and is less likely to respond to atropine.** It is more likely to lead to symptomatic, irreversible bradyarrhythmias that require permanent pacing.
- **Cardiac transplant and bradyarrhythmias[6,7]:**
  - Following cardiac transplant, **denervation** causes donor hearts to generate faster sinus rates due to loss of vagal input, particularly if the donor was young.
  - Bradyarrhythmias have been reported to occur as well, with sinus node dysfunction being the most common presentation. Potential causes include surgical trauma, perioperative ischemia, pretransplant medications, and rejection. AV conduction abnormalities are much less common.
  - Bicaval anastomosis, now more common than atrial anastomosis, decreases the likelihood of surgical trauma to the sinoatrial (SA) node or SA nodal artery and therefore decreases the incidence of postoperative bradyarrhythmias.
  - **If AV conduction blocks develop, suspicion for rejection or coronary vasculopathy should be high.**

- **Right bundle branch block** (RBBB) is a common conduction disturbance following transplant, often due to the need for periodic endomyocardial biopsy of the RV septum to ensure appropriate immunosuppression. Permanent pacing is not required.
- **Infection and bradycardia:**
  - Although infections and febrile illness typically cause resting tachycardia, there are some infectious syndromes that can be complicated by bradyarrhythmias.
  - In patients with suspected or known **endocarditis**, ECGs should be ordered and carefully reviewed daily for prolongation of the PR interval or higher-degree AV block, which can signal the presence of an underlying or developing aortic root abscess.
  - **Lyme disease**, a tick-borne illness caused by *Borrelia burgdorferi* and endemic to the northeastern United States, can present with a constellation of findings that includes myocarditis, conduction abnormalities, and rarely, LV failure. AV conduction blocks are the most common.[8] These dysrhythmias typically resolve spontaneously within days to weeks, rarely requiring permanent pacing. However, symptomatic bradycardia and marked PR prolongation (>300 milliseconds) seem to predict a more ominous prognosis with higher likelihood of progression to complete heart block.[9]
  - **Chagas disease**, a protozoan illness endemic to South America, presents with cardiac involvement in over 90% of cases. In addition to heart failure, patients can present with all degrees of AV block.
- **Increased intracranial pressure:**
  - The presence of **bradycardia, hypertension, and respiratory depression (Cushing triad or reflex)** should raise significant suspicion for dangerously elevated intracranial pressure.
  - Clinical situations that could lead to intracranial hypertension include hepatic failure, central nervous system tumors, trauma, and hydrocephalus.
  - These are medical emergencies that require immediate treatment to avoid catastrophic neurologic compromise.
- **Drug toxicity:**
  - **Digoxin** toxicity should be suspected in any patient taking digoxin, the elderly, patients with renal insufficiency, or patients taking new medications such as amiodarone. Digoxin toxicity classically presents with enhanced automaticity and increased AV block (paroxysmal atrial tachycardia with AV block ["PAT with block"] is a hallmark of digoxin toxicity). Therapy is supportive, with temporary pacing and discontinuation of digoxin.
    - In life-threatening situations, **Digibind**, the Fab fragments of digoxin antibodies, can be used.[10]
    - Digibind can precipitate heart failure and severe hypokalemia and carries significant expense. It should be reserved for situations where significant overdose (>10 mg) is suspected, extreme serum digoxin levels (>10 ng/mL) are discovered, or life-threatening bradyarrhythmias are present.
  - If **β-blocker** toxicity is suspected, **atropine** (up to 2 mg IV), IV fluids, and **glucagon** (50 to 150 μg/kg IV over 1 minute, followed by 1 to 5 mg/hour in 5% dextrose) can be used to bypass the β-adrenergic receptor blockade and act downstream to improve contractility and heart rate.
    - If bradycardia and hypotension persist, escalation of management would sequentially include IV insulin/glucose, calcium, isoproterenol, and vasopressors (norepinephrine or dopamine).
    - Hemodialysis may be useful with sotalol, atenolol, acebutolol, and nadolol but not with metoprolol, propranolol, or timolol. Transvenous pacing can be used for high-grade AV block unresponsive to initial management.

- ○ If **Calcium channel-blocker (CCB)** overdose is suspected, glucagon and calcium should be administered. Transvenous pacing can be used for heart block refractory to noninvasive management.
  - ▪ The non-dihydropyridines (diltiazem and verapamil) are more likely to cause severe bradycardia, sinus pauses, and high-grade AV block. Dihydropyridines (amlodipine, nifedipine, and nicardipine) will cause hypotension and, more commonly, a reflex tachycardia.
  - ▪ CCB toxicity tends to be less responsive to atropine.

REFERENCES

1. Mangrum JM, Dimarco JP. The evaluation and management of bradycardia. *N Engl J Med* 2000;342:703-709.
2. Epstein AE, DiMarco JP, Ellenbogen KA, et al. ACC/AHA/HRS 2008 guidelines for device-based therapy of cardiac rhythm abnormalities. *J Am Coll Cardiol* 2008;51;e1-e62.
3. Epstein AE, DiMarco JP, Ellenbogen KA, et al. 2012 ACCF/AHA/HRS focused update incorporated into the ACCF/AHA/HRS 2008 guidelines for device-based therapy of cardiac rhythm abnormalities. *J Am Coll Cardiol* 2013;61:e6-e75.
4. Bernstein AD, Daubert JC, Fletcher RD, et al. The revised NASPE/BPEG generic code for anti-bradycardia, adaptive-rate, and multisite pacing. *Pacing Clin Electrophysiol* 2002;25:260-264.
5. Lamas GA, Ellenbogen KA. Evidence base for pacemaker mode selection: from physiology to randomized trials. *Circulation* 2004;109:443-451.
6. Thajudeen A, Stecker EC, Shahata M, et al. Arrhythmias after heart transplantation: mechanism and management. *J Am Heart Assoc* 2012;1:e001461.
7. Leonelli FM, Pacifico A, Young JB. Frequency and significance of conduction defects early after orthotopic heart transplant. *Am J Cardiol* 1994;73:175-179.
8. McAlister HT, Klementowicz PT, Andrews C, et al. Lyme carditis: an important cause of reversible heart block. *Ann Intern Med* 1989;110:339-345.
9. Steere AC, Batsford WP, Weinberg M, et al. Lyme carditis: cardiac abnormalities of Lyme disease. *Ann Intern Med* 1980;93:8-16.
10. Antman, EM, Wenger, TL, Butler, VP, et al. Treatment of 150 cases of life-threatening digitalis intoxication with digoxin-specific Fab antibody fragments. Final report of a multicenter study. *Circulation* 1990;81:1744-1752.

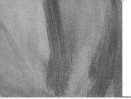

Sudden Cardiac Death

25

Marye J. Gleva and Jefferson Lee

GENERAL PRINCIPLES

Definition

Sudden cardiac death (SCD) is unexpected, abrupt natural death from cardiac causes within 1 hour of symptom onset. It is overwhelmingly due to ventricular arrhythmias, specifically ventricular fibrillation (VF), and ventricular tachycardia (VT).

Classification

- Ventricular arrhythmias:
  - Monomorphic VT
  - Polymorphic VT
  - VF
- Bradyarrhythmias:
  - Asystole
  - Pulseless electrical activity (PEA)

Epidemiology[1,2]

- **SCD accounts for roughly 15% of all deaths and 50% of cardiac-related deaths**.
- American Heart Association estimates that there are 300,000 to 350,000 SCDs per year in the United States.
- Overall incidence of SCD is 1 to 2 per 1,000 people each year (0.1% to 0.2%) (Figure 25-1).[2]
- Mean survival rate of out-of-hospital cardiac arrest is <10% to 20%.
- In selected high-risk groups (e.g., coronary artery disease [CAD]), the yearly incidence of SCD has been reported as high as 100 to 120 per 1,000 per year (10% to 12%).
- **However, more than two-thirds of patients who die from SCD are considered "low risk" with either no known cardiac risk factors or "low-risk" CAD.**

Etiology[1]

- Eighty percent of SCDs are associated with CAD.
- A total of 10% to 15% of SCDs are caused by various nonischemic cardiomyopathies (NICMs).
- A total of 5% to 10% of SCDs are due to ion channelopathies, valvular, or inflammatory causes (Figure 25-2).
- Ventricular tachyarrhythmias are more closely associated with myocardial ischemia and inherited ion channel diseases.
- Bradyarrhythmias (e.g., asystole and PEA) are less common causes of SCD but are associated with multiple organ failure.
- Tension pneumothorax, cardiac tamponade or severe heart failure can lead to PEA.

Pathophysiology

The "perfect storm" of cardiac structural abnormalities, biochemical alterations, and electrical instability conspires to bring about the arrhythmia that causes SCD (Table 25-1 and Figure 25-3).[3,4]

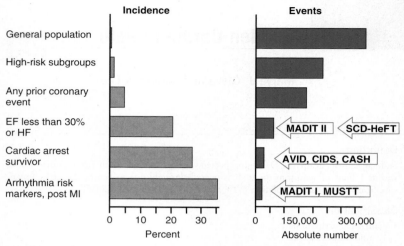

FIGURE 25-1. Absolute numbers of events and event rates of sudden cardiac death in the general population and in specific subpopulations over 1 year. "General population" refers to an unselected population of age ≥35 years and high-risk subgroups of those with multiple risk factors for a first coronary event. Clinical trials that include specific subpopulations of patients are shown at the right side of the figure. AVID, Antiarrhythmics Versus Implantable Defibrillators; CASH, Cardiac Arrest Study Hamburg; CIDS, Canadian Implantable Defibrillator Study; EF, ejection fraction; HF, heart failure; MADIT, Multicenter Automatic Defibrillator Implantation Trial; MI, myocardial infarction; MUSTT, Multicenter UnSustained Tachycardia Trial; SCD-HeFT, Sudden Cardiac Death in Heart Failure Trial. (Modified from Myerburg RJ, Kessler KM, Castellanos A. SCD. Structure, function, and time-dependence of risk. *Circulation* 1992;85:I2-I10, with permission.)

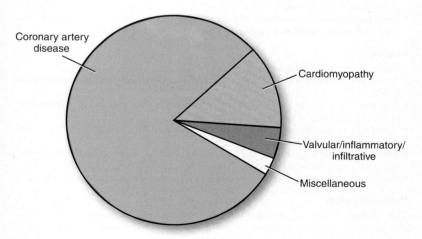

FIGURE 25-2. Etiology of sudden cardiac death.

TABLE 25-1	ABNORMALITIES ASSOCIATED WITH SUDDEN CARDIAC DEATH

Myocardial disease
- Ischemic cardiomyopathy—chronic and acute myocardial infarction
- Nonischemic cardiomyopathy—dilated, alcoholic, postpartum

Coronary artery
- Coronary arteritis
- Coronary atherosclerosis—ischemia/infarct
- Coronary artery embolism and other mechanical obstructions (e.g., dissection and spasm)
- Congenital coronary abnormalities

Hypertrophic states
- Hypertensive heart disease
- Left ventricular hypertrophy
- Obstructive and nonobstructive hypertrophic cardiomyopathy
- Pulmonary hypertension

Valvular abnormalities
- Aortic regurgitation/stenosis
- Infective endocarditis
- Prosthetic valve dysfunction

Inflammatory, infiltrative, neoplastic, and degenerative processes
- Amyloidosis
- Arrhythmogenic right ventricular dysplasia
- Chagas disease
- Hemochromatosis
- Neuromuscular disorders—muscular dystrophy, myotonic dystrophy, Friedreich ataxia
- Sarcoidosis
- Viral myocarditis

Congenital heart disease
- Congenital aortic and pulmonic stenosis
- Postsurgical repair
- Right-to-left shunts

Electrophysiologic abnormalities
- Conduction system abnormalities—Wolff–Parkinson–White syndrome, His-Purkinje fibrosis
- Repolarization abnormalities—congenital and acquired long QT syndromes (see drugs below), Brugada syndrome

Commotio cordis (chest wall trauma)

(Continued)

TABLE 25-1	ABNORMALITIES ASSOCIATED WITH SUDDEN CARDIAC DEATH (*Continued*)

Central nervous system (e.g., intracranial hemorrhage and severe stress/emotion) and neurohormonally mediated abnormalities (catecholamines)

Drug-induced—antiarrhythmic (classes Ia, Ic, III), psychotropics (haloperidol and tricyclics) and other QT-prolonging medications

Sudden infant death syndrome

Toxin/metabolic disturbances—hypomagnesemia, hypo/hyperkalemia, hypocalcemia, acidemia, cocaine

Other conditions—tamponade, aortic dissection, rapid blood loss, massive pulmonary embolism, sudden complete airway obstruction

Modified from: Myerburg RJ, Castellanos A. Cardiac Arrest and Sudden Cardiac Death. In: Bonow RO, Mann DL, Zipes DP, Libby P, eds. *Braunwald's Heart Disease: A Textbook of Cardiovascular Medicine*, 9th ed. Philadelphia, PA: Elsevier; 2012:845-884.

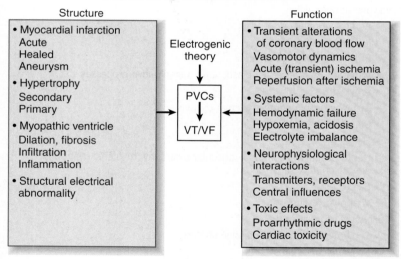

FIGURE 25-3. Biologic model of sudden cardiac death (SCD). Structural cardiac abnormalities are commonly defined as the causative basis for SCD. However, functional alterations of the abnormal anatomic substrate are usually required to alter stability of the myocardium, permitting a potentially fatal arrhythmia to be initiated. In this conceptual model, short-term or long-term structural abnormalities interact with functional modulations to influence the probability that premature ventricular contractions (PVCs) initiate ventricular tachycardia or fibrillation (VT/VF). (From Myerburg RJ, Kessler KM, Bassett AL, et al. A biological approach to sudden cardiac death: structure, function, and cause. *Am J Cardiol* 1989;63:1512-1516, with permission.)

Risk Factors

- Among patients with CAD and other select cardiomyopathies, a **significantly reduced left ventricular ejection fraction (LVEF) is the single most powerful independent predictor for SCD**, though its specificity for predicting SCD is low.
- Electrical instability, manifested by frequent premature ventricular contractions (PVCs) or runs of nonsustained VT, portends an increased risk of SCD in patients with reduced LVEF, but this finding is not specific enough to be clinically useful.
- As most SCD events are related to CAD, other risk factors for SCD closely mirror those of atherosclerosis[1]:
  - Age: 1 in 100,000 per year for adolescents; 1 in 1,000 per year for middle-aged adults; and 1 in 500 per year for older adults.
  - Gender: In younger people, SCD is much more likely among men; this risk is nearly even between genders after age 65.
  - Hypercholesterolemia
  - Hypertension
- Left ventricular hypertrophy (LVH), often as a consequence of hypertension, increases SCD risk beyond that of CAD alone.
- Lifestyle factors: Cigarette smoking and obesity. These carry higher than expected rates of SCD when adjusted for the risk related to CAD.
- Large population studies have also demonstrated modestly increased SCD risk in the morning hours, on Mondays, during winter months, and with acute psychosocial stressors.
- While survivors of cardiac arrest represent a high-risk population, the number of patients who are at risk for SCD but have not yet suffered an arrest is substantially higher (Figure 25-1).[2]

Associated Conditions (Table 25-1)[3]

- **Ischemic cardiomyopathy (ICM):**
  - Primary prevention of sudden death is strongly influenced by six recent trials in post-MI patients with reduced LVEF (MADIT I, CABG-PATCH, MUSTT, MADIT II, DINAMIT, and SCD-HeFT; see Table 25-2).[5-10]
  - **Implantable cardioverter-defibrillators (ICDs) prevent SCD. In patients with ICM, the number of ICDs needed to save one life over 8 years is 6.**
  - With the possible exception of β-blockers, **antiarrhythmic drug (AAD) therapy does not prevent SCD.**
  - In an effort to identify the highest-risk patients, early studies enrolled patients with background arrhythmias (NSVT) who had inducible arrhythmia during electrophysiologic study (EPS) (MADIT I, MUSTT); this likely explains the large benefit of ICD in these trials (54% to 60% relative risk reduction [RRR] in all-cause mortality).[5,7]
  - The two largest trials (MADIT II and SCD-HeFT) enrolled patients based on reduced LVEF alone and found a 23% to 31% RRR in all-cause mortality with an ICD.[8,10]
  - Current recommendation regarding the timing of ICD implantation for ICM is **>1 month post-MI or >3 months post-revascularization.**[1,11]
  - Although patients are at the highest risk of arrhythmic death at the time of the myocardial infarction (MI), **many of the arrhythmias that occur around the time of an MI are not predictive of long-term mortality.**
  - Mortality benefit of ICD for patients in MADIT II was greatest for those with more remote MI.
  - ICD trials enrolling patients who had recent coronary revascularization or recent MI (CABG-PATCH, DINAMIT) did not demonstrate a mortality benefit for early ICD placement.[6,9]
  - Current recommendations for primary prevention of SCD specify that patients with ICM should be treated with **appropriate heart failure medications** (β-blocker, angiotensin-converting enzyme inhibitor, angiotensin receptor blocker,

TABLE 25-2	THE TEN MOST CITED IMPLANTABLE CARDIOVERTER-DEFIBRILLATOR TRIALS ORGANIZED BY THE TYPE OF CARDIOMYOPATHY AND TYPE OF SUDDEN CARDIAC DEATH PREVENTION		
Combined ICM and NICM	Secondary Prevention	AVID[22]	1,016 patients resuscitated from VF or sustained VT with syncope or other serious cardiac symptoms and an LVEF ≤40% ICD (75.4%) versus antiarrhythmic drugs (64.1%) alive at 3 years	31% RRR mortality ($P = 0.02$)
		CASH[23]	288 survivors of cardiac arrest due to ventricular arrhythmias ICD (65.4%) versus amiodarone or metoprolol (55.6%) alive average 57 months	23% RRR mortality ($P =$ NS, 0.08)
		CIDS[24]	659 survivors of cardiac arrest or syncope secondary to arrhythmia ICD (76.7%) versus amiodarone (73.0%) alive at 3 years	20% RRR mortality ($P =$ NS, 0.142)
ICM	Primary Prevention	SCD-HeFT[10]	2,521 patients with NYHA class 2–3 HF and LVEF ≤35% ICD (78%) versus amiodarone (72%) versus placebo (71%) alive average 45 months	23% RRR mortality ($P = 0.007$)
		CABG-PATCH[6]	900 patients undergoing elective CABG, LVEF <35% abnormal SAECG ICD (77.4%) versus conventional therapy (79.1%) alive average 32 months	7% RRI mortality ($P =$ NS, 0.64)
		DINAMIT[9]	674 patients with a recent MI (6–40 days), LVEF ≤35%, NYHA class 1–3 HF, abnormal HRV, or elevated average heart rate. ICD (81.3%) versus conventional therapy (83%) alive average 30 months Death from arrhythmia reduced 58% ($P = 0.009$)	8% RRI mortality ($P =$ NS, 0.66)
		MUSTT[7]	704 patients with prior MI, LVEF ≤40%, NSVT, and inducible VT on EPS ICD +AAD (76%) versus AAD (45%) versus conventional therapy (52%) alive at 5 years	55–60% RRR mortality ($P ≤0.001$)

TABLE 25-2		THE TEN MOST CITED IMPLANTABLE CARDIOVERTER-DEFIBRILLATOR TRIALS ORGANIZED BY THE TYPE OF CARDIOMYOPATHY AND TYPE OF SUDDEN CARDIAC DEATH PREVENTION (*Continued*)	
ICM	Primary Prevention	**MADIT I**[5]	196 patients with prior MI, LVEF ≤0.35%, NYHA class 1–3 HF, NSVT, and inducible VT on EPS ICD (84.2%) versus conventional therapy (61.4%) alive average 27 months	54% RRR mortality (*P* = 0.009)
		MADIT II[8]	1,232 patients with a prior MI and LVEF ≤30% ICD (85.8%) versus conventional therapy (80.2%) alive average 20 months	31% RRR mortality (*P* = 0.016)
NICM		**DEFINITE**[12]	458 patients with NICM, an LVEF ≤35%, and PVCs or NSVT ICD (87.8%) versus standard therapy (82.5%) alive at 2 years ICD reduced the risk of sudden death from arrhythmia specifically	35% RRR mortality (*P* = NS, 0.08)

AAD, antiarrhythmic drug; ICD, implantable cardioverter-defibrillator; AVID, Antiarrhythmic Drug versus Defibrillator; CASH, cardiac arrest survival in Hamburg; CIDS, Canadian Implantable Defibrillator Study; SCD-HeFT, Sudden Cardiac Death in Heart Failure Trial; CABG-PATCH, Coronary Artery Bypass Graft Patch Trial; DINAMIT, Defibrillator in Acute Myocardial Infarction Trial; MUSTT, Multicenter Unsustained Tachycardia Trial; MADIT I, Multicenter Automatic Defibrillator Implantation Trial; MADIT II, Multicenter Automatic Defibrillator Implantation Trial; DEFINITE, Defibrillators in Non-Ischemic Cardiomyopathy Treatment Evaluation; ICM, ischemic cardiomyopathy; NICM, nonischemic cardiomyopathy; VF, ventricular fibrillation; VT, ventricular tachycardia; LVEF, left ventricular ejection fraction; NYHA, New York Heart Association; HF, heart failure; SAECG, signal-averaged ECG; MI, myocardial infarction; HRV, heart rate variability; PVC, premature ventricular contraction; NSVT, nonsustained ventricular tachycardia; EPS, electrophysiologic study; RRR, relative risk reduction; RRI, relative risk increase.

and aldosterone antagonist), **antiplatelet medications** (aspirin), and **atherosclerotic medications** (statins).
- **Viable ischemic myocardium should be revascularized** if indicated.
- After above measures are performed, an ICD is indicated for patients with severe left ventricular (LV) dysfunction who have an expected survival with good functional status of >1 year.[1]
- **NICM:**
  - Although NICM is less common than ICM, patients with NICM are also at risk for SCD.
  - Two major trials have examined the use of ICDs in this patient population (Table 25-2) with the following conclusions:
    - The SCD-HeFT trial reported a 23% RRR in all-cause mortality, which was similar among its patients with ICM and NICM.[10]
    - The largest study of exclusively NICM patients (DEFINITE) demonstrated a nonsignificant trend toward reduction in mortality and a significant 80% reduction in arrhythmic death with an ICD.[12]

- A meta-analysis of all NICM primary prevention trials revealed a **31% RRR in all-cause mortality with an ICD. The number needed to treat to prevent one SCD in patients with NICM at 2 years is 25.**[13]
- Because some cases of NICM resolve with treatment over time, the Centers for Medicare and Medicaid Services approved **ICD implantation for NICM patients with reduced LVEF after a minimum of 3 months of medical treatment**.
  - Syncope, regardless of etiology, confers a higher risk of SCD in patients with NICM.
  - Management of patients with NICM at risk for SCD starts with **appropriate heart failure therapy** (see Chapters 14 and 15).
  - **Reassessment of LV function with noninvasive cardiac imaging** after 3 to 9 months of treatment determines whether an ICD is to be recommended.
- **Hypertrophic cardiomyopathy (HCM)**: Some patients with HCM are at an increased risk for SCD (see Chapter 16).[14]
- **Arrhythmogenic right ventricular cardiomyopathy** (ARVC)[15,16]:
  - ARVC has been implicated as a cause of SCD in both the young and old patients.
  - Classic pathology is a fibrofatty replacement of right ventricular myocardium, although it can occur in either ventricle.
  - Genetic and molecular studies have demonstrated ARVC to be a disease of the desmosome cardiac structural complex.
  - Overt structural abnormalities are not always present, and the disease often presents with syncope, tachycardia (monomorphic or polymorphic VT, often left bundle branch block pattern), or SCD.
  - ARVC, like HCM, is associated with SCD in young athletes.
  - Evidence suggests that strenuous cardiopulmonary exercise contributes to an accelerated disease process in ARVC.
  - Incidence of SCD in patients varies, with reported values ranging from 0.8% to 9%.
  - Observational studies have identified clinical risk factors that may predict an increased risk of SCD:
    - Family of history of SCD
    - History of unexplained syncope
    - Left heart failure
  - **ICD is generally recommended for patients with ARVC for primary prevention of SCD if these risk factors are present as well as for secondary prevention regardless of risk factors**.[1,11]
- **Inflammatory and infiltrative cardiomyopathies:**
  - Inflammatory and infectious cardiomyopathies can induce SCD via complete heart block or ventricular tachyarrhythmias.
  - Most common inciting agents are thought to be viral, but many other infective agents have been implicated, including bacterial, fungal, protozoal, parasitic, spirochetal, and rickettsial.
  - Noninfective agents have been implicated as well, including toxins, radiation, and chemotherapeutics.
  - Management of SCD in the acute setting is largely supportive, but drug therapy, catheter ablation, or device placement may be necessary in the face of persistent arrhythmias.
  - **Immunomodulation with steroids does not appear to alter outcome**.
  - Infiltrative cardiomyopathy encompasses a heterogeneous mix of diseases, including sarcoidosis, amyloidosis, hemochromatosis, and Fabry disease.
  - On the whole, management of infiltrative and inflammatory diseases generally involves the treatment of the underlying condition.
  - Indication for an ICD in chronic cardiomyopathy secondary to inflammatory diseases is the same as that in NICM.
- **Cardiac sarcoidosis**[17]:
  - SCD may be the first manifestation of sarcoidosis.

- One-quarter of patients with cardiac sarcoidosis will develop complete heart block and up to 70% will have SCD as the terminal event.
  - Corticosteroids may reduce the burden of granuloma formation and subsequent arrhythmias as well as attenuate but not completely obviate the incidence of SCD.
  - Presence of spontaneous VT, severe LV dysfunction, and severe intraventricular conduction disturbance warrant therapy with an ICD and/or a pacemaker.
- **Cardiac amyloidosis**[18]:
  - **Cardiac amyloidosis is associated with a poor outcome**.
  - Several markers of mortality exist, including cardiac troponins; detectable cardiac troponins carry a median survival of 6 to 8 months versus 21 to 22 months in patients with undetectable levels.
  - Regardless, an ICD **does not** appear to affect long-term outcome with the exception of those with familial amyloidosis awaiting cardiac transplantation.
- **Primary electrical abnormalities** (inherited arrhythmogenic diseases/channelopathies):
  - Long QT syndrome (LQTS, see Chapter 27)
  - Short QT syndrome (see Chapter 27)
  - Idiopathic VF
  - Early repolarization syndrome
- **Brugada syndrome**[19,20]:
  - This is **a rare cause of SCD associated with right bundle branch block and persistent ST-segment elevation in the early precordial leads** (V1, V2).
  - It is largely due to alterations in sodium channel function (SCN5A).
  - Risk appears to be higher in Asian populations and has been implicated as the cause of death in Lai Tai (death during sleep) in Thailand, Bangungut (to rise and moan in sleep followed by death) in the Philippines, and Pokkuri (unexpected sudden death at night) in Japan.
  - Ninety percent of the patients are male.
  - Risk factors for SCD include syncope and ST-segment elevation.
  - ST elevation can be observed either spontaneously or induced by the administration of sodium channel blockers, such as flecainide, procainamide, and ajmaline.
  - Role of EPS remains less well established in risk stratification.
  - Treatment with quinidine or isoproterenol may be useful in patients with arrhythmia storm even in the presence of an ICD.
  - Long-term prevention of SCD involves the placement of an ICD for patients with a history of syncope, sustained VT, or prior cardiac arrest.
- **Commotio cordis**[21]:
  - Low-impact trauma to the anterior chest at a specific time during ventricular repolarization (15 to 30 milliseconds before the T-wave peak) can cause VF and SCD.
  - In the United States, this occurs almost exclusively in young men playing sports involving a high-speed projectile (e.g., baseball, lacrosse, and hockey).
  - Witnesses to commotio cordis events typically report a seemingly inconsequential impact to the victim's chest with some victims collapsing immediately while others participating for several seconds before collapsing.
  - Immediate cardiopulmonary resuscitation (CPR) and defibrillation have been associated with improved survival.
  - On-site automated external defibrillators have reduced the time to defibrillation and have been credited with dramatic survival stories.
  - **Historically, out-of-hospital defibrillation within 3 minutes of a witnessed adult arrest produces survival rates of >50%.**
  - **Every 1-minute delay in defibrillation beyond the first 3 minutes decreases the likelihood of survival by approximately 10%.**
  - Most bystanders underestimate the severity of the trauma or believe that the wind has been knocked out of the person, which delays CPR efforts.

DIAGNOSIS

Clinical Presentation

- Prodrome: Nearly one-quarter of patients have chest pain, palpitations, dyspnea, or fatigue in the days or months leading up to the SCD event.
- Onset of terminal event: Change in clinical status from seconds to an hour in duration.
- Cardiac arrest: Abrupt loss of consciousness due to lack of cerebral blood flow. Successful resuscitation will depend on the type of arrhythmia (VF/VT survival is better than PEA/asystole), setting of the arrest (access to a defibrillator and personnel trained in CPR), and underlying clinical status.
- Biologic death: No return of spontaneous circulation, with progression to irreversible organ dysfunction after resuscitation.

Differential Diagnosis

Sudden loss of blood pressure can also occur from severe septic or anaphylactic shock, massive intravascular fluid loss, and acute adrenal insufficiency.

Diagnostic Testing

Laboratory Testing

- The clinical utility of laboratory testing is usually retrospective and not as a first-line diagnostic modality; specificity can also be poor.
- Cardiac biomarker (i.e., troponin and creatine kinase-MB) can be increased hours later if myocardial infarct was the inciting event for arrhythmia.
- Arterial blood gas and basic metabolic panel can be grossly abnormal, particularly in asystole and PEA.
- Any of the aforementioned lab tests can be abnormal with prolonged hypoperfusion of vital organs, thereby impairing diagnostic specificity.

Electrocardiography

Telemetry or 12-lead electrocardiogram (ECG) should immediately identify the culprit arrhythmia for SCD:

- Wide complex tachycardia in VT or VF
- Narrow complex QRS rhythm in PEA
- Absence of any electrical activity in asystole. Evaluate two or more electrocardiography leads for low amplitude or "fine" VF.

Imaging

- Portable chest radiography may show acute lung pathology leading to SCD arrhythmia (e.g., tension pneumothorax and PEA).
- Bedside transthoracic echocardiography may show new wall-motion abnormalities if myocardial infarct or cardiac tamponade precipitated the culprit arrhythmia.

TREATMENT

- **Acute management**[25]:
  - Rapid recovery efforts are critical, as the time between onset and resuscitation has a dramatic effect on the rate of success; irreversible brain damage begins within 5 minutes of the arrest.
  - **Initial assessment:** Witnesses to the arrest should assess for loss of consciousness and pulse. If SCD is suspected, immediate activation of the emergency medical system is the first priority.

- **Basic life support:** Using the CAB mnemonic (circulation, airway, breathing), trained rescuers can clear the airway, establish ventilation, and begin chest compressions; **because timely defibrillation of VF/VT is the most effective treatment for SCD, requesting a defibrillator is an important early step**.
- **Advanced cardiac life support (ACLS):** Goals of ACLS are to establish a perfusing cardiac rhythm, maintain ventilation, and support circulation. Algorithms for various cardiac rhythms can be found in Chapter 7; **the importance of early defibrillation for VT/VF cannot be overstated.**
- **Stabilization:** Further stabilization and a search for reversible underlying cause for the arrest should take place in an intensive care unit setting. Appropriate tests include ECG (for ischemia, infarction, or LQTS); **blood work** (particularly potassium, magnesium, and cardiac biomarkers); **evaluation of LV structure and function** with either two-dimensional echocardiography, radionuclide testing, and/or cardiac magnetic resonance imaging. Noncardiac causes, such as pulmonary embolus, should be excluded when appropriate. Because of the high prevalence of CAD, most treatment plans include an urgent **evaluation for cardiac ischemia with coronary angiography**. For most episodes of resuscitated SCD, an IV **Antiarrhythmics drug (AAD)** is given (see below).
- **Long-term management**:
  - Correct reversible causes
  - Prevention of a second event with ICD
  - AAD therapy and/or percutaneous catheter ablation

Medications

- **Acute setting**[25]:
  - **Amiodarone** may be given during the early resuscitation (150 mg IV over 10 minutes) and continued as an IV infusion (1 mg/kg for 6 hours, 0.5 mg/kg for the next 18 hours).
  - **Lidocaine** and, less frequently, procainamide are alternative IV drugs that are occasionally used.
  - **β-Blocker** therapy is reasonable for most patients with VT; however, patients with bradycardia-induced VT/VF should not be given β-blockers, as these patients benefit from an increase in heart rate with atropine, isoproterenol, or pacing.
  - **IV magnesium** is useful in the setting of polymorphic VT and long QT intervals.
- Long-term management:
  - AADs are generally used to reduce arrhythmia burden for patients with recurring tachyarrhythmias that result in ICD shocks.
  - Commonly used oral AADs for secondary prevention of VT include amiodarone, sotalol, mexiletine, and β-blockers such as metoprolol, atenolol, and acebutolol.

Surgical Management

- **ICDs:**
  - The ICD is an implantable device that is programmed to recognize life-threatening arrhythmias and deliver therapies to restore sinus rhythm.
  - Most ICDs are implanted subcutaneously in the upper chest with leads placed transvenously into the right heart chambers. Rarely, an ICD can be implanted in the abdomen and leads can be placed on the epicardium surgically.
  - ICDs can have one lead (single-chamber system), two leads (dual-chamber system), or three leads in the heart (biventricular cardiac resynchronization system).
  - From randomized trials (AVID, CIDS, CASH; see Table 25-2) comparing ICDs with AAD in VT/VF survivors, an ICD confers a 28% RRR in mortality and a 51% RRR in arrhythmic death.[22-24]

- The device can be programmed to perform various therapies (rapid antitachycardia pacing or electrical shocks) at specific heart rates (zones).
  - Prospective randomized controlled ICD trials in patients at increased risk for VT/VF have demonstrated a mortality benefit due to delivering shock therapy.
  - Success rates of terminating VT and VF exceed 95%.
- **ICD therapy has become the standard of care for most survivors of cardiac arrest.**
- Catheter ablation:
  - Catheter ablation serves an adjuvant role for patients who experience recurring VT despite AAD therapy.
  - With recurrent VT in the context of a ventricular aneurysm, surgical ventricular restoration (Dor procedure) may decrease VT burden if catheter ablation and AADs prove unsuccessful.

SPECIAL CONSIDERATIONS

When the ICD procedure is contraindicated (e.g., active bacteremia), an external LifeVest may be worn as a bridge to eventual ICD placement.

REFERENCES

1. Zipes DP. ACC/AHA/ESC 2006 guidelines for management of patients with ventricular arrhythmias and the prevention of sudden cardiac death. *J Am Coll Cardiol* 2006;48:e247-e346.
2. Myerburg RJ, Kessler KM, Castellanos A. SCD. Structure, function, and time-dependence of risk. *Circulation* 1992;85:I2-I10.
3. Myerburg RJ, Castellanos A. Cardiac Arrest and Sudden Cardiac Death. In: Bonow RO, Mann DL, Zipes DP, Libby P, eds. *Braunwald's Heart Disease: A Textbook of Cardiovascular Medicine*, 9th ed. Philadelphia, PA: Elsevier; 2012:845-884.
4. Myerburg RJ, Kessler KM, Bassett AL, Castellanos A. A biological approach to sudden cardiac death: structure, function and cause. *Am J Cardiol* 1989;63:1512-1516.
5. Moss AJ, Hall WJ, Cannom DS, et al. Improved survival with an implanted defibrillator in patients with coronary disease at high risk for ventricular arrhythmia. Multicenter Automatic Defibrillator Implantation Trial Investigators. *N Engl J Med* 1996;335:1933-1940.
6. Bigger JT Jr. Prophylactic use of implanted cardiac defibrillators in patients at high risk for ventricular arrhythmias after coronary-artery bypass graft surgery. Coronary Artery Bypass Graft (CABG) Patch Trial Investigators. *N Engl J Med* 1997;337:1569-1575.
7. Buxton AE, Lee KL, Fisher JD, et al. A randomized study of the prevention of sudden death in patients with coronary artery disease. Multicenter Unsustained Tachycardia Trial Investigators. *N Engl J Med* 1999;341:1882-1890.
8. Moss AJ, Zareba W, Hall WJ, et al. Prophylactic implantation of a defibrillator in patients with myocardial infarction and reduced ejection fraction. *N Engl J Med* 2002;346:877-883.
9. Hohnloser SH, Kuck KH, Dorian P, et al., on behalf of the DINAMIT Investigators. Prophylactic use of an implantable cardioverter-defibrillator after acute myocardial infarction. *N Engl J Med* 2004;351:2481-2488.
10. Bardy GH, Lee KL, Mark DB, et al. Sudden Cardiac Death in Heart Failure Trial (SCD-HeFT) Investigators. Amiodarone or an implantable cardioverter-defibrillator for congestive heart failure. *N Engl J Med* 2005;352:225-237.
11. Epstein AE. ACC/AHA/HRS 2008 guidelines for device-based therapy of cardiac rhythm abnormalities. *Circulation* 2008;117:e350-e408.
12. Kadish A, Dyer A, Daubert JP, et al. Prophylactic defibrillator implantation in patients with nonischemic dilated cardiomyopathy. *N Engl J Med* 2004;350:2151-2158.
13. Desai AS, Fang JC, Maisel WH, Baughman KL. Implantable defibrillators for the prevention of mortality in patients with nonischemic cardiomyopathy: a meta-analysis of randomized controlled trials. *JAMA* 2004;292:2874-2879.
14. Maron BJ, Spirito P, Shen WK, et al. Implantable cardioverter-defibrillators and prevention of sudden cardiac death in hypertrophic cardiomyopathy. *JAMA* 2007;298:405-412.

15. Gemayel C, Pelliccia A, Thompson PD. Arrhythmogenic right ventricular cardiomyopathy. *J Am Coll Cardiol* 2001;38:1773-1781.

16. Corrado D, Leoni L, Link MS, et al. Implantable cardioverter-defibrillator therapy for prevention of sudden death in patients with arrhythmogenic right ventricular cardiomyopathy/dysplasia. *Circulation* 2003;108:3084-3091.

17. Mitchell DN, du Bois RM, Oldershaw PJ. Cardiac sarcoidosis. *BMJ* 1997;314:320-321.

18. Dispenzieri A, Kyle RA, Gertz MA, et al. Survival in patients with primary systemic amyloidosis and raised serum cardiac troponins. *Lancet* 2003;361:1787-1789.

19. Brugada P, Brugada J. Right bundle branch block, persistent ST segment elevation and sudden cardiac death: a distinct clinical and electrocardiographic syndrome. A multicenter report. *J Am Coll Cardiol* 1992;20:1391-1396.

20. Priori SG, Napolitano C, Gasparini M, et al. Natural history of Brugada syndrome: insights for risk stratification and management. *Circulation* 2002;105:1342-1347.

21. Link MS, Estes NA III. Mechanically induced ventricular fibrillation (commotio cordis). *Heart Rhythm* 2007;4:529-532.

22. The Antiarrhythmics versus Implantable Defibrillators (AVID) Investigators. A comparison of antiarrhythmic-drug therapy with implantable defibrillators in patients resuscitated from near-fatal ventricular arrhythmias. *N Engl J Med* 1997;337:1576-1583.

23. Kuck KH, Cappato R, Siebels J, et al. Randomized comparison of antiarrhythmic drug therapy with implantable defibrillators in patients resuscitated from cardiac arrest: the Cardiac Arrest Study Hamburg (CASH). *Circulation* 2000;102:748-754.

24. Connolly SJ, Gent M, Roberts RS, et al. Canadian Implantable Defibrillator Study (CIDS): a randomized trial of the implantable cardioverter defibrillator against amiodarone. *Circulation* 2000;101:1297-1302.

25. Field JM, Hazinski MF, Sayre MR, et al. 2010 American Heart Association Guidelines for Cardiopulmonary Resuscitation and Emergency Cardiovascular Care. *Circulation* 2010;122:s640-s656.

Atrial Fibrillation

26

Thomas K. Kurian and Mitchell N. Faddis

GENERAL PRINCIPLES

- Atrial fibrillation (AF) is the most common sustained arrhythmia, accounting for over one-third of hospitalizations for cardiac arrhythmias.
- AF is associated with thromboembolic stroke, heart failure, and increased all-cause mortality.
- AF can be classified by frequency and duration of symptoms into paroxysmal, persistent, long-standing persistent, and permanent categories.
- The management for AF includes rate control, rhythm control, and anticoagulation to prevent thromboembolism.
- Rate control is achieved with β-blockers, calcium channel blockers, or digoxin.
- Rhythm control is achieved with antiarrhythmic drugs and synchronized direct current (DC) cardioversion. Surgical and catheter-based therapies are available for select patients.
- The overall goal of preventing thromboembolic events with oral anticoagulation must be balanced against the bleeding risks. The $CHADS_2$ risk score estimates yearly stroke risk based on underlying risk factors.[1]

Definition

- AF is a supraventricular arrhythmia characterized by uncoordinated, chaotic electrical activity and deterioration of proper atrial mechanical function, with an irregular ventricular response.
- Mechanism of AF is likely multifactorial; however, it primarily involves focal electrical "triggers" that originate predominantly from the pulmonary veins (PVs) and an anatomic substrate capable of initiation and perpetuation of AF.

Classification[2,3]

- **Paroxysmal AF:** ≥2 episodes lasting ≤7 days, often self-terminating within 24 hours.
- **Persistent AF:** Lasts >7 days and fails to stop spontaneously. Persistent AF requires medical and/or electrical intervention to achieve sinus rhythm. Persistent AF may be the first presentation, the culmination of several episodes of paroxysmal AF, or **long-standing persistent AF** (>1 year).
- **Permanent AF:** Continuous AF where cardioversion has failed or has not been attempted, lasting >1 year. Refers to patients in whom a decision has been made not to pursue restoration of sinus rhythm by any means, including catheter or surgical ablation.
- **Lone AF:** Paroxysmal, persistent, or permanent AF in younger patients (<60 years old) with a structurally normal heart.

Epidemiology

- AF afflicts 2.2 million people in North America alone, but it is frequently asymptomatic and diagnosed only after a complication, such as a stroke. AF often coexists with other conditions, including hypertension, heart failure, coronary heart disease, and valvular/structural heart disease.[2,4-6]
- AF is strongly associated with increasing age.

TABLE 26-1	**FACTORS THAT PREDISPOSE PATIENTS TO ATRIAL FIBRILLATION ("PIRATES" MNEMONIC)**

- P—pericarditis, pulmonary disease, pulmonary embolism, postoperative
- I—ischemia, infection
- R—rheumatic heart disease (particularly mitral valve disease)
- A—alcohol ("holiday heart"), atrial myxoma
- T—thyrotoxicosis, theophylline
- E—enlargement (particularly left atrial enlargement)
- S—systemic hypertension, sick sinus syndrome, sleep apnea, and size (obesity)

- The estimated prevalence of AF is approximately 1% in the general population, with a wide range from 0.1% among adults <55 years to over 9% among octogenarians.[2]
- The lifetime risk of developing AF is nearly 1 in 4.[5]

Etiology

There are many common etiologies and risk factors that predispose to the development of AF, only some of which are reversible. The **mnemonic PIRATES** can be a helpful way to remember the causes (Table 26-1).

Pathophysiology

- The mechanisms underlying AF are diverse ranging from repetitive firing of ectopic sites to multiple reentrant loops. In most AF patients, these ectopic foci are located within or near the PVs.
- The mechanism of AF is thought to involve a **combination of multiple reentrant wavelets, mostly initiated by focal triggers at or near PVs** and possibly maintained by high-frequency reentrant rotors in the posterior left atrium.[2,3,7,8]
- The conduction properties of the atrium are influenced by underlying structural disease, cardiac autonomic tone, the size of the atria, and the degree of atrial fibrosis.
- Restoration of sinus rhythm has a higher success rate when it is achieved rapidly; there is increasing stability of AF the longer the arrhythmia is present.
- The axiom "a-fib begets a-fib" refers to **atrial electrical remodeling that reinforces the mechanisms underlying AF** such as shortening of the atrial action potential duration and refractory period.[2]

DIAGNOSIS

Clinical Presentation

History

- Common symptoms include **palpitations, shortness of breath, fatigue, decreased exertional capacity**, and **chest discomfort**.
- Less commonly, orthopnea and edema from heart failure can occur. In the setting of sick sinus syndrome (SSS), patients may present with syncope.
- An embolic event can cause focal neurologic symptoms or organ/limb ischemia.
- **Many occurrences of AF are asymptomatic.**[9]
- It is important to obtain the clinical pattern of AF, including time of onset, precipitating cause, and duration and frequency of symptoms, along with complications and coexisting disorders. In addition, a past medical history can assess for underlying cardiac disease, and social habits can be helpful to identify risk factors.

Physical Examination

- Significant findings may be absent if AF is paroxysmal. If present, there can be an irregular pulse, tachycardia, or the absence of a venous *a* wave. For more severe cases, heart failure signs may be present.
- It is important to identify possible etiologies such as valvular murmurs or wheezing for underlying pulmonary disease. A goiter may be present, indicating hyperthyroidism. Other findings may include focal neurologic deficits demonstrating recent thromboembolism.

Diagnostic Testing

Laboratories

If appropriate, thyroid function tests and cardiac biomarkers should be checked.

Electrocardiography

- AF can be identified on electrocardiogram (ECG) or rhythm strip with an **irregular ventricular rhythm that is void of P waves** (Figure 26-1).
- The ventricular response will vary according to different properties of the atrioventricular (AV) node and conduction system, vagal and sympathetic tone, and the presence of accessory pathways.
- AF may occur with additional arrhythmias, including atrial flutter and other atrial tachycardias.
- The **Ashman phenomenon** refers to wide complex beats that arise due to transient block in one bundle branch—usually right bundle-branch block—of the atrial impulses at varying cycle lengths, often preceded by a "long–short" interval.
- Ambulatory cardiac rhythm monitoring is indicated for outpatients in whom AF is suspected. It is helpful to identify the frequency and duration of paroxysmal AF.

Imaging

- Chest radiography can be helpful to identify intrinsic pulmonary pathology and assess cardiac borders.
- **Echocardiography:**
  - The transthoracic echocardiogram can evaluate the size of the atria and ventricles and detect valvular heart disease.

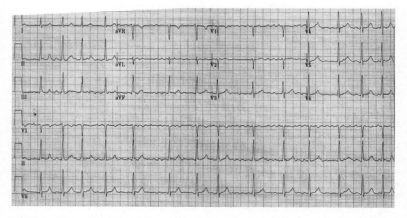

FIGURE 26-1. Typical ECG demonstrating AF. Note the irregular ventricular rhythm and fibrillatory waves have replaced P waves.

- Transesophageal echocardiography (TEE) is much more sensitive for identifying thrombi in the left atrium and is useful to assess if cardioversion can occur without the need for prior anticoagulation.[2]
- Echocardiographic features associated with the development of AF include left atrial enlargement, left ventricular (LV) hypertrophy, and reduced LV fractional shortening.[10]

TREATMENT

- Patients with new-onset AF do not always need admission to the hospital. Indications for admission include active ischemia, rapid heart rate, significant ST-segment changes, associated medical problems, elderly patients, underlying heart disease with hemodynamic compromise, or the need for the initiation of certain antiarrhythmic medications in patients receiving cardioversion therapy.
- The three main goals to be considered in the treatment of AF are[2]
  - **Rate control**
  - **Rhythm control**
  - **Anticoagulation to prevent thromboembolism**
- The appropriate choice of therapy is tailored to each patient based on the type of AF, safety factors, symptoms, and patient preference. Refer to the management overview and algorithm for evaluating newly diagnosed AF, recurrent paroxysmal AF, recurrent persistent AF, and permanent AF (Figures 26-2 through 26-4).[1,2]

Medications

Rate Control

- Appropriate rate control allows time for proper ventricular filling in diastole, avoids rate-related ischemia, and generally improves cardiac hemodynamics.
- Strict rate control (<80 beats per minute [bpm] at rest or <110 bpm during 6-minute walk) is not beneficial compared with lenient rate control (resting heart rate <110 bpm) in patients with persistent AF who have ejection fraction >40 % (RACE II Rate Control Efficiency in permanent atrial fibrillation).[11]
- No benefit has been shown for use of a routine strategy of rhythm control in patients with AF and systolic heart failure compared with a strategy of rate control in patients who are not symptomatic with AF.[2,12-16]
- Ventricular rate control is important for avoiding hemodynamic instability associated with a rapid rate, relieving patient symptoms, and preventing tachycardia-associated cardiomyopathy.
- Correction of associated causes (hypoxia and hyperthyroidism infection) dramatically improves the success of rate control.
- **Medically, rate control is accomplished by depressing AV nodal conduction** with the use of a β-blocker or nondihydropyridine calcium channel blocker or with nodal blocking and vagal tone enhancement using digoxin.[2,17]
  - **β-Blocker:**
    - Preferred drug for AF associated with thyrotoxicosis, acute myocardial infarction, and high adrenergic tone in the postsurgical state. It is reasonable for most other causes of AF.
    - Caution should be used in administering β-blockers to patients with acute decompensated heart failure or with reactive airway disease.
  - **Calcium channel blockers** (nondihydropyridine):
    - Reasonable for most causes of AF.
    - These should also be used cautiously in patients with heart failure or hypotension.
  - **Digoxin**:
    - Preferred in patients with AF and symptomatic heart failure with reduced LV ejection fraction.

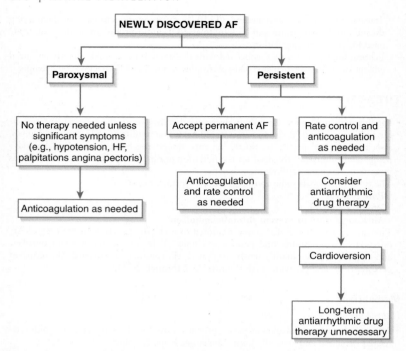

FIGURE 26-2. Management overview and algorithm with pharmacologic therapy for patients with newly diagnosed atrial fibrillation (AF). (From Fuster V, Rydén LE, Cannom DS, et al. 2011 ACCF/AHA/HRS focused updates incorporated into the ACC/AHA/ESC 2006 guidelines for the management of patients with atrial fibrillation. *J Am Coll Cardiol* 2011;57:e101-e198, with permission.)

- Less effective for ambulatory, active patients.
- Digoxin should be avoided in the setting of acute renal failure or chronic kidney disease.
  - **Amiodarone:**
    - Amiodarone is a class III antiarrhythmic that has AV nodal-blocking properties along with sympatholytic and calcium channel antagonist properties.
    - It should be considered a **secondary agent**, used primarily for refractory rate control or in hypotensive patients.
    - It has the potential of converting the patient into sinus rhythm, thus increasing the risk of thromboembolism in those with prolonged AF who are not anticoagulated.
    - Amiodarone causes an increase in digoxin levels and inhibits warfarin metabolism, so appropriate adjustments to those medications should be made.
  - Combined therapy may be necessary for some patients but one should be mindful of the increased potential for significant bradycardia.

Rhythm Control
- There are multiple antiarrhythmic medications used to achieve and maintain rhythm control; appropriate selection is based on safety, comorbidities, and the pattern of AF diagnosed (Figure 26-5).[2,18]

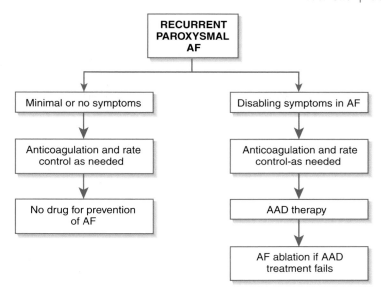

FIGURE 26-3. Management overview and algorithm with pharmacologic therapy for patients with recurrent paroxysmal atrial fibrillation (AF). AAD, antiarrhythmic drug. (From Fuster V, Rydén LE, Cannom DS, et al. 2011 ACCF/AHA/HRS focused updates incorporated into the ACC/AHA/ESC 2006 guidelines for the management of patients with atrial fibrillation. *J Am Coll Cardiol* 2011;57:e101-e198, with permission.)

- Pharmacologic cardioversion is less effective than DC cardioversion, although there is evidence that pretreatment with certain antiarrhythmic medications (e.g., amiodarone, flecainide, ibutilide, propafenone, and sotalol) can enhance the success of DC cardioversion.[2]
- The choice of medication varies, but in general **flecainide**, **sotalol**, **propafenone**, and **dronedarone** are preferred in patients with no or minimal heart disease, while **amiodarone or dofetilide** can be used in patients with reduced LV function or heart failure.[2,17,19-21]
- **Proarrhythmic side effects** require some of the medications to be initiated and titrated on an inpatient basis with continuous telemetry monitoring and routine ECGs.[2,19]
- **Potential organ toxicity** requires frequent outpatient follow-up and monitoring.
- Despite rhythm control, many patients with AF experience a recurrence. Of those who are successfully cardioverted, only 20% to 30% continue in sinus rhythm for more than 1 year without antiarrhythmic therapy.
- Risk factors for recurrence include advanced age, heart failure, left atrial enlargement, obesity, hypertension, and rheumatic heart disease.[2]
- Pertinent findings of rhythm-control strategies:
  ○ When compared with a rate-control strategy in large trials with mostly older patients with asymptomatic persistent AF, there was **no mortality benefit to a rhythm-control strategy and trends toward improved survival and stroke risk with the rate-control strategy** were present (Atrial Fibrillation Follow-up Investigation of Rhythm Management [AFFIRM] and RACE trials).[12,15]
  ○ Most patients with symptomatic AF prefer a rhythm-control strategy to achieve sinus rhythm. In asymptomatic patients, the differences in quality of life between the two strategies are not demonstrable in large studies.[2,12-16]

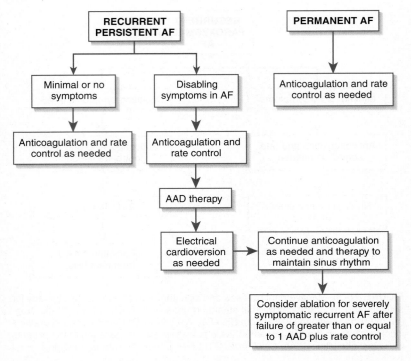

FIGURE 26-4. Management overview and algorithm with pharmacologic therapy for patients with recurrent persistent or permanent atrial fibrillation (AF). AAD, antiarrhythmic drug. (From Fuster V, Rydén LE, Cannom DS, et al. 2011 ACCF/AHA/HRS focused updates incorporated into the ACC/AHA/ESC 2006 guidelines for the management of patients with atrial fibrillation. *J Am Coll Cardiol* 2011;57:e101-e198, with permission.)

- ○ Embolic events take place with equal frequency in both methods of treatment, usually occurring when the patient is not taking warfarin or when the anticoagulation is subtherapeutic.[12,15]

Anticoagulation
- • Preventing a stroke
  - ○ There is a significant risk of stroke in patients with AF due to the formation of a thrombus secondary to stasis of blood in the left atrial appendage.
  - ○ The annual risk of stroke from AF has been estimated at 1.5% in patients 50 to 59 years old and 23.5% in patients 80 to 89 years old.[22]
  - ○ Risk factors for thromboembolic events related to AF and yearly risk of stroke without anticoagulation can be estimated using the CHADS2 scoring system (Table 26-2).[1] More recently, an expanded scoring system has been introduced (CHA$_2$DS$_2$-VASc) which includes female gender, vascular disease and age 65-74 years as additional risk factors and increases the value of age >75 years (Table 26-2). (reference: Lip GY, et al. Improving stroke risk stratification in atrial fibrillation. Am J Med. 2010;123(6):484-8.)

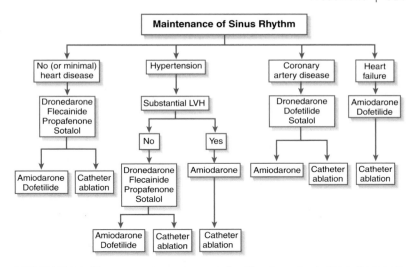

FIGURE 26-5. Management overview and algorithm for antiarrhythmic therapy to maintain normal sinus rhythm, based on various disease states, for patients with recurrent paroxysmal or persistent AF. (From Fuster V, Rydén LE, Cannom DS, et al. 2011 ACCF/AHA/HRS focused updates incorporated into the ACC/AHA/ESC 2006 guidelines for the management of patients with atrial fibrillation. *J Am Coll Cardiol* 2011;57:e101-e198, with permission.)

- ○ The overall goal of preventing thromboembolic events must be balanced with avoiding bleeding complications with oral anticoagulation. Because the risk/benefit ratio for oral anticoagulation is unique to each individual, variation exists in recommended anticoagulation strategies. The American College of Cardiology/American Heart Association/European Society of Cardiology recommendations are shown in Table 26-3.
  - ○ Using the simplified CHADS2 scoring for patients at increased risk for stroke (CHADS2 score ≥2), anticoagulation therapy is recommended. For patients with a lower risk for stroke (CHADS2 score 0), the risks of full anticoagulation outweigh the benefit; thus aspirin is reasonable. Intermediate-risk patients (CHADS2 score 1) may use either aspirin or oral anticoagulants.
- • Warfarin
  - ○ Warfarin inhibits vitamin K-dependent coagulation factor synthesis in the liver.
  - ○ The anticoagulation effect of warfarin is highly variable with genetic polymorphisms, oral intake of vitamin K, and interactions with other drugs.
  - ○ The anticoagulation effect can be monitored with the International Normalized Ratio (INR) blood test which is a standardized way to report the prothrombin time (PT). In most patients, the goal INR is 2.0-3.0, though some clinical situations may call for higher goals.
  - ○ When starting warfarin, INR blood tests should be performed every week with the expectation of dose modulation to achieve a regular goal INR. Once a steady-state has been achieved and several INRs are in the goal range, blood tests can be performed less frequently.
  - ○ It is often helpful to educate patients to maintain a rather consistent diet to best regulate the warfarin dose. Elimination of foods containing vitamin K is a common mistake that patients make and is not necessary to dose warfarin successfully.

TABLE 26-2	STROKE RISK IN PATIENTS WITH NONVALVULAR ATRIAL FIBRILLATION

CHADS$_2$ Risk Criteria	Score
Congestive Heart Failure	1
Hypertension	1
Age ≥75 Years	1
Diabetes Mellitus	1
Stroke or TIA in the past	2

CHADS$_2$ Score	Recommended Therapy
0	Aspirin (81 to 325 mg daily) or no therapy*
1	Aspirin (81 to 325 mg daily) or oral anticoagulant**
≥2	Oral anticoagulant**

CHA$_2$DS$_2$-VASc Risk Criteria[3,4]	Points
Congestive Heart Failure/LV Dysfunction	1
Hypertension	1
Age >75 Years	2
Diabetes Mellitus	1
Prior **S**troke, TIA, thromboembolism	2
Peripheral **V**ascular Disease or Coronary Artery Disease	1
Age 65–74 Years	1
Sex Category (i.e., Female Sex)	1

CHA$_2$DS$_2$-VASc Score	Recommended Therapy
0	No therapy preferred
1	Aspirin, 81 to 325 mg daily, or oral anticoagulant**
≥2	Oral anticoagulant**

Score	Adjusted stroke rate (%/year) based on CHADS$_2$ score[5]	Adjusted stroke rate (%/year) based on CHA$_2$DS$_2$-VASc score[6]
0	1.9	0
1	2.8	1.3
2	4.0	2.2
3	5.9	3.2
4	8.5	4.0
5	12.5	6.7
6	18.2	9.8
7		9.6
8		6.7
9		15.2

*No therapy is acceptable for patients <65 years old and no heart disease (lone AF).

**If warfarin is the oral anticoagulant used, INR should be 2.0 to 3.0, with a target of 2.5. INR <2.0 is not effective at preventing strokes. If mechanical valve, target INR >2.5.

TABLE 26-3	ANTITHROMBOTIC THERAPY FOR PATIENTS WITH ATRIAL FIBRILLATION		
	Dabigatran	**Apixaban**	**Rivaroxaban**
Mechanism of Action	Direct thrombin inhibitor	Direct factor Xa inhibitor	Direct factor Xa inhibitor
Pro-Drug	Yes	No	No
Food Effect	No	No	No
Dosing (PO)	75-150mg bid*	2.5-5mg bid▲	15-20mg qd**
Renal Clearance	85%	~27%	~33%
Mean Half Life ($t_{1/2}$)	14-17 hrs	~12 hrs	5-13 hrs
Time to peak effect	0.5-2 hrs	3-4 hrs	2-4 hrs

*150mg bid for patients with CrCl >30mL/min; 75mg bid for patients with CrCl 15-30mL/min. Discontinue use in patients who develop acute renal failure. Do not use in patients with mechanical heart valves.

▲5 mg bid is recommended dose. 2.5mg bid is recommended for patients with at least two of the following: age of 80 yrs or more, body weight of 60 kg or less, SCr of 1.5 mg/dL or more. Not recommended for use in patients with severe hepatic impairment.

**20 mg with evening meal for patients with CrCl >50mL/min; 15mg with evening meal for patients with CrCl 15-50mL/min. Do not use in patients with moderate and severe hepatic impairment or with hepatic disease associated with coagulopathy.

Data from individual drug package inserts.

- Warfarin Alternatives
  - Important Considerations (Table 26-3)
    - As a rule, warfarin alternatives do not require frequent blood tests to adjust the dose. This is considered a major convenience for patients and physicians alike.
    - Dosing for all warfarin alternatives MUST be adjusted for renal insufficiency. Unanticipated over-anticoagulation is a major cause of life-threatening bleeding complications.
    - It is important to know there are no reliably effective reversal agents for warfarin alternatives. Agents such as prothrombin complex concentrate (PCC) or recombinant factor VIIa (rFVIIa) may be considered, but these have not been studied in clinical trials.
  - **Dabigatran**
    - The direct thrombin inhibitor Dabigatran has been approved to reduce the risk of stroke and systemic embolism in patients with non-valvular AF based largely on a direct trial against warfarin (RE-LY).[23]
    - The 150mg BID dose was superior to warfarin for stroke prophylaxis, though it had similar rates of important bleeding events.
    - The 110mg BID dose (not currently available in the U.S.) was non-inferior to warfarin for stroke prevention, with lower rates of bleeding events.
    - The 75mg BID dose that is currently available was not formally studied.
    - The most common side effect is **dyspepsia or gastric ulcers**, attributed to the acidic nature of the medication.

- ○ **Apixaban**
  - ▪ Apixaban is an oral factor Xa inhibitor that has been approved to reduce the risk of stroke and systemic embolism in patients with nonvalvular atrial fibrillation
  - ▪ Apixaban was superior to warfarin for stroke prophylaxis, and it was associated with lower bleeding events and an improvement in overall mortality. (reference: Granger CB, et al. Apixaban versus warfarin in patients with atrial fibrillation. N Engl J Med. 2011 Sep 15;365(11):981-92.)
  - ▪ There is an increased risk of stroke when apixaban is stopped. If apixaban is to be stopped, consider coverage with another anticoagulant for at least one week.
  - ▪ The most common side effect is bleeding complications.
- ○ **Rivaroxaban**
  - ▪ Rivaroxaban is an oral factor Xa inhibitor that has been approved to reduce the risk of stroke and systemic embolism in patients with nonvalvular atrial fibrillation. It has approval for other thromboembolic diseases, such as treatment and prevention of deep vein thrombosis (DVT) and pulmonary embolism (PE)
  - ▪ Rivaroxaban was noninferior to warfarin in the pivotal clinical trial, with similar overall major bleeding events and fewer intracranial and fatal bleeding events (reference: Patel MR, et al. Rivaroxaban versus warfarin in nonvalvular atrial fibrillation. N Engl J Med. 2011;365(10):883-91.)
  - ▪ Rivaroxaban is marketed with once-daily dosing.
  - ▪ There is an increased risk of stroke when rivaroxaban is stopped. If rivaroxaban is to be stopped, consider coverage with another anticoagulant for at least one week.
  - ▪ The most common side effect is bleeding complications.
- ○ **Clopidogrel**
  - ▪ In general, aspirin plus clopidogrel is not a substitute for other oral anticoagulants.
  - ▪ The bleeding risk is similar between warfarin and aspirin + clopidogrel, however warfarin has been shown to be superior in preventing vascular events in AF patients.

Other Non-pharmacologic Therapies

- Cardioversion can be performed with **synchronized DC electrical current and/or antiarrhythmic medications**.[2,17]
- Because of the increased risk of thromboembolic events in the first several weeks after cardioversion, elective cardioversions should generally be performed with anticoagulation and continued for a minimum of 4 weeks thereafter.[2,17]
- If the patient is hemodynamically unstable, urgent synchronized DC cardioversion is warranted without anticoagulation.[2,17]
- Other situations where cardioversion can be performed without anticoagulation include short-duration AF (<48 hours) or after a TEE demonstrates the absence of a left atrial thrombus.[2,17]
- In the stable patient, if the AF has lasted longer than 48 hours, is of unknown duration, or there is coexisting mitral stenosis or a history of a thromboembolism, cardioversion should be delayed until anticoagulation can be maintained at appropriate levels (international normalized ratio [INR] of 2.0 to 3.0) for 3 to 4 weeks or until TEE evaluation for thrombi of the left atrial appendage is performed.[2,17]
- An additional option to minimize stroke risk is obliteration of the left atrial appendage, removing the most common site for thrombus formation. This procedure is performed surgically as adjunctive therapy during a Cox-Maze procedure, but percutaneous left atrial occluder devices are under investigation.

Surgical Management

- **Catheter-based ablation**[2,3]:
  - ○ Because the triggers for AF are frequently found in or around the PVs, **percutaneous pulmonary vein isolation (PVI) procedures** targeting this area have been developed.

- Advantages of a PVI procedure over the Cox-Maze procedure include quicker recovery and lower procedural mortality.
- The main disadvantage is a considerably lower success rate (>60% with single procedures, >70% with multiple procedures for paroxysmal AF).
- Because of the modest risk profile associated with this complex procedure, **catheter ablation for the treatment of AF is recommended for symptomatic patients with AF that is refractory to at least one class I or class III antiarrhythmic medication**.
- **Surgical-based ablation**[2,3]:
  - The gold-standard surgical treatment for AF is the **Cox-Maze procedure**, which aims to eliminate all macroreentrant circuits that may develop in the atria.
  - Initially, this procedure involved many surgical incisions across both the right and left atria ("cut and sew") but more refined variations have used linear ablation lines with various energy systems, including radiofrequency energy, microwave, cryoablation, laser, and high-intensity focused ultrasound. Long-term success is reported to be 70% to >95%.
  - It is generally performed for patients undergoing concomitant cardiac surgery but has been more recently used as a stand-alone procedure and in patients in whom catheter ablation has been unsuccessful.

LIFESTYLE/RISK MODIFICATION

- For obese patients, weight loss can reduce the burden of AF.
- Sleep-disordered breathing can trigger AF and evaluation with a sleep study is appropriate in select patients.
- Activity restriction has not been shown to reduce AF burden.

SPECIAL CONSIDERATIONS

- **Wolff–Parkinson–White (WPW) syndrome**[2]:
  - **AF in the setting of WPW can be a life-threatening arrhythmia** in the presence of very rapid AV conduction across an accessory pathway.
  - **Calcium channel blockers are contraindicated** in WPW, as they increase the ventricular rate via the accessory pathway, leading to hypotension or ventricular fibrillation.
  - If the patient is hypotensive, DC cardioversion can be performed. In hemodynamically stable patients, intravenous procainamide or amiodarone can be given.
- **SSS:**
  - Patients with AF associated with SSS often have rapid AF alternating with significant sinus bradycardia and sinus pauses.
  - The use of AV nodal agents to control the rate of AF is difficult; in some cases, a permanent pacemaker may be needed.
- **Medically refractory AF:** When pharmacologic therapy cannot control the heart rate and symptoms, alternative options include an ablation of the AV node with placement of a permanent pacemaker ("ablate and pace" strategy) or more aggressive rhythm-control measures, such as PVI, are appropriate.

REFERENCES

1. Gage BF, Waterman AD, Shannon W, et al. Validation of clinical classification schemes for predicting stroke: results from the National Registry of Atrial Fibrillation. *JAMA* 2001;285:2864-2870.
2. Fuster V, Rydén LE, Cannom DS, et al. 2011 ACCF/AHA/HRS focused updates incorporated into the ACC/AHA/ESC 2006 guidelines for the management of patients with atrial fibrillation. *J Am Coll Cardiol* 2011;57:e101-e198.
3. Calkins H, Kuck KH, Cappato R, et al. 2012 HRS/EHRA/ECAS expert consensus statement on catheter and surgical ablation of atrial fibrillation: recommendations for patient selection,

procedural techniques, patient management and follow-up, definitions, endpoints, and research trial design. *Heart Rhythm* 2012;9:632-696.

4. Cameron A, Schwartz MJ, Kronmal RA, et al. Prevalence and significance of atrial fibrillation in coronary artery disease (CASS Registry). *Am J Cardiol* 1988;61:714-717.

5. Go AS, Hylec, EM, Philips KA, et al. Prevalence of diagnosed atrial fibrillation in adults: national implications for rhythm management and stroke prevention: The Anticoagulation and Risk Factors in Atrial Fibrillation (ATRIA) study. *JAMA* 2001;285:2370-2375.

6. Krahn AD, Manfreda J, Tate RB, et al. The natural history of atrial fibrillation: incidence, risk factors, and prognosis in the Manitoba follow-up study. *Am J Med* 1995;98:476-484.

7. Chen SA, Hsieh MH, Tai CT, et al. Initiation of atrial fibrillation by ectopic beats originating from the pulmonary veins: electrophysiological characteristics, pharmacological responses, and effects of radiofrequency ablation. *Circulation* 1999;100:1879.

8. Haïssaguerre M, Jais P, Shah DC, et al. Spontaneous initiation of atrial fibrillation by ectopic beats originating in the pulmonary veins. *N Engl J Med* 1998;339:659-666.

9. Page RL, Wilkinson WE, Clair WK, et al. Asymptomatic arrhythmias in patients with symptomatic paroxysmal atrial fibrillation and paroxysmal supraventricular tachycardia. *Circulation* 1994;89:224-227.

10. Vaziri SM, Larson MG, Benjamin EJ, et al. Echocardiographic predictors of nonrheumatic atrial fibrillation: The Framingham Heart Study. *Circulation* 1994;89:724-730.

11. Van Gelder IC, Groenveld HF, Crijns HJ, et al. Lenient versus strict rate control in patients with atrial fibrillation. *N Engl J Med* 2010;362:1363-1373.

12. Van Gelder IC, Hagens VE, Bosker HA, et al. A comparison of rate control and rhythm control in patients with recurrent persistent atrial fibrillation. *N Engl J Med* 2002;347:1834-1840.

13. Wyse DG, Waldo AL, DiMarco JP, et al. A comparison of rate control and rhythm control in patients with atrial fibrillation. The Atrial Fibrillation Follow-up Investigation of Rhythm Management (AFFIRM) investigators. *N Engl J Med* 2002;347:1825.

14. Carlson J, Miketic S, Wendeler J, et al. Randomized trial of rate-control versus rhythm-control in persistent atrial fibrillation: the Strategies of Treatment of Atrial Fibrillation (STAF) study. *J Am Coll Cardiol* 2003;41:1690-1696.

15. Opolski G, Torbicki A, Kosior DA, et al. Rate control vs rhythm control in patients with nonvalvular persistent atrial fibrillation: the results of the Polish How to Treat Chronic Atrial Fibrillation (HOT CAFE) Study. *Chest* 2004;126:476-486.

16. Honloser SH, Kuck KH, Lilienthal J. Rhythm or rate control in atrial fibrillation—Pharmacological Intervention in Atrial Fibrillation (PIAF): a randomised trial. *Lancet* 2000;356:1789-1794.

17. Anderson JL, Halperin JL, Albert NM, et al. Management of patients with atrial fibrillation (compilation of 2006 ACCF/AHA/ESC and 2011 ACCF/AHA/HRS recommendations): a report of the American College of Cardiology/American Heart Association Task Force on Practice Guidelines. *J Am Coll Cardiol* 2013;61:1935-1944.

18. Nichol G, McAlister F, Pham B, et al. Meta-analysis of randomized controlled trials of the effectiveness of antiarrhythmic agents at promoting sinus rhythm in patients with atrial fibrillation. *Heart* 2002;87:535-543.

19. Echt DS, Liebson PR, Mitchell LB, et al. Mortality and morbidity in patients receiving encainide, flecainide, or placebo. The Cardiac Arrhythmia Suppression Trial. *N Engl J Med* 1991;324:781-788.

20. Torp-Pedersen C, Moller M, Bloch-Thomsen PE, et al. Dofetilide in patients with congestive heart failure and left ventricular dysfunction. Danish Investigations of Arrhythmia and Mortality on Dofetilide Study Group. *N Engl J Med* 1999;341:857-865.

21. Singh SN, Fletcher RD, Fisher SG, et al. Amiodarone in patients with congestive heart failure and asymptomatic ventricular arrhythmia. Survival Trial of Antiarrhythmic Therapy in Congestive Heart Failure. *N Engl J Med* 1995;333:77-82.

22. Wolf PA, Abbott RD, Kannel WB. Atrial Fibrillation as an independent risk factor for stroke: the Framingham Study. *Stroke* 1991;22:983-988.

23. Connlly SJ, Ezekowitz MD, Yusuf S, et al. Dabigatran versus warfarin in patients with atrial fibrillation. *N Engl J Med* 2009;361:1139-1151.

24. Patel MR, Mahaffey KW, Garg J, et al. Rivaroxaban versus warfarin in Nonvalvular atrial fibrillation. *N Engl J Med* 2011;365:883-891.

QT Syndromes

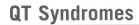

27

Andrew J. Krainik and Preben Bjerregaard

Long QT Syndromes

GENERAL PRINCIPLES

- **Long QT syndromes** (LQTSs) are characterized by prolongation of the QT interval on the surface electrocardiogram (ECG).[1] Syncope and sudden cardiac arrest are usually the result of ventricular arrhythmias (especially **torsades de pointes**).
- Although the LQTS was initially described as a rare inheritable condition, acquired prolongation of the QT interval (through pharmacologic effect) is now commonly recognized as an important etiology.
- Congenital LQTS is a genetic **cardiac ion channelopathy**, whereas acquired LQTS represents alteration of a functioning ion channel by an exogenous factor, typically a drug or electrolyte abnormality.
- The first cases of LQTS were reported in 1957 by Jervell and Lange-Nielsen, who described arrhythmogenic prolongation of the QT interval in association with congenital deafness (**Jervell** and **Lange-Nielsen syndrome**). Subsequently, Romano and Ward described the complex in the presence of normal hearing (**Romano–Ward syndrome**).
- Prior to genotyping, two additional syndromes, Andersen–Tawil syndrome and Timothy syndrome, have been classified as LQTS, though with vastly different clinical features.
- The genetic basis of congenital LQTS was determined in the 1990s, when mutations in cardiac Na^+ and K^+ channels were found to result in prolongation of the QT interval.[2]
- The mechanism of arrhythmia and sudden cardiac arrest is similar in both forms.

Definition

- The syndrome is defined by electrocardiographic measurement of the QT interval on the 12-lead surface ECG (Figure 27-1).
  - The QT is usually measured in lead II or lead V_5 but should reflect the **longest QT interval found in any lead**.
  - Because of the direct influence of heart rate on the QT, it is advisable to correct the measurement (QTc), as with **Bazett formula** (QTc $= QT/\sqrt{RR}$**).** This method, however, is known to underestimate the QT interval in bradycardia and to overestimate the QT interval in tachycardia.
- **Upper limits of normal** for the QTc interval are often less than 440 milliseconds for men and 460 milliseconds for women. A **shorthand rule for estimating QTc** has been described: At heart rates of 70 and greater, the QTc is not prolonged if the QT is less than one-half of the RR interval.[3]
- The syndrome may also be defined by the **presence of mutations in specific ion channels** (see Classification), even in the presence of normal QT intervals. Furthermore, a subset of patients are thought to have **"latent" LQTS**, whereby prolongation of the QT is seen only with sympathetic stimulation, exercise, or specific triggers.

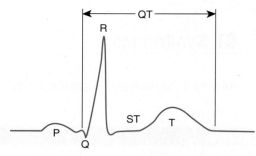

FIGURE 27-1. Surface electrocardiogram with identified deflections and measurement of the QT interval. (From Morita H, Wu J, Zipes DP. The QT syndromes: long and short. *Lancet* 2008;372:750-763, with permission.)

- The acquired form of LQTS requires the involvement of a characteristic pharmacologic agent or electrolyte abnormality.

Classification
- Prolongation of the QT interval is broadly categorized etiologically as **inherited or congenital** or **acquired**.
- The congenital LQTS is categorized by the specific genetic mutation involved in the patient (see Diagnostic Testing). There are at least 10 described subtypes at present.
- Other medical conditions that may be accompanied by a prolonged QT interval include **post-myocardial infarction**, **hypertrophic cardiomyopathy**, **dilated cardiomyopathy**, **myocarditis**, **hypothyroidism**, **pheochromocytoma**, **subarachnoid hemorrhage**, and **takotsubo cardiomyopathy**.

Epidemiology
- Initial estimates of the **prevalence** of congenital LQTS ranged from 1:5,000 to 1:10,000. However, with the development of mutation-specific genotyping, recent studies have suggested significantly higher rates, with one study of neonates suggesting a prevalence approaching 1:2,000.[4]
- Studies have estimated the **incidence** of sudden cardiac death as between 1,000 and 2,000 events in the United States annually. Estimates of aborted arrest and syncope are difficult to ascertain.

Pathophysiology
- The duration of the QT interval represents the duration of ventricular depolarization and repolarization and is related to the duration of the action potentials of the ventricular myocardial cells.
- The **cardiac action potential** is related to the transmembrane flux of ion currents through specific channels, especially the inward flow of Na^+ and Ca^{2+} currents and the outward flow of K^+ currents (Figure 27-2).
- Clinically, prolongation of the QT interval is a reflection of prolonged cardiac action potentials caused by either a **loss of function of potassium channels** or a **gain of function of sodium channels**.
  - Lengthening of the action potential, which is often inhomogeneous, can lead to perturbation of repolarization in the form of **early after depolarizations** (EADs).

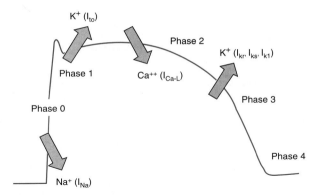

FIGURE 27-2. Phases of the cardiac action potential with associated ion currents. Downward-facing arrows indicate inward (depolarizing) currents and upward-facing arrows indicate (repolarizing) outward currents. (From Morita H, Wu J, Zipes DP. The QT syndromes: long and short. *Lancet* 2008;372:750-763, with permission.)

- ○ EADs can initiate a triggered activity, which may stimulate neighboring myocytes and lead to a ventricular premature depolarization (VPD). Such a VPD occurring very early can create local reentrant excitation.
- ○ In a heart with QT prolongation and dispersion of repolarization, such a local reentrant excitation can then propagate into **polymorphic ventricular tachycardia** often in the form of **torsades de pointes**.[5]
- Torsades de pointes is usually seen following a sequence of **long–short R-R interval**, where a VPD (the short interval) follows a pause (the long interval) which may be compensatory, following another VPD.
- Another phenomenon connected to torsades de pointes is beat-to-beat amplitude variation in the T-waves **(T-wave alternans)** during variable time prior to the arrhythmic event and therefore a sign of a high risk of torsades de pointes.
- **Repolarization reserve** is a concept that has been proposed to explain the interplay of various congenital and acquired factors in determining the variable clinical manifestations of the syndrome.[6]
  - ○ It suggests that redundancy in ion channels and their respective currents involved in repolarization provides a measure of safety.
  - ○ Patients with "poor" repolarization reserve may be especially susceptible to arrhythmia when exposed to QT-prolonging agents or sympathetic stimulation.

DIAGNOSIS

Clinical Presentation

- Patients may present in adolescence and early adulthood with variable complaints related to ventricular arrhythmia, often with **unexplained syncope** and **sudden cardiac arrest**.
- Congenital LQTS is now known, via postmortem molecular genetic studies, to affect a significant portion of infants who die unexpectedly (sudden infant death syndrome).[7]
- A history of seizures, often representing a missed diagnosis of ventricular fibrillation, should increase suspicion.
- A thorough family history, including unexpected sudden cardiac death, syncope, diagnoses of LQTS, and defibrillator implantation, is necessary.

- Medications, especially those recently prescribed, should be reviewed for potential QT-prolonging effect. Patients with acquired LQTS are often taking multiple medications with QT-prolonging effects. Prompt recognition of common QT-prolonging agents is critical in preventing arrhythmia in patients with **polypharmacy**.

Diagnostic Criteria

- Recognition of the syndrome is based on ECG characteristics (see Definition).
- Diagnostic criteria that incorporate ECG findings, clinical history, and family history were published before the advent of genetic testing and are listed in Table 27-1.[8] This involves a point-scoring system in which greater than 3 points indicates high probability of LQTS, 2 to 3 points indicates intermediate probability, and 0 to 1 indicates low probability.

Diagnostic Testing

- **Mutation-specific genotyping** is commercially available and should be considered in patients with appropriate ECG criteria and history.
  - Opinion still varies with regard to the appropriate use of genetic testing. In the author's experience, patients should have at least intermediate probability of LQTS and be well acquainted with the information garnered from testing, as well as how it will be used.

TABLE 27-1	DIAGNOSTIC CRITERIA FOR LONG QT SYNDROME

ECG findings	Points
QTc	
≥480 ms	3
460–470 ms	2
450 ms (in men)	2
Torsades de pointes	2
T-wave alternans	1
Notched T-waves (three leads)	1
Low heart rate for age	0.5
Clinical history	
Syncope	
With stress	2
Without stress	1
Congenital deafness	0.5
Family history	
Family member with definite LQTS	1
Unexplained sudden cardiac death before age 30 in immediate family members	0.5

ECG, electrocardiogram; LQTS, long QT syndrome.
Modified from Schwartz PJ, Moss AJ, Vincent GM, Crampton RS. Diagnostic criteria for the long QT syndrome. An update. *Circulation* 1993;88:782-784, with permission.

○ If a familial mutation is known to exist, genetic testing can be tailored to the specific mutation.

○ Patients with borderline QT intervals (440 to 460 milliseconds) and a highly suspicious history may be further tested with epinephrine infusion and continuous electrocardiographic monitoring, with the goal to unmask latent QT prolongation.[9]

○ The majority of cases of LQTS are classified as LQT1, LQT2, or LQT3. Phenotypic features of each specific genetic mutation are reviewed in the following sections.

○ Specific genes, ion channels, and phenotypic features are listed in Table 27-2.[10]

○ **LQT1 is the most common genetic variant** of LQTS, comprising approximately 33% to 45% of genotyped cases.

  ▪ Clinical features involve syncope and **adrenergic-triggered arrhythmia** including **exercise. Swimming** is a commonly reported situation preceding events. Because of the association with adrenergic stimulation, epinephrine infusion may be particularly useful in "unmasking" patients with latent LQT1 for diagnostic purposes.

  ▪ The characteristic T-wave in LQT1 is **broad-based** and **monophasic.**

  ▪ The gene involved in LQT1 is **KCNQ1** and the affected channel is believed to be the **voltage-gated potassium ion channel Ik_s,** responsible for the delayed rectifier current of the action potential. Mutations in KCNQ1 can be inherited in an autosomal-dominant or autosomal-recessive pattern. The autosomal-recessive form is sometimes associated with profound deafness; this is referred to as the Jervell and Lange-Nielsen syndrome.

○ **LQT2 is the second most common genetic variant**, comprising 25% to 35% of genotyped patients.

  ▪ Clinically, events are often triggered by **loud sounds and cognitive stress,** believed to result in sudden changes in sympathetic discharge.

  ▪ The characteristic T-wave of LQT2 is **flat and bifid.**

  ▪ The gene involved in LQT2 is **KCNH2** (sometimes referred to as HERG), responsible for the rapid component of **potassium-rectifying current Ik_r.**

TABLE 27-2 CHANNELOPATHIES AND THE LONG QT SYNDROME

LQTS	Chromosome	Gene	Protein	Current
1	11p15.5	KCNQ1	KvLQT1	I_{Ks}
2	7q35-36	KCNH2	HERG	I_{Kr}
3	3p24-21	SCN5A	Nav1.5	I_{Na}
4	4q24-27	ANK2	Ankyrin-B	I_{Na-K}, I_{Na-Ca}, I_{Na}
5	21q22	KCNE1	MinK	I_{Ks}
6	21q22	KCNE2	MiRP1	I_{Kr}
7	17q23	KCNJ2	Kir2.1	I_{K1}
8	12p13.3	CACNA1C	Cav1.2	I_{Ca}
9	3p25.3	CAV3	Caveolin-3	I_{Na}
10	11q23.3	SCN4B	NaVβ4	I_{Na}

LQTS, long QT syndrome.
Modified from Morita H, Wu J, Zipes DP. The QT syndromes: long and short. *Lancet* 2008;372: 750-763.

Normally, the Ik_r current is involved in the terminal portion of the action potential and allows protection against EADs.

- ○ **LQT3** occurs in 2% to 8% of genotyped patients with LQTS.
  - ▪ Clinically, events leading to sudden cardiac arrest occur during **rest, especially at night**. Adrenergic stimulation is involved in about 20% of cardiac events in LQT3.
  - ▪ Characteristic ECG changes in LQT3 include a **long isoelectric ST segment, followed by a narrow-peaked T-wave**.
  - ▪ The gene involved in LQT3 is **SCN5A**, resulting in a **gain-of-function** Na$^+$ current, resulting in prolongation of the plateau of the cardiac action potential.
- • The **risk of subsequent event** (syncope or sudden cardiac arrest) following the diagnosis of LQTS is variable, and high-risk features have been reported (Table 27-3).
  - ○ **Length of QT interval is a powerful predictor of events**, with risk of arrhythmia increasing exponentially with QT prolongation.
  - ○ When QT interval measurement is combined with genetic mutation, risk stratification is greatly enhanced and is valuable in guiding therapy (Table 27-4).[11]

TREATMENT

- • In all patients with prolongation of the QT interval, **electrolyte abnormalities** should be sought and corrected as possible, especially low serum **potassium** and **magnesium**. Patients with chronically low levels of serum potassium and magnesium should be prescribed oral supplements.

TABLE 27-3	HIGH-RISK FACTORS PREDICTING VENTRICULAR ARRHYTHMIA OR EXCESSIVE QT PROLONGATION

ECG changes
   Long QT interval
   Increased QT variance (QTc > 500 ms)
   Increased interval from peak to end of T-wave
   T-wave alternans
   T-U waves
Electrolyte abnormalities
   Hypokalemia
   Hypomagnesemia
Female gender
Older age
HIV disease
LV systolic dysfunction
Previous history of drug-induced long QT or torsades de pointes
Relatives with history of drug-induced long QT

ECG, electrocardiogram; HIV, human immunodeficiency syndrome; LV, left ventricular.

TABLE 27-4	RISK STRATIFICATION FOR EVENTS BEFORE AGE 40, USING GENETIC AND ELECTROCARDIOGRAM DATA
High risk (≥50%)	QTc >500 ms and LQT1 or LQT2, and LQT3 (males)
Intermediate risk (30–49%)	QTc <500 ms and LQT2 (females) and LQT3 (male or females) QTc ≥500 ms and LQT3 (females)
Low risk (<30%)	QTc <500 ms and LQT1 (males) and LQT2 (males)

Data from Priori SG, Schwartz PJ, Napolitano C, et al. Risk stratification in the long-QT syndrome. *N Engl J Med* 2003;348:1866-1874.

- In patients with congenital LQTS, **strict avoidance of any medications with known QT-prolonging effects** should be endorsed. Patients should be educated and given access to this information, for instance, via the website www.qtdrugs.org (last accessed 8/5/13), which is managed and updated by the University of Arizona College of Pharmacy.
- In patients with acquired prolonged QT, suspected medications should be **discontinued** as soon as they are recognized.
- Often patients with acquired LQTSs require no further therapy beyond avoidance if the QT interval regresses to normal after discontinuation of the medication or correction of electrolyte abnormalities.
- **Exercise restriction** is generally recommended for any patient with congenital LQTS.

Medications

- **Pharmacologic arrhythmia suppression** is the pillar of therapy for patients with congenital LQTS.
- **β-Adrenergic blockade** has been demonstrated to be very effective in certain genetic variants (LQT1), but less effective in others (LQT2).[12]
  - β-Blockers may be **particularly useful in preventing symptoms in LQT1**.
  - β-Blockers have mixed results in the prevention of events in LQT2, producing the competing effects of adrenergic suppression (antiarrhythmic) and bradycardia (proarrhythmic).
  - β-Adrenergic blockade is less effective in LQT3.
  - Propranolol and nadolol, titrated to tolerated doses, are the β-blockers of choice.
- **Mexiletine and flecainide may both be beneficial in the treatment of LQT3.**
  - **Mexiletine**, a Vaughan-Williams class IB Na⁺ channel-blocking antiarrhythmic drug, may have clinical efficacy.
  - In patients with specific SCN5A mutations, **flecainide**, a class IC Na⁺ channel-blocking antiarrhythmic, may also provide benefit, though Brugada syndrome pattern ECGs have been reported in some patients.

Other Non-pharmacologic Therapies

- **Implantable cardioverter defibrillators** (ICDs) provide an effective means of terminating arrhythmia and are potentially life-saving in patients with LQTS.
- Defibrillator implantation should be considered in patients who are at **high risk for subsequent events** or who have experienced **resuscitated cardiac arrest**.
- Patients with **events despite optimal treatment** with medications should be considered for defibrillator implantation.

Surgical Management

- **Surgical interruption of the left cervical sympathetic chain** (stellate ganglionectomy) is a modality for suppression of arrhythmia that is currently under evaluation.
- The rationale for this procedure stems from the sympathetic/adrenergic component that often precedes events in patients with LQTS.
- Surgical interruption of the cardiac sympathetic nerve may also be effective for LQT1.

Acquired Prolongation of the QT Interval

- Knowledge of the proarrhythmic effects of certain medications like **quinidine** has long preceded the understanding brought about by the genetic and molecular studies of patients with LQTS.
- Variable risk of QT prolongation has been explained by the concept of **repolarization reserve** (see Pathophysiology). One of the extensions of this concept is the existence of different levels of susceptibility to excessive QT prolongation and torsades de pointes.
- Medications with QT-prolonging effects are exceedingly common, and clinicians should familiarize themselves with some of the most prescribed medications (Table 27-5).
  - Websites like www.qtdrugs.org (last accessed 8/5/13) maintain a comprehensive list of QT-prolonging agents.
  - A total of 2% to 3% of all medications have known QT-prolonging effects.
- **Torsades de pointes is more common with antiarrhythmic drugs**, occurring in 1% to 5%. With other QT-prolonging medications, torsades de pointes is rare, occurring in <0.1% of patients.
- Several clinical characteristics that predict drug-induced torsades de pointes have been described. These include **female gender, hypokalemia, bradycardia, recent conversion from atrial fibrillation (especially with a QT-prolonging antiarrhythmic drug), heart failure, digitalis use, baseline QT prolongation, subclinical congenital LQTS**, and **hypomagnesemia**.[13]
- Increasingly, the decision as to whether a QT-prolonging medication needs to be prescribed is being made by noncardiologists.

TABLE 27-5	COMMON MEDICATIONS KNOWN TO PROLONG THE QT INTERVAL

Antiarrhythmic drugs

Dofetilide, amiodarone, sotalol, quinidine, disopyramide, ibutilide

Antipsychotics

Chlorpromazine, haloperidol, thioridazine, clozapine, risperidone

Anti-infective agents

Clarithromycin, erythromycin, amantadine, azithromycin, gatifloxacin

Anti-emetics

Droperidol, ondansetron, granisetron

Antidepressants

Some serotonin reuptake inhibitors

Other

Cisapride, methadone, arsenic

○ If one of these medications is deemed necessary, it is important to warn the patient of the risk and instruct them to promptly report any symptoms of palpitations, dizziness, syncope, or presyncope.

○ Additionally, changes in condition that predispose to electrolyte abnormalities such as new medications (especially diuretics), nausea, vomiting, and diarrhea need to be reported.

Short QT Syndrome

GENERAL PRINCIPLES

- **Short QT syndrome** (SQTS) is a rare inherited condition characterized by abnormally short QT interval (Figure 27-3) and an increased risk of atrial and ventricular arrhythmia.[14]
- Originally described in 2000 (http://shortqtsyndrome.org, last accessed 8/5/13), only 53 patients in 14 families have been published. Of the 14 families, 9 of the probands presented with sudden cardiac arrest.

Definitions

- Like LQTS, SQTS is defined primarily by the ECG measurement of the QT interval on the 12-lead surface ECG (Figure 27-1).
- **Lower limit of normal for the QTc interval is 360 milliseconds in males and 370 milliseconds in females.**
- In patients diagnosed with SQTS, the **QTc interval has been** ≤345 milliseconds and the QT interval often <300 milliseconds.
- In addition to such a short QT interval, a family history of SQTS, or sudden cardiac death, documented atrial or ventricular fibrillation or symptoms suggesting atrial or ventricular fibrillation are important for making the diagnosis of SQTS.
- **Because the QT interval in SQTS is minimally affected by heart rate, Bazett formula will overcorrect the QT interval at heart rates >60 beats per minute (bpm), which in some cases (especially in children with faster heart rates) may lead to missing a diagnosis of SQTS.** The best way to make the ECG diagnosis of a short QT is, therefore, to measure the QT interval at a heart rate as close to 60 bpm as possible.

Pathophysiology

- SQTS has variable inheritance pattern just like LQTS and so far **mutations** responsible for SQTS have been found in the **KCNH2, KCNQ2,** and **KCNJ2** genes. This has

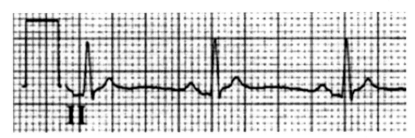

FIGURE 27-3. Lead II in the first patient described with SQTS; heart rate is 60 and QT interval is 230 milliseconds.

led to the definition of three syndromes, SQT1, SQT2, and SQT3, all with a gain of function of potassium currents (I_{Kr}, I_{Ks}, and I_{K1}) leading to shortened action potentials and thereby shortened QT interval. Many patients with the disease have not yet been genetically categorized.

- Shortening of the action potentials leads to shortened refractory periods and increased dispersion of refractoriness which in turn creates a substrate for reentry and tachyarrhythmias such as atrial and ventricular fibrillation.
- Some patients have shown various conduction system diseases in terms of right-bundle-branch block, left anterior hemiblock, and atrioventricular (AV) block.
- A special subcategory of SQTS is children born with atrial fibrillation and very slow ventricular response.
- QTc intervals between 345 and 360 milliseconds have been seen in some patients with **early repolarization, idiopathic ventricular fibrillation**, and **Brugada syndrome**, all of which convey an increased risk of sudden cardiac arrest.

Epidemiology

- **Very short QT intervals are very rare** in the general population. In a recent study of 106,432 hospitalized patients, none had a QTc of less than 300 milliseconds.[15]
- In the Framingham Study, 2 standard deviations below the mean QTc was 332 milliseconds in males and 344 milliseconds in females.[16]

Etiology

- SQTS is primarily an inherited condition; however, causes of secondary shortening of the QT are known.
- **Hypercalcemia** is a common cause of shortened QT intervals, often as an effect of **hyperparathyroidism, malignancy, renal disease**, and **medications**.
- Short QT intervals have also been reported in **chronic fatigue syndrome** and as reaction to **atropine** administration, **digoxin** intoxication, **enhanced catecholaminergic state**, and **hyperthermia**.

DIAGNOSIS

Clinical Presentation

- In the absence of a family history and ECG, historical information compatible with a diagnosis of SQTS is often nonspecific and is more likely to represent other processes.
- If the patient is **known to have a short QT interval**, complaints consistent with **atrial** or **ventricular tachyarrhythmia** strongly favor a diagnosis of SQTS.
- Patients may complain of **palpitations** and unheralded **syncope**.
- **Sudden cardiac arrest** is a possible presentation.

Diagnostic Testing

- Diagnosis is entirely reliant on successful **ECG recognition**. A short QT (**<360 milliseconds in males and <370 milliseconds in females**) is a rare finding and should prompt additional investigation into the etiology. **In SQTS patients the QTc has so far been ≤345 milliseconds.**
- **Tall, peaked T-waves** especially in left precordial leads are characteristic for some forms of SQTS.
- The lack of changes in QT interval with changes in heart rate is a typical feature in patients with SQTS.
- Effective refractory periods are very short in both atria and ventricles.
- Ventricular fibrillation is easily induced during electrophysiologic studies, often during positioning of the electrode catheter in the right ventricle.

- There are no clear guidelines on the evaluation of patients with suspected SQTS.
  - It is important to identify and treat secondary causes (see Etiology) of QT shortening when possible.
  - **Genetic testing** for known mutations can confirm the diagnosis of SQTS.
  - The utility of additional studies, including ambulatory monitoring and stress testing for assessment of QT/RR slope and invasive electrophysiologic testing for assessment of refractory periods, and inducibility of tachyarrhythmias are not well defined.

TREATMENT

- Currently, the only established treatment for SQTS is ICD implantation for the prevention of sudden cardiac death. The tall peaked T-waves have in some cases been problematic for sensing of the intracardiac electrogram causing double counting and inappropriate shocks.
- At present, no medications are thought to be reliable enough to forestall defibrillator placement in patients with confirmed SQTS.
  - The addition of antiarrhythmic drugs to device-based therapy may prove useful in patients with recurrent defibrillator shocks.
  - **Quinidine** has been proposed as possible treatment of SQTS. It is thought to be effective through blockade of I_{Kr} producing channels, thus prolonging the action potential.
  - **Flecainide and propafenone** have been suggested as a second choice of drugs for the treatment of atrial fibrillation due to their effect of prolonging the refractory period in both the atria and ventricles.

REFERENCES

1. Moss AJ, Schwartz PJ, Crampton RS, et al. The long QT syndrome: prospective longitudinal study of 328 families. *Circulation* 1991;84:1136-1144.
2. Splawski I, Shen J, Timothy KW, et al. Spectrum of mutations in long QT syndrome genes: KCNQ1, HERG, SCN5A, KCNE1, and KCNE2. *Circulation* 2000;102:1178-1185.
3. Phoon CK. Mathematic validation of a shorthand rule for calculating QTc. *Am J Cardiol* 1998;82:400-402.
4. Schwartz PJ, Stramba-Badiale M, Crotti L, et al. Prevalence of the congenital long QT syndrome. *Circulation* 2009;120:1761-1767.
5. Viskin S, Alla SR, Barron HV, et al. Mode of onset of torsade de pointes in congenital long QT syndrome. *J Am Coll Cardiol* 1996;28:1262-1268.
6. Roden DM. Taking the "idio" out of "idiosyncratic": predicting torsades de pointes. *Pacing Clin Electrophysiol* 1998;21:1029-1034.
7. Arnestad M, Crotti L, Rognum TO, et al. Prevalence of long-QT syndrome gene variants in sudden infant death syndrome. *Circulation* 2007;115:361-367.
8. Schwartz PJ, Moss AJ, Vincent GM, Crampton RS. Diagnostic criteria for the long QT syndrome. An update. *Circulation* 1993;88:782-784.
9. Vyas H, Hejlik J, Ackerman MJ. Epinephrine QT stress testing in the evaluation of congenital long-QT syndrome diagnostic accuracy of the paradoxical QT response. *Circulation* 2006;113:1385-1392.
10. Morita H, Wu J, Zipes DP. The QT syndromes: long and short. *Lancet* 2008;372:750-763.
11. Priori SG, Schwartz PG, Napolitano C, et al. Risk stratification in the long-QT syndrome. *N Engl J Med* 2003;348:1866-1874.
12. Priori SG, Napolitano C, Schwartz PJ, et al. Association of long QT syndrome loci and cardiac events among patients treated with β-blockers. *JAMA* 2004;292:1341-1344.
13. Roden DM. Drug-induced prolongation of the QT interval. *N Engl J Med* 2004;350:1013-1022.
14. Bjerregaard P, Nallapaneni H, Gussak I. Short QT interval in clinical practice. *J Electrocard* 2010;43:390-395.
15. Reinig MG, Engel TR. The shortage of short QT intervals. *Chest* 2007;132:246-249.
16. Sagie A, Larson MG, Goldberg RJ, et al. An improved method for adjusting the QT interval for heart rate (the Framingham Heart Study). *Am J Cardiol* 1992;70:797-801.

Peripheral Arterial Disease

C. Huie Lin and Jasvindar Singh

- Importance of peripheral arterial disease (PAD) has been increasingly recognized: Prevalence of the disease may be as high as 29% in patients with risk factors.[1]
- PAD is associated with 4% to 5% per year risk of myocardial infarction (MI), cerebrovascular accident (CVA), and vascular death.[1]
- This chapter will primarily focus on vascular disease processes that lead to ischemia of the lower extremity, kidney, and carotid artery territories.
- PAD consists of a group of disorders that lead to progressive stenosis, occlusion, or aneurysmal dilation of the aorta and its noncoronary branch arteries, including the carotid artery, upper extremity, visceral, and lower extremity arterial branches.

Lower Extremity Peripheral Arterial Disease

GENERAL PRINCIPLES

Classification

- Patients with lower extremity PAD range from those who are asymptomatic to those with acute limb-threatening emergencies. The clinician must differentiate between the severity of symptoms in deciding on further workup and the urgency of a treatment plan.
- Lower extremity PAD is commonly defined by presentation:
  - Asymptomatic
  - Claudication
  - Critical limb ischemia (CLI)
  - Acute limb ischemia (ALI)

Epidemiology

- Prevalence of PAD has been estimated at 3% to 10% of the population, based on ankle–brachial testing. This increases to 15% to 20% in persons aged greater than 70 years.[2]
- In a high-risk patient population aged greater than 50 to 69 years with a history of cigarette smoking or diabetes, the prevalence of PAD is estimated at 29%.[3]

Etiology

The most common cause of PAD is atherosclerosis (Table 28-1).

Risk Factors

- **The major cause of lower extremity PAD is atherosclerosis**, with identified risk factors of smoking, diabetes, hypertension, hyperlipidemia, hyperhomocysteinemia, and family history of coronary artery disease (CAD).

| TABLE 28-1 | ETIOLOGY OF PERIPHERAL ARTERIAL DISEASE |

- Atherosclerosis
- Connective tissue diseases
  - Marfan syndrome
  - Ehlers–Danlos syndrome
- Dysplastic disease
  - Fibromuscular dysplasia
- Vasculitic diseases
  - Large vessels: Giant-cell (temporal) arteritis, Takayasu arteritis
  - Medium-sized vessels: Kawasaki disease, polyarteritis nodosa
  - Small vessel disease (arterioles and microvessels), Wegener granulomatosis, microscopic polyangiitis, Churg–Strauss syndrome, Henoch–Schönlein purpura, cryoglobulinaemic vasculitis
  - Thromboangiitis obliterans (Buerger disease)
- Prothrombotic diseases
- Vasospastic diseases

- Cigarette smoking is a significant dose-dependent contributor to the development of lower extremity PAD. **More than 80% of patients are current or former smokers,** and a cigarette smoker is two to three times more likely to have lower extremity PAD than detectable CAD.[1]

Associated Conditions

- Although PAD can cause significant morbidity, the shared pathophysiology and risk factors between PAD and CAD mean that the **majority of these patients will die from cardiovascular diseases such as MI or ischemic stroke.**
- Patients with lower extremity PAD have a twofold to sixfold increased risk of death due to coronary heart disease events and are four to five times more likely to have a stroke or transient ischemic attack (TIA).[1]

DIAGNOSIS

Clinical Presentation

- **Asymptomatic** lower extremity PAD:
  - Limb function is not necessarily normal.
  - Patients may not have classic exertional limb discomfort but may have less typical symptoms, such as decreased walking speed or poor balance.
- **Claudication:**
  - Claudication symptoms are due to exercise-induced ischemia.
  - Symptoms of chronic lower extremity atherosclerotic occlusion are variable but are frequently described as **reproducible cramping or fatigue with walking**, with resolution shortly after rest.

○ Symptoms may occur anywhere in the lower extremity, including buttocks, thighs, or calves.
- **Critical limb ischemia:**
  ○ CLI is limb pain that occurs at rest (**rest pain**) or **impending limb loss** that is caused by severe compromise of blood flow to the affected extremity.
  ○ This term should be used to describe all patients **with chronic pain at rest, ulcers, or gangrene** attributable to objectively proven arterial occlusive disease.
- **Acute limb ischemia:**
  ○ ALI is caused by a sudden decrease in limb perfusion that threatens tissue viability. Symptoms occur as a result of thrombosis of an atherosclerotic plaque or a lower extremity embolism, frequently of cardiac or aortic origin.
  ○ The typical symptoms and signs of ALI include "the six P's:" **pain, paralysis, paresthesias, pulselessness, pallor,** and **polar (cold).**

History

- Asymptomatic patients aged ≥50 years with cardiovascular risk factors and all patients ≥70 years should be asked about walking impairment, rest pain, and nonhealing wounds. If positive, further testing should be initiated.
- Claudication can be confused with pseudoclaudication from spinal stenosis. Classically, limb discomfort associated with spinal stenosis is not reliably reproduced with exertion; it is exacerbated by standing and relieved only by sitting.
- CLI usually presents with rest pain that is worse while lying in a supine position. Patients with CLI will often maintain limbs in a dependent position and are frequently unable to walk.
- As described above, typical symptoms and signs of ALI include "the six P's:" **pain, paralysis, paresthesias, pulselessness, pallor,** and **polar (cold).**

Physical Examination

- Visualization:
  ○ Capillary refill
  ○ Nonhealing wounds or ulcers
  ○ Livedo reticularis (for atheroembolization)
  ○ Calf atrophy
  ○ Alopecia over the dorsum of the foot
- Auscultation and palpation: Bruits over major vascular beds as well as palpation of peripheral pulses over the femoral, popliteal, posterior tibial, and dorsalis pedis arteries (Figure 28-1). The presence of a bruit or a thrill only describes turbulent flow but does not confirm arterial stenosis. In addition, both the volume and the quality of the peripheral pulses should be noted.
- **Elevation-dependency test:**
  ○ This is a screening maneuver, which can be performed by elevating the lower extremities to 60 degrees above horizontal while the patient is supine. Development of pallor in the sole of the foot indicates arterial disease in that extremity.
  ○ After the patient is sitting upright with legs hanging off the examination table, delayed return of color and venous engorgement in either lower extremity may confirm inadequate circulation.
  ○ With more advanced disease, a deep red color develops along with dependent edema, so-called **dependent rubor.**

Diagnostic Testing

- All patients with symptomatic claudication should undergo measurement of the **ankle-brachial index** (ABI) to confirm the diagnosis and to establish a baseline result (Figure 28-2).[1,2,4-6]

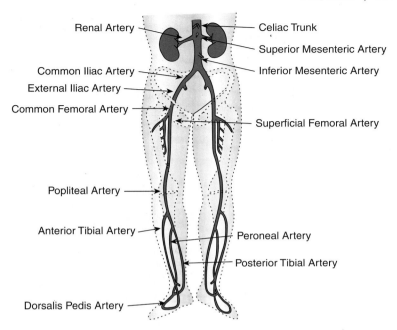

FIGURE 28-1. Diagram of major branches of lower extremity peripheral arterial anatomy.

- ○ Advanced age and diabetes mellitus contribute to vessel rigidity and make the ABI test less reliable. When this occurs, a toe-brachial index (TBI) can be used instead.
  - ▪ Toe pressures <30 mmHg indicate ischemia, impaired wound healing, and increased risk of amputation.
  - ▪ An ABI <0.9 and a TBI of <0.7 are considered diagnostic of lower extremity PAD.
  - ▪ For the purposes of coronary risk estimation and lipid management, an ABI <0.90 is considered a coronary risk equivalent even in asymptomatic patients.[7]
- ○ If the resting ABI is normal and clinical suspicion is high, ABI can be repeated after exercise or **plantar flexion test**. While standing, the patient raises his or her heels off the ground, standing on tip-toe and then returns to the normal position. When symptoms develop or after 50 repetitions, the ABI is repeated.
- ○ **Segmental limb pressure examination** may be helpful to further identify the location and extent of lower extremity PAD. Cuffs are placed on the upper thigh, lower thigh, and upper calf. A drop of 20 mmHg in the systolic pressure between segments is consistent with arterial stenosis.
- ○ **Pulse volume recordings** use pneumoplethysmography to identify changes in pulse contour and amplitude. In the presence of arterial disease, the slope flattens, the pulse width widens, and the dicrotic notch is lost.
- • **Duplex ultrasonography:**
  - ○ Duplex ultrasonography combines Doppler velocity and waveform analysis with gray-scale visualization of the arterial wall.
  - ○ A normal waveform is triphasic, with forward flow in cardiac systole followed by a brief flow reversal in early diastole followed by forward flow in late diastole.

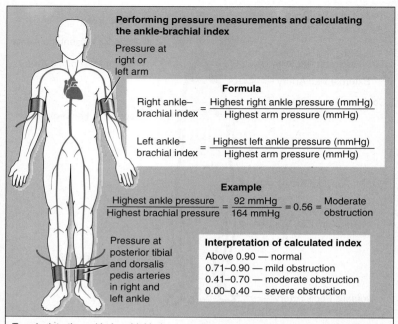

To calculate the ankle-brachial index, systolic pressures are determined in both arms and both ankles with the use of a hand-held Doppler instrument. The highest readings for the dorsalis pedis and posterior tibial arteries are used to calculate the index.

FIGURE 28-2. Performing pressure measurements and calculating the ankle-brachial index. (From White C. Intermittent claudication. *N Engl J Med* 2007;356:1241-1250, with permission.)

- ○ With arterial stenosis, distal blood flow velocities increase. In severe stenosis, the flow-reversal component is absent as well (Figure 28-3).[8] The degree of stenosis is determined by combining waveform analysis and measurement of the peak systolic velocity.
- For specific anatomic delineation to guide revascularization, additional imaging with **computed tomography (CT)**, **magnetic resonance angiography (MRA)**, or **digital subtraction angiography** can be used.
  - ○ **Digital subtraction angiography** (Figure 28-4) remains the gold standard test but it is invasive and carries risks related to the use of contrast and radiation exposure.
  - ○ **CT angiography** is rapid and noninvasive but carries similar contrast and radiation risks. Calcium found in atherosclerotic lesions can create so-called blooming artifacts, rendering images less accurate.
  - ○ **MRA** carries fewer risks and gives detailed information, although prior stent placement can affect image quality.

TREATMENT

- The primary goal should be prevention of the development of PAD through **risk-factor modification**, especially smoking cessation.[1,2,5,6]

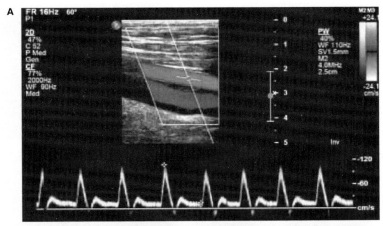

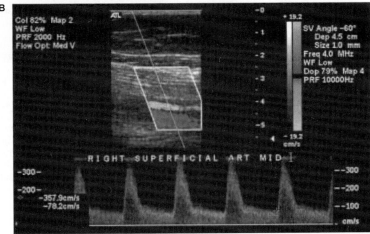

FIGURE 28-3. Doppler arterial waveforms from patients without **(A)** and with **(B)** PAD. In the setting of PAD, the peak systolic velocity increases and the diastolic flow reversal is lost. (From Begelman SM, Jaff MR. Noninvasive diagnostic strategies for peripheral arterial disease. *Cleve Clin J Med* 2006;73:S22-S29, with permission.)

- When prevention fails, early detection and lifestyle modification, along with medical and, in some cases, mechanical reperfusion therapy should be combined to maintain and improve quality of life and to avoid limb- and life-threatening progression.

Medications
- Antiplatelet therapy:[1,2,5,6,9]
  - **Aspirin** (75 to 325 mg daily) or
  - **Clopidogrel** (75 mg daily)

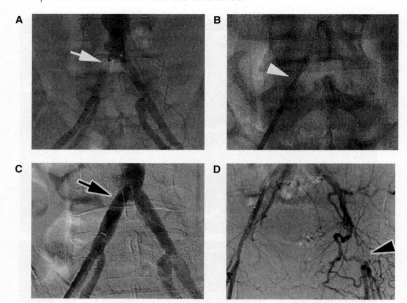

FIGURE 28-4. Lower extremity peripheral arterial disease angiography and percutaneous intervention. **(A)** Severe hazy lesion in the ostial right common iliac artery (white arrow). A marker pigtail has been used to perform angiography to allow assessment of lesion length. **(B)** Deployment of a 7.0 × 16-mm Racer bare metal stent (Medtronic, Minneapolis) in the right common iliac lesion (white arrowhead). **(C)** Post–stent digital subtraction angiography demonstrates brisk flow through the stent (black arrow) and patency of the right common iliac artery. **(D)** Digital subtraction angiography demonstrating a chronic total occlusion of the left common femoral artery (black arrowhead) with well-developed collaterals in the same patient.

- **Cilostazol**, a phosphodiesterase type 3 inhibitor, has both vasodilatory and platelet-inhibitory properties and has been shown to improve walking distance by about 50% compared with placebo.[1,2,5,6,10] Because other phosphodiesterase inhibitors are associated with an increased mortality in patients with heart failure, care should be taken to avoid cilostazol in patients with left ventricular dysfunction.
- The efficacy of pentoxifylline remains uncertain.[11]
- **Lipid-lowering therapy** (statins) for a goal low-density-lipoprotein cholesterol level <100 mg/dL.[1,2,5,6]
- **Antihypertensive therapy** (angiotensin-converting enzyme [ACE] inhibitor and/or β-blocker) for a goal blood pressure <140/90 mmHg or <130/80 mmHg with diabetes.[1,2,5,6]
- **Glucose control** with goal hemoglobin A1c <7%.[1,2,5,6]

Other Nonpharmacologic Therapies

- Smoking cessation[1,2,5,6]
- Daily foot inspection and proper foot care

- **S**upervised **exercise program**: Improvements in functional capacity occur over several months. Trials of ≥30 minutes of exercise three times per week led to a 150% improvement in maximal walking ability.[1,12]

Surgical Management

- For symptomatic patients with claudication that causes limitations in quality of life or vocational ability and who do not respond adequately to a supervised exercise program and medical management, a **revascularization procedure** may be considered.
- **Endovascular treatments** such as percutaneous transluminal angioplasty (PTA) with or without stenting (Figure 28-4), catheter-based thrombolysis, mechanical thrombectomy, and open surgical procedures are reasonable treatment options based on comorbidities and vascular anatomy.
- Approximately 5% of patients with intermittent claudication will require a revascularization intervention for severe symptoms or progression to CLI, and only 2% will ultimately require amputation for distal ischemia. In contrast, nearly half of patients with CLI will require revascularization for limb salvage.[1]

REFERRAL

- For rapid disease progression, urgent referral to a vascular specialist is warranted to limit the extent of tissues necrosis and increase the chance of limb salvage.
- If signs of ALI are present (the six P's), the vascular consult is emergent, and immediate concerns should address anticoagulation to prevent the propagation of thrombus material and initiate plans for urgent or emergent revascularization.

MONITORING/FOLLOW-UP

- Clinically stable patients should be regularly evaluated with history and physical examination as well as noninvasive studies such as ABI.
- Patients with progressive symptoms may require more intense evaluation including imaging or invasive angiography.
- All patients with PAD require regular follow-up for continued medical management of both the primary disease and secondary cardiovascular disease.

Renal Artery Stenosis

GENERAL PRINCIPLES

Epidemiology

- Renovascular hypertension resulting from renal artery stenosis (RAS) is the **most common correctable cause of secondary hypertension**.
- In patients undergoing cardiac catheterization, the prevalence of RAS may be as high as 30%, with lesions >50% found in 11% to 18%.[1]

Etiology

- **Atherosclerotic disease is the cause of most RAS.** Less common causes of RAS are listed in Table 28-2.
- Fibromuscular dysplasia (FMD) is the second most common cause of RAS. Although occurring in both genders, the typical presentation of FMD is that of hypertension in a young woman.

TABLE 28-2	CAUSES OF RENAL ARTERY STENOSIS

- Atherosclerosis
- Fibromuscular dysplasia
- Renal artery aneurysms
- Aortic or renal artery dissection
- Vasculitis
- Thrombotic or cholesterol embolization
- Collagen vascular disease
- Retroperitoneal fibrosis
- Trauma
- Posttransplantation stenosis
- Postradiation

Pathophysiology

- Renal hypoperfusion leads to **activation of the renin–angiotensin system**. The vasoactive properties of aldosterone and angiotensin II lead to volume expansion and elevated systemic blood pressures.
- Progression of high-grade RAS can result in **loss of renal function**, mass, and ultimately ischemic nephropathy.
- Atherosclerotic RAS tends to involve the ostium of the renal arteries and the aorta.
- FMD involves the mid- and distal renal artery and may extend into the side branches. The characteristic "string of beads" appearance (Figure 28-5) and location within the renal artery help to differentiate FMD from atherosclerotic RAS. FMD can also affect other arterial beds, especially the carotid and vertebral arteries.

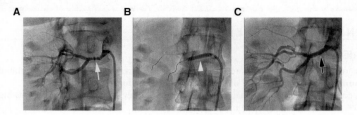

FIGURE 28-5. Fibromuscular dysplasia of the renal artery in a patient with severe refractory hypertension. **(A)** Invasive angiography of the right renal artery with classic "beads-on-a-string" stenotic appearance (white arrow) of the right renal artery. **(B)** Inflation of a 4.0 × 20 mm Angiosculpt (Angioscore, Freemont) scoring angioplasty balloon (white arrowhead) to treat the stenotic lesion. **(C)** Final postintervention angiography reveals brisk flow through the right renal artery lesion (black arrow) following further dilatation with a noncompliant angioplasty balloon.

DIAGNOSIS

Clinical Presentation

- RAS may be clinically silent in many individuals.
- **Severe hypertension** and **fluid retention** are the hallmark findings of RAS. Clinical features that should prompt evaluation for RAS include[1]:
  - Onset of hypertension before the age of 30 years
  - Onset of severe hypertension after the age of 55 years
  - Accelerated hypertension (sudden and persistent worsening of previously controlled hypertension)
  - Resistant hypertension (refractory despite three drugs, one of which must be a diuretic)
  - Malignant hypertension (coexistent evidence of acute end-organ damage)
  - Worsening renal function after the administration of an ACE inhibitor or angiotensin receptor blocker (ARB)
  - An unexplained atrophic kidney or >1.5-cm size discrepancy between the two kidneys
  - Sudden unexplained pulmonary edema

Diagnostic Testing[1]

- **Duplex ultrasonography** with Doppler is recommended as an initial test for the detection of RAS.
- **CT or MRA** can define lesion characteristics and is helpful in imaging patients in whom ultrasonography proves difficult.
  - CT uses nephrotoxic contrast, which can be particularly risky in a RAS population.
  - MRA uses gadolinium contrast, traditionally thought to be less nephrotoxic than CT contrast. However, an association with gadolinium and nephrogenic systemic fibrosis has raised concerns in patients with significant renal impairment.
- If initial tests are inconclusive or considered too risky, **catheter angiography** could be considered for definitive diagnosis.
- Owing to the **high prevalence of atherosclerotic RAS in patients with lower extremity PAD and CAD**, a renal angiogram should be considered in patients with CAD and clinical suspicion for RAS who are already undergoing invasive angiography.[13]
- Because of the association with cerebral aneurysms, all patients with renal FMD should undergo MRA screening or CT angiography of the head.

TREATMENT

Medications

- Medical treatment for atherosclerotic RAS focuses mainly on **controlling renovascular hypertension**.[1]
- ACE inhibitors and ARBs should be avoided in bilateral RAS, as these drugs may contribute to worsening the physiologic consequences of RAS.

Surgical Management

- A revascularization strategy may be considered for **hemodynamically significant RAS**, defined as (1) ≥50% to 70% diameter stenosis by visual estimation with a peak translesional gradient of >20 mmHg or a mean gradient ≥10 mmHg with 5-Fr catheter or pressure wire or (2) any stenosis ≥70% diameter stenosis or (3) ≥70% diameter stenosis by intravascular ultrasound.[1,5,6]
- In particular, intervention in the following scenarios may be desired[1,5,6]:
  - Accelerated, refractory, or malignant hypertension
  - Hypertension with an unexplained unilateral small kidney
  - Hypertension with intolerance to medication

- Chronic kidney disease with bilateral RAS or a RAS to a solitary functioning kidney
- Recurrent, sudden unexplained pulmonary edema
- Recurrent angina in the setting of severe hypertension
- The type of revascularization strategies for RAS are the subject of ongoing clinical trials.
  - PTA (Figure 28-5) with provisional stenting has resulted in a higher clinical success rate and lower restenosis rate, especially for ostial lesions.
  - Patients with FMD are an exception; in such individuals, balloon angioplasty alone is the therapy of choice.
  - In some situations, specifically macroaneurysmal disease and small, multiple renal arteries, the anatomy is unfavorable for percutaneous therapy and vascular surgical reconstruction may be the treatment of choice.

Lifestyle/Risk Modification

Cardiovascular risk-factor reduction may aid in treatment of RAS, but is more likely to affect the risks of other cardiovascular diseases. These include:
- Smoking cessation
- Blood pressure control (<140/80)
- Goal serum lipid levels
- Goal serum glucose control

Carotid Artery Stenosis

GENERAL PRINCIPLES

- Stroke is the third leading cause of death in the United States and represents a major cause of long-term disability.
- The detection of carotid artery stenosis presents an opportunity to identify patients at high risk for stroke and prevent cerebrovascular events and other adverse cardiovascular events.
- **Nearly half of patients with atherosclerotic carotid artery disease have severe CAD.** As a result, although recent trials have focused on the role of percutaneous carotid intervention versus carotid endarterectomy in the prevention of stroke, the management of carotid artery disease must be multimodal and include the treatment of modifiable risk factors such as hypertension, dyslipidemia, diabetes, and tobacco abuse.

Classification

- Asymptomatic carotid stenosis is defined as identifiable carotid artery plaque in the absence of neurologic symptoms such as amaurosis fugax, TIA, or CVA.
- Symptomatic carotid stenosis in contrast is the presence of neurologic symptoms suggestive of embolic or ischemic disease.
- Transcranial Doppler studies have demonstrated that embolic events may be present in asymptomatic carotid stenosis and is associated with a higher rate of symptomatic events.

Epidemiology

- Carotid stenosis >50% is present in 7% of the men and 5% of the women aged >65 years.
- Although strokes and TIAs have multiple etiologies, approximately 80% are ischemic in origin. Of the ischemic strokes about 25% are due to a vascular stenosis or occlusion.[14]
- Modifiable risk factors for stroke include hypertension, tobacco use, dyslipidemia, and diabetes.
- In general, relative risk of stroke increases as the degree of stenosis progresses and with the development of symptoms.

Pathophysiology

- Carotid artery stenosis is most commonly the result of atherosclerotic plaque formation, although less commonly fibromuscular dysplasia, cystic medial necrosis, or arteritis may play a role.
- Atherosclerotic carotid artery disease may result in cerebrovascular ischemic events via two mechanisms:
  - **Flow limitation:** Although collateral circulation via the Circle of Willis may compensate, severe stenosis or acute plaque rupture of the internal carotid can potentially cause ischemia/infarction of the affected hemisphere.
  - **Cerebral embolic event:** Embolization of thrombus or atheromatous debris from the carotid plaque can result in stroke.

DIAGNOSIS

Clinical Presentation

History

- Atherosclerotic carotid artery stenosis can present as an asymptomatic carotid bruit, TIA, or stroke.
- Focal neurologic symptoms suggestive of cerebrovascular ischemia or infarction include, but are not limited to, unilateral weakness, paresthesia, or sensory loss, neglect, abnormal visual-spatial ability, monocular blindness, hemianopsia, aphasia, ataxia, cranial nerve deficits, visual field loss, dizziness, imbalance, and incoordination.

Physical Examination

- Auscultation: Patients presenting to a cardiovascular specialist should undergo auscultation of the carotid arteries. Most bruits detected will be during systole; if the bruit extends into diastole, this indicates a significant gradient in the carotid artery with stenosis of about 80%.
- Neurologic evaluation: Patients with a carotid bruit should be evaluated for neurologic signs via a brief neurologic examination for strength, sensation, and orientation. Pre-existing neurologic deficits should be examined and documented in patients who have previously had a CVA.

Diagnostic Testing

Laboratories

Routine evaluation of patients with asymptomatic and symptomatic carotid stenosis should include factors important for the medical management of systemic atherosclerosis:

- Fasting lipid profile
- Renal function studies
- Fasting glucose and hemoglobin A1$_C$
- Although biomarkers such as C-reactive protein (CRP) and matrix metalloproteinase (MMP) have held promise for prediction of vulnerable carotid plaque, their reliability has not been clearly demonstrated.

Imaging

- **Ultrasound with Doppler:**
  - Ultrasound has been reported to have a sensitivity of 87% to 99% and specificity of 69% to 96% in the identification of >50% stenosis.[14]
  - Asymptomatic patients should undergo carotid ultrasound if any of the following are true[14]:
    - Audible carotid bruit
    - Known or suspected carotid stenosis
    - Evidence of systemic atherosclerosis (e.g., PAD or CAD)

- All symptomatic patients with ischemic focal neurologic symptoms should undergo carotid ultrasound.
- **MRI/MRA:**
  - MRI/MRA allows high-resolution imaging of the carotid anatomy as well as the aortic arch vessels up to the Circle of Willis.
  - Contrast MRA improves imaging of high-grade stenosis and slowly flowing blood.
  - Sensitivity of MRA has been reported as 97% to 100% and sensitivity of 82% to 96%, although a weakness of MRA has been the overestimation of degree of stenosis.[14]
- **CT angiography:**
  - CT angiography allows imaging of the carotid as well as the arch vessels and cerebral vessels.
  - Multidetector imaging with three-dimensional reconstruction has improved the quality of imaging significantly and now may be near comparable to the resolution of invasive angiography with a sensitivity of 100% and specificity of 63%.[14]
  - Heavily calcified lesions as well as metallic dental or cranial implants can cause significant imaging artifacts.
  - Iodinated contrast is required, which can be nephrotoxic to individuals with pre-existing renal insufficiency.
- **Invasive angiography:**
  - Angiography offers excellent resolution of vascular anatomy, though the invasive nature of this technique incurs significant risk, in part dependent on variations in carotid and aortic arch anatomy and potential stroke risk.
  - Outside of a planned catheter-based intervention, the use of routine diagnostic angiography has generally fallen out of favor with the exception of resolving conflicting noninvasive test results.

TREATMENT

Medications

- Medical treatment should focus on control of the modifiable risk factors of cerebrovascular events.
- Antiplatelet medications[14]:
  - If not contraindicated, antiplatelet therapy with **aspirin** (75 to 325 mg daily) should be administered.
  - **Clopidogrel** (75 mg daily) may be considered instead of aspirin.
  - **Dipyridamole** may be considered in conjunction with aspirin in select patients.
- For patients with a history of TIA or stroke, control of risk factors including hypertension, diabetes, and cholesterol (with a **statin** medication) should be initiated.

Surgical Management

- Revascularization of the carotid artery continues to be the subject of ongoing clinical investigation.
- **Asymptomatic carotid artery stenosis**[14]:
  - Recently published guidelines suggest considering prophylactic carotid endarterectomy in highly selected patients with high-grade asymptomatic carotid stenosis performed by surgeons with <3% morbidity/mortality rates and in patients with a low perioperative risk.
  - Carotid artery stenting may be considered in select asymptomatic patients with >70% stenosis by noninvasive imaging and >60% by invasive imaging.
- **Symptomatic carotid artery stenosis**[14]:
  - For patients with a recent (<6 months) TIA or ischemic stroke within the last 6 months with ipsilateral severe (>70% by noninvasive or >50% by invasive imaging)

carotid stenosis, endarterectomy by a surgeon with a perioperative morbidity and mortality of <6% is recommended.

○ Revascularization may be performed earlier (<2 weeks after the index event) if there are no contraindications.

○ Carotid artery stenting may be an alternative in patients with an average or low risk of complications associated with endovascular intervention.

○ The decision for stenting versus endarterectomy should be undertaken on a case-by-case basis factoring in operator experience, patient clinical scenario, vessel anatomy, and lesion complexity.

REFERENCES

1. Hirsch AT, Haskal ZJ, Hartzer NR. ACC/AHA 2005 practice guidelines for the management of patients with peripheral arterial disease (lower extremity, renal, mesenteric, and abdominal aortic). *Circulation* 2006;113:e463-e654.
2. Norgren L, Hiatt WR, Dormandy JA, et al. TASC II Working Group. Inter-Society Consensus for the Management of Peripheral Arterial Disease (TASC II). *J Vasc Surg* 2007;45:S5-S68.
3. Hirsch AT, Criqui MH, Treat-Jacobson D, et al. Peripheral arterial disease detection, awareness, and treatment in primary care. *JAMA* 2001;286:1317-1324.
4. White C. Intermittent claudication. *N Engl J Med* 2007;356:1241-1250.
5. Rooke TW, Hirsch AT, Misra S, et al. 2011 ACCF/AHA focused update of the guideline for the management of patients with peripheral artery disease (updating the 2005 guideline). *Circulation* 2011;124:2020-2045.
6. Rooke TW, Hirsch AT, Misra S, et al. Management of patients with peripheral artery disease (compilation of 2005 and 2011 ACCF/AHA guideline recommendations): a report of the American College of Cardiology Foundation/American Heart Association Task Force on Practice Guidelines. *J Am Coll Cardiol* 2013;61:1555-1570.
7. National Institutes of Health. National Heart, Lung, and Blood Institute. National Cholesterol Education Program. Third Report of the National Cholesterol Education Program (NCEP) Expert Panel on Detection, Evaluation, and Treatment of High Blood Cholesterol in Adults (Adult Treatment Panel III). Final Report. NIH Publication No. 02-5215. September, 2002.
8. Begelman SM, Jaff MR. Noninvasive diagnostic strategies for peripheral arterial disease. *Cleve Clin J Med* 2006;73:S22-S29.
9. Robless P, Mikhailidis DP, Stansby GP. Cilostazol for peripheral arterial disease. *Cochrane Database Syst Rev* 2008;1:CD0003748.
10. Salhiyyah K, Senanayake E, Abdel-Hadi M, et al. Pentoxifylline for intermittent claudication. *Cochrane Database Syst Rev* 2012;1:CD005262.
11. Wong PF, Chong LY, Mikhailidis DP, et al. Antiplatelet agents for intermittent claudication. *Cochrane Database Syst Rev* 2011;11:CD001272.
12. Watson L, Ellis B, Leng GC. Exercise for intermittent claudication. *Cochrane Database Syst Rev* 2008;4:CD000990.
13. Weber-Mzell D, Kotanko P, Schumacher M, et al. Coronary anatomy predicts presence or absence of renal artery stenosis. A prospective study in patients undergoing cardiac catheterization for suspended coronary artery disease. *Eur Heart J* 2002;21:1684-1691.
14. Brott TG, Halperin JL, Abbara S, et al. 2011 ASA/ACCF/AHA/AANN/AANS/ACR/ASNR/CNS/SAIP/SCAI/SIR/SNIS/SVM/SVS guideline on the management of patients with extracranial carotid and vertebral artery disease. *Circulation* 2011;124:e54-e130.

Diseases of the Aorta

29

Jay Shah and Alan C. Braverman

- The aorta is composed of three separate layers:
  - The **intima** is the thin innermost lining, comprising primarily endothelium.
  - The **media** is the muscular middle layer, comprising smooth muscle cells and elastin.
  - The **adventitia** is the fibrous outer layer.
- The nutrient supply to the vessel wall is a combination of passive diffusion from the lumen and the vasa vasorum, which supplies most of the aorta, with the exception of the infrarenal abdominal aorta.
- Aortopathies, or diseases of the aorta, are a spectrum of diseases that usually involve the intima or media of the aorta, and the pathophysiology will depend upon the underlying disease state.
- Some basic principles of physiology, however, are pertinent to the understanding of all aortopathies.
  - The smooth intimal layer and elastic media allow the aorta to have low vascular resistance and a natural distensibility.
  - The elasticity of the aorta is directly related to blood pressure; **the higher the pressure, the stiffer the walls of the aorta become,** as the load is borne less by elastin and more by collagen.
  - With age, there is an increase in the collagen/elastin ratio in the aortic wall, resulting in a less compliant structure.
  - Atherosclerosis also serves to lessen the elasticity of involved aortic segments, and may disrupt the intimal layer as well.
  - Genetically triggered aortic diseases usually lead to abnormalities of the aortic media, with decreased distensibility, cystic medial degeneration (CMD), progressive wall weakness, and aneurysmal enlargement or dissection.
  - Though the underlying pathophysiologic processes that cause aortic diseases vary, the clinical consequences are usually severe.

Abdominal Aortic Aneurysms

GENERAL PRINCIPLES

- An abdominal aortic aneurysm (AAA) is defined as an **abdominal aortic diameter >3.0 cm**.
- It is the most common form of aortic aneurysm.
- About 3% to 9% of men aged more than 50 years have AAA and it is fivefold more common in men than women.[1,2]
- It is thought to relate to a chronic inflammatory state in the aortic wall, which over time, degrades the elastin and smooth muscle cells, weakening the vessel wall, and leading to dilation.
- Risk factors include smoking, atherosclerosis, emphysema, hypertension, and hyperlipidemia.

DIAGNOSIS

Clinical Presentation

- Most commonly (90%) located in the infrarenal aorta.
- AAAs have an insidious course over years, with relative paucity of symptoms.
  - The vast majority of AAAs are small.
  - Gradual enlargement may cause abdominal or back pain.
  - Complications include mural thrombus formation, distal thromboembolism, rapid expansion, or rupture.
- **Size of the aneurysm predicts 5-year risk of rupture[3]:**
  - 5% for AAA 3.0 to 4.0 cm in diameter
  - 10% to 20% for AAA 4.0 to 5.58 cm in diameter
  - 30% to 40% for AAA 5.5 to 6.0 cm in diameter
  - 80% for AAA >7 cm in diameter
  - Enlargement of the aneurysm is also nonlinear; the larger the diameter, the faster the growth rate.
- Aneurysm rupture:
  - A total of 30% to 50% of patients with ruptured AAA die before reaching hospital.
  - Symptoms include abdominal or back pain; hypotension when ruptures into peritoneal cavity.
  - Rupture is associated with >40% to 50% operative mortality.

Diagnostic Testing

Imaging

- Ultrasound:
  - It is widely available, relatively accurate, inexpensive, and involves no radiation.
  - Limited by body habitus, overlying bowel and gas, and operator.
  - The United States Preventive Services Task Force (USPSTF) has recommended routine screening for AAA in men aged 65 to 75 years with a history of smoking.[4]
- CT:
  - Computed tomography (CT) angiography is highly accurate and allows for visualization of the proximal and distal aorta and branch vessels.
  - It provides valuable information such as presence of mural thrombus, calcification, and coexisting anatomic abnormalities.
  - It has replaced angiography for the routine imaging of AAA.
  - Limited by the need for intravenous contrast and radiation.
- MRI:
  - Magnetic Resonance Imaging (MRI) and MR angiography (MRA) are highly accurate for diagnosing and sizing AAA.
  - It does not utilize intravenous iodinated contrast.
  - No radiation exposure.
  - Limited by availability.

TREATMENT

Medications

The following modifications and therapy are beneficial in preventing AAA growth.
- Control of hypertension
- Control of hyperlipidemia and statin therapy
- Angiotensin-converting enzyme inhibitors, angiotensin receptor blockers (ARBs), and doxycycline have beneficial effects in animal models, but have not been proven to modify the disease course in humans.[5-7]

Other Nonpharmacologic Therapies

• Smoking cessation
• Moderate exercise

Surgical Management

• For AAA <5.0 to 5.5 cm, surgery is not indicated unless a complication occurs.[1-3]
• For AAA >5.0 to 5.5 cm, or those with complications, surgical or endovascular **treatment is indicated**.[1-3]
  ○ Open repair involves directly visualizing the AAA and excision of the aneurysm, followed by a graft sewn end-to-end to the proximal and distal aorta.
  ○ Endovascular aortic repair (EVAR) involves a catheter-based approach, through which a stent-graft is placed across the aneurysmal portion of the aorta, excluding it from exposure to arterial blood flow and pressures.
    ▪ Stent-grafts are fabric (woven polyester, similar to material used in open repair) that is suspended on a metal (usually stainless steel) frame.
    ▪ The proximal and distal ends of the stent-graft lie outside of the aneurysm, and therefore it excludes the aneurysm from the lumen of the aorta, without resection of the aneurysm itself.
    ▪ The anatomy must allow enough space for deployment, with appropriate "landing zones" proximally and distally to anchor the stent-graft.
    ▪ Complications of EVAR include leaks through or around the fabric ("endo-leak"), stent migration or fracture, and infections.

Thoracic Aortic Aneurysm

GENERAL PRINCIPLES

Definition

• Generally, an **aortic size >4.0 cm in the thorax** is considered abnormal. Age, body surface area, and gender must be considered when diagnosing a thoracic aortic aneurysm (TAA).
• Nomograms relating body surface area, age, and aortic root and ascending aortic diameter are readily available.

Epidemiology

• TAAs are less common than AAAs, with an incidence of about 10 in 100,000 person-years.
• Most commonly involves the ascending aorta (60%), followed by the descending aorta (30% to 35%) and the aortic arch (5% to 10%).

Etiology

• TAAs involving the aortic root are caused by a variety of pathogenic mechanisms, including degenerative, atherosclerotic, infectious, inflammatory, and genetic diseases (Table 29-1).[8]
• **CMD** is a histologic finding of bland, mucoid-appearing, basophilic-staining cysts in the media that represents degeneration of the elastin and collagen fibers, and smooth muscle cell loss.
  ○ CMD appears in the elderly, to varying degrees, and is exacerbated by chronic hypertension.

TABLE 29-1	CAUSES OF THORACIC AORTIC ANEURYSMS

- CMD
  - Aging and hypertension accelerate CMD
- Genetic disorders[a]
  - Marfan syndrome
  - Loeys–Dietz syndrome
  - Familial thoracic aortic aneurysm/dissection syndrome
  - Vascular Ehlers–Danlos syndrome
- Congenital conditions
  - Bicuspid aortic valve[a]
  - Turner syndrome
  - Aortic coarctation
  - Congenital heart disease
- Atherosclerosis
- Prior aortic surgery
  - Especially prior repair of aortic dissection
- Inflammatory/infectious conditions
  - Giant cell arteritis
  - Takayasu arteritis
  - Behçet disease
  - Syphilitic aortitis
  - Bacterial aortitis

[a]First-degree relatives of patients with these conditions should be screened for aortic disease.
CMD, cystic medial degeneration.

- It is also seen in genetic diseases, such as Marfan syndrome (MFS), Loeys–Dietz syndrome (LDS), familial thoracic aortic aneurysm (FTAA), Turner syndrome, and bicuspid aortic valve (BAV) disease.
- The loss of the main components that provide the load-bearing support for the aortic wall leads to progressive dilation and aneurysm formation.
- **Atherosclerosis** involves the descending aorta more commonly than the ascending aorta. Risk factors for atherosclerotic aneurysms are the same as those for coronary artery disease.
- **MFS** is a genetically triggered autosomal dominant disease that affects 1 in 5,000 to 10,000 individuals.
  - Caused by a mutation in *FBN1* on chromosome 15, which encodes fibrillin-1, a structural protein that is the major component of the microfibrils.
  - Aortic root aneurysms in MFS typically involve the aortic root and are largest at the sinuses of Valsalva.
  - MFS is a **phenotypically variable** disease, affecting the skeleton, eyes (ectopia lentis), skin, dura (dural ectasia), and lung (spontaneous pneumothorax).
  - Overactivation of transforming growth factor-β (TGF-β) is observed in tissues affected in MFS, and drugs that block TGF-β, such as ARBs, are known to attenuate aneurysm formation in Marfan mice.[9] Prospective trials of these agents in people with MFS are ongoing.
- **LDS** is an autosomal dominant aortic aneurysm syndrome due to mutations in *TGFBR1* and *TGFBR2* and is characterized by the triad of hypertelorism (wide-set eyes), bifid or wide uvula, and generalized arterial tortuosity. Patients may have cleft palate, velvety, translucent skin, pectus deformities, club feet, and arachnodactyly.[10]
  - Patients have a high risk of aortic dissection (AD) or rupture at an earlier age and with smaller aortic sizes than in MFS.
  - LDS can cause aneurysms in the ascending aorta, arch, and in other medium–large arteries, and commonly affects the arch vessels with aneurysm or dissection.

- ○ One clinical distinguishing feature between LDS and MFS is the absence of lens dislocation in LDS.
- • **Familial thoracic aortic aneurysm and dissection syndrome** (FTAA/D) is a group of disorders characterized by an autosomal dominant inheritance of and dissection, which have variable phenotypic expression and age of onset, and no features of MFS or LDS. BAV and/or cerebral aneurysms may be present in some individuals.
  - ○ Livedo reticularis, moya-moya, and patent ductus arteriosus may be present.
  - ○ Mutations in the vascular smooth muscle gene, *ACTA2*, occur in 14% and in *MYH11* in 1%.[9]
  - ○ Gene mutations in *FBN1* and *TFGBR1* and *TGFBR2* are also described.
  - ○ Up to 20% of first-degree relatives of the individual with unexplained TAA or dissection will also have thoracic aortic disease. Thus, it is imperative to screen family members.
- • **Vascular Ehlers–Danlos syndrome** (vEDS) is a rare, but severe disorder caused by a mutation in the *COL 3A1* gene.[9]
  - ○ Inherited in an autosomal dominant pattern, vEDS is characterized by spontaneous rupture or dissection of medium–large arteries.
  - ○ Arterial rupture or dissection may occur in the aorta or in medium-sized arteries in the absence of significant aneurysm formation.
  - ○ Surgical repair of the vessel is very difficult due to poor vascular connective tissue the lack of appropriate collagen to provide support for sutures.
- • **Bicuspid aortic Valve (BAV)** occurs in approximately 1% to 2% of the population and is associated with increased risk of ascending aortic aneurysm, dissection, and coarctation of the aorta.[11]
  - ○ Over half of patients with BAV have aortic dilatation, generally of the ascending aorta and root, independent of valvular stenosis or regurgitation. The aortic aneurysms in BAV typically involve the ascending aorta.
  - ○ Dissection is 10 times more common with BAV than in the normal population because of abnormalities of elastic tissue in the aortic media.
  - ○ BAV may be familial in about 10% of cases, and may be inherited as an autosomal dominant trait with reduced penetrance; patients with BAV and aneurysm should have their first-degree relatives screened for BAV and/or TAA.
- • **Turner syndrome** is a genetic disorder caused by complete or partial loss of the second sex chromosome (XO or Xp), and is associated with BAV or aortic coarctation.
  - ○ CMD can occur in Turner syndrome, which may lead to TAA.
  - ○ Because Turner syndrome is associated with short stature, aortic size must be corrected for body surface area.
- • **Inflammatory aortitis** is caused by diseases such as giant cell arteritis, Takayasu arteritis, and the HLA-B27 spondyloarthropathies.
- • **Infectious aneurysms**, also called mycotic aneurysms, can be caused by acute infections involving *Staphylococcus, Streptococcus,* or *Salmonella* species.
  - ○ Patients present with fever, pain, and bacteremia.
  - ○ Infected aneurysms tend to be saccular, may progress rapidly, and have high risk or rupture.
  - ○ Syphilitic aortitis is very rare and involves the ascending aorta.

DIAGNOSIS

Clinical Presentation
- • **Most TAAs are asymptomatic, and incidentally found** on radiologic studies or echocardiograms done for other reasons.
- • When they occur, symptoms are related to enlarging aneurysms, which may cause chest or back pain.

- ○ Aortic root dilation may lead to significant AR.
- ○ Mural thrombus formation may lead to a thromboembolism.
- The most serious complications are aortic rupture or dissection.
- The natural history and progression of TAA depends upon the etiology.
  - ○ While age-related CMD or atherosclerosis may cause an aneurysm to slowly grow over years, a TAA related to LDS or vEDS may grow rapidly or lead to acute dissection in the setting of a relatively small aneurysm.
  - ○ The rate of dilation and risk of rupture are also dependent on the size of the aorta.
    - ■ Similar to AAA, the relationship of size and risk of rupture is nonlinear.
    - ■ The yearly risk of rupture or dissection for TAAs <5 cm is approximately 2%; for TAAs 5 to 6 cm is approximately 3%; and for TAAs >6 cm is about 7%.[12]

Diagnostic Testing

Imaging

- **Chest radiography** (CXR) may show a wide mediastinum or prominent aortic knob. Small aneurysms may not be appreciable on CXR, and CXR is not a useful test to exclude the presence of TAA.
- **Transthoracic echocardiogram** (TTE) is useful for defining the dimensions of the aortic root, as well as the proximal ascending aorta.
  - ○ TTE also provides information about the structure and function of the aortic valve.
  - ○ The ascending and proximal descending aorta may be seen but with less quality and accuracy than CT or MRI.
- **Transesophageal echocardiogram** (TEE) is an excellent modality to image the aortic root, arch, and descending aorta.
  - ○ There is a small blind spot at the level of the mid-high ascending aorta that may be missed by TEE.
  - ○ It provides useful information about cardiac and valve function.
- **CT with angiography** (CTA) and **MRI/MRA** are excellent tests to image the entire thoracic aorta.
  - ○ Measurement of aneurysms needs to be carefully done, especially if the aorta is tortuous, because the axial slices may image the aorta at an oblique angle, which may provide inaccurate measurements of the true transverse dimension of the aorta.
  - ○ MRI/MRA may be preferred as the imaging modality of choice for chronic surveillance, due to lack of radiation and iodinated contrast.

TREATMENT

Medications

- Aggressive blood pressure (BP) control (goal <120/60 mmHg) is critical to minimize the risk of progressive dilation, rupture, and dissection by lowering the shear forces on the aorta.
- β-Blockers lower BP, as well as lessen the rate of change in pressure with each systole (dP/dt), and are therefore indicated in TAA.
- ARBs, by antagonizing TGF-β, may have a role in slowing aortic dilation in patients with MFS (and possibly LDS), and prospective trials addressing this possibility are ongoing.[9]

Other Nonpharmacologic Therapies

- Smoking cessation is imperative.
- Lifestyle modifications that limit stress on the aorta are recommended, such as avoiding heavy weight lifting and participation in certain jobs and sports.
- Pregnancy in the setting of genetically triggered aneurysm syndromes can cause a rapid enlargement of TAA, and increases the risk of rupture or dissection, so contraception and timing of pregnancy must be discussed with patients.

Surgical Treatment

- Ascending thoracic aortic aneurysm:
  - Surgical resection and repair of the aorta is the treatment of choice.
  - Involvement of the aortic root and presence of AR are two factors that impact the surgical procedure.
  - When there is significant AR from an abnormal aortic valve and aortic root involvement, the modified Bentall procedure is performed.
    - After resection of the aortic valve, root and proximal ascending aorta, a prosthetic valve is suspended in a tube made of woven Dacron polyester, which is sutured in an end-to-end fashion.
    - The coronary arteries are preserved with "buttons" of native aortic wall, and are reimplanted into the aortic graft.
  - If the aortic valve itself is normal, it may be possible to resuspend the patient's native aortic valve in the graft; this is termed a valve-sparing surgery.
- Descending thoracic aortic aneurysms:
  - Surgical resection of the aneurysm is followed by an end-to-end anastomosis of a graft.
    - Small branches of the descending aorta are ligated.
    - Cardiopulmonary bypass is necessary.
    - The operative morbidity and mortality may be very significant, depending upon comorbidities.
  - Thoracic endovascular aortic aneurysm repair (TEVAR) is often possible, and is performed in patients with the appropriate anatomy.
    - There is a significantly lower procedure-related mortality with TEVAR compared to traditional open repair.[13,14]
    - Stent-grafts are fabric (woven polyester, similar to material used in open repair) that is suspended on a metal (usually stainless steel) frame.
    - The proximal and distal ends of the stent-graft lie outside of the aneurysm, and therefore it excludes the aneurysm from the lumen of the aorta, without resection of the aneurysm itself.
    - The anatomy must allow enough space for deployment, with appropriate landing zones proximally and distally to anchor the stent-graft.
    - Complications of TEVAR include leaks through or around the fabric ("endo-leak"), stent migration or fracture, and infections.

MONITORING/FOLLOW-UP

- Long-term surveillance must be performed even after definitive repair, and the imaging modality (TTE, CTA, or MRI) and timing depends upon the location, size, and underlying etiology of the TAA.
- In general, after the initial diagnosis, imaging should be performed at more frequent intervals (every 6 months), until the TAA is deemed to be stable. Thereafter, imaging should be performed every 1 to 2 years.

Aortic Dissection And Variants

GENERAL PRINCIPLES

Definition

- **Classic Aortic Dissection (AD)** is a tear in the intima, which allows blood to enter the aortic wall and propagate in an anterograde or retrograde fashion, creating a false lumen or channel.

- **Aortic intramural hematoma** (IMH) results from a spontaneous rupture of the vasa vasorum, creating a hematoma in the media without an intimal flap.
- **Penetrating aortic ulcer** (PAU) results from an atherosclerotic lesion that can penetrate through the media, and may lead to aortic rupture, dissection, or pseudoaneurysm.

Classification

- There are several classification systems for ADs, and involvement of the ascending aorta is the defining characteristic (Figure 29-1).[15]
- DeBakey types I and II, and Stanford type A dissections involve the ascending aorta.
- DeBakey type III or Stanford type B dissections do not involve the ascending aorta.

DeBakey Type I	Type II	Type III
Stanford	Type A	Type B

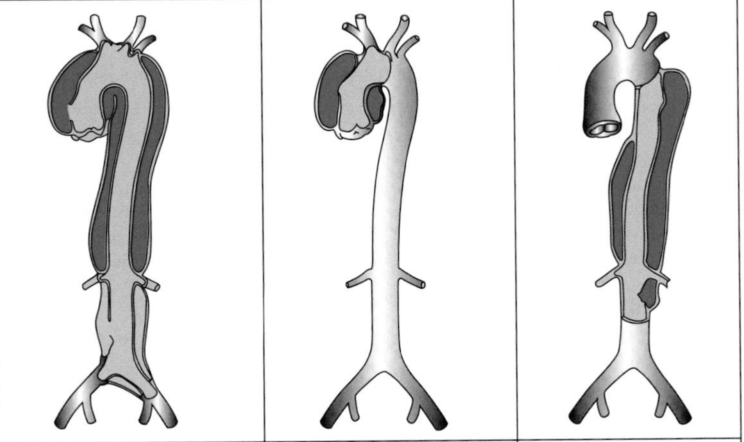

DeBakey

Type I   Originates in the ascending aorta, propagates at least to the aortic arch and often beyond it distally.

Type II   Originates in and is confined to the ascending aorta.

Type III   Originates in the descending aorta and extends distally down the aorta or, rarely, retrograde into the aortic arch and ascending aorta.

Stanford

Type A   All dissections involving the ascending aorta, regardless of the site of origin

Type B   All dissections not involving the ascending aorta

FIGURE 29-1. Classification systems for aortic dissection: Stanford and DeBakey. (From Nienaber CA, Eagle KA. Aortic dissection: new frontiers in diagnosis and management. Part I: from etiology to diagnostic strategies. *Circulation* 2003;108:628-635, with permission.)

TABLE 29-2	RISK FACTORS FOR AORTIC DISSECTION

- Hypertension
- Genetic disorders[a]
  - Marfan syndrome
  - Loeys–Dietz syndrome
  - Familial thoracic aortic aneurysm/dissection syndrome
  - Vascular Ehlers–Danlos syndrome
- Congenital conditions
  - Bicuspid aortic valve
  - Turner syndrome
  - Aortic coarctation
  - Supravalvular aortic stenosis
- Cocaine/methamphetamine use
- Atherosclerosis/penetrating aortic ulcer
- Trauma—blunt or iatrogenic
  - Catheter induced
  - Aortic valve surgery
  - Coronary artery bypass grafting
  - Deceleration injury (e.g., motor vehicle crash)
- Inflammatory/infectious conditions
  - Giant cell arteritis
  - Takayasu arteritis
  - Behçet disease
  - Syphilitic aortitis
- Pregnancy

[a]First-degree relatives of patients with these conditions should be screened for aortic disease.

- Classification of the anatomy is important because the decision regarding surgical or medical management is dependent on the location of the dissection. Dissections of the ascending aorta (types I, II, and A) require immediate surgical repair, while those involving the descending aorta (type III or B) are initially treated medically.

Epidemiology

AD is a rare, but life-threatening condition, with an incidence of 5 to 30 per million people per year.

Etiology

- Several conditions predispose the aorta to dissection, most as a result of abnormalities in the arterial wall composition (Table 29-2).
- Approximately 75% of patients with AD have hypertension.[16]
- Patients with genetic disorders such as the MFS, LDS, vEDS, BAV, or familial aortic aneurysm syndrome are particularly prone to aortic dilation and dissection.[17]
- Cocaine or methamphetamine-induced hypertension, inflammatory conditions such as giant cell arteritis, or direct trauma from catheterization or aortic surgery can disrupt the aortic intima and lead to dissection.

DIAGNOSIS

Clinical Presentation

- The clinical presentation of AD may be quite variable, and one must maintain a high index of suspicion for the diagnosis.
- Significant morbidity and mortality from dissection are attributed to end-organ damage and aortic rupture (Table 29-3).
- Organ systems may be compromised by compression of branch vessels by an expanding false lumen, or direct extension of a dissection into the vessel.
- Cardiovascular and neurologic manifestations are two particularly devastating complications of AD.

TABLE 29-3 COMPLICATIONS OF AORTIC DISSECTION

- Aortic rupture
- Myocardial ischemia/infarction
- Neurologic deficits: stroke, coma, altered consciousness, syncope, and paraplegia
- Malperfusion: coronary, mesenteric, limb, spinal cord, renal, and hepatic
- Hypotension/shock
- Hemothorax
- Cardiac tamponade/hemopericardium
- Acute aortic regurgitation and congestive heart failure
- Subsequent aneurysm formation

- ○ When the ascending aorta is involved, **acute AR** may lead to heart failure.
- ○ **Cardiac tamponade, aortic rupture, or myocardial infarction** from coronary artery involvement may lead rapidly to hemodynamic shock and death.
  - ■ Dissection complicated by acute hemopericardium may lead to cardiac tamponade.
  - ■ Poor outcomes have been reported from pericardiocentesis secondary to recurrent bleeding and acute decompensation. Therefore, pericardiocentesis should generally be avoided in favor of emergent surgery.
- ○ Neurologic sequelae may result from acute dissection involving the carotid or vertebral arteries, and cerebral hypoperfusion may lead to syncope, altered mental status, and stroke. Transverse myelitis, myelopathy, paraplegia, or quadriplegia may result from spinal malperfusion.
- Mesenteric ischemia may occur, which may be difficult to diagnose and can be fatal.

History
- In contrast to the crescendo discomfort of angina pectoris, the pain of acute dissection is maximal at its onset, usually sudden and severe, often described as a sharp, tearing pain in the chest, neck, or interscapular areas.
- In addition to the dissection itself, presenting symptoms may also be related to malperfusion or complications involving various organ systems.

Physical Examination
- Physical examination should include a complete pulse exam and BP in both arms and legs, as there may be pulse or pressure deficits.
- Cardiac auscultation may reveal an AR murmur.
- Pulse differentials and an AR murmur are present in the minority of patients and physical examination alone is not sufficient to rule out AD.

Diagnostic Testing

Laboratories
- D-dimer may be of assistance in the evaluation; it is usually elevated in acute AD, and, when normal, has been shown to have a modestly high negative predictive value.
- Importantly, in IMH, the D-dimer may not be elevated and in the setting of a high clinical index of suspicion a negative D-dimer does not rule out an acute AD.
- A clear role for the D-dimer in evaluation of AD has not been established.[18]

Imaging

- CXR:
  - It may demonstrate a widened mediastinum or abnormal aortic contour.
  - Pleural effusion may represent hemothorax and displaced calcium at the aortic knob may occasionally be present.
  - Up to 10% to 20% of ADs are associated with an unremarkable chest radiograph. Therefore, **a normal CXR does not rule out an AD.**[18,19]
- Given the critical nature of ADs, immediate diagnostic confirmation and definition of the extent of the dissection are imperative. The choice of imaging should be made on the basis of sensitivity, specificity, clinical stability, and operator availability and experience (Table 29-4).[18]

TABLE 29-4	COMPARISON OF DIAGNOSTIC IMAGING MODALITIES FOR AORTIC DISSECTION			
Test	Sensitivity (%)	Specificity (%)	Advantages	Disadvantages
TEE	98–99	94–97	Excellent evaluation of aortic root and descending thoracic aorta, aortic valve, and pericardium	Requires esophageal intubation; limited to thoracic aorta, little information about branch vessels
CT	96–100	96–100	Widely and rapidly available; superior imaging of entire aorta, heart, branch vessels, and complications such as rupture, hemopericardium, and malperfusion	Nephrotoxic iodinated contrast required
MRI	>98	>98	Superior accuracy, sensitivity, and specificity for all types of dissection	Limited availability, time-consuming procedure, less monitoring during scan

TEE, transesophageal echocardiogram; CT, computed tomography.

- ○ **If the patient presents with hemodynamic instability or hypotension, rapid evaluation by TEE or CT scan should be performed** to assess for complications of dissection, including pericardial effusion, AR, or aortic rupture.
- ○ CT is widely and rapidly available. Intravenous contrast is required to evaluate for dissection and offers superior imaging of the entire aorta, aortic arch, and branch vessels.
- ○ TEE requires an experienced operator and esophageal intubation to perform the procedure; however, it can be performed at the bedside and visualizes the aortic valve, aortic root, and pericardium well.
- ○ Because of the time delay and difficulties with hemodynamic monitoring, MRI is usually not the first test of choice.
- ○ While TTE may diagnose an AD, the sensitivity and specificity of this approach is far less than other diagnostic modalities.

TREATMENT

Medications

- **When AD is suspected, immediate initiation of β-blocker therapy** to reduce shear forces is paramount while pursuing confirmation of the diagnosis (Table 29-5).[18]
- **BP should be reduced to as low a level as possible** without compromising organ perfusion.
- β-Blocker therapy is recommended to achieve a **target heart rate <70 beats per minute**.

TABLE 29-5	**SELECTED PHARMACOLOGIC THERAPY FOR AORTIC DISSECTION**[a]

Intravenous β-blocker (preferred negative inotrope)[b]

- Esmolol: Give 500 μg/kg IV bolus, then continuous IV infusion at 50–200 μg/kg/minute, titrated to effect. Short half-life allows rapid titration
- Labetalol: Give 20 mg IV over 2 minutes, then 40–80 mg IV every 15 minutes until adequate response (maximum 300 mg), then continuous IV infusion at 2–10 mg/minute IV, titrated to effect

Intravenous vasodilator (*after* initiation of β-blockade)

- Sodium nitroprusside: Start continuous infusion with no bolus at 20 μg/minute, titrate 0.5–5 μg/kg/minute with a maximum of 800 mcg/minute. **Use only in presence of β-blockers**

  Caution: Thiocyanate toxicity may occur in patients with renal impairment or prolonged infusions

- Enalaprilat: Give 0.625–1.25 mg IV, then increase by 0.625–1.25 mg every 6 hours to a maximum of 5 mg every 6 hours, titrated to effect

---

[a]Goal of therapy is heart rate less than 70 beats/minute and blood pressure as low as possible without compromising organ perfusion.

[b]If contraindication to β-blockers, use diltiazem: 0.25 mg/kg IV over 2 minutes, then continuous IV infusion at 5–15 mg/hour, titrated to effect.

- Nondihydropyridine calcium channel blockers (i.e., diltiazem, verapamil) may be considered if β-blocker therapy is contraindicated.
- Care should be taken to **avoid vasodilators**, such as sodium nitroprusside, in the absence of negative chronotropic medications, as they may induce reflex tachycardia, thereby increasing dP/dt, which may extend the dissection.

Surgical Management

- **Emergent surgery is indicated with any ascending AD.**[16,19]
  - Medical therapy alone is associated with >50% 14-day mortality rate.
  - Surgery is associated with an approximate 25% 14-day mortality rate.
  - Surgical repair involves excising the intimal tear when possible, obliterating entry into the false channel proximally and distally, and placing a graft in an end-to-end fashion to replace the ascending aorta.
  - If significant AR complicates AD, the aortic valve is either resuspended or the valve is replaced, depending upon the underlying condition of the valve and aortic root. Composite valve graft placement or valve-sparing surgery may be required depending upon the circumstances.
  - Endovascular repair for AD involving the ascending aorta is currently not performed.
- Surgical treatment for **descending AD**:
  - In the absence of complications (Table 29-6), descending aortic (type B) dissections are initially managed medically.
  - Surgical intervention in the acute setting of a type B AD is associated with >30% mortality, compared to a mortality of about 10% for medical therapy alone.[16,19]
  - Long-term complications of descending ADs include aneurysm formation, rupture, and retrograde dissection. Long-term follow-up requires surveillance by CT or MRI.
  - Surgical or endovascular repair in descending (type B) AD is reserved for complications such as end-organ ischemia, refractory pain, uncontrolled hypertension, rupture, or a rapidly expanding aortic diameter.
  - There is growing experience managing acute complications of descending ADs with endovascular therapy using stent-grafting. Occasionally, a branch vessel is supplied by the false lumen, and significant ischemia may develop due to slow flow through the false lumen. In these settings, stenting or balloon fenestration of the false lumen to relieve ischemia may also be performed.

TABLE 29-6	INDICATIONS FOR SURGERY FOR AORTIC DISSECTION

- Type I, II, or type A dissection
- Type III or type B dissection with[a]
  - Rupture
  - Branch vessel compromise/organ ischemia
  - Refractory hypertension
  - Aneurysmal dilation
  - Refractory pain

---

[a]Complications of type B dissection may be treated with surgery or endovascular intervention.

SPECIAL CONSIDERATIONS

Aortic Intramural Hematoma

- Aortic IMH is a variant of AD in which there is no intimal tear or false lumen, but instead a primary hematoma occurs in the aorta wall, possibly related to rupture of the vasa vasorum (Figure 29-2).[20]
- IMH may be focal or may propagate anterograde or retrograde through the aorta. Classification of location is the same as that of AD (types A and B).
- Symptoms are also similar to those of AD, predominantly sudden onset of chest or back pain.
- Complications include progression to classic AD, aortic rupture, hemopericardium, and AR.

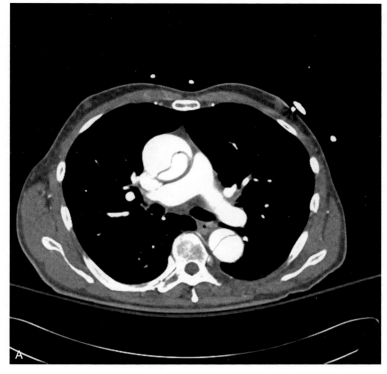

FIGURE 29-2. Types of acute aortic syndromes. (**A**) Classic aortic dissection. (**B**) Intramural hematoma (IMH) of the aorta. Black arrows indicate IMH in ascending aorta; white arrows denote crescentic IMH in descending aorta. (**C**) Penetrating atherosclerotic ulcer (PAU) of the aorta (black arrow). White arrows point to associated contained hematoma. (Modified with permission from Braverman AC, Thompson RW, Sanchez LA. Diseases of the aorta. In: Bonow RO, Mann DL, Zipes DP, Libby P, eds. *Braunwald's Heart Disease*, 9th ed. Philadelphia, PA: Elsevier; 2011:1309-1337.)

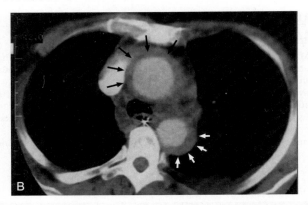

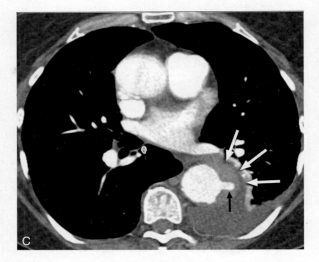

FIGURE 29-2. (Continued)

- Natural history of IMH may include:
  - Progression to AD (in type A IMH, may be as high as 25% to 50%)[21]
  - Complete resolution of the hematoma
  - Persistence and stabilization of the hematoma
  - Progression to aortic aneurysm
- Diagnostic modalities include TEE, contrast CT, or MRI/MRA. The classic appearance is a smooth-walled lumen with a crescentic or circumferential thickening of the media.
- Surgery is recommended for IMH involving the ascending aorta and careful observation and medical management is recommended for IMH of the descending aorta.

Penetrating Aortic Ulcer

- PAU results from an atherosclerotic plaque that penetrates the media, and forms an ulceration, or crater in the aortic wall (Figure 29-2).[20,22] PAUs may be isolated, or associated with multiple atheroma and ulcers, and are usually located in the descending and abdominal aorta.
- Classically, it involves an elderly person with significant atherosclerotic aortic and vascular disease and multiple coronary risk factors.
- Symptoms are very similar to classic AD, including sudden onset of chest, back, or abdominal pain.
- PAU may lead to aortic rupture, dissection, pseudoaneurysm, and late aneurysm formation. AD caused by PAU is likely to be a focal dissection, with a thick-walled flap.
- Diagnostic modalities include TEE, CT, and MRI/MRA, and aortography.
  - ○ The classic appearance is a focal, crater-like appearance of the atherosclerotic plaque, and displacement of the intima.
  - ○ Contrast studies will demonstrate an "outpouching" that constitutes the ulcer crater.
- Surgical treatment is generally recommended for PAU in the ascending aorta.
- In the descending aorta, intervention is reserved for persistent pain, significant dilation of the aorta, rupture, or pseudoaneurysm formation.
  - ○ In the descending and abdominal aorta, PAU and its complications are especially amenable to endovascular treatment, given the relatively short segment of the aorta that is usually affected.
  - ○ Patients with PAU are often high-risk candidates for open surgical procedures.

REFERENCES

1. Chaikof EL, Brewster DC, Dalman RL, et al. The care of patients with an abdominal aortic aneurysm: the Society for Vascular Surgery practice guidelines. *J Vasc Surg* 2009;50:S2-S49.
2. Moll FL, Powel JT, Fraedrich G, et al. Management of abdominal aortic aneurysms clinical practice guidelines of the European society for vascular surgery. *Eur J Vasc Endovasc Surg* 2011;41:S1-S58.
3. Brewster DC, Cronenwett JL, Hallett JW, et al. Guidelines for the treatment of AAA: report of a subcommittee of the Joint Council of the American Association for Vascular Surgery and Society for Vascular Surgery. *J Vasc Surg* 2003;37:1106-1117.
4. U.S. Preventive Services Task Force. Screening for abdominal aortic aneurysm: recommendation statement. *Ann Intern Med* 2005;142:198-202.
5. Habashi JP, Judge DP, Holm TM, et al. Losartan, an AT1 antagonist, prevents aortic aneurysm in a mouse model of Marfan syndrome. *Science* 2006;312:117-121.
6. Xiong W, Knispel RA, Dietz HC, et al. Doxycycline delays aneurysm rupture in a mouse model of Marfan syndrome. *J Vasc Surg* 2008;47:166-172.
7. Dodd BR, Spence RA. Doxycycline inhibition of abdominal aortic aneurysm growth: a systematic review of the literature. *Curr Vasc Pharmacol* 2011;9:471-478.
8. Boyer JK, Gutierrez F, Braverman AC. Approach to the dilated aortic root. *Curr Opin Cardiol* 2004;19:563-569.
9. Gillis E, Van Laer L, Loeys BL. Genetics of thoracic aortic aneurysm: at the crossroad of transforming growth factor-β signaling and vascular smooth muscle cell contractility. *Circ Res* 2013;113:327-340.
10. Loeys BL, Schwarze U, Holm T, et al. Aneurysm syndromes caused by mutations in the TGF-β receptor. *N Engl J Med* 2006;355:788-798.
11. Braverman AC, Guven H, Beardslee MA, et al. The bicuspid aortic valve. *Curr Probl Cardiol* 2005;30:470-522.
12. Davies RR, Goldstein LJ, Coady MA, et al. Yearly rupture or dissection rates for thoracic aortic aneurysms: simple prediction based on size. *Ann Thorac Surg* 2002;73:17-28.
13. Matsumura JS, Cambria RP, Dake MD, et al. International controlled clinical trial of thoracic endovascular aneurysm repair with the Zenith TX2 endovascular graft: 1-year results. *J Vasc Surg* 2008;47:247-257.

14. Walsh SR, Tang TY, Sadat U, et al. Endovascular stenting versus open surgery for thoracic aortic disease: systematic review and meta-analysis of perioperative results. *J Vasc Surg* 2008;47:1094-1098.

15. Nienaber CA, Eagle KA. Aortic dissection: new frontiers in diagnosis and management. Part I: from etiology to diagnostic strategies. *Circulation* 2003;108:628-635.

16. Tsai TT, Trimarchi S, Nienaber CA. Acute aortic dissection: perspectives from the International Registry of Acute Aortic Dissection (IRAD). *Eur J Vasc Endovasc Surg* 2009;37:149-159.

17. Braverman AC. Acute aortic dissection: clinician update. *Circulation* 2010;122:184-188.

18. Hiratzka LF, Bakris GL, Beckman JA, et al. 2010 ACCF/AHA/AATS/ACR/ASA/SCA/SCAI/SIR/STS/SVM guidelines for the diagnosis and management of patients with thoracic aortic disease. *J Am Coll Cardiol* 2010;55:1509-1544.

19. Hagan PG, Nienaber CA, Isselbacher EM, et al. The international registry of acute aortic dissection (IRAD). New insights into an old disease. *JAMA* 2000;283:897-903.

20. Braverman AC, Thompson RW, Sanchez LA. Diseases of the Aorta. In: Bonow RO, Mann DL, Zipes DP, Libby P, eds. *Braunwald's Heart Disease*, 9th ed. Philadelphia, PA: Elsevier; 2011;1309-1337.

21. Estrera A, Miller C, Lee T, et al. Acute type A intramural hematoma: analysis of current management strategy. *Circulation* 2009;120:S287-S291.

22. Braverman AC. Penetrating atherosclerotic ulcers of the aorta. *Curr Opin Cardiol* 1994;9:591-597.

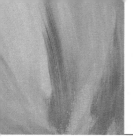

Standard Imaging and Diagnostic Testing Modalities: Nuclear Cardiology

30

Chirayu Gor and Sudhir K. Jain

GENERAL PRINCIPLES

Definitions

- **Single-photon emission computed tomography** (SPECT) is the most commonly utilized modality for the assessment of myocardial perfusion and viability.
- Uses include
  - Myocardial perfusion imaging (MPI)
    - Most common clinical application of SPECT
    - In the setting of a stress test (images at rest compared to those at stress)
    - In patients with active anginal symptoms, as resting images only
  - Assessment of myocardial viability
  - Measurement of left ventricular (LV) volume and function

Physics

- Radiotracer is administered intravenously. The isotope is extracted from the blood by viable myocytes and retained for a given period of time.
- As the isotope decays, a gamma camera (Figure 30-1) captures the emitted photons and uses them to produce a digital image by rotating in an orbital path around the patient.[1]
  - The camera is rotated to different positions to collect photons from different views.
  - Multiple images, each comprising 20 to 25 seconds of emission data, are collected.
  - Imaging information from each view is back-projected onto an imaging matrix, creating a reconstruction of the heart (Figure 30-2).[1]
  - The images are then acquired electronically.
- The long axis of the left ventricle is identified by special techniques, and then tomographic images in three standard planes (Figure 30-3) are derived[1]:
  - **Short-axis images** are obtained by cutting perpendicular to the long axis of the heart.
    - This produces doughnut-like slices.
    - These images are similar to the parasternal short-axis view on two-dimensional echocardiography.
  - **Vertical long-axis images** are obtained by cutting parallel to the long axis of the heart.
  - **Horizontal long-axis images** are also cut parallel to the long axis of the heart, but they are orthogonal to the vertical long-axis image.
- Representative images are presented in Figures 30-4, 30-5, and 30-6.[2]

Radiotracers[3]

- The majority of SPECT studies use agents based on either **technetium-99m** (^{99m}Tc) (^{99m}Tc-sestamibi, ^{99m}Tc-tetrofosmin, and ^{99m}Tc-teboroxime) or **thallium-201** (^{201}Tl).
- Understanding SPECT MPI requires understanding the properties of these tracers.

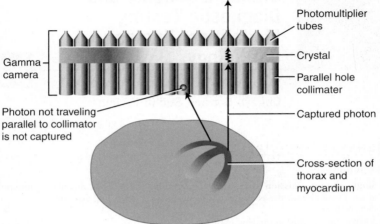

FIGURE 30-1. Transmission of photons emitted from myocardium to a gamma camera. (From Braunwald E, Zipes DP, Libby P, et al., eds. *Braunwald's Heart Disease: A Textbook of Cardiovascular Medicine*, 9th ed. Philadelphia, PA: Elsevier; 2004, with permission.)

- Thallium-201:
  - Similar properties to potassium:
    - Both are mobilized into cells via active transport (utilization of an ATPase).
    - Both are absent in scar tissue due to an inability to mobilize into the cell.
    - Lack of uptake of ^{201}Tl in a region of myocardium can differentiate infarcted versus viable (normal or ischemic) myocardium.
  - The half-life of this agent is approximately 73 hours.
  - It emits 80 keV of photon energy.
  - Early myocardial uptake of ^{201}Tl is primarily related to regional blood flow.
  - A region of myocardium that is poorly perfused will only take up a small degree of ^{201}Tl initially (first 5 to 10 minutes).
  - Perfusion subsequent to that is primarily due to concentration gradient (redistribution phase).
  - Since blood vessels with atherosclerosis do not perfuse myocardium as well as blood vessels of normal caliber, the initial uptake under peak stress will be low.
- 99mTc is a relatively newer agent.
  - The half-life is 6 hours.
  - Emits 140 keV of photon energy
  - First-pass absorption is only 60%, and there is very little redistribution.
  - Most common protocol when using ^{99m}Tc is the dual-isotope method.
- Washington University/Barnes-Jewish Hospital uses a 1-day **dual-radionuclide SPECT protocol**.[4]
  - It consists of an injection of 3.0 to 3.5 mCi of ^{201}Tl at rest and an injection of 25 to 30 mCi of ^{99m}Tc at peak stress.

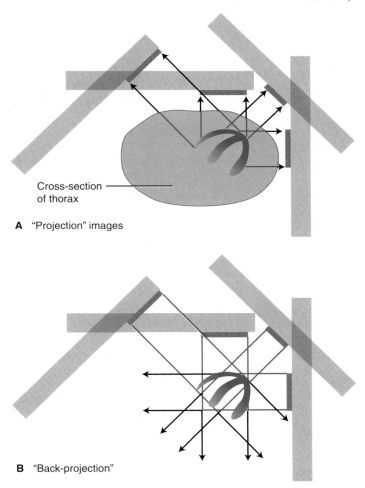

A "Projection" images

Cross-section
of thorax

B "Back-projection"

FIGURE 30-2. Detection of photons by a gamma camera. The camera is rotated to different angles to enable image acquisition from multiple views. (From Braunwald E, Zipes DP, Libby P, et al., eds. *Braunwald's Heart Disease: A Textbook of Cardiovascular Medicine*, 9th ed. Philadelphia, PA: Elsevier; 2004, with permission.)

- SPECT imaging starts immediately after the initial injection of ^{201}Tl at rest. This takes advantage of ^{201}Tl high first-pass absorption.
- Immediately following ^{201}Tl imaging, the patient undergoes the stress test.
- At peak exercise or vasodilator infusion, 25 to 30 mCi of ^{99m}Tc is injected. SPECT imaging is repeated 15 to 30 minutes later.
- The entire examination takes approximately 90 minutes.

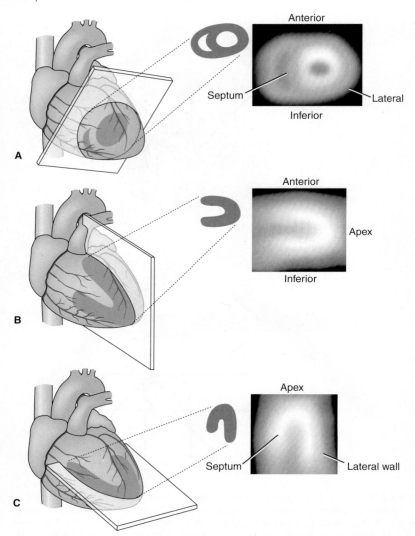

FIGURE 30-3. Tomographic views of the left ventricle. Short-axis view, vertical long-axis view, and horizontal long-axis view (top to bottom). (From Braunwald E, Zipes DP, Libby P, et al., eds. *Braunwald's Heart Disease: A Textbook of Cardiovascular Medicine*, 9th ed. Philadelphia, PA: Elsevier; 2004, with permission.)

Interpretation and Image Analysis

- SPECT myocardial scan analysis involves describing:
  - The presence and location of perfusion defects
  - The size and severity of the perfusion abnormality

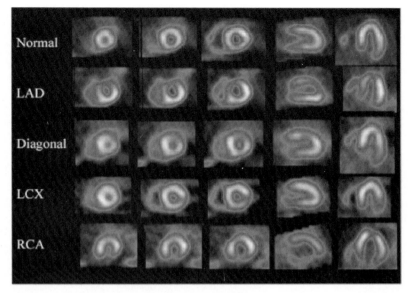

FIGURE 30-4. [99m]Tc stress images showing perfusion defects in each of the respective coronary distributions. (From Fuster V, Alexander RW, O'Rourke RA, et al., eds. *Hurst's The Heart*, 13th ed. New York, NY: McGraw-Hill; 2005, with permission.)

- ○ The reversibility of defects seen on stress images
- ○ The presence of any infarct (the size and severity also should be mentioned)
- **A defect seen in at least two tomographic planes is more likely to represent a true abnormality compared with a defect seen on one plane.**
- Similar regions of myocardium are compared at rest and at stress
  - ○ **An ischemic region will show a normal perfusion pattern at rest but reduced uptake of scintillation counts during stress.**
  - ○ **An infarcted area will demonstrate reduced perfusion at rest and at stress.**
  - ○ If a persistent defect is present (suggesting infarction), it is important to pay attention to the adjacent myocardium. One may see a fixed defect on both stress and rest images, but the stress images may show **peri-infarct ischemia** that is not demonstrated on resting images.
- The extent (size) and the severity of the perfusion abnormality are independently associated with the risk of adverse events over time.[5-15]
- **Transient ischemic dilatation** (TID) refers to the appearance of LV cavity enlargement on stress images when compared to resting pictures.
  - ○ It is suggestive of diffuse subendocardial ischemia and is a marker for severe and extensive coronary artery disease (CAD). TID suggests that the patient may have multi-vessel disease.
  - ○ Detection of lung uptake of radiotracer also suggests multivessel disease.

Artifacts

- **Breast tissue** can reduce the scintillation counts registered on the gamma camera. May cause a mild to moderately severe fixed defect of the anterior and anterolateral wall.

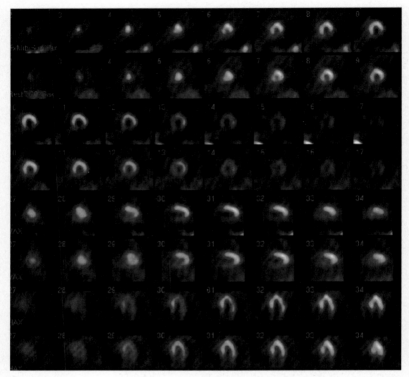

FIGURE 30-5. Rest and SPECT MPI images. Upper row represents stress images; lower row represents rest images. There is a large transmural infarction of the inferior wall and large, moderately severe ischemia of the inferolateral and lateral walls.

- Electrocardiogram (ECG) gating allows assessment of wall motion abnormalities. Evaluate wall motion abnormality associated with the areas that appear to be fixed defects.
- Fixed defects more likely represent breast attenuation artifacts rather than true infarct when associated with preserved wall motion.
- Attenuation artifacts of the inferior wall can be caused by extracardiac structures that interfere with scintillation count measurements.
  - The **diaphragm** overlaps the inferior wall and can lead to the interpretation of a fixed defect in that region.
  - Placing the patient in a prone position can shift the diaphragm off of the inferior wall.

APPLICATIONS

Stable Chest Pain Syndromes
- The goal of MPI is to identify normally perfused, ischemic, and infarcted myocardium.
- The most common way of performing SPECT MPI is as a stress test (see next page).

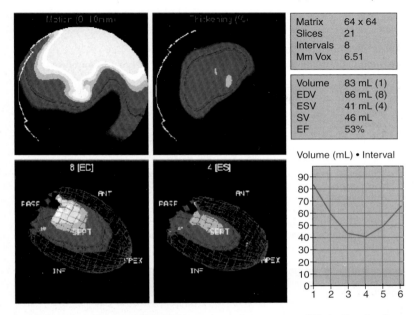

Matrix	64 x 64
Slices	21
Intervals	8
Mm Vox	6.51

Volume	83 mL (1)
EDV	86 mL (8)
ESV	41 mL (4)
SV	46 mL
EF	53%

FIGURE 30-6. ECG-gated SPECT images used to measure LV ejection fraction, wall motion, and volume.

- There is a strong relationship between the extent of ischemia and the risk of cardiac death or myocardial infarction (MI)—the greater the extent of ischemia, the higher the event risk.[8,11]
- SPECT MPI gives incremental prognostic information regarding the risk of cardiac death or nonfatal MI.[15]
- The likelihood of cardiac death or nonfatal MI is very low with normal MPI, ≤1% per year over extended follow-up (13 to 89 months).[16]

Suspected Acute Coronary Syndromes

- Patients presenting to the emergency department with symptoms suggestive of an acute coronary syndrome (ACS) (but nondiagnostic ECG and cardiac biomarkers) can undergo ^{99m}Tc-based MPI.
  - The patient is injected with ^{99m}Tc at rest and then scanned in 45 to 60 minutes.
  - As there is little redistribution of radiotracer, the images obtained in a patient with symptoms due to active ischemia reflect myocardial blood flow at the time of injection (during the ischemic state).
- The presence of perfusion defects by ^{99m}Tc pain imaging suggests either active ischemia or infarction, immediately placing the patient at a higher risk for CAD.

Assessment after Acute Myocardial Infarction

- In stable patients following ST-segment elevation MI (STEMI), SPECT MPI can help to risk stratify patients for future cardiac events.

- An MPI study that does not demonstrate reversible defects has been associated with lower risk cardiac death and non-fatal MI.

Assessment of Myocardial Viability

- **Myocardial viability can be assessed by using either ^{201}Tl or 18-fluorodeoxyglucose (FDG).**
- ^{201}Tl is an excellent agent for viability due its long half-life and ability to redistribute.
  - Myocardial viability assessment should ideally be performed 24 hours after ^{201}Tl injection, as this can detect additional viable segments, which may be missed by 1-day rest–stress SPECT MPI alone.
  - The presence of ^{201}Tl after redistribution implies preserved myocyte activity.
- FDG is a positron emission tomography (PET) radiotracer that can be used with SPECT.
  - Two studies have demonstrated similar sensitivity to resting ^{201}Tl SPECT at detecting viable myocardium but increased specificity with FDG SPECT.
  - Although the image quality and resolution of PET is clearly superior to those of SPECT, several studies have shown good correlations of viability between FDG PET and FDG SPECT (Figure 30-7).[17-19]
  - The magnitude of tracer uptake is proportional to the magnitude of preserved tissue viability.

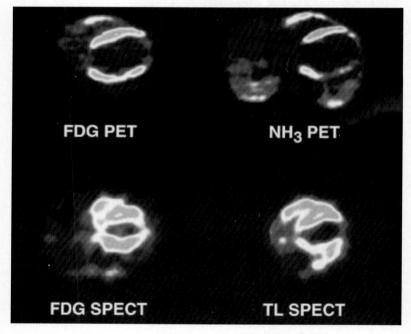

FIGURE 30-7. Comparison of myocardial viability by both PET and SPECT. Both modalities demonstrate apical infarction with metabolically active myocardium in the other walls. Note the improved spatial resolution of PET over SPECT. (From Schiepers C, ed. *Diagnostic Nuclear Medicine*, 2nd ed. New York, NY: Springer; 2005, with permission.)

INDICATIONS

Exercise Stress Testing

- Exercise stress testing is discussed in detail in Chapter 10.
- In patients who are able to exercise to an adequate workload (at least 85% of age-adjusted maximal predicted heart rate and 5 metabolic equivalents), treadmill (or bicycle) stress is the preferred modality.

Pharmacologic Stress Testing

- Pharmacologic stress testing is discussed in detail in Chapter 10.
- Indications for the use of pharmacologic stress testing include
  - Inability to perform adequate exercise (e.g., pulmonary disease, peripheral vascular disease, and musculoskeletal or mental conditions)
  - Baseline ECG abnormalities including left bundle branch block (LBBB), ventricular preexcitation, and permanent ventricular pacing
  - Risk stratification of clinically stable patients into low- and high-risk groups very early after acute MI (more than 1 day) or presentation to the emergency department with a presumptive ACS
- There are three vasodilator agents currently used: **dipyridamole, adenosine**, and **regadenoson**.[3]
  - Adenosine and regadenoson cause coronary vasodilation through A2A receptors. There is greater a vasodilation in normal coronary blood vessels than in those with atherosclerotic lesions.
  - Undesirable effects of adenosine are mediated through its activation of the A1 (AV block), A2B (peripheral vasodilation), and A3 (bronchospasm) receptors.
  - Regadenoson has a higher avidity for the A2A receptor and less for the A1, A2B, and A3 receptors. Its side-effect profile is more favorable than adenosine.
- Methylxanthines (e.g., caffeine, theophylline, and theobromine) are competitive inhibitors of both adenosine and regadenoson and must be held prior to testing. Aminophylline 50 mg to 250 mg IV is used to reverse the bronchospastic effect of the vasodilator agents.

Appropriateness Use Criteria

- As per the Appropriateness Use Criteria for Cardiac Radionuclide Imaging[20,21]:
  - "An appropriate imaging study is one in which the expected incremental information, combined with clinical judgment, exceeds the expected negative consequences by a sufficiently wide margin for a specific indication that the procedure is generally considered acceptable care and a reasonable approach for the indication."
  - "Expected negative consequences include the risks of the procedure (i.e., radiation or contrast exposure) and the downstream impact of poor test performance such as delay in diagnosis (false negatives) or inappropriate diagnosis (false positives)."
- There are 52 criteria rated in these guidelines:
  - Criteria are rated as A (appropriate), I (inappropriate), and U (uncertain or possibly appropriate).
  - An example of appropriate use criteria for the detection of CAD in symptomatic patients[20,21]:
    - Appropriate use of MPI: Low pretest probability of CAD (ECG uninterpretable) OR unable to exercise.
    - Inappropriate use of MPI: Low pretest probability of CAD (ECG interpretable) AND able to exercise.

○ A detailed explanation and the full list of criteria are available online (my.americanheart .org, last accessed 9/5/2013).

Limitations

- MPI is unable to quantify absolute myocardial blood flow:
  ○ May underestimate severity of CAD in patients with so-called balanced ischemia.[15]
  ○ Potential for false-negative stress test with triple-vessel CAD where myocardial perfusion will appear identical in all three coronary distributions.
- Prone to attenuation artifact:
  ○ Emitted photons scatter in different directions as they travel through tissue in the body rather than moving directly in their initial trajectory.
  ○ This decreases the spatial resolution of MPI.

Radiation Safety

- The most important determinant of appropriate use criteria for cardiac radionuclide imaging is often radiation exposure.
- Physicians should be guided by the principle of "as low as reasonably achievable" (ALARA) to reduce lifetime biological risk from radiation exposure.
- Table 30-1 outlines the relative radiation exposures with various cardiac imaging modalities.[22,23]

TABLE 30-1	RADIATION EXPOSURE OF CARDIAC IMAGING MODALITIES
Imaging	Estimates of effective doses (in mSV)
Pacemaker insertion	1.5
Background level of radiation absorbed from natural sources in the U.S.	≤3.0
Cardiac computed tomography (without contrast, for assessment of coronary calcium)	3.0
Comprehensive electrophysiological evaluation	5.7
Diagnostic coronary angiography	7
Cardiac blood pool imaging, gated equilibrium; planar single study at rest or stress	7.8
Percutaneous coronary intervention	15
Myocardial perfusion imaging study with ejection fraction	15.6
Cardiac computed tomography (with contrast, for assessment of coronary arteries, without assessment for coronary calcium)	16

REFERENCES

1. Bonow, RO, Mann, DL, Zipes, DP, et al., eds. Braunwald's Heart Disease: A Textbook of Cardiovascular Medicine, 9th ed. Philadelphia, PA: Elsevier; 2012.

2. Fuster V, Walsh RA, Harrington RA, et al., eds. Hurst's The Heart, 13th ed. New York, NY: McGraw-Hill; 2011.

3. Henzlova MJ, Cerqueira MD, Hansen CL, Taillefer R, Yao S. ASNC Imaging guidelines for nuclear cardiology procedures: stress protocols and tracers. J Nucl Cardiol 2009. Available at: http://www.asnc.org/imageuploads/ImagingGuidelinesStressProtocols021109.pdf, last accessed 9/4/2013.

4. Berman DS, Kiat H, Friedman JD, et al. Separate acquisition rest thallium-201/stress technetium-99m sestamibi dual-isotope myocardial perfusion single-photon emission computed tomography: a clinical validation study. J Am Coll Cardiol 1993;22:1455-1464.

5. Berman DS, Hachamovitch R, Kiat H, et al. Incremental value of prognostic testing in patients with known or suspected ischemic heart disease: a basis for optimal utilization of exercise technetium-99m sestamibi myocardial perfusion single-photon emission computed tomography. J Am Coll Cardiol 1995;26:639-647.

6. Hachamovitch R, Berman DS, Kiat H, et al. Exercise myocardial perfusion SPECT in patients without known coronary artery disease: incremental prognostic value and use in risk stratification. Circulation 1996;93:905-914.

7. Parisi AF, Hartigan PM, Folland ED. Evaluation of exercise thallium scintigraphy versus exercise electrocardiography in predicting survival outcomes and morbid cardiac events in patients with single- and double-vessel disease. Findings from the Angioplasty Compared to Medicine (ACME) Study. J Am Coll Cardiol 1997;30:1256-1263.

8. Hachamovitch R, Berman DS, Shaw LJ, et al. Incremental prognostic value of myocardial perfusion single photon emission computed tomography for the prediction of cardiac death: Differential stratification for risk of cardiac death and myocardial infarction. Circulation 1998;97:535-543.

9. Jain S, Baird JB, Fischer KC, Rich MW. Prognostic value of dipyridamole thallium imaging after acute myocardial infarction in older patients. J Am Geriatr Soc 1999;47:295-301.

10. Sharir T, Berman DS, Lewin HC, et al. Incremental prognostic value of rest-distribution Tl-201 single photon emission computed tomography. Circulation 1999;100:1964-1970.

11. Vanzetto G, Ormezzano O, Fagret D, et al. Long-term additive prognostic value of thallium-201 myocardial perfusion imaging over clinical and exercise stress test in low to intermediate risk patients : study in 1137 patients with 6-year follow-up. Circulation 1999;100:1521-1527.

12. Gibbons RJ, Hodge DO, Berman DS, et al. Long-term outcome of patients with intermediate-risk exercise electrocardiograms who do not have myocardial perfusion defects on radionuclide imaging. Circulation 1999;100:2140-2145.

13. Diaz J, Brunken RC, Blackstone EH, et al. Independent contribution of myocardial perfusion defects to exercise capacity and heart rate recovery for prediction of all-cause mortality in patients with known or suspected coronary heart disease. J Am Coll Cardiol 2001;37:1558-1564.

14. Hachamovitch R, Berman DS, Kiat H, et al. Value of stress myocardial perfusion single photon emission computed tomography in patients with normal resting electrocardiograms: an evaluation of incremental prognostic value and cost-effectiveness. Circulation 2002;105:823-829.

15. Bourque JM, Beller GA. Stress myocardial perfusion imaging for assessing prognosis: an update. JACC Cardiovasc Imaging 2011;4:1315-1319.

16. Metz LD, Beattie M, Hom R, et al. The prognostic value of normal exercise myocardial perfusion imaging and exercise echocardiography: a meta-analysis. J Am Coll Cardiol 2007;49:227-237.

17. Schiepers C, ed. Diagnostic Nuclear Medicine, 2nd ed. New York, NY: Springer; 2005.

18. Bax JJ, Visser FC, Blanksma PK, et al. Comparison of myocardial uptake of fluorine-18-fluorodeoxyglucose imaged with PET and SPECT in dyssynergic myocardium. J Nucl Med 1996;37:1631-1636.

19. Martin WH, Delbeke D, Patton JA, et al. FDG-SPECT: correlation with FDG-PET. J Nucl Med 1995;36:988-995.

20. Hendel RC, Berman DS, Di Carli MF, et al. 2009 Appropriate use criteria for cardiac radionuclide imaging. J Am Coll Cardiol 2009;53:2201-2229.
21. Hendel RC, Berman DS, Di Carli MT, et al. ACCF/ASNC/ACR/AHA/ASE/SCCT/SCMR/SNM 2009 appropriate use criteria for cardiac radionuclide imaging. Circulation 2009;119:e561-e587.
22. Mettler FA Jr, Huda W, Yoshizumi TT, Hahesh H. Effective doses in radiology and diagnostic nuclear medicine: a catalog. Radiology 2008;248:254-263.
23. Gerber TC, Carr JJ, Arai AE, et al. Ionizing radiation in cardiac imaging: a science advisory from the American Heart Association Committee on Cardiac Imaging of the Council on Clinical Cardiology and Committee on Cardiovascular Imaging and Intervention of the Council on Cardiovascular Radiology and Intervention. Circulation 2009;119:1056-1065.

Echocardiography

31

Majesh Makan and Mohammed Saghir

GENERAL PRINCIPLES

Definition
- Echocardiography is ultrasound imaging of the heart.
- Images are acquired by placing the ultrasound probe on the chest (transthoracic) or by intubating the esophagus with a modified probe (transesophageal).

Physics
- High-frequency sound waves (20,000 Hz) are emitted by a transducer which are modified by the body and reflected back to the transducer.
- Ultrasound can pass easily through fluids but poorly through bones and air.
- Hyperechoic structures:
  - Black regions on ultrasound where waves are attenuated.
  - Blood, pleural effusions, and pericardial effusions
- Hypoechoic structures:
  - Gray areas of varying brightness
  - Often depend on how well the structure reflects ultrasound waves
  - Myocardium, valves, vessel walls, masses, thrombi, and vegetations

Modalities
- Color Doppler:
  - Graphical display of blood flow
  - Flow toward the transducer is displayed in red.
  - Flow away is displayed in blue.
- Pulse-wave Doppler:
  - Allows displaying, over time, the full range of velocities and flows within a gated area.
  - Useful in assessing severity of valvular lesions and assessing pressure gradients.
- Continuous-wave Doppler:
  - Allows displaying, over time, all velocities and flows along a single trajectory from the transducer
  - Differs from pulse-wave that examines a fixed area
- Continuous- and pulse-wave are complementary in hemodynamic assessment.
- Tissue Doppler:
  - Assesses myocardial velocity instead of blood velocity
  - Useful for assessing diastolic function
  - Also used for constriction/restriction and efficacy of cardiac resynchronization therapy
- Strain imaging:
  - Measures myocardial deformation within a cardiac cycle
  - Useful for quantifying regional myocardial function about multiple axes
  - Used in the diagnosis of certain cardiomyopathies (i.e., hypertrophic obstructive cardiomyopathy and hypertensive heart disease)

- Contrast echocardiography:
  - Contrast is lipid microspheres filled with perfluorocarbon gas that permits for excellent delineation of the endocardial border.
  - Uses:
    - Difficult image acquisition
    - Assessment of wall motion abnormalities
    - Detection of left ventricular (LV) thrombus
- Agitated saline echocardiography:
  - Created by mixing normal saline with a small volume of air
  - Resultant microbubbles injected intravenously and well visualized in the right-sided cardiac chambers.
  - Bubbles are larger than red blood cells and cannot cross the pulmonary microvasculature.
  - Appearance of saline bubbles in the left-sided cardiac chambers within three heartbeats of visualization in the right chambers consistent with intracardiac shunt.
  - Visualization after three heartbeats may suggest intrapulmonary shunt.
- Three-dimensional echocardiography:
  - Technological improvements now allow for real-time 3D volumetric acquisition and display.
  - Detailed measurements of LV volume and mass, right ventricular (RV) volume and function, congenital malformations, and valvular pathology (particularly involving the mitral valve).

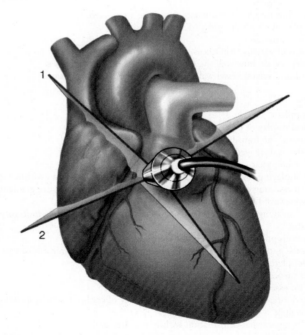

FIGURE 31-1. Transducer orientation used for acquiring parasternal views. Plane 1 represents a parasternal long-axis view. Scanning plane 2 is obtained by rotating the transducer 90 degrees and can be used to obtain a family of short-axis views of the heart. (From Feigenbaum H. *Echocardiography*, 4th ed. Malvern, PA: Lea & Febiger; 1986, with permission.)

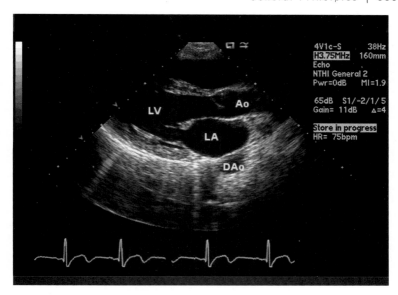

FIGURE 31-2. Parasternal long-axis view. Ao, aortic root; LA, left atrium; LV, left ventricle; DAo, descending aorta.

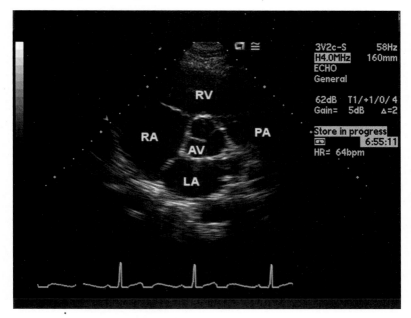

FIGURE 31-3. Short-axis 2D echocardiogram at the level of the aortic valve. AV, aortic valve; LA, left atrium; PA, pulmonary artery; RA, right atrium; RV, right ventricle.

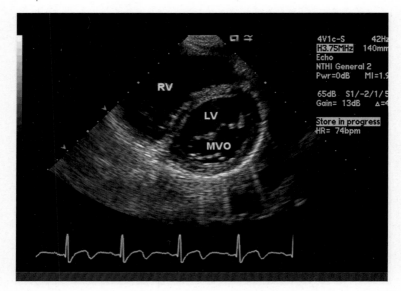

FIGURE 31-4. Short-axis 2D echocardiogram at the level of the mitral valve. LV, left ventricle; MVO, mitral valve orifice; RV, right ventricle.

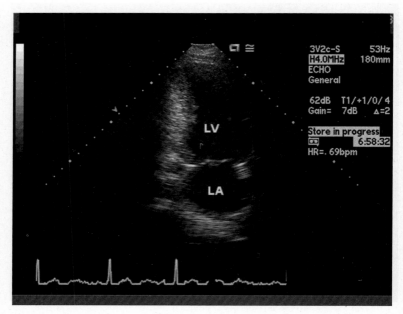

FIGURE 31-5. Apical two-chamber view of the left ventricle. LA, left atrium; LV, left ventricle.

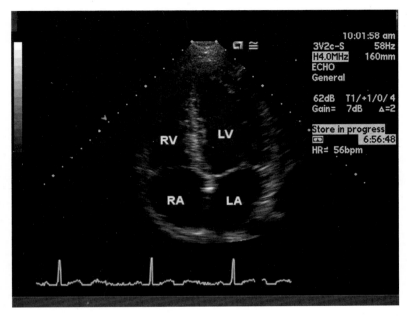

FIGURE 31-6. Apical four-chamber view of the heart. LA, left atrium; RA, right atrium; LV, left ventricle; RV, right ventricle.

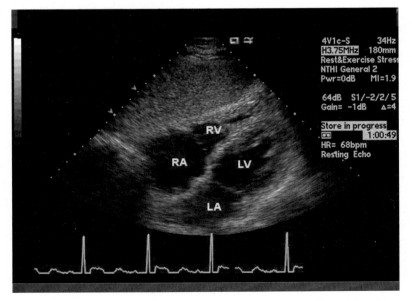

FIGURE 31-7. Subcostal four-chamber view. RA, right atrium; RV, right ventricle; LA, left atrium; LV, left ventricle.

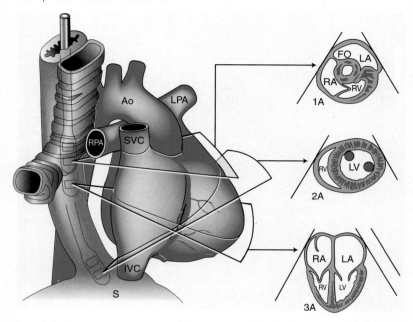

FIGURE 31-8. TEE views obtained in the horizontal transducer position. 3A is recorded in the gastric position, 2A from the midesophagus, and 1A from the upper esophagus. Ao, aorta; IVC, inferior vena cava; LA, left atrium; LAA, left atrial appendage; LUPV, left upper pulmonary vein; LV, left ventricle; RA, right atrium; RPA, right pulmonary artery; RV, right ventricle; S, stomach; SVC, superior vena cava. (From Feigenbaum H. *Echocardiography*, 4th ed. Malvern, PA: Lea & Febiger; 1986, with permission.)

APPLICATIONS

- The American Society of Echocardiography has developed **appropriateness criteria** that may be obtained at http://www.asecho.org/clinical-information/guidelines-standards/ (last accessed 9/6/2013).
- Common indications for transthoracic echocardiography (TTE) are
  - Dyspnea
  - Shock
  - Respiratory failure
  - Murmur
  - Fever
  - Chest pain
  - Congenital heart disease
  - Stroke
  - Assessment of LV function with regards to heart failure or implantable cardioverter defibrillator (ICD) placement

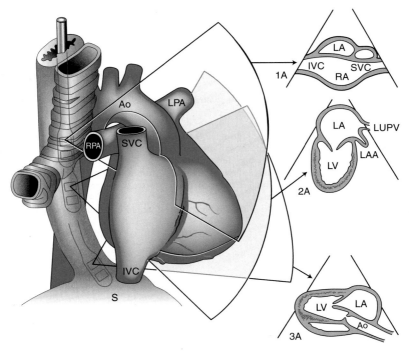

FIGURE 31-9. TEE views obtained in the longitudinal transducer position. 3A is recorded in the gastric position, 2A from the midesophagus, and 1A from the upper esophagus. Ao, aorta; IVC, inferior vena cava; LA, left atrium; LAA, left atrial appendage; LUPV, left upper pulmonary vein; LV, left ventricle; RA, right atrium; RPA, right pulmonary artery; RV, right ventricle; S, stomach; SVC, superior vena cava. (From Feigenbaum H. *Echocardiography*, 4th ed. Malvern, PA: Lea & Febiger; 1986, with permission.)

- Common indications for transesophageal echocardiography (TEE) (similar to TTE with the following):
  - Assessment of aortic pathology
  - Evaluation of LA appendage for thrombus
  - Assessment of valvular pathology
- TTE Advantages:
  - Portable, non-invasive, affordable, and able to answer most cardiac clinical questions
  - Provides accurate assessment of structure, hemodynamics, and physiology
- TTE Disadvantages:
  - Can be limited by body habitus
  - Obesity and chronic obstructive pulmonary disease can limit image quality.
- TEE advantages:
  - Better at visualizing posterior structures such as the atria, atrial appendage, aortic valve, and mitral valve
  - Effective in evaluation of the aorta

- Higher frequency transducer can give better visualization of the valves and non-biologic structures (i.e., pacemaker leads).
- TEE disadvantages:
  - Semi-invasive procedure
  - Poor visualization of distal structures such as the LV apex
- TTE is very good with hemodynamics and function, whereas TEE is very good with structure and anatomy.
- TEE will give excellent pictures of a stenotic aortic valve, whereas TTE will provide more accurate valvular gradients.
- Stress echocardiography:
  - TTE that is performed before, during, and after cardiovascular stress looking for new or worsening regional myocardial wall motion abnormalities.
  - Exercise or chemical stress such as dobutamine
  - More specific but less sensitive than myocardial perfusion imaging (see Chapter 30) A greater degree of myocardial ischemia is needed to see a wall motion defect compared to a perfusion defect.
  - Dobutamine stress testing with low- and high-dose dobutamine can be use to assess for myocardial viability.

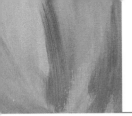

Cardiac Computed Tomography and Magnetic Resonance Imaging

32

Mohammed Saghir and Ravi Rasalingam

Cardiac Computed Tomography

GENERAL PRINCIPLES

Definitions

- Computed tomography coronary angiography (CTCA) involves imaging the coronary arteries.
- It also allows the evaluation of cardiac chambers and surrounding structures.
- Coronary calcium screening has a role in the risk stratification for primary prevention of coronary artery disease.

Physics

- Multidetector technology allows for multiple CT slices to be taken per rotation of the computed tomography (CT) tube allowing for finer spatial resolution.
- The thinnest image that can be reconstructed from the data collected is determined by the slice thickness of the scanner.
- The 64-slice scanner's ability to obtain thinner slice thickness makes it superior to the traditional scanners (4- or 16-slice detector technology). Imaging of sub-millimeter coronary vasculature requires very high spatial resolution.
- CT radiation differs from that of a standard X-ray as the source of ionizing radiation rotates around the body.
- Potential radiation effects and magnitude of dose are dependent on many factors.
- The effective dose or dose equivalent, defined in Sieverts (Sv), is the weighted sum of the radiation dose to a number of body tissues (Table 32-1).

Interpretation and Image Analysis

- Image acquisition must be timed with the cardiac cycle.
- Image acquisition is coupled with electrocardiogram (ECG) triggering.
- Retrospective gating:
  - X-rays applied throughout the cardiac cycle
  - Desired images are selected post-acquisition.
  - Results in increased radiation exposure
- Prospective gating:
  - Application of X-rays only at specific times in the cardiac cycle
  - Preferred as it minimizes radiation exposure
  - The gating is often timed with end-diastole and end-systole when the heart is relatively still to minimize motion artifacts.
- Imaging of the heart during a complete cardiac cycle allows cine imaging is useful for measuring ejection fraction, wall motion, and valvular orifice area.

TABLE 32-1	COMPARISON OF EFFECTIVE RADIATION DOSES IN CARDIAC IMAGING
Yearly background radiation	1 mSv
Standard chest radiograph	0.1 mSv
Diagnostic cardiac catheterization	5 mSv
Nuclear myocardial perfusion stress test	10–35 mSv
Nongated chest CT	8 mSv
Coronary calcium CT scan	1–1.5 mSv
Retrospective gated angiography (64-slice)	18–22 mSv
Prospective dose-modulation gated coronary CT angiography (64-slice)	2–5 mSv

CT, computed tomography.

APPLICATIONS

Coronary CT Angiography

- Define cardiac anatomy:
  - Congenital anomalies
  - Pulmonary vein configuration
  - Bypass graft location
  - Tumors/thrombi
  - Coronary anomalies
  - Vein or arterial mapping
- Chest pain syndrome in the intermediate risk patient with either indeterminate ECG or inability to exercise:
  - Ability of CTCA to assess severity and extent of atherosclerosis in comparison to conventional angiography has been validated in multiple studies with both 16- and 64-slice scanners.[1-8]
  - Strong negative predictive value to exclude significant coronary stenosis
- Assessment of both the lumen and arterial wall for positive remodeling and plaque vulnerability:
  - Positive remodeling:
    - Expansion of the arterial cross-sectional area in an attempt to preserve the luminal area in response to increasing plaque burden
    - Not well appreciated on conventional angiography (Figure 32-1)
  - Plaque vulnerability:
    - Most plaques associated with myocardial infarction are non-obstructive in nature.
    - Often non-calcified and more prone to rupture than their obstructive, more calcified counterparts
- Acute chest pain in the intermediate risk patient with normal ECG and negative serial enzymes. Excellent negative predictive value in ruling out ACS among patients where no coronary lesions were seen.
- Appropriateness criteria have been developed regarding the use of CTCA.[9]

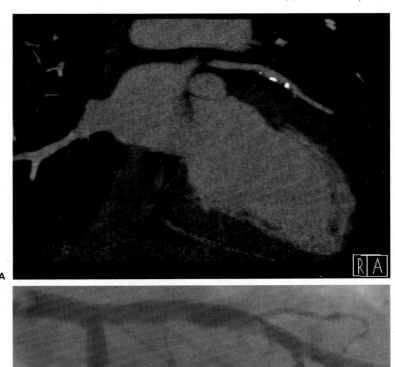

FIGURE 32-1. Atherosclerosis of the proximal LAD with positive remodeling. **(A)** CTCA. **(B)** Conventional angiography.

Coronary Artery Calcification

- Coronary artery calcification (CAC) imaging can be applied to specific stenoses or calculated as an overall calcium score.
- Overall atherosclerotic burden can be correlated with CAC.
- There is a strong correlation of atherosclerotic burden with CAC.[10-14]
  - Predictive of long-term cardiovascular events. The results of one such study of over 6,000 persons followed for a median of 3.8 years are presented in Table 32-2.[11]
  - Overall atherosclerotic burden, rather than a specific stenosis, that can be important in the prediction of long-term cardiovascular events.
- Quantification of CAC is performed as a CAC score or Agatston score.[15]
  - Computer-generated by multiplying the calcium plaque area (in square millimeters) by the calcium plaque density (Hounsfield number)
  - A high CAC score does not equate to a severely stenotic lesion but rather to a high atherosclerotic burden and a higher risk of cardiovascular events.[10-14]
- CAC may have a role in the risk stratification of asymptomatic individuals at an intermediate risk for cardiovascular event by Framingham criteria.[12,16]

TABLE 32-2	CORONARY CALCIUM SCORE AND CARDIOVASULAR RISK[a]	
Coronary calcium score	Major coronary event[b] (HR)	Any coronary event (HR)
0	1.00	1.00
0–100	3.89	3.61
101–300	7.08	7.73
>300	6.84	9.67

HR, hazard ratio.

[a]After adjustment for standard coronary risk factors.

[b]Myocardial infarction or death from coronary artery disease.

Modified from Detrano R, Guerci AD, Carr JJ, et al. Coronary calcium as a predictor of coronary events in four racial or ethnic groups. *N Engl J Med* 2008;358:1336-1345.

- More aggressive cardiovascular management may be indicated in those individuals scoring higher than the 75th percentile of CAC score.
- Disadvantages of CAC include relatively moderate specificity for predicting significant coronary artery lesions.

Limitations

- Contraindications:
  - Serum creatinine >1.5 mg/dL
  - Pregnancy
  - Breastfeeding
  - History of severe allergy to IV contrast
- Image quality will be reduced in patients with the following conditions:
  - Irregular heart rhythms (atrial fibrillation/flutter and/or frequent premature atrial/ventricular contractions) with improper ECG triggering. Can result in slice misregistration and/or errors in radiation dose modulation.
  - High regular heart rates (>70 bpm) refractory to rate-lowering agents causes motion artifact.
  - Extreme obesity (BMI >40 kg/m²) leads to excessive radiation attenuation with a subsequent reduction in the signal-to-noise ratio.
- Metallic objects (e.g., surgical clips, mechanical heart valves, or the wires of a pacer/automatic implanted cardiac defibrillator) are prone to radiation scatter, producing streaking artifacts. Coronary stent patency assessment is possible but not always reliable.

Cardiac Magnetic Resonance Imaging

GENERAL PRINCIPLES

Definitions

- The high resolution of cardiovascular magnetic resonance (CMR) allows the detailed examination and measurement of cardiac anatomy.
- Uses a strong magnetic field and radiofrequency waves to provide detailed images of internal organs and tissues.

Physics

- Hydrogen nuclei align their magnetic moments when exposed to an electromagnetic field.
- The quantity of nuclei in alignment depends on the duration and intensity of the applied field.
- When the field is deactivated, the nuclei return to their normal state and release detectable photons that correlate with their resonating frequency.
- Magnetic resonance provides markedly detailed images by exploiting the difference in water content in soft tissue. The relation between applied field strength and detected frequency allows for imaging of soft tissue that has high water content and, correspondingly, a high proportion of hydrogen atoms.
- Lack of radiation exposure is particularly important in cases where serial studies are needed.
- Simple breath-holding techniques and cardiac gating have improved image quality and reduce motion artifact during imaging of the heart and coronary arteries.

APPLICATIONS

Congenital Heart Disease[17-19]

- The ability to delineate complex cardiac anatomy and without radiation exposure is advantageous in young patients who need sequential studies.
- Can quantify cardiac shunt to assist in treatment and prognosis.
- Particularly helpful for postoperative follow-up where right ventricular assessment and complex post-operative anatomy can pose difficulties for 2D echocardiography.

Cardiomyopathies[17]

- CMR is well established in the evaluation of left ventricular (LV) and right ventricular (RV) mass and function.
- Can distinguish between ischemic and non-ischemic cardiomyopathy with gadolinium enhancement including
  - Arrhythmogenic RV dysplasia
  - Infiltrative cardiomyopathies such as
    - Amyloid heart disease
    - Hemochromatosis
    - Sarcoidosis
  - Focal inflammatory changes in myocarditis
  - Serial assessment of rejection episodes following heart transplantation
  - Pericardial thickening in the evaluation of constrictive pericarditis (Figure 32-2)
- Identification of fibrotic areas linked to the risk of sudden cardiac death and development of heart failure
- Quantification of infracted myocardium and determination of viability in ischemic cardiomyopathy
- LV noncompaction, the failure of loosely arranged muscle fibers to form mature compacted myocardium during the embryonic development, which is increasingly recognized during high-resolution magnetic resonance (MR) studies.
- Tumor infiltration into the pericardium with differentiation of cystic tumors, fatty tumors, melanoma metastasis, hemorrhage, and vascular tumors (Figure 32-3)

Valvular Heart Disease

- Allows for morphologic and functional assessment of cardiac valves.[17,20-23]
  - Not prone to poor acoustic windows that may be encountered in transthoracic echocardiography.
  - Valuable alternative when a transesophageal echocardiography procedure is not desired by the patient.

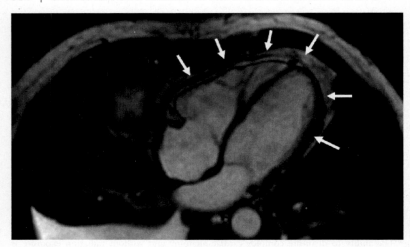

FIGURE 32-2. Pericardial constriction: concentric pericardial thickening and constriction around the LV and RV (*white arrows*).

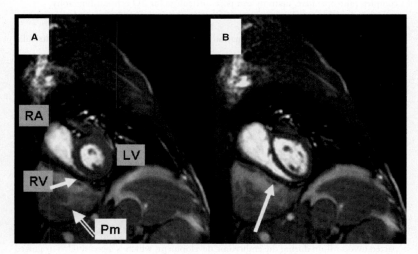

FIGURE 32-3. RV compression. **A:** Pericardial mass (Pm; *double arrow*) compressing the RV (*white arrow*) during systole. Right atrium is enlarged. **B:** Ability of the RV to fill during diastole is significantly impaired (*white arrow*).

- Measure peak velocity.
- Estimate the pressure gradient to evaluate the severity of stenosis.
- Volume quantification permits accurate assessment of valvular regurgitation.
- Most prosthetic valves are safe for imaging but focal artifacts may obscure the images.

Vascular Disease[24]

- CMR can image many aspects of the vessel wall, including the assessment of dissection, thrombus, inflammation, and atherosclerotic plaque.
- Magnetic resonance angiography (MRA) may be done without contrast injection using "time-of-flight" techniques or with intravenous gadolinium. This is useful in patients with contraindications to X-ray contrast.
- A rare but significant side effect of gadolinium contrast agents, **nephrogenic systemic fibrosis** (NSF), has been described in patients with severe renal insufficiency; therefore, caution is warranted in these patients (see below).[17,24]
- MRA combined with vascular wall imaging is valuable in the detection and serial monitoring of thoracic and abdominal aortic aneurysms.

Coronary Artery Disease

- The direct visualization of coronary arteries with coronary MRA has improved in recent years but still faces technical challenges, mainly due to motion artifacts. CT or cardiac catheterization is preferable.
- Ischemia[25,26]:
  - Gadolinium-enhanced CMR incorporated with a pharmacological agent such as adenosine.
  - Visualize ischemia as areas of myocardial hypoperfusion as the contrast washes through the myocardium.
- Infarction: Delayed imaging of late gadolinium enhancement is highly sensitive for the detection of myocardial fibrosis.
- The combination of these two techniques allows the determination of myocardial viability and prediction of myocardial recovery following revascularization.

Contrast Enhancement

- MR imaging (MRI) benefits from the use of contrast agents.
- These agents generate effects by altering the local magnetic field and relaxation parameters within the imaged tissue.
- The most commonly used contrast agents are gadolinium chelates.
  - Gadolinium is an extracellular contrast agent that is normally not retained in myocardium.
  - It is retained by infarcted myocardium where it is seen as a bright signal on imaging.
- Anaphylactoid reactions with these agents have been observed in less than 0.1% of cases.[17,24]
- NSF:
  - A rare but serious complication
  - Described with administration of certain gadolinium chelates.
  - Gadolinium-based contrast agents should be avoided unless the diagnostic information is essential and not available with non–contrast-enhanced MRI in the following patients:
    - Acute or chronic severe renal insufficiency
    - Renal dysfunction of any severity due to the hepatorenal syndrome
    - In the perioperative liver transplantation period
    - Dialysis patients should receive gadolinium agents only when this is essential and if so, dialysis should be performed as soon as possible after scan.

Contraindications

- Absolute:
  - Pacemakers/implanted cardiac defibrillators (ICDs) and other electronic implants. This is primarily due to inappropriate electronic function rather than the magnetic field's effect on the implant.[17,27]

- Metallic fragments in the eye are not held in place by scar. An orbital X-ray should be performed prior to MRI if a metal fragment is suspected to be in the eye.
  - Aneurysm clips in the brain are not protected by scar.
- Relative:
  - Cochlear implants, insulin pumps, and nerve stimulators
  - Mechanical cardiac valves, if dehiscence is suspected.[17,27]
  - Cardiac lead wires
  - Orthopedic implants are usually stable if embedded for several weeks but cause artifacts when adjacent to the area of interest.
  - Staples are considered safe when embedded for several weeks.
- Acoustic noise is due to the currents in the wires of the gradient magnets:
  - In 3T scanners, depending on the imaging techniques, the noise can reach more than 130 dB.
  - Appropriate ear protection is mandatory.
- Pregnancy:
  - Not enough data exist on the effects of MR on the developing fetus.
  - Current guidelines recommend that a pregnant woman should undergo MR imaging only when essential and ideally after the first trimester after organogenesis is completed.
  - Although no harmful effects on the fetus have been demonstrated, the fetus may be more sensitive to the effects of heating and noise.
  - Gadolinium compounds cross the placenta and are not recommended for use in pregnancy.

REFERENCES

1. Budoff MJ, Dowe D, Jollis JG, et al. Diagnostic performance of 64-multidetector row coronary computed tomographic angiography for evaluation of coronary artery stenosis in individuals without known coronary artery disease: results from the prospective multicenter ACCURACY (Assessment by Coronary Computed Tomographic Angiography of Individuals Undergoing Invasive Coronary Angiography) trial. J Am Coll Cardiol 2008;52:1724-1732.
2. Garcia MJ, Lessick J, Hoffmann MH, et al. Accuracy of 16-row multidetector computed tomography for the assessment of coronary artery stenosis. JAMA 2006;296:403-411.
3. Hoffmann U, Truong QA, Schoenfeld DA, et al. Coronary CT angiography versus standard evaluation in acute chest pain. N Engl J Med 2012;367:299-308.
4. Meijboom WB, Meijs MF, Schuijf JD, et al. Diagnostic accuracy of 64-slice computed tomography coronary angiography: a prospective, multicenter, multivendor study. J Am Coll Cardiol 2008;52:2135-2144.
5. Miller JM, Rochitte CE, Dewey M, et al. Diagnostic performance of coronary angiography by 64-row CT. N Engl J Med 2008;359:2324-2336.
6. Ollendorf DA, Kuba M, Pearson SD. The diagnostic performance of multi-slice coronary computed tomographic angiography: a systematic review. J Gen Intern Med 2011;26:307-316.
7. Paech DC, Weston AR. A systematic review of the clinical effectiveness of 64-slice or higher computed tomography angiography as an alternative to invasive coronary angiography in the investigation of suspected coronary artery disease. BMC Cardiovasc Disord 2011;11:32. doi:10.1186/1471-2261-11-32.
8. Stein PD, Yaekoub AY, Matta F, Sostman HD. 64-slice CT for diagnosis of coronary artery disease: a systematic review. Am J Med 2008;121:715-725.
9. Taylor AJ, Cerqueira M, Hodgson JM, et al. ACCF/SCCT/ACR/AHA/ASE/ASNC/NASCI/SCAI/SCMR 2010 Appropriate use criteria for cardiac computed tomography. Circulation 2010;122:e525-e555.
10. Bundoff MJ, Hokanson JE, Nasir K, et al. Progression of coronary artery calcium predicts all-cause mortality. JACC Cardiovasc Imaging 2010;3:1229-1236.
11. Detrano R, Guerci AD, Carr JJ, et al. Coronary calcium as a predictor of coronary events in four racial or ethnic groups. N Engl J Med 2008;358:1336-1345.
12. Greenland P, LaBree L, Azen SP, et al. Coronary artery calcium score combined with Framingham score for risk prediction in asymptomatic individuals. JAMA 2004;291:210-215.

13. O'Rourke RA, Brundage BH, Froelicher VF, et al. American College of Cardiology/American Heart Association Expert Consensus document on electron-beam computed tomography for the diagnosis and prognosis of coronary artery disease. Circulation 2000;102:126-140.

14. Taylor AJ, Bindeman J, Feuerstein I, et al. Coronary calcium independently predicts incident premature coronary heart disease over measured cardiovascular risk factors: mean three-year outcomes in the Prospective Army Coronary Calcium (PACC) project. J Am Coll Cardiol 2005;46:807-814.

15. Agatston AS, Janowitz WR, Hildner FJ, et al. Quantification of coronary artery calcium using ultrafast computed tomography. J Am Coll Cardiol 1990;15:827-832.

16. Greenland P, Alpert JS, Beller GA, et al. 2010 ACCF/AHA guideline for assessment of cardiovascular risk in asymptomatic adults: executive summary. Circulation 2010;122:2748-2764.

17. Hundley WG, Bluemke DA, Finn JP, et al. ACCF/ACR/AHA/NASCI/SCMR 2010 expert consensus document on cardiovascular magnetic resonance. Circulation 2010;121:2462-2508.

18. Weber OM, Higgins CB. MR evaluation of cardiovascular physiology in congenital heart disease: flow and function. J Cardiovasc Magnet Res 2006;8:607-617.

19. Wood JC. Anatomical assessment of congenital heart disease. J Cardiovasc Magnet Res 2006;8:595-606.

20. Djavidani B, Debl K, Lenhart M, et al. Planimetry of mitral valve stenosis by magnetic resonance imaging. J Am Coll Cardiol 2005;45:2048-2053.

21. McVeigh ER, Guttman MA, Lederman RJ. Real-time interactive MRI-guided cardiac surgery: aortic valve replacement using a direct apical approach. Magn Reson Med 2006;56:958-964.

22. Reant P, Lederlin M, Lafitte S, et al. Absolute assessment of aortic valve stenosis by planimetry using cardiovascular magnetic resonance imaging: comparison with transesophageal echocardiography, transthoracic echocardiography, and cardiac catheterization. Eur J Radiol 2006;59:276-283.

23. Suzuki J, Caputo GR, Kondo C, et al. Cine MR imaging of valvular heart disease: display and imaging parameters affect the size of the signal void caused by valvular regurgitation. Am J Roentgenol 1990;155:723-727.

24. Kramer CM, Budoff MJ, Fayad ZA, et al. ACCF/AHA Clinical Competence Statement on Vascular Imaging with Computed Tomography and Magnetic Resonance. A report of the American College of Cardiology Foundation/American Heart Association/American College of Physicians Task Force on Clinical Competence and Training. J Am Coll Cardiol 2007;50:1097-1114.

25. Lee DC, Johnson NP. Quantification of absolute myocardial blood flow by magnetic resonance perfusion imaging. JACC Cardiovasc Imaging 2009;2:761-770.

26. Nandalur KR, Dwamena BA, Choudhri AF, et al. Diagnostic performance of stress cardiac magnetic resonance imaging in the detection of coronary artery disease. J Am Coll Cardiol 2007;50:1343-1353.

27. Levine GN, Gomes AS, Arai AE, et al. Safety of magnetic resonance imaging in patients with cardiovascular devices. Circulation 2007;116:2878-2891.

Positron Emission Tomography

33

Jiafu Ou and Robert J. Gropler

GENERAL PRINCIPLES

Definitions

While single-photon emission computed tomography (SPECT) has been the dominant nuclear modality in clinical practice, positron emission tomography (PET) has transitioned from a valuable research technique to an important clinical modality.

Physics

- Positron emission is a type of β-decay of an unstable radionuclide.
- In this unstable radionuclide, a proton undergoes spontaneous decay into a neutron, a neutrino, and a β^+ particle (positron).
- After a high-energy positron is emitted from a nucleus, it travels a few millimeters in the tissue losing kinetic energy until it ultimately collides with an electron (a negatively charged β particle).
- This collision results in complete annihilation of both the positron and the electron, with conversion to energy in the form of electromagnetic radiation composed of two high-energy gamma rays, each with an energy of 511 keV.
- The discharged gamma rays travel in opposite directions (180 degrees from each other).
- These gamma rays can be simultaneously detected by a PET scanner, which is referred to as coincidence detection.
- The PET scanner consists of multiple stationary detectors that encircle the thorax and can be programmed to register only events with temporal coincidence of photons that strike at directly opposing detectors using electronic collimation (Figure 33-1).[1]
- By determining where these gamma rays originated, the PET scanner can create an image showing where in the body the annihilation occurred.
- Coincidence detection offers **greater sensitivity and spatial resolution compared with SPECT scans**.
- Three FDA-approved PET tracers are available for cardiovascular applications: rubidium-82 (^{82}Rb) and ^{13}N-ammonia for perfusion and fluorine-18 radiolabeled fluorodeoxyglucose (^{18}F-FDG) for metabolism.
- Rubidium-82:
  - Rubidium is a potassium analog with kinetics similar to thallium-201 whose uptake correlates with blood flow.
  - It has a high myocardial extraction fraction over a wide range of coronary blood flow.
  - Its short half-life of 75 seconds means that any trapped ^{82}Rb quickly disappears from the myocardium by physical decay.
  - ^{82}Rb is produced from strontium-82 via a commercially available generator that can be purchased and kept on site.
  - The generator costs approximately $30,000 per unit and due to the half-life of the strontium-82 requires 13 units per year.
- ^{13}N-ammonia:
  - Nitrogen-13 is cyclotron produced and used to radiolabel ammonia to yield ^{13}N-ammonia.

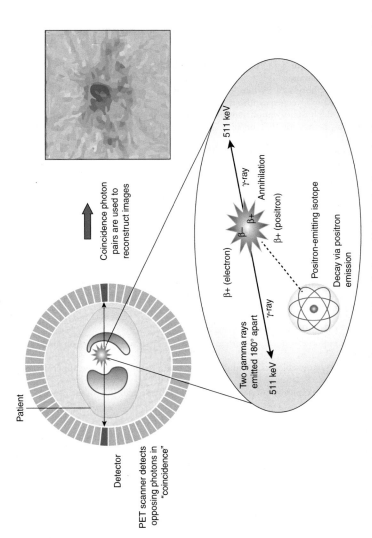

FIGURE 33-1. Schematic of positron and electron beta particle emission, with detection by a coincidence camera, as the basis of positron-emission tomography imaging. (From Udelson JE, Dilsizian V, Bonow RO. Nuclear Cardiology. In: Libby P, Bonow RO, Mann DL, Zipes DP, eds. *Braunwald's Heart Disease: A Textbook of Cardiovascular Medicine,* 8th ed. Philadelphia, PA: Elsevier; 2008:345-391, with permission.)

- ◦ ^{13}N-ammonia is a partially extractable perfusion tracer whose uptake is proportion to myocardial perfusion.
- ◦ It has a 9.9-minute half-life and favorable myocardial kinetics.
- ◦ Its image quality is generally superior to that obtained with the shorter half-life of ^{82}Rb.
- ◦ The main limitation with ^{13}N-ammonia is the requirement of an on-site cyclotron.
- ^{18}F-FDG:
  - ◦ ^{18}F is cyclotron produced and used to radiolabel fluorodeoxyglucose to yield ^{18}F-FDG.
  - ◦ ^{18}F has a half-life of about 110 minutes.
  - ◦ Following injection of 5 to 10 mCi, ^{18}F-FDG rapidly exchanges across the capillary and cellular membranes.
  - ◦ It is then phosphorylated by hexokinase to FDG-6-phosphate and not metabolized further or used in glycogen synthesis.
  - ◦ Because the dephosphorylation rate of ^{18}F-FDG is slow, it becomes trapped in the myocardium, permitting PET or SPECT imaging of regional glucose metabolism.

Interpretation and Image Analysis
- Similar to SPECT, emission data are displayed as tomograms in the horizontal and vertical long-axis and short-axis views.
- If the data are acquired in dynamic mode, with appropriate mathematical modeling, myocardial perfusion and metabolic data can be displayed in absolute terms:
  - ◦ Milliliters per gram per minute (mL/g/minute) for blood flow
  - ◦ Moles per gram per minute for metabolism

APPLICATIONS

Clinically available cardiac PET radiotracers fall within two broad categories: myocardial perfusion imaging (MPI) and myocardial metabolism.

Myocardial Perfusion Imaging
- MPI requires radiotracer injection both at rest and after stress. Images are obtained after each injection.
- Stress is usually pharmacologically induced vasodilatation with adenosine, dipyridamole, or regadenoson.
- Exercise stress test is typically not performed due to the short half-lives of the radiotracers.
- Clinical uses:
  - ◦ Detect myocardial ischemia and infarction.
  - ◦ Assess left ventricular (LV) systolic function.
  - ◦ Relative regional differences of radiotracer uptake can be detected and quantified by PET to identify the regions of ischemia or infarction (similar to SPECT).
  - ◦ Absolute regional coronary blood flow at rest and during stress (in mL/g/minute) can be obtained.
    - ▪ Detection and evaluation of extensive multi-vessel CAD with balanced ischemia on qualitative images
    - ▪ Evaluation of the significance of a given lesion
    - ▪ Monitoring of therapeutic strategies
  - ◦ Diagnostic test of choice in patients who may be prone to artifacts that could lead to an indeterminate SPECT test, such as severely obese patients.
- Advantages[2,3]:
  - ◦ **Better sensitivity and specificity compared with SPECT**[4,5]
  - ◦ Provides ischemic burden data and higher diagnostic accuracy

- ○ Increased procedure efficiencies and patient throughput as stress and rest perfusion protocols completed in less time than with SPECT
- ○ Lower radiation exposure compared with SPECT
- Limitations:
  - ○ The expense of both scanners and the radiopharmaceuticals. Some studies, however, suggest that it can be cost saving in specific patient populations.[6,7]
  - ○ Inability to routinely perform treadmill stress test.

Myocardial Viability

- ^{18}F-FDG is most commonly used for assessing myocardial viability.
- Ischemic myocardium that is viable remains metabolically active (utilizes glucose).
- Assessed either by administering ^{18}F-FDG with ^{13}N-ammonia or [82]Rb or by utilizing a SPECT MPI study.

Myocardial Metabolism[13]

- Myocardium requires a continuous supply of oxygen and metabolic substrates to meet its energy demands.
  - ○ Fatty acids are the preferred energy source for overall oxidative metabolism under normal conditions.
  - ○ Fatty acids cannot be oxidized in ischemic myocardium, and glucose becomes the preferred energy source.[8]
  - ○ This metabolic phenomenon is useful for the identification of myocardium that is under-perfused but still viable.
    - Such tissue is often hypokinetic or akinetic but will exhibit improved function if blood flow is restored.
    - MPI with either PET or SPECT should accompany ^{18}F-FDG cardiac PET imaging so that the areas of hypoperfusion are identified.
  - ○ Stress MPI may be performed to identify the presence and amount of reversible perfusion defects unless there is a contraindication for stress testing.
  - ○ ^{18}F-FDG PET imaging should be performed following a 6- to 12-hour fast followed by a glucose load and supplemental insulin administered as needed to favor metabolism of glucose over fatty acids by the heart.
  - ○ ^{18}F-FDG images are typically compared with resting MPI.
- Clinical implications:
  - ○ **Cardiac ^{18}F-FDG PET imaging has been considered a gold standard for the assessment of myocardial viability.**[3,9]
  - ○ Useful in patients with LV dysfunction due to coronary artery disease who are eligible for coronary revascularization and have resting myocardial perfusion defects in order to differentiate viable (i.e., hibernation or stunning) from non-viable myocardium (i.e., scar).[10,11]
  - ○ Three major patterns of perfusion metabolism comparisons can be seen and quantified (Figure 33-2)[12]:
    - Normal myocardial perfusion with normal or enhanced ^{18}F-FDG uptake.
    - **Reduced myocardial perfusion with preserved ^{18}F-FDG uptake represents predominantly viable myocardium**.
    - Reduced myocardial perfusion with reduced ^{18}F-FDG uptake represents predominantly non-viable myocardium or scar.
  - ○ Potential for improved heart failure symptoms following revascularization correlates with the magnitude of the PET mismatch pattern.
- The presence of viable myocardium is a marker of an increased CV risk.
- Patients with preserved myocardial viability who undergo revascularization have reduction in the risk of cardiac death.[10,11]

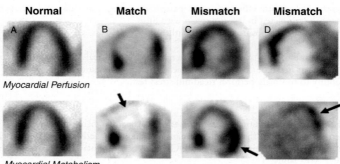

Normal	Match	Mismatch	Mismatch

Myocardial Perfusion

Myocardial Metabolism

FIGURE 33-2. Patterns of myocardial perfusion (upper panel) and metabolism (with ^{18}F-FDG lower panel). (From Schelbert HR. Positron Emission Tomography for the Noninvasive Study and Quantitation of Myocardial Blood Flow and Metabolism in Cardiovascular Disease. In: Fuster V, O'Rourke R, Walsh R, Poole-Wilson R. eds. *Hurst's the Heart*, 12th ed. New York, NY: McGraw Hill; 2007, with permission.)

- Revascularization conferred no natural history advantage in patients without substantial myocardial viability.
- Advantages:
  - Detection scheme yields higher image quality in obese patients.
  - More accurate than thallium-201 SPECT, more sensitive the dobutamine echocardiography, and contraindications to ferromagnetic objects as is the case with magnetic resonance imaging.
  - Most experience in patients with severe ischemic cardiomyopathy.
- Disadvantages:
  - Glucose pre-loading with adequate insulin availability is required for successful results.
  - Expensive

REFERENCES

1. Udelson JE, Dilsizian V, Bonow RO. Nuclear Cardiology. In: Libby P, Bonow RO, Mann DL, Zipes DP, eds. Braunwald's Heart Disease: A Textbook of Cardiovascular Medicine, 8th ed. Philadelphia, PA: Elsevier; 2008:345-391.
2. Heller GV, Calnon D, Dorbala S. Recent advances in cardiac PET and PET/CT myocardial perfusion imaging. J Nucl Cardiol 2009;16:962-969.
3. Bengel FM, Higuchi T, Javadi MS, Lautamäki R. Cardiac positron emission tomography. J Am Coll Cardiol 2009;54:1-15.
4. Nandalur KR, Dwamena BA, Choudhri AF, et al. Diagnostic performance of positron emission tomography in the detection of coronary artery disease: a meta-analysis. Acad Radiol 2008;15:444-451.
5. Di Carli MF, Hachamovitch R. New technology for noninvasive evaluation of coronary artery disease. Circulation 2007;115:1464-1480.
6. Merhige ME, Breen WJ, Shelton V, et al. Impact of myocardial perfusion imaging with PET and (82)Rb on downstream invasive procedure utilization, costs, and outcomes in coronary disease management. J Nucl Med 2007;48:1069-1076.
7. Patterson RE, Eisner RL, Horowitz SF. Comparison of cost-effectiveness and utility of exercise ECG, single photon emission computed tomography, positron emission tomography, and coronary angiography for diagnosis of coronary artery disease. Circulation 1995;91:54-65.

8. Peterson LR, Gropler RJ. Radionuclide imaging of myocardial metabolism. Circ Cardiovasc Imaging 2010;3:211-222.

9. Schinkel AF, Bax JJ, Poldermans D, et al. Hibernating myocardium: diagnosis and patient outcomes. Curr Probl Cardiol 2007;32:375-410.

10. Allman K, Shaw L, Hachamovitch R, Udelson JE. Myocardial viability testing and impact of revascularization on prognosis in patients with coronary artery disease and left ventricular dysfunction: a meta-analysis. J Am Coll Cardiol 2002;39:1151-1158.

11. Boehm J, Haas F, Bauernschmitt R, et al. Impact of preoperative positron emission tomography in patients with severely impaired LV-function undergoing surgical revascularization. *Int J* Cardiovasc Imaging 2010;26:423-432.

12. Dilsizian V, Bacharach SL, Beanlands RS, et al. PET myocardial perfusion and metabolism clinical imaging. J Nucl Cardiol 2009;16:651-680.

13. Schelbert HR. Positron Emission Tomography for the Noninvasive Study and Quantitation of Myocardial Blood Flow and Metabolism in Cardiovascular Disease. In: Fuster V, O'Rourke R, Walsh R, Poole-Wilson R, eds. Hurst's the Heart, 12th ed. New York, NY: McGraw Hill; 2007.

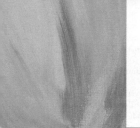

Coronary Angiography, Intravascular Ultrasound, and Intracardiac Echocardiography

34

Alok Bachuwar and John M. Lasala

Cardiac Catheterization and Angiography

GENERAL PRINCIPLES

Definitions

Cardiac catheterization/angiography is one of the most widely used and comprehensive modalities of cardiac imaging that provides

- Visual information
- Pressure measurement and oximetry
- Direct mechanical intervention of coronary and valvular lesions

Physics

- Catheter-based angiography is performed using a **cinefluorographic system** (Figure 34-1).[1]
  - The system produces an X-ray beam that projects through the patient at a desired angle.
  - The projected X-ray beam is then detected after it passes through the patient.
  - The beam is then transduced into a visible light image.
- Basic components of a cinefluorographic system are a generator, an X-ray tube, and an image intensifier (II).
  - The generator controls and delivers electrical power to the X-ray tube.
  - The X-ray tube contains a filament that is heated by the generator to ultimately form the X-ray beam.
  - The X-ray beam attenuates as it passes through the tissue.
  - The degree of attenuation varies with the tissue density, projection angle, and distance.
  - After passing through the patient, the attenuated X-ray enters the II.
  - The II converts the attenuated X-ray beam into a visible light image.
  - The image X-ray tube and II are positioned 180 degrees apart on a rotating gantry. Thus, the II always remains opposite to the X-ray tube at various angles.
  - It is convenient to think of the II as the camera that is taking pictures.
- Cinefluorographic systems operate in two modes: **fluoroscopy and acquisition**.
  - Fluoroscopy mode (often referred to as "fluoro") provides a real-time X-ray image with adequate quality for guiding catheter manipulation.
  - The acquisition mode (known as "cine") generates images of much greater visual quality, which are then recorded.
  - Most cinefluorographic systems are calibrated to give an X-ray dose that is 15 times greater during cine when compared with fluoro.
  - Fluoro is used for catheter positioning, and cine is then used to record dye injection after catheter placement.

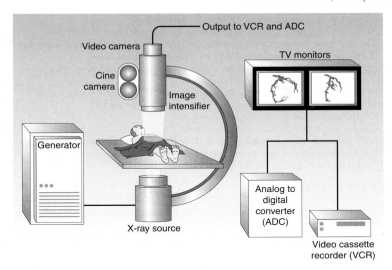

FIGURE 34-1. The cinefluorographic system. (From Zipes DP, Libby P, Bonow RO, Braunwald E, eds. *Braunwald's Heart Disease: A Textbook of Cardiovascular Medicine*, 7th ed. Philadelphia, PA: Elsevier; 2004, with permission.)

Technique

- Catheter placement requires **arterial or venous access**.
  - Arterial access is typically obtained through the femoral, radial, or brachial arteries.
  - Venous access is typically obtained through the femoral, internal jugular, or subclavian veins.
- Classically, an 18-gauge needle is inserted into the vessel at a 45-degree angle. After blood return is seen, a J-tipped wire is advanced into the vessel. The needle is then removed. A **sheath–dilator** combination is advanced over the wire into the vessel. The dilator is then removed leaving the sheath in place. The sheath secures the access site and acts as a door, allowing catheter insertion and removal.
- Many different catheters are used for the various anatomic structures that are targets of contrast injection.
- Common targets include
  - Left main (LM) coronary artery (Judkins left and Amplatz left catheters)
  - Right coronary artery (Judkins right, Amplatz right, and WRP catheters)
  - Left ventricle (pigtail catheter)
  - Aortocoronary venous grafts (Judkins right, Amplatz right, right coronary bypass, left coronary bypass, and multipurpose catheters)
  - Left internal mammary artery (LIMA) (LIMA catheter and Judkins right catheter) and aorta (pigtail catheter)
- Less common targets include the right internal mammary artery, right ventricle, pulmonary artery, pulmonary veins, and surgical conduits for the treatment of congenital heart disease.
- After the target is successfully cannulated by the catheter, **contrast** is injected.
  - Contrast is a radiopaque substance that appears dark when viewed on a white fluoroscopic background.
  - The purpose of contrast is to allow delineation of cardiac structures by temporarily opacifying them.

- ○ All modern X-ray contrasts are exclusively iodine-based.
- ○ Although the current generation of contrast is fairly safe, there are still risks.
- ○ The two most common risks of using contrast are **contrast-induced nephropathy (CIN) and allergic reactions**, which are discussed in detail below.
- Angiograms are obtained at various angles to allow more complete visualization of 3D structures (Figures 34-2 and 34-3).[1]
- The nomenclature used describes the position of the II in relation to the patient.
  - ○ AP (anteroposterior) means that the II is directly over the patient.
  - ○ Cranial means that the II is angled superiorly.
  - ○ Caudal means that the II is angled inferiorly.
  - ○ LAO (left angle oblique) means that the II is angled to the patient's left.
  - ○ RAO (right angle oblique) means that the II is angled to the right of the patient.
  - ○ Lateral means that II is placed fully lateral to the patient.

APPLICATIONS

- The primary uses of cardiac catheterization are to assess the presence and/or severity of
  - ○ Coronary artery disease (CAD)
  - ○ Valvular heart disease
  - ○ Cardiomyopathy
  - ○ Congenital heart disease
  - ○ Pulmonary hypertension
  - ○ Aortic disease (aneurysm and dissection)
- Cardiac catheterization is considered the diagnostic gold standard for the first five indications. Spatial and temporal resolution is superior to cardiac computer tomography (CT) and magnetic resonance imaging (MRI) for these purposes.

LIMITATIONS

- Major complications are uncommon[2-5]:
  - ○ Death (0.10% to 0.14%)
  - ○ Myocardial infarction (0.05% to 0.07%)
  - ○ Contrast agent reactions (0.23% to 0.37%)
  - ○ Local vascular complications (0.2% to 0.43%)
  - ○ **CIN** (5%)[6]:
    - ▪ CIN is transient rise in serum creatinine following coronary angiography.
    - ▪ The mechanism remains unclear but may involve vasoconstriction-induced acute tubular necrosis and/or a direct cytotoxic effect on the tubular cells.[7]
    - ▪ It is the third most common cause of hospital-acquired kidney failure.[8]
    - ▪ **Risk factors** include volume depletion, preexisting chronic kidney disease, diabetes, heart failure, hypotension, ST-elevation myocardial infarction, larger doses of contrast, and the use of hyperosmolar contrast media.[7,9]
    - ▪ Most creatinine elevations are nonoliguric, peak within 1 to 2 days, and return to baseline in 7 days.
    - ▪ Rare to require chronic dialysis[10]
    - ▪ Associated with increased length of hospital stay and in-hospital mortality
    - ▪ The main measures to prevent CIN are to limit contrast volume and prehydration of the patient.[7,9,11-15]
    - ▪ The use of diuretics in the absence of adequate hydration results in worse renal outcomes.[11]
    - ▪ There may be benefit to using sodium bicarbonate rather than saline for prehydration.[16-18]
    - ▪ The free radical scavenger *N*-acetylcysteine may have benefit as well; however, data from individual studies and meta-analyses have been conflicting.[19]

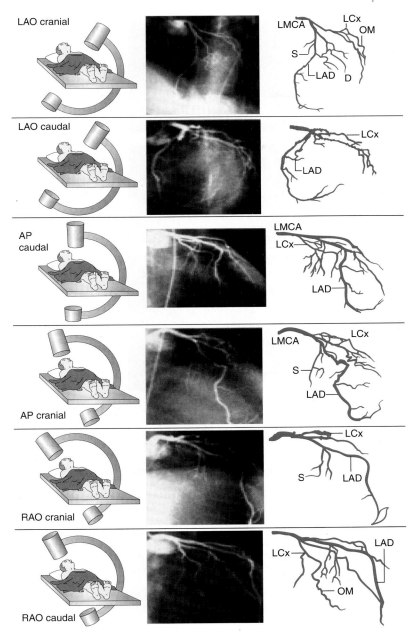

FIGURE 34-2. Angiographic views of the left coronary circulation. (From Zipes DP, Libby P, Bonow RO, Braunwald E, eds. *Braunwald's Heart Disease: A Textbook of Cardiovascular Medicine*, 7th ed. Philadelphia, PA: Elsevier; 2004, with permission.)

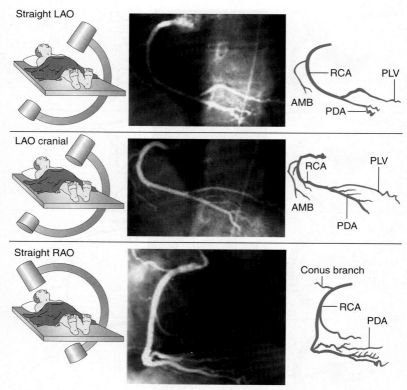

FIGURE 34-3. Angiographic views of the right coronary circulation. (From Zipes DP, Libby P, Bonow RO, Braunwald E, eds. *Braunwald's Heart Disease: A Textbook of Cardiovascular Medicine*, 7th ed. Philadelphia, PA: Elsevier; 2004, with permission.)

- ○ **Allergic reactions** to three materials: local anesthetic, iodinated contrast, and protamine sulfate.
  - ■ Most common allergic reactions (<1% of procedures) are caused by contrast.
  - ■ Symptoms vary on a spectrum including sneezing, urticaria, angioedema, bronchospasm, and even anaphylactic shock.
  - ■ Severe reactions should be treated with 10 μg boluses of epinephrine.
  - ■ Premedication with prednisone (20 mg PO tid × 24 to 48 hours), diphenhydramine (25 mg PO tid × 24 to 48 hours), and an H2 blocker (cimetidine or ranitidine) can reduce the risk of a second reaction to 5% to 10% and a severe reaction (bronchospasm or shock) to <1%.
  - ■ Use for patient with known or suspected history of a contrast reaction.
- • Another limitation of coronary angiography is its inability to assess extraluminal manifestations of CAD.
  - ○ Luminal involvement is often the final stage of the progression of CAD.
  - ○ This drawback can be overcome by performing cardiac catheterization with intravascular ultrasound (IVUS) to assess for extraluminal involvement.

○ Nevertheless, cardiac CT and cardiac MRI both allow extraluminal assessment of the coronary arteries without additional cost.

Intravascular Ultrasound

GENERAL PRINCIPLES

Definitions

- IVUS is a catheter-based ultrasound modality that provides a high-resolution, tomographic evaluation of coronary and other arteries.
- A typical IVUS setup is shown in Figure 34-4.
- The reconstruction of ultrasound data into a 2D image allows for
  ○ Circumferential evaluation of the vessel
  ○ Assessment of lumen diameter and area
  ○ Plaque size and composition
- This technique complements angiography and may be used to confirm, refute, or supplement angiographic data.
- It is also able to provide additional characterization of the vessel wall.

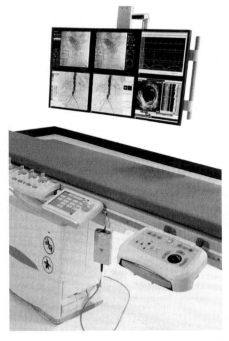

FIGURE 34-4. Example setup of intravascular ultrasound display and controls within a typical cardiac catheterization lab. (Image provided courtesy of Volcano Corporation.)

Physics

- Incorporates a miniaturized ultrasound probe within a catheter. Ultrasound waves are emitted from the device in a range of 20 to 40 MHz and received through a fixed or rotating array.
- The catheter is pulled back through a vessel, and data are reconstructed into cross-sectional images and displayed in real time.
- Catheters range in size from 2.9 to 3.2 Fr and can be utilized in 5- to 75-Fr guide catheters.
- Resolution is 150 to 250 μm.
- Catheters typically utilize either solid-state or mechanically rotating transducers (Figure 34-5).
  - Solid-state transducer:
    - Circumferential phased array that is activated serially to provide cross-sectional image in real time.
    - Ring down artifact: A zone immediately surrounding the catheter where interference creates an area of essentially no information.
    - Solid-state devices have increased flexibility and may track through tortuous vessels more easily than mechanical systems.
  - Mechanically rotating transducer:
    - Single transducer that is rotated inside the tip of a catheter along a central drive cable connected to an external motor drive.
    - Guide wire artifact: The guide wire creates a shadow artifact in the images produced as the IVUS catheter runs over the wire.
    - Mechanical catheters have improved near-field resolution.

Interpretation and Image Analysis

- IVUS-produced images:
  - The catheter occupies a null area in the center of the coaxial 2D image.
  - The dark (echolucent) area surrounding this ring represents the lumen of the artery.
  - The three layers of vessel wall can be identified as bright–dark–bright, given the higher reflectivity of the intima and adventitia layers relative to the media.
- The intima is not as well seen within a normal vessel without significant atherosclerotic plaque seen secondary to its limited thickness.

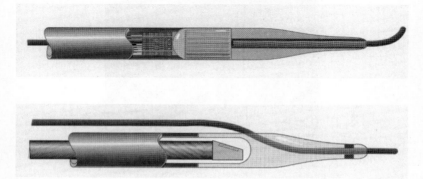

FIGURE 34-5. Catheter types. (**A**) Solid-state/phased array transducer (**B**) mechanical transducer. (Image provided courtesy of Volcano Corporation.)

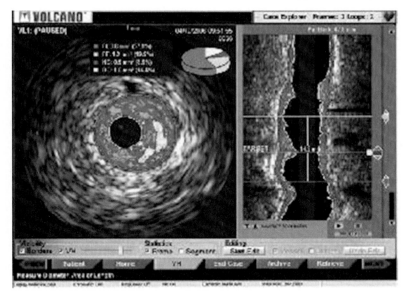

FIGURE 34-6. An IVUS image of a coronary artery (**A**) and a 2D map of the vessel by pullback (**B**). The length of a given target segment can be measured for choosing the appropriate stent length. (Image provided courtesy of Volcano Corporation. Volcano and the Volcano Logo are registered trademarks of Volcano Corporation.)

- The primary clinically relevant differentiation rests in identifying the transition from the lumen to the intima media. This allows for quantification of vessel stenosis and plaque characterization.
- Cross-sectional IVUS measurements have been well-validated.
- Motorized transducer pullback through a stationary imaging sheath allows for accurate length and volume measurements (Figure 34-6).
- Virtual histology utilizes backscatter radiofrequency data acquired during IVUS imaging to improve upon tissue characterization.[20]

APPLICATIONS

IVUS can be utilized to assess lesion size and morphology, serve as an adjunct to percutaneous, and characterize atherosclerotic disease.[21]

Evaluation of Coronary Lesions
- Frequently used to determine the degree of stenosis in situations where angiographic imaging is considered unreliable or equivocal such as
  - LM stenosis
  - Ostial coronary lesions
  - Bifurcation lesions
  - Overlapped segments
  - Intermediate lesions
- Lesion significance can be determined with a few simple measurements and calculations (Figure 34-6).

- **Percent lumen area stenosis**: Cross-sectional area of the lumen at the site of a lesion compared to the reference luminal area.
- **Minimum lumen area** (MLA)[22]:
  - Luminal area of the lesion at its narrowest site
  - Ischemic MLA is the threshold at which a given MLA is considered significant.
    - Varies with respect to the artery involved.
    - <4 mm^2 for epicardial arteries.
    - <6 mm^2 to 7 mm^2 for LM.
- **Plaque burden**:
  - Cross-sectional area of the vessel (media-to-media) minus the cross-sectional area of the lumen.
  - A large burden of plaque may be present even without an evidence of significant obstruction.
  - IVUS has been found to demonstrate 35% to 51% of cross-sectional area occupied by plaque in a reference segment of a vessel, which is believed to be angiographically normal.[23,24]
- **Remodeling**:
  - IVUS can be utilized to distinguish between positive and negative remodeling.[25,26]
  - Positive remodeling is originally described as the Glagov phenomenon.
    - Localized expansion of a vessel in response to atherosclerotic plaque to preserves the lumen diameter.
    - Often associated with large, soft, lipid-laden plaque and inflammation.
  - Negative remodeling signifies constriction of the lumen at the site of atherosclerotic plaque.
  - This implies that some segments of a vessel demonstrate outward vessel expansion, while others constriction at the site of any given plaque.
  - Lesions demonstrating positive remodeling have been correlated with acute coronary syndromes.[26,27]
  - The finding of positive remodeling in IVUS predicts target lesion revascularization rates after intervention

Adjunct to Percutaneous Coronary Intervention[28]

- Evaluation of complex lesions before percutaneous coronary intervention (PCI):
  - Measurements of lesion length and vessel size can be utilized in decision-making regarding the sizing of stents.
  - Adjunctive atheroablative procedures such as cutting balloon angioplasty and rotational or directional atherectomy may be utilized based on IVUS assessment. As an example, IVUS identification of superficial calcification within a given plaque may lead to use of rotational atherectomy over directional coronary atherectomy.[29]
- Identify side-branch involvement or unusual lesion morphology.

Quality Assurance Following Stent Deployment

- Apposition of a stent is confirmed by IVUS with visualization of stent struts against the vessel wall.
- A stent is considered fully expanded if the lumen area following stenting is at least 90% of the lumen area of a proximal or distal reference point. There is an increased risk of restenosis and thrombosis if a stent is inadequately expanded or lacks apposition against the vessel wall.
- IVUS guidance in the setting of PCI has been demonstrated to reduce total lesion revascularization rates and stent thrombosis.[30]
- IVUS can be utilized to identify marginal tears occurring at the edge of stents following deployment. Marginal tears have been shown to increase the risk of adverse cardiac events.

Plaque Composition and Characterization[31]

- Calcifications:
  - Regions of calcification appear bright (echogenic) with shadows and reverberations extending peripherally from the lesion.
  - May be superficial or deep, determined by the distance of the calcification from the center of the lumen.
  - Quantified by the percentage of the circumference arc that it encompasses around the lumen of a vessel and its length measured axially.
  - May identify a lesion that is less extensive based on its arc of coverage when fluoroscopy identifies significant calcification.
  - Higher sensitivity over traditional modalities at identifying calcified plaque.[24,32]
- Fibrous: The fibrous components appear as bright as or brighter than adventitia (hyperechoic) with some properties similar to calcification.
- Fat:
  - Plaque that is predominantly lipid-laden is less echogenic than fibrous plaque.
  - Areas of plaque that are darker (hypoechoic) than adventitia are more suggestive of fat.
  - Caution must be taken as these hypoechoic areas can also be artifact created by nearby calcification or branch vessels.
- Thrombus versus soft plaque:
  - Thrombus and soft plaque appear less dark (hypoechoic) than adventitia.
  - Thrombus is more likely to have irregular morphology and mobility independent of its vessel wall.

LIMITATIONS

Peri-procedural complications include
- Dissection
- Intramural or extramural hematoma
- Pericardial effusion/tamponade

Intracardiac Echocardiography

GENERAL PRINCIPLES

Definitions

Intracardiac echocardiography (ICE) is used to provide imaging of intracardiac structures during structural heart disease interventional procedures.

Physics

- ICE incorporates a small transducer within a catheter, utilizing either a fixed, phased-array or a mechanically rotating transducer.
- A phased array is also able to provide Doppler data and a more thorough structural evaluation of the heart.
- Frequencies between 5 to 10 MHz provide further tissue penetration up to 15 cm, which is on par with the scale necessary to evaluate cardiovascular structures.

Interpretation and Image Analysis

- Transseptal puncture is necessary among a variety of structural heart disease procedures, notably atrial septal defect (ASD) and patent foramen ovale (PFO) closures and in some electrophysiologic ablation procedures.[33]

• The probe may be flexed anteriorly, posteriorly, or side-to-side, allowing control similar to transesophageal echocardiography.

APPLICATIONS

ICE can serve as an adjunct to other imaging modalities to provide further anatomic evaluation[34]:
• Valvuloplasty procedures
• Evaluation of prosthetic valves
• ASD/PFO closure[35]

LIMITATIONS

• Expense:
  ○ The cost of IVUS catheters ranges from $600 to $900 each.
  ○ IVUS imaging consoles cost an estimated $150,000 to $200,000.
• Procedure time: Associated increase in total procedural time given the additional steps and equipment necessary to utilize ICE.
• Safety:
  ○ Coronary spasm—2.9%
  ○ Risk of other significant complications (e.g., dissection, thrombosis, and abrupt closure) is approximately 0.4%.
• Availability is somewhat limited as this procedure is performed predominantly by interventional cardiologists.
• Requires frequent use to overcome its learning curve.

REFERENCES

1. Zipes DP, Libby P, Bonow RO, et al., eds. *Braunwald's Heart Disease: A Textbook of Cardiovascular Medicine*, 7th ed. Philadelphia, PA: Elsevier; 2004.
2. Popma JJ. Coronary Arteriography. In: Bonow RO, Mann DL, Zipes DP, et al., eds. *Braunwald's Heart Disease: A Textbook of Cardiovascular Medicine*, 9th ed. Philadelphia, PA: Elsevier; 2011:406-440.
3. Scanlon P, Faxon D, Audet A, et al. ACC/AHA guidelines for coronary angiography. *J Am Coll Cardiol* 1999;33:1756-1824.
4. Noto TJ Jr, Johnson LW, Krone R, et al. Cardiac catheterization 1990: a report of the Registry of the Society for Cardiac Angiography and Interventions (SCA&I). *Cathet Cardiovasc Diagn* 1991;24:75-83.
5. Johnson, LW, Lozner EC, Johnson S, et al. Coronary arteriography 1984-1987: a report of the Registry of the Society for Cardiac Angiography and Interventions. I. Results and complications. *Cathet Cardiovasc Diagn* 1989;17:5-10.
6. Tommaso CL. Contrast-induced nephrotoxicity in patients undergoing cardiac catheterization. *Cathet Cardiovasc Diagn* 1994;31:316-321.
7. Barrett BJ, Parfrey PS. Preventing nephropathy induced by contrast medium. *N Engl J Med* 2006;354:379-386.
8. Nash K, Hafeez A, Hou S. Hospital-acquired renal insufficiency. *Am J Kidney Dis* 2002;39:930-936.
9. Solomon R, Dauerman HL. Contrast-induced acute kidney injury. Circulation 2010;122:2451-2455.
10. McCullough PA, Wolyn R, Rocher LL, et al. Acute renal failure after coronary intervention: incidence, risk factors and relationship to mortality. *Am J Med* 1997;103:368-375.
11. Solomon R, Werner C, Mann D, et al. Effects of saline, mannitol, and furosemide to prevent acute decreases in renal function induced by radiocontrast agents. *N Engl J Med* 1994;331:1416-1420.
12. Briguori C, Visconti G, Focaccio A, et al. Renal Insufficiency After Contrast Media Administration Trial II (REMEDIAL II): RenalGuard System in high-risk patients for contrast-induced acute kidney injury. *Circulation* 2011;124:1260-1269.

13. Trivedi HS, Moore, Nasr S, et al. A randomized prospective trial to assess the role of saline hydration on the development of contrast nephrotoxicity. *Nephron Clin Pract* 2003;93:C29-C34.

14. Mueller C, Buerkle G, Buettner HJ, et al. Prevention of contrast media-associated nephropathy: randomized comparison of 2 hydration regimens in 1620 patient undergoing coronary angioplasty. *Arch Intern Med* 2002;162:329-336.

15. Hiremath S, Akbari A, Shabana W, et al. Prevention of contrast-induced acute kidney injury: is simple oral hydration similar to intravenous? A systematic review of the evidence. *PLoS One* 2013;8:e60009.

16. Birck R, Krzossok S, Markowetz F, et al. Acetylcysteine for prevention of contrast induced nephropathy: meta-analysis. *Lancet* 2003;362:598-603.

17. Zoungas S, Nonomiya T, Huxley R, et al. Systematic review: sodium bicarbonate treatment regimens for the prevention of contrast-induced nephropathy. *Ann Intern Med* 2009;151:631-638.

18. Merten GJ, Burgess WP, Gray LV, et al. The prevention of radiocontrast-agent-induced nephropathy with sodium bicarbonate: a randomized control trial. *JAMA* 2004;291:2328-2334.

19. ACT Investigators. Acetylcysteine for prevention of renal outcomes in patients undergoing coronary and peripheral vascular angiography: main results from the randomized Acetylcysteine for Contrast-induced nephropathy Trial (ACT). *Circulation* 2011;124:1250-1259.

20. Diethrich EB, Irshad K, Reid D. Virtual histology and color flow intravascular ultrasound in peripheral interventions. *Sem Vasc Surg* 2006;19:155-162.

21. Bourantas C, Naka K, Garg S, et al. Clinical indications for intravascular ultrasound imaging. *Echocardiography* 2010;27:1282-1290.

22. Brigouri, C, Anzuini A, Airoldi F, et al. Intravascular ultrasound criteria for the assessment of the functional significance of intermediate coronary artery stenosis and comparison with fractional flow reserve. *Am J Cardiol* 2001;87:136-141.

23. Mintz GS, Painter JA, Pichard AD, et al. Atherosclerosis in angiographically "normal" coronary artery reference segments: an intravascular ultrasound study with clinical correlations. *J Am Coll Cardiol* 1995;25:1479-1485.

24. St. Goar FG, Pinto FJ, Alderman EL, et al. Intravascular ultrasound imaging of angiographically normal coronary arteries: an in vivo comparison with quantitative angiography. *J Am Coll Cardiol* 1991;18:952-958.

25. Schoenhagen P, Ziada KM, Vince DG, et al. Arterial remodeling and coronary artery disease: the concept of "dilated" versus "obstructive" coronary atherosclerosis. *J Am Coll Cardiol* 2001;38:297-306.

26. Nicholls SJ, Tuzcu EM, Sipathi I, et al. Intravascular ultrasound in cardiovascular medicine. *Circulation* 2006;114:e55-e59.

27. Schoenhagen P, Ziada KM, Dapadia SR, et al. Extent and direction of arterial remodeling in stable versus unstable coronary syndromes: an intravascular ultrasound study. *Circulation* 2000;101:598-603.

28. Bonello L, Labriolle A, Lemelse G, et al. Intravascular ultrasound-guided percutaneous coronary interventions in contemporary practice. *Arch Cardiovasc Dis* 2009;102:143-151.

29. Mintz GS, Potkin BN, Keren G, et al. Intravascular ultrasound evaluation of the effect of rotational atherectomy in obstructive atherosclerotic coronary artery disease. *Circulation* 1992;86:1383-1393.

30. Roy, P, Torguson R, Okabe T, et al. Angiographic and procedural correlates of stent thrombosis after intracoronary implantation of drug-eluting stents. *J Interv Cardiol* 2007;20:307-313.

31. Nair A, Kuban BD, Tuzcu EM, et al. Coronary plaque classification with intravascular ultrasound radiofrequency data analysis. *Circulation* 2002;106:2200-2206.

32. Mintz GS, Popma JJ, Pichard AD, et al. Patterns of calcification in coronary artery disease: A statistical analysis of intravascular ultrasound and coronary angiography in 1155 lesions. *Circulation* 1995;91:1959-1965.

33. Dravid SG, Hope B, McKinnie JJ. Intracardiac echocardiography in electrophysiology: a review of current applications in practice. *Echocardiography* 2008;25:1172-1175.

34. Kort S. Intracardiac echocardiography: evolution, recent advances, and current applications. *J Am Soc Echocardiogr* 2006;19:1192-1201.

35. Salome N, Braga P, Goncalves M, et al. Transcatheter device occlusion of atrial septal defects and patent foramen ovale under intracardiac echocardiographic guidance. *Rev Port Cardiol* 2004;23:709-717.

Adult Congenital Heart Disease

35

Elisa A. Bradley and Ari M. Cedars

Introduction

GENERAL PRINCIPLES

- Congenital heart diseases (CHDs) are those malformations of the heart or great vessels that have been present since birth.
- Three factors bear particular consideration when caring for an adult patient with CHD:
  - The original congenital cardiac lesion
  - The specific surgical repair(s) that the patient has undergone.
  - The anticipated natural history associated with both the condition and the repair

Classification

A classification of CHD is presented in Table 35-1. Select conditions are described in more detail later in this chapter.

Epidemiology

- Eighty-five percent of patients with CHD survive into adulthood.[1]
- There are approximately one million adults living with CHD.
- Gender prevalence varies by cardiac lesion.

Etiology

- Genetic:
  - Chromosomal abnormalities and congenital syndromes are present in almost 20% of patients with congenital heart defects.
  - 40% to 50% of patients with trisomy 21 have CHD.
  - 15% of patients with tetralogy of Fallot (ToF) or conotruncal defects have 22q11.2 deletion.
  - Other genetic disorders are DiGeorge syndrome, velocardiofacial syndrome, and conotruncal anomaly face syndrome.
- Environmental:
  - Maternal infections (e.g., rubella)
  - Medications/drugs (e.g., lithium, thalidomide, alcohol)
  - Maternal conditions (e.g., diabetes, lupus)

TABLE 35-1   CLASSIFICATION OF CHDs

- Septal defects
  - ASD
    - Secundum ASD
    - Primum ASD
    - Sinus venosus ASD
    - Unroofed coronary sinus
  - VSD
  - AVSD
- PDA
- Partial and total anomalous pulmonary venous connection (PAPVC) and (TAPVC)[a]
- Left-sided heart obstructive lesions
  - AS
  - BAV
  - SubAS
  - Supravalvular AS
  - Coarctation of the aorta (CoA)
  - Interrupted aortic arch (IAA)
- RVOT obstruction
  - Pulmonary atresia
  - Pulmonary stenosis
- Pulmonary hypertension and Eisenmenger syndrome
- Tetralogy of Fallot (ToF)[a]

- TGA
  - d-transposition[a]
  - l-transposition ("congenitally corrected")
- Persistent truncus arteriosus[a]
- Single ventricle
  - Double inlet left ventricle (DILV)
  - Double outlet right ventricle (DORV)
  - Hypoplastic left heart syndrome (HLHS)
  - Hypoplastic right heart syndrome (HRHS)
  - Tricuspid atresia[a]
- Heterotaxy syndromes (polysplenia, asplenia)
  - Coronary artery abnormalities
  - Dextrocardia
- Ebstein anomaly
- Multiple lesion syndromes
  - Tetralogy of Fallot
  - Shone syndrome (supravalvular mitral membrane, parachute mitral valve, SubAS, and CoA)
  - Williams Syndrome
  - Noonan syndrome

[a]Cyanotic lesions.

Atrial Septal Defect

GENERAL PRINCIPLES

Classification

- The types of atrial septal defects (ASDs) are illustrated in Figure 35-1.
- **Secundum ASD**:
  - Defect of the true fossa ovalis due to either enlarged ostium secundum or insufficient septum secundum tissue
  - Most common form of ASD, about 75%
  - Occurs more frequently in women
  - Can be associated with mitral valve prolapse
- **Primum ASD**:
  - Defect in lower atrial septum due to defective fusion of septum primum with the endocardial cushions

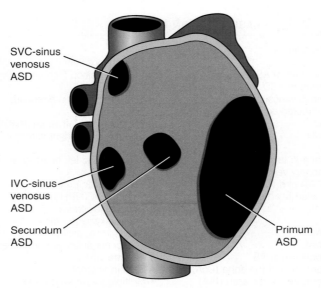

FIGURE 35-1. Anatomic location of common ASDs.

- ○ Accounts for 15% of ASDs
- ○ Associated with trisomy 21, AV canal defects, and cleft mitral valve
- **Sinus venosus ASD**:
  - ○ Defect where the superior vena cava (SVC) or inferior vena cava (IVC) meets the right atrium (RA) at the intra-atrial septum.
  - ○ Commonly due to unroofing of pulmonary veins as they pass behind the RA on their way to the left atrium (LA).
  - ○ Accounts for 10% of ASDs[2]
  - ○ Associated with partially anomalous pulmonary venous return (PAPVR)
- Unroofed coronary sinus (1%) is associated with persistent left SVC.
- Other associated defects are valvular pulmonic stenosis (PS) and coronary artery abnormalities.

Pathophysiology

- Under normal conditions, there is left-to-right (L-to-R) shunting from the higher pressure LA to the lower pressure RA.
- Over time, the right-sided chambers can dilate secondary to volume overload, which can lead to atrial arrhythmias.
- In a small percentage of patients (10% to 15%, predominantly females), continued volume overload to the right heart can lead to pulmonary hypertension and eventually shunt reversal.

DIAGNOSIS

Clinical Presentation

History

- Majority are asymptomatic.[2]
- Gradual onset of symptoms often leads to late diagnosis.
- Early symptoms: dyspnea on exertion and/or fatigue

- Late symptoms: atrial arrhythmias (third to fourth decade)
- End-stage symptoms: In a small percentage of patients, there is the development of **pulmonary hypertension and Eisenmenger syndrome**.

Physical Examination
- **Fixed split S2**
- Loud P2 present with elevated pulmonary pressures
- Soft systolic murmur at the left upper sternal border secondary to increased flow across the right ventricular outflow tract (RVOT) and pulmonary valve (PV)
- Right ventricle (RV) heave or pulmonary artery (PA) tap with large shunts or the development of pulmonary hypertension
- Large shunts may result in a diastolic rumble at the left lower sternal border.

Diagnostic Testing
- Electrocardiogram (ECG):
  - Incomplete right bundle branch block (RBBB) pattern (rSR') and atrioventricular (AV) block
  - Patients with any ASD except primum may have right axis deviation with right atrial enlargement (RAE) and right ventricular hypertrophy (RVH) and may have AV block
  - Patients with primum ASD may have left axis deviation (or extreme right axis) and first-degree AV block
  - Sinus venosus ASD may have an abnormal p-wave axis (leftward).
- Chest radiography: enlarged cardiac silhouette with RA and RV enlargement and increased pulmonary vascular markings
- Transthoracic echocardiogram (TTE):
  - Two-dimensional imaging of the atrial septum (parasternal, apical, subcostal views) employing color Doppler to display shunting.
  - Contrast echo with agitated saline (bubble study) to confirm an R-to-L shunt if color Doppler is negative/inconclusive.
  - Tricuspid regurgitation (TR) jet should be used to estimate PA pressure.
- Transesophageal echocardiogram (TEE) improves lesion definition particularly in the case of sinus venosus and coronary sinus defects.
- Magnetic resonance imaging (MRI): useful with unclear or inconclusive TTE results.
- Cardiac catheterization:
  - Generally not required for uncomplicated ASD if there is acceptable non-invasive imaging.
  - Used for the measurement of pulmonary vascular resistance, associated valvular disease, pulmonary to systemic flow ratio (Qp:Qs) and for coronary artery evaluation in patients being evaluated for closure.
  - Often is done at the time of percutaneous closure.

TREATMENT

Medications
- Antiarrhythmic therapy and electrical cardioversion are recommended in the presence of atrial fibrillation.[1]
- Anticoagulation is warranted in the presence of atrial fibrillation.
- Rate control can be used in combination with anticoagulation in the patient for whom sinus rhythm cannot be maintained.[1]

Surgical Management
- Indications for closure[1,2]:
  - RA or RV enlargement (with or without symptoms) due to an atrial level shunt as demonstrated by:
    - Pulmonary flow: systemic flow ratio >1.5:1 (Qp:Qs) (Class Ia, IIa, etc)

- ASD >10 mm by echocardiography (Class Ia)
- Evidence of paradoxical embolism (Class IIa)
    - ○ Orthodeoxia–platypnea (dyspnea and deoxygenation as a result of changing from a recumbent position to sitting/standing) (Class IIa).
    - ○ Pulmonary hypertension with pulmonary pressures or resistance <2/3 systemic, or who are responsive to pulmonary vasodilators or test occlusion of the ASD (Class IIb).
    - ○ Concomitant with Maze operation for atrial arrhythmias (Class IIb).
- Contraindication to closure: irreversible severe pulmonary arterial hypertension (PAH) with no net left-to-right (L-to-R) shunt.
- Catheter-based versus surgical intervention (Class I indications):
    - ○ Catheter-based closure in uncomplicated secundum ASD as defect size permits
    - ○ Primum ASD, sinus venosus ASD, and coronary sinus ASD should be closed surgically.

Lifestyle/Risk Modification

- Endocarditis prophylaxis: indicated the first 6 months after closure, in patients with net R-to-L shunting, and degenerated closure in the presence of prosthetic material.[1,3]
- Pregnancy: generally well tolerated, risk of transmission in women with sporadic ASD is 8% to 10%.[2]
- Activity[1]:
    - ○ Small defect, normal right heart volume, no PAH: no limitations
    - ○ Large defect with normal pulmonary pressures: no limitations
    - ○ Presence of mild pulmonary hypertension: low-intensity competitive sports (Class IA; 36th Bethesda Conference, Table 35-2)[4,5]
    - ○ Cyanosis or large R-to-L shunt: no participation in competitive sports
    - ○ Symptomatic arrhythmias: preparticipation screening
    - ○ Post-closure: no limitations as long as pulmonary pressures are normal, and there is no evidence of arrhythmia, no second- or third-degree AV block, and no myocardial dysfunction.
- Thromboembolic prophylaxis:
    - ○ Aspirin for the first 6 months after surgical or device closure
    - ○ Warfarin after the documented thromboembolic cerebrovascular event

Ventricular Septal Defect

GENERAL PRINCIPLES

- Ventricular septal defects (VSDs) are the most common congenital heart defect in infants (0.5% to 5%).[6]
- The majority of VSDs close spontaneously (approximately 80%).

Classification[1]

- **Type 1**: (so-called conal, subpulmonary, infundibular, supracristal, doubly committed juxta-arterial):
    - ○ Accounts for 6% of VSDs in non-Asians, but up to 33% in Asians.
    - ○ It is located near the outflow portion of the RV.
    - ○ Frequently associated with aortic insufficiency (AI).
- **Type 2**: (so-called perimembranous, paramembranous, conoventricular):
    - ○ Overall the most common type of VSD, about 80%
    - ○ Located in the membranous septum adjacent to tricuspid septal leaflet.

TABLE 35-2	BETHESDA EXERCISE CLASSIFICATION		
		Dynamic	
Static	**A. Low** (<40% Max O_2)	**B. Moderate** (40-70% Max O_2)	**C. High** (>70% Max O_2)
I. Low (<20% MVC)	IA Billiards, bowling, cricket, curling, golf riflery	IB Baseball, softball, fencing, table tennis, volleyball	IC Badminton, cross-country skiing (classic technique), field hockey, orienteering, race walking, racquetball, squash, running (long distance), soccer, tennis
II. Moderate (20-50% MVC)	IIA Archery, auto racing, diving, equestrian, motorcycling	IIB American football, field events (jumping), figure skating, rodeoing, rugby, running (sprint), surfing, synchronized swimming	IIC Basketball, ice hockey, cross-country skiing (skating technique), lacrosse, running (middle distance), swimming, team handball
III. High (>50% MVC)	IIIA Bobsledding, luge, field events (throwing), gymnastic, martial arts, sailing, sport climbing, water skiing, weight lifting, windsurfing	IIIB Body building, downhill skiing, skateboarding, snowboarding, wrestling	IIIC Boxing, Canoeing, Kayaking, cycling, decathlon, rowing, speed-skating, triathlon

MaxO$_2$, maximal oxygen uptake; MVC, maximal voluntary contraction.
Adapted from Mitchell JH, Haskell W, Snell P, Van Camp SP. Task Force 8: Classification of sports. *J Am Coll Cardiol* 2005;45:1364-1367, with permission.

○ May be associated with AI.
○ May be closed by septal leaflet of the tricuspid valve (TV) leading to a "septal aneurysm."
○ Rarely may be a Gerbode defect between the left ventricle (LV) and the RA.
○ May be associated with subvalvular pulmonary stenosis.
- **Type 3**: (so-called inlet, AV canal type):
  ○ Accounts for 5% to 8% of VSDs.
  ○ Common in patients with Trisomy 21.
  ○ In the lower RV adjacent to the TV.
- **Type 4**: (muscular):
  ○ Accounts for 20% of VSDs in infants but less in adults.
  ○ Central, apical, or at margin of the septum and free wall of the RV.
  ○ Spontaneous closure is common in childhood.
  ○ Often seen without other defects.
  ○ Can occur as part of a multilesion syndrome (i.e., ToF, transposition of the great arteries [TGA]).

Pathophysiology

- Blood flows preferentially from the high-pressure LV into the RV.
- A sufficiently large Qp:Qs can result in LV volume overload and heart failure.
- Over time, an uncorrected VSD with an L-to-R shunt may cause pulmonary vascular remodeling and eventual reversal of the shunt (Eisenmenger syndrome).
- Small: <1/3 size of aortic annulus with a small L-to-R shunt, no LV volume overload, and no PAH.
- Moderate: 1/3 to 2/3 size of aortic diameter with a small-to-moderate L-to-R shunt, mild-to-moderate LV volume overload, and mild/no PAH. Qp:Qs is approximately 1.5 to 1.9.
- Large: 2/3 size of aortic diameter, a large L-to-R shunt, LV volume overload and RV pressure overload, and PAH is typical. Qp:Qs >2.0.

DIAGNOSIS

Clinical Presentation

- The presentation varies from an asymptomatic murmur to fulminant heart failure.
- When symptomatic, the history is significant for dyspnea on exertion and fatigue.
- The examination is characterized by a **loud, harsh holosystolic murmur** (as long as the RV pressure is low). As RV pressure rises, the murmur becomes softer.

Diagnostic Testing

- ECG: left atrial (LA) and LV enlargement/hypertrophy with isolated LV volume overload; RV hypertrophy with progressive pulmonary hypertension.
- Chest radiography: cardiomegaly and increased pulmonary vascular markings with a moderate-to-large defect and Qp:Qs >1.5.
- TTE:
  ○ Diagnostic study of choice to confirm diagnosis, location, size, and shunting present at VSD
  ○ Evaluation of pulmonary pressures
  ○ Identification of associated lesions (i.e., AI)
- MRI: to assess anatomy and the presence of other lesions
- Cardiac catheterization:
  ○ More accurately assesses both Qp:Qs and pulmonary vascular pressures and resistance than other imaging modalities.

○ Confirm VSD anatomy and number, to define coronary anatomy and the presence of valvular lesions preoperatively.

TREATMENT

Surgical Management

- Open surgical closure[1,6]:
  - ○ Indicated with Qp:Qs > 2.0 and evidence of LV volume overload or history of infective endocarditis (Class I indication).
  - ○ Reasonable in the setting of pulmonary hypertension if Qp:Qs >1.5 with:
    - PA pressure <2/3 systemic pressure and
    - Pulmonary vascular resistance (PVR) <2/3 systemic vascular resistance (Class IIa indication).
  - ○ Reasonable if Qp:Qs >1.5 in the presence of LV systolic or diastolic dysfunction (Class IIa indication).
- Percutaneous closure[1,6]:
  - ○ Can be considered with a type 4 VSD where there is significant left-sided chamber enlargement or PAH and the VSD is remote from aorta and TV (Class IIb indication).
  - ○ VSD closure is contraindicated in patients with severe, irreversible pulmonary hypertension.
- In absence of the above findings, the VSD is termed "restrictive" and can be observed.

Lifestyle/Risk Modification

- Endocarditis prophylaxis: indicated 6 months following closure, degeneration of closure with prosthetic material, and R-to-L shunting as with Eisenmenger syndrome.[1,3]
- Pregnancy: generally well tolerated, should be avoided if there is presence of Eisenmenger syndrome, and the risk of transmission is about 1% to 5%.[1]
- Activity[1,4]:
  - ○ No restrictions with normal PA pressures.
  - ○ Post repair:
    - Asymptomatic patients with small residual defect and no PAH, arrhythmia, or myocardial dysfunction can resume normal activity 3 to 6 months after repair.
    - Avoid competitive sports if persistent severe PAH.

Atrioventricular Septal Defect

GENERAL PRINCIPLES

Definition

Atrioventricular septal defect (AVSD) is also known as AV canal defect and endocardial cushion defect or common atrioventricular canal.

Etiology

- Due to defective fusion of septum primum with endocardial cushions
  - ○ Complete: primum ASD, type 3 VSD, and common AV valve
  - ○ Incomplete: primum ASD, no VSD, and cleft anterior mitral leaflet
  - ○ Partial: cleft anterior mitral leaflet
- Often seen with trisomy 21 (one-third of AVSDs)[1]
- Partial AVSD is not associated with trisomy 21.
- Associated defects: ToF, conotruncal anomalies, heterotaxy syndromes, and subaortic stenosis (SubAS).[1]

Pathophysiology

- The abnormal connection between the atria and ventricles causes blood from the right and left heart to mix. This can lead to low systemic oxygen saturation and cyanosis.
- The common AV valve is often incompetent, leading to regurgitant flow returning to the atria, increasing pulmonary congestion and pressures.
- Initially low pulmonary vascular resistance leads to increased Qp:Qs, volume overload and LV failure.
- A nonrestrictive VSD leads to RV pressure overload and failure.

DIAGNOSIS

Clinical Presentation

- Most AVSDs are repaired in childhood but unrepaired in adults who typically present with Eisenmenger syndrome and symptoms of heart failure, cyanosis, or atrial arrhythmias.
- The physical findings in an unrepaired AVSD are similar to those in ASD and VSD. There may also be cardiac findings of PAH, Eisenmenger syndrome, and cyanosis.
- An apical systolic murmur from persistent mitral regurgitation (MR) via the cleft mitral leaflet is present in those with a repaired AVSD.

Diagnostic Testing

- ECG: left axis deviation, with or without first-degree AV block; signs of any chamber enlargement.
- TTE: diagnostic study of choice to confirm the location, size, and severity. Typically sufficient for complete characterization.
- MRI: evaluate for associated lesions.
- Cardiac catheterization used to evaluate PA pressures when considering operation/reoperation.

TREATMENT

Surgical Management[1]

- Often done in infancy, but reoperation may be required.
- Reoperation recommended (all Class I indications):
  - Presence of left AV valve regurgitation/stenosis resulting in symptoms, arrhythmias, increase in LV dimensions, or reduction in LV function.
  - Left ventricular outflow tract (LVOT) obstruction with mean gradient >50 mmHg or peak >70 mmHg or lower gradient if associated with MR or AI.
  - Residual ASD or VSD with a significant L-to-R shunt (as mentioned earlier).
- Regular evaluation of AV conduction system (ECG and Holter monitor) is necessary in repaired patients as surgical repair can lead to AV node and conduction system disease.

Lifestyle/Risk Modification

- Endocarditis prophylaxis: indicated with concomitant prosthetic valve, cyanosis, residual defect near prosthetic patch (thus inhibiting endothelialization of graft), within 6 months of repair, and peripartum in patients with prosthetic valve or cyanosis.[1,3]
- Pregnancy: usually well tolerated in repaired patient with no residual PAH; in the patient with trisomy 21, there is a 50% risk of transmission to offspring.[1,7]
- Activity: no restrictions in repaired patient if there is no valvular regurgitation, arrhythmia, or LVOT obstruction.

Patent Ductus Arteriosis

GENERAL PRINCIPLES

Definition
- Persistent connection between the proximal descending aorta and the roof of the PA.
- Associated defects: ASD and VSD, maternal rubella infection, fetal valproate syndrome, and chromosomal abnormalities.

Pathophysiology
- Allows L-to-R blood flow across the patent ductus arteriosus (PDA).
- Patent shunt can lead to left chamber volume overload and increased pulmonary flow.
- May cause remodeling and subsequent pulmonary hypertension/Eisenmenger physiology.

DIAGNOSIS

Clinical Presentation
- The presentation largely depends on the size of the PDA, ranging from dyspnea and fatigue to cyanosis/clubbing with Eisenmenger physiology.[8]
- The examination is characterized by a **continuous machinery-type murmur** best at left infraclavicular area.
- The pulse is increased, and there is a wide pulse pressure if the PDA is large with a large L-to-R shunt.
- There may be differential cyanosis with clubbing/cyanosis of the feet due to an R-to-L shunt allowing deoxygenated blood to preferentially be sent to the lower extremities. This occurs when pulmonary pressures meet or exceed systemic pressures.

Diagnostic Testing
- ECG: normal or with left atrial enlargement (LAE) and left ventricular hypertrophy (LVH) if significant L-to-R shunt; RV hypertrophy with pulmonary hypertension.
- TTE: used to diagnose PDA, evaluate net shunt direction, and for estimation of PA pressure
- Chest radiography: typically demonstrates left heart enlargement and increased pulmonary vascularity until the development of Eisenmenger syndrome.

TREATMENT

Surgical Management[1,8]
- Class I indications for closure:
  - LA or LV enlargement
  - Prior endarteritis
  - **Catheter-based closure is preferred** unless deemed impossible after consultation with an adult congenital interventional cardiologist.
- Class IIa indications for closure:
  - Asymptomatic small PDA closure via catheter
  - Patient with PAH and net L-to-R shunt
- Class III indication for closure: not indicated in PAH with net R-to-L shunt

Lifestyle/Risk Modification
- Endocarditis prophylaxis: not recommended unless the patient is cyanotic.[1,3,8]
- Pregnancy: generally well tolerated, exceptions include large degree of shunting and in the presence of PAH.[7]

- Activity: generally no restrictions with a small defect or post closure; larger defects warrant a restriction in activity.[4]

Partially Anomalous Pulmonary Venous Return

GENERAL PRINCIPLES

Definition

- PAPVR occurs when some portion of the pulmonary venous drainage is to systemic venous structures or to the RA.
- Typical sites of connection include
  - Innominate vein in cases of left-sided PAPVR
  - SVC or IVC with associated sinus venosus ASD with right-sided PAPVR
  - May connect to coronary sinus in cases of persistent left-sided SVC
  - May have anomalous connection to subdiaphragmatic veins.
- Scimitar syndrome:
  - PAPVR to IVC, hepatic veins, or subdiaphragmatic veins
  - Associated with pulmonary sequestration, aorto pulmonary collaterals to the right lung, and right-branch PA stenosis

Pathophysiology

- The pathophysiology is similar to ASD, predominantly due to L-to-R shunting of blood. Eisenmenger physiology will not result in R-to-L shunting.
- This is a frequently isolated congenital defect but may be associated with many other congenital heart abnormalities such as polysplenia-type heterotaxy.

DIAGNOSIS

Clinical Presentation

History

- PAPVR is typically asymptomatic if the shunt is small.
- Exercise intolerance and edema occur with larger shunts.
- Symptoms compatible with RV failure, severe TR, and/or PAH can also occur.

Physical Examination

- RV heave with a large shunt
- Right-sided S3 in cases of RV failure
- Palpable PA pulsation with a PV opening snap
- Right-sided S4 in cases of pulmonary hypertension
- Edema may be present in cases of RV failure or severe TR.
- Systolic TR murmur in cases of TR
- Diastolic tricuspid flow murmur in cases of a large shunt

Diagnostic Testing

- ECG: RA and RV enlargement and RVH in patients with PAH
- Chest radiography: RA and RV enlargement and increased pulmonary vascular markings
- TTE: RA/RV enlargement, TR, and PAH
- CT/MRI will identify anatomy of anomalous pulmonary venous return
- Catheterization will quantify degree of shunt and identify location of shunt and presence and degree of pulmonary hypertension.

TREATMENT

Surgical Management

- Criteria similar to those for secundum ASD repair.
- After surgical repair, 10% of patients will develop pulmonary venous stenosis at the site of reanastomosis, which may require stenting or repeat surgery if physiologically significant.

Lifestyle/Risk Modification

- Endocarditis prophylaxis: indicated only for other associated lesions[3]
- Pregnancy: well tolerated unless there is severe TR or RV dysfunction
- Activity: no restrictions

Totally Anomalous Pulmonary Venous Return

GENERAL PRINCIPLES

Definition

- Totally anomalous pulmonary venous return (TAPVR) is due to failure of fusion of pulmonary venous confluence with the posterior wall of the LA.
- Confluence occurs behind RA with a decompressing vein draining to a systemic venous structure such as the IVC, SVC, innominate vein, coronary sinus, and subdiaphragmatic veins.
- Cor triatriatum: partial fusion with a residual perforated membrane between the pulmonary venous confluence and the LA.

Epidemiology

- 80% to 90% of patients with asplenia-type heterotaxy have TAPVR.
- TAPVR is also associated with other congenital heart lesions.

Pathophysiology

- All pulmonary venous return passes to systemic veins and then to the RA and RV.
- Patients depend on atrial, ventricular, or PDA-level R-to-L shunts to survive.
- Must be repaired or palliated in childhood or death will ensue unless there is sufficient mixing at the level of the R-to-L shunt.
- There may be stenosis at the site of anastomosis between the pulmonary veins and systemic veins.
- The overall situation is worse with connections to subdiaphragmatic structures.

DIAGNOSIS

Clinical Presentation

- Almost universally recognized in childhood
- Cyanosis is present in patients without obstruction of the decompressing vein that connects the pulmonary and systemic veins but with sufficient anatomical R-to L-shunting
- Shock may be present in cases with anastomotic vein stenosis or with insufficient R-to-L shunting.
- Adult patients will almost all have had repair or palliation.
- May be no physical findings if the patient has had prior repair.

- Signs and symptoms of pulmonary hypertension and RV pressure overload may occur if there is pulmonary venous obstruction after repair.
- With palliated patients (those who have an ASD or VSD without complete repair), there will be signs and symptoms of RV volume overload and failure, TR, and edema.

Diagnostic Testing

- Chest radiography: RA and RV enlargement, pulmonary hypervascularity in unrepaired or palliated patient; repaired patient may be normal.
- ECG: RA and RV enlargement, RV hypertrophy in unrepaired or palliated patient; repaired patient may be normal.
- TTE
  ○ RA and RV volume overload
  ○ There will be an evidence of R-to-L shunting at the atrial, ventricular, or PDA level if palliated or unrepaired.
  ○ Repaired patient may be normal.
- CT/MRI: useful to identify anastomosis between the pulmonary and systemic veins prior to surgical repair
- Catheterization: useful to identify pulmonary vein stenosis in patients who have had repair.

TREATMENT

Lifestyle/Risk Modification

- Endocarditis prophylaxis: indicated for only for other associated lesions if repair is complete; indicated due to cyanosis if repair is palliative[3]
- Pregnancy: well tolerated in the absence of pulmonary venous stenosis if repaired, contraindicated if palliated
- Activity: normal if repaired

Surgical Management

- TAPVR is typically repaired in childhood.
- Postoperative monitoring for an evidence of pulmonary venous stenosis should be regularly performed, particularly in asymptomatic patients with poor exercise tolerance or pulmonary hypertension.
- Surgery or stenting is indicated to relieve pulmonary venous stenosis in repaired patients.
- Complete repair should be considered in patients who are palliated.

Bicuspid Aortic Valve

GENERAL PRINCIPLES

Epidemiology

- Bicuspid aortic valve (BAV) is the most common congenital cardiac malformation, present in one in 80 adults.[9]
- Men are affected more than women (4:1).
- Autosomal dominant with reduced penetrance
- Associated with an increased risk of aortic dissection
- Associated defects: SubAS, parachute mitral valve, VSD, PDA, and coarctation[1,8]
- Increased risk of cerebral aneurysms (up to 10%)[10]

Pathophysiology

- Right-to-non-coronary cusp fusion is associated with a higher risk of developing aortic stenosis (AS) and AI.[11]
- Abnormal aortic tissue similar to cystic medial necrosis of Marfan syndrome

DIAGNOSIS

Clinical Presentation

- Two-thirds of patients develop symptoms of AS by the fifth decade.
- Systolic ejection sound due to valve opening (usually disappears by fourth decade due to calcification)
- **Crescendo–decrescendo midsystolic murmur at the upper sternal border with radiation to the neck** (in the presence of AS)
- With more significant AS, the murmur becomes more late peaking, and peripheral pulses are diminished and delayed (pulsus parvus et tardus).

Diagnostic Testing

- ECG: may or may not have LVH, LAE, or ST-T repolarization.
- TTE:
  - Qualify the lesion (anatomy of cusp fusion)
  - Quantify degree of AS
  - Assess the aortic root
  - May require TEE if difficult to visualize on transthoracic echo
  - Should be done yearly for AS when mean gradient >30 mmHg or peak gradient >50 mmHg, every 2 years if gradients are less
  - Screening TTE: first-degree relatives of patients with BAV, fetus of all pregnant women with BAV in the second trimester
- MRI/CT:
  - Can be beneficial to evaluate the thoracic aorta
  - Serial imaging for aorta should be done every 2 years if <40 mm and every year if >40 mm.

TREATMENT

Medications

- β-Blockers are indicated for patients with BAV and aortic dilatation (Class IIa indication).[1,8,9]
- Statins can be used to delay valve sclerosis (Class IIb indication).[1,7]
- Angiotensin-receptor-blockers are currently under evaluation; they may reduce the rate of aortic dilatation.[1,8]

Surgical Management

- **Balloon valvuloplasty**[1,9]:
  - Indicated in young adults/adolescents if there is no valve calcification and no AR and:
    - Patients have symptoms (angina, dyspnea, and syncope) AND peak-to-peak gradient at of >50 mmHg (Class I indication).
    - ST or T wave abnormalities with rest or exercise AND peak-to-peak gradient >60 mmHg (Class I indication)
    - Peak-to-peak gradient >50 mmHg in preparation for pregnancy or activity in competitive sport (Class IIa indication)

○ In older adults, valvuloplasty can be considered a bridge to aortic valve replacement (Class IIb indication) but is otherwise generally contraindicated.
- **Surgical repair/replacement** indications are similar to those for AS or AI with a normal valve (see Chapter 19).[1,12]
- Historical note: The Ross procedure involves excision of the aortic valve, autograft of the PV and pulmonary trunk into the aortic valve position, coronary artery re-implantation, and placement of an allograft PV.

Lifestyle Modifications

- Endocarditis prophylaxis: not required unless previous valve replacement[3]
- Pregnancy: generally well tolerated unless there is AS or aortic root dilatation.[1]
- Activity: limitations are based on the degree of AS; avoidance of competitive sports and isometric exercises with severe AS and/or dilated aorta is indicated.[1]

Subaortic Stenosis

GENERAL PRINCIPLES

- SubAS favors males 2:1 and is usually a solitary lesion.
- Other associated abnormalities include VSD (37%), BAV (23%), and AVSD.[1,9]
- SubAS is due to a fibrous ring or fibromuscular ring in the LVOT.
- Subvalvular accelerated turbulent flow causes aortic valvular damage in the form of obstruction or AI.
- Physiology may be similar to valvular AS if severe.

DIAGNOSIS

Clinical Presentation

- Patients are asymptomatic early but as the disease progresses, symptoms of AS (valvular or subvalvular) or AI may be present.
- SubAS often presents with a murmur, a crescendo–decrescendo murmur at left parasternal apical border.
- Murmur of AI may also be appreciated.

Diagnostic Testing

TTE: the diagnostic study of choice to illustrate the anatomy, gradient, and associated findings (i.e., AI, mitral involvement, systolic function, etc.).

TREATMENT

Surgical Management[1,9]

- Class I indications for surgery:
  ○ Mean gradient >30 mmHg or peak gradient >50 mmHg
  ○ Progressive AI and LV end-diastolic diameter >50 mm or left ventricular ejection fraction <55%
- Class IIb indications for surgery:
  ○ Mean gradient 30 mmHg with progressive AI or AS
  ○ Peak gradient <50 mmHg and mean <30 mmHg and LVH
- There is recurrence of the fibromuscular band after surgery is present in at least one-third of the patients.

Lifestyle Modifications

Pregnancy and engagement in competitive sports should be planned and discussed with the treating physician.

Supravalvular Aortic Stenosis

GENERAL PRINCIPLES

- Supravalvular AS is a fixed obstruction immediately distal to the sinus of Valsalva.
- The coronary arteries arise proximal to the obstruction (thus they receive high systolic pressure and low diastolic flow).
- Typically seen in **Williams Syndrome** (autosomal dominant mutation on chromosome 7 elastin gene): elfin facies, cognitive disorders, joint abnormalities, and behavioral problems[1,9]
- All first-degree relatives should have screening for this heritable condition.
- Aortic valve abnormalities are found in 50% of the patients.
- PA abnormalities (peripheral PA stenoses) are also seen.
- The pathophysiology is similar to AS, except that there is sometimes coronary artery involvement.

DIAGNOSIS

Clinical Presentation

- The clinic presentation may include symptoms of outflow obstruction (dyspnea, angina, and syncope), hypertension, and coronary ischemia.
- Coanda effect: preferential flow up the right portion of the ascending aorta can lead to discordant amplitude of carotid and upper extremity arterial pulses. There may also be differential blood pressures in upper extremities.
- Suprasternal notch thrill may be heard.
- Crescendo–decrescendo murmur at left upper sterna border with radiation to the right neck.

Diagnostic Testing

- TTE: used to characterize the anatomy of the proximal aorta, obstruction, and associated defects.
- MRI/CT: may be required to define the anatomy and associated defects.
- Proximal renal artery and main and branch PA flow should be evaluated.
- Myocardial perfusion imaging can be used if there is suspicion for coronary ischemia. Periodic screening may be indicated.

TREATMENT

Surgical Management[1,9]

Class I indications for surgery:
- Symptoms AND/OR mean gradient >50 mmHg and peak gradient >70 mmHg
- Lesser gradients AND symptoms, LVH, planned pregnancy or competitive sports, or LV systolic dysfunction

Lifestyle/Risk Modifications

- Pregnancy: not advised
- Activity: should avoid competitive sports and isometric exercises

Coarctation of the Aorta

GENERAL PRINCIPLES

- Coarctation of the aorta (CoA) is due to a narrowing near the level of the ligamentum arteriosum.
- These patients also have an intrinsic aortic wall abnormality similar to the aorta of BAV. This predisposes to aortic dilatation and rupture.
- Associated defects:
  - BAV, brachiocephalic vessel anomalies, SubAS, VSD, arch hypoplasia, circle of Willis cerebral artery aneurysm (10%)[9]
  - One-third of the patients with Turner syndrome have CoA.
- Evidence of hypoperfusion distal to the site of obstruction depends on the degree of narrowing.

DIAGNOSIS

Clinical Presentation

- CoA is typified by systemic hypertension and inconsistent upper and lower extremity pulses (weaker femoral pulse).
- Other symptoms include headache, epistaxis, and claudication.
- Assess for brachial–femoral pulse delay in all hypertensive patients (Class I).[1]
  - Assess the brachial and femoral pulses for timing and amplitude.
  - Measure the brachial and popliteal blood pressures as well.
- A left infrascapular murmur is classical.

Diagnostic Testing

- Chest radiography: "Figure 3" sign due to indentation at the CoA and post-obstructive dilation; rib notching (present on the inferior rib borders)
- TTE: Suprasternal notch window with color flow and continuous wave may show turbulence in the descending aorta and continuous forward diastolic flow.
- Stress testing: to determine the rest and exercise gradient as well as rest/exercise hypertension

TREATMENT

Surgical Management[1,9]

- Class I indications for replacement or balloon valvuloplasty:
  - Peak-to-peak CoA gradient >20 mmHg
  - Peak-to-peak CoA gradient <20 mHg when anatomic or radiologic evidence of significant collateral flow
  - Recurrent discreet CoA and peak-to-peak gradient of >20 mmHg.
- Recurrence rate after balloon angioplasty is 7%.
- Stent placement for long-segment CoA can be considered (Class IIb).

Lifestyle/Risk Modification

- Endocarditis prophylaxis: indicated for patients in whom repair or stenting has been performed in the past 6 months.[1,3]
- Pregnancy: risk varies according to associated lesions and the presence/absence of aortic root dilatation.[1]

- Activity[1,4]:
  - Unrepaired CoA should avoid contact sports, isometric exercises, and most competitive sport.
  - Stress testing can be used before allowing low-to-moderate intensity sports if no associated lesions and low gradients.

MONITORING/FOLLOW-UP

- All patients with CoA should have one MRI or CT of the thoracic aorta and cerebral vasculature.[1]
- CoA repair site should be evaluated at least every 5 years (irrespective of repair status).

Pulmonary Hypertension/Eisenmenger Physiology

GENERAL PRINCIPLES

- Pulmonary hypertension: CHD-related PAH occurs due to one or a combination of:
  - Pulmonary over-circulation
  - Exposure of the pulmonary vasculature to systemic pressures
- Eisenmenger physiology[13]:
  - This is an end-stage complication for many congenital heart defects.
  - **Reversal of blood flow across a defect** at the level of the pulmonary and systemic ventricles or arteries resulting in **pulmonary-to-systemic shunting** of blood.
  - Occurs when **pulmonary blood pressures meet or exceed systemic**.
  - Associated conditions are ventricular arrhythmias (50%), hemoptysis (20%), pulmonary embolism (10%), syncope (10%), and endocarditis (10%).
  - Hyperviscosity syndrome due to polycythemia (fatigue, headache, dizziness). Hypoxia leads to increased cell turnover and polycythemia.
  - High cell turnover also leads to increased uric acid (gout) and pigmented gallstones (cholelithiasis). Decreased urate clearance can lead to renal disease.
  - Neurologic disease (cerebral hemorrhage, embolus, abscess)
- PAH can be caused by many forms of CHD: L-to-R shunts (ASD, VSD, AVSD, PDA), TAPVR, PAPVR, truncus arteriosus, TGA, and single ventricle disorders

DIAGNOSIS

Clinical Presentation

- Symptoms may include dyspnea on exertion (most common), palpitations, edema, hemoptysis, and progressive cyanosis.
- Physical findings may include central cyanosis, clubbing, and signs of right heart failure (prominent jugular venous pulsations, increased a-waves, ascites, RV impulse, PA impulse, palpable P2, cessation of previous shunt murmur).

Diagnostic Testing

- The initial work-up should include additional testing for other causes of PAH (e.g., pulmonary function tests, CT of the chest for identification of pulmonary emboli, etc.)
- ECG: RAE, RVH, and right axis deviation
- TTE demonstrates defect with bidirectional or pulmonary to systemic shunting and increased PA pressure. Agitated saline bubble study is contraindicated, as it can result in air embolism.
- Yearly blood counts, iron level, creatinine, and uric acid are recommended.[1]
- Yearly digital oximetry and treatment with oxygen if responsive.[1]

TREATMENT

- Pulmonary vasodilators may improve quality of life.[1]
- Warfarin may be used for the prevention of pulmonary emboli/cerebral emboli (contraindicated with active hemoptysis).
- Iron deficiency anemia should be treated.
- Therapeutic phlebotomy for erythrocytosis is generally not done but may be considered if the hemoglobin is >20 g/dL and if there is hyperviscosity in the absence of dehydration.
- Endocarditis prophylaxis is indicated due cyanotic nature of this lesion (Class IIa).[3]
- Pregnancy should be avoided and early termination is recommended (Class I indication).[1]
- Activity: avoid strenuous exercise, acute exposure to excessive heat (i.e., a hot tub), and dehydration.[1]

Tetralogy of Fallot

GENERAL PRINCIPLES

Definition

- The primary defect of ToF is anterior deviation of the infundibular septum.
- Consists of four major defects (Figure 35-2):
  - Subpulmonary infundibular stenosis
  - VSD
  - Aorta overriding (posterior malalignment) VSD
  - RVH
- 5% of patients also have an associated ASD (pentalogy of Fallot).[14]
- 25% will have a right-sided aortic arch, and coronary artery anomalies can also occur.[1]

Epidemiology

- ToF represents 5% to 10% of all CHD and it is the most common cyanotic heart disease.[14]
- Sudden death occurs in 1.5% per decade of follow-up in repaired patients (thought to be mediated by ventricular arrhythmia).
- Associated syndromes are 22q11 deletion, Alagille syndrome, CHARGE syndrome, VACTERL association (or VATER syndrome).

Pathophysiology

- Narrowed RVOT restricts systemic venous blood flow to the pulmonary vasculature.
- Dynamic infundibular subpulmonic stenosis is exacerbated during periods of increased myocardial contractility.
- Leads to further increases in resistance to pulmonary blood flow, and to preferential shunting of blood from the RV to the LV, producing a cyanotic so-called tet spells.

DIAGNOSIS

Clinical Presentation

- Most patients undergo primary surgery in the first year of life.
- Palliative repair varies based on when this was completed.

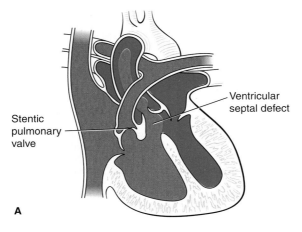

Ventricular
septal defect

Stentic
pulmonary
valve

A

Tetralogy of Fallot—repair of small PV Tet

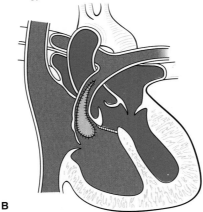

B

FIGURE 35-2. ToF, with (1) stenotic PV, (2) VSD, (3) RVH, and (4) overriding aorta with mixing of oxygenated and deoxygenated blood. (From: American Heart Association, with permission.)

- Repair typically includes patching of VSD and ASD (if present) with enlargement of the RVOT. The extent of which will depend on the degree and extent of obstruction.
- Patients with prior repair are typically left with severe PI.

History

- Severe PI or residual PS may lead to exertional dyspnea, edema, or other symptoms of RV failure.
- Unrepaired adult patients typically present similar to a non-restrictive VSD without pulmonary hypertension. This is due to protection of the pulmonary vasculature by subpulmonic stenosis.

Physical Examination

- Post-repair:
  - Systolic murmur from RVOT
  - May or may not have diastolic murmur of PI or residual PS.
  - Pansystolic may indicate a VSD patch leak.
- Arterial-to-pulmonary shunt (i.e., Blalock-Taussig shunt) may lead to reduced/absent pulses on the ipsilateral side.

Diagnostic Testing

- Chest radiography: boot-shaped horizontal heart is classic in unrepaired ToF; right-sided aortic arch may be seen; RA and RV enlargement in repaired ToF.
- ECG: RVH and RBBB common in repairs prior to 1990s; there is an increased risk of sustained ventricular arrhythmias and sudden death if the QRS is >180 milliseconds.
- TTE: useful for routine follow-up of PI, RVH/RV enlargement, and systolic function; assess for degeneration of repair.

TREATMENT

Surgical Management[1]

- Severe PI and symptoms or decreased exercise tolerance are a Class I indication for surgical repair.
- Pulmonic valve replacement reasonable with prior ToF, severe PI, and any of the following (Class IIa):
  - Moderate-to-severe RV dysfunction
  - Moderate-to-severe RV enlargement
  - Symptomatic or sustained atrial or ventricular arrhythmias
  - Moderate-to-severe TR
- Patients with residual RVOT obstruction and any of the following (Class IIa indication)[1]:
  - Peak gradient >50 mmHg
  - RV/LV pressure ratio >0.7
  - Progressive or severe dilation of the RV with dysfunction
  - Residual VSD with an L-to-R shunt >1.5:1
  - Severe AI with symptoms or more than mild LV dysfunction
  - Combination of multiple remaining lesions leading to RV enlargement or reduced function

Lifestyle/Risk Modification

- Endocarditis prophylaxis: not indicated in the repaired patient unless within 6 months of repair or there is an evidence of degeneration of prior repair.[1,3]
- Pregnancy[1]:
  - Post repair with good functional capacity and without residual defect
  - Genetic prenatal counseling is recommended. 4% to 6% of fetuses born to women with ToF will have a congenital heart defect (in the absence of 22q11 deletion syndrome).
- Activity[1,4]:
  - In the repaired ToF patient, there are no restrictions, given that the following are met: normal RV pressure, mild to no RV volume overload, no residual shunt, and no evidence of arrhythmia on ambulatory ECG or exercise testing.

○ Patients with PI, RV hypertension, or arrhythmias may only participate in low-intensity sports (Class IA sports per 36th Bethesda Conference, Table 35-2).[5]

MONITORING/FOLLOW-UP

- Yearly cardiology follow-up with TTE or MRI (Class I indication)
- Annual ECG to assess rhythm and QRS duration
- Arrhythmia prevention
  ○ Risk factors include prior palliative shunt, infundibulotomy/RV scar, QRS duration >180 ms, inducible ventricular tachycardia (VT) on electrophysiologic study, nonsustained VT documented on ambulatory monitoring, LV end-diastolic pressure >12 mmHg, cardiothoracic ratio of >0.6 on chest radiography, and age >18.
  ○ Referral to EP specialist is recommended for high risk patients.

Transposition of the Great Arteries

GENERAL PRINCIPLES

Classification

- There are two types of TGA:
  ○ Dextro-TGA (d-TGA)
  ○ Levo-TGA (l-TGA), also known as congenitally corrected TGA (CCTGA) or double switch
- Associated defects:
  ○ d-TGA: coronary anomalies, PDA, VSD (45%), LVOT obstruction (25%), and CoA (5%)[1,15]
  ○ CCTGA: VSD (70%, perimembranous), subvalvular/valvular PS (40%), AI (90%, of the systemic semilunar valve), AV block (2% yearly rate), ventricular dysfunction (near universal by adulthood), and Ebstein-like anomaly of TV[15]

Pathophysiology

- d-TGA:
  ○ Path of blood: RA to RV to aorta
  ○ Septal defect or PDA allows for mixing of deoxygenated/oxygenated blood and thus survival.
  ○ Presents with cyanosis in infancy. One-third die in first week without intervention (90% die at 1 year without intervention).
- CCTGA:
  ○ Path of blood: RA to LV (first switch) to PA (second switch) to LA to RV to aorta
  ○ RV functions as the systemic ventricle

DIAGNOSIS

Clinical Presentation

d-TGA

- Clinical presentation in adulthood is often based on complications associated with the type of repair (Table 35-3).
- Atrial switch operations (i.e., Mustard and Senning procedures) (Figure 35-3)[15]:
  ○ An intra-atrial baffle is used to redirect blood across the atrium from the SVC and IVC to the mitral valve.

TABLE 35-3 COMMON SURGICAL PROCEDURES PERFORMED IN ADULTS WITH TGA

Name	Description	Advantage	Disadvantage	Consequences
Mustard procedure (atrial switch)	Intra-atrial baffle (pericardium or PTFE)	Low mortality	Arrhythmia, sinus node dysfunction Baffle leak or obstruction. Ventricular Failure.	Most common TGA seen in adults, although supplanted by ASO
Senning procedure (atrial switch)	Intra-atrial baffle (atrial septum)	Low mortality	Arrhythmia, sinus node dysfunction Baffle leak or obstruction Ventricular Failure.	Supplanted by ASO
Jatene procedure (arterial switch operation, ASO)	Arterial switch operation, PA and aortic root	Establishes LV as systemic ventricle Less arrhythmia than atrial switch	Coronary artery closure Neoaortic root dilatation	Surgery of choice for TGA repair
Rastelli procedure	Ventricular switch (RV to PA conduit and LV to aorta baffle)	Establishes LV as systemic ventricle	High risk	Used when a VSD and pulmonary stenosis are present with d-TGA
Rashkind procedure	Balloon atrial septostomy	Rapidly creates an ASD to allow mixing of arterial and venous blood	Palliative	Used in first few days of life to allow for mixing of blood in d-TGA
Blalock-Hanlon procedure	Off pump surgical atrial septostomy	Off pump procedure, allows mixing of arterial and venous blood	Palliative	Used prior to the advent of Rashkind to allow early mixing of blood in d-TGA

PTFE, polytetrafluoroethylene; TGA, transposition of the great arteries; PA, pulmonary artery; LV, left ventricle; RV, right ventricle; VSD, ventricular septal defect.

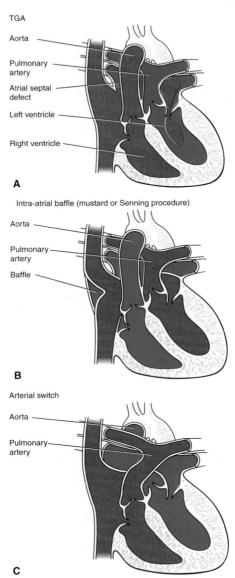

FIGURE 35-3. (**A**) Dextrotransposition of the great arteries (d-TGA). Note the systemic and venous systems in parallel, with mixing only through an ASD. (**B**) Atrial switch procedure, bringing venous blood to the morphologic left ventricle and out to the lungs. The RV is the systemic ventricle, which is the cause of many of the long-term sequelae in this repair. (**C**) Arterial switch procedure, maintaining the left ventricle as the systemic ventricle.

- Dacron graft or pericardium (Mustard procedure)
- Atrial septum (Senning procedure)
  ○ Common problems:
    - Systemic pressure results in RV failure and severe TR
    - Baffle obstruction or leak occurs in 25% of patients, which may cause paradoxical embolus. Obstruction is more common in the SVC limb.
    - Arrhythmia: 50% develop sinus node dysfunction and 30% develop intra-atrial reentry tachycardia (IART) by age 20.
    - Pulmonary hypertension
  ○ Atrial switch procedures result in a loud A2. If there is RV failure there may be TR and RV heave.
- Arterial switch operation (ASO or Jatene procedure) (Figure 35-3)[15]:
  ○ PA and aorta trunks are transected and sewn to the contralateral root with transposition of the coronary arteries to the neoaorta. This preferable as the LV remains the systemic ventricle.
  ○ Common problems: dilation of the neoaortic root leading to AI, stenosis near anastomosis sites (leads to PS or AS physiology), coronary artery ostia stenosis, supravalvular AS or PS
  ○ Arterial switch procedure usually results in a normal physical examination.

CCTGA

- >50% are diagnosed in adulthood.
- Presentation varies from asymptomatic to advanced (heart failure, arrhythmias).
- Often these patients present with systemic AV valve regurgitation and subsequent systemic ventricular dysfunction.
- Physical findings include medial point of maximal impulse (PMI), indicating a rotated heart, single S2, and possible murmur of VSD, AI, or PS.

Diagnostic Testing

- ECG:
  ○ Atrial switch: RVH, sinus bradycardia, or junctional escape
  ○ Arterial switch: normal
  ○ CCTGA:
    - First-degree AV block (50%) and reversal of precordial Q-wave pattern due to reversed septal activation
    - Complete heart block may be evidence (2% per year).[15]
- Chest radiography: "egg on its side" in uncorrected d-TGA patients; cardiomegaly in CCTGA due to left-sided RV enlargement.
- TTE:
  ○ d-TGA: parallel great arteries, aorta anterior, and to the right
  ○ Arterial switch may identify suture lines for great vessels or coronary buttons.
  ○ CCTGA: parallel great arteries, aorta is located anterior, and to the left
  ○ May be difficult to identify the morphologic ventricle, these are some clues: RV has a trabeculated apex, RV has moderator band, TV is displaced apically in the RV, LV is attached to a bileaflet AV valve.
- MRI: standard for assessing function
- Diagnostic catheterization:
  ○ Further assess baffle leaks, presumed stenosis in conduits/baffles/great vessels, or unanticipated sources for ventricular dysfunction
  ○ Assess coronary anatomy after Jatene operation

TREATMENT

Other Nonpharmacologic Therapies

Interventional catheterization (Class IIa indications)[1]:
- Occlusion of baffle leak
- Dilation or stenting of obstruction at SVC or IVC
- Dilation or stenting pulmonary obstruction
- Can be used to dilate or stent conduit obstruction if RV pressure >50% systemic pressure or peak-to-peak gradient >30 mmHg following Rastelli repair.
- Dilation or stenting of pulmonary arterial stenoses or coronary arterial stenoses after Jatene procedure

Surgical Management[1]

- d-TGA post-baffle (Mustard and Senning procedures) (Class I indications):
  - Moderate to severe systemic AV valve regurgitation (morphologic TV).
  - Baffle leak with an L-to-R shunt >1.5:1, an R-to-L shunt with arterial desaturation rest/exercise, symptoms, and progressive LV enlargement.
  - SVC or IVC baffle stenosis not amenable to percutaneous treatment
  - Pulmonary obstruction not amenable to percutaneous intervention
  - Symptomatic severe subpulmonary stenosis
- d-TGA post-ASO (Jatene procedure) (Class I indications):
  - RVOT obstruction peak-to-peak gradient >50 mmHg or RV/LV pressure ratio >0.7 not amenable to percutaneous intervention
  - Coronary artery abnormality with myocardial ischemia not amenable to percutaneous treatment
  - Severe neoaortic valve regurgitation
  - Severe neoaortic root dilatation (>55 mm)
- d-TGA post-Rastelli procedure:
  - Conduit stenosis meeting criteria for surgery for PS
  - Conduit regurgitation meeting criteria for surgery for PI
  - Residual VSD meeting criteria for surgery for VSD
  - Subaortic baffle stenosis with mean gradient of 50 mmHg or less in the presence of AI
- CCTGA (Class I indications):
  - Severe AV valve regurgitation
  - Anatomic repair (arterial and atrial switch) when LV has been functioning at systemic pressures
  - VSD closure when LV-to-AO baffle is not possible.
  - LV-to-PA conduit in cases of LV dysfunction and severe LV outflow obstruction
  - Moderate to progressive AV valve regurgitation
  - Conduit obstruction with high RV pressures or RV dysfunction after anatomic repair
  - Conduit obstruction and high LV pressures in patients with non-anatomic correction
  - Moderate-to-severe AR/neo-AR and ventricular dysfunction
- Electrophysiology/pacing:
  - d-TGA: symptomatic sinus bradycardia or sick sinus syndrome warrants pacemaker implantation (Class I indication)
  - CCTGA: regular ECG monitoring for evidence of heart block and pacemaker implantation in patients with symptomatic bradycardia

Lifestyle/Risk Modification

- Endocarditis prophylaxis: indicated for prosthetic valve, cyanotic shunt, degeneration of prior repair with prosthetic material, and within 6 months of repair.[1,3]
- Pregnancy: requires in-depth evaluation prior to determining if there is ventricular dysfunction or arrhythmia.[15]

- Activity[1,4]:
  - d-TGA:
    - Atrial baffle or Rastelli repair: avoid isometric activity, can participate in Class IA and IIA sports if no history of heart failure, arrhythmia, or syncope
    - Post-ASO: generally no restrictions unless there are hemodynamic abnormalities.
  - CCTGA: asymptomatic patients can participate in Class IA and IIA sports in the absence of significant chamber enlargement or arrhythmia.

MONITORING/FOLLOW-UP

Patients with TGA should have TTE and/or MRI yearly (Class I indication).

Ebstein Anomaly

GENERAL PRINCIPLES

Classification

- Ebstein anomaly is rare accounting for only 1% of congenital heart defects.[16]
- It has been linked to maternal lithium use.
- It consists of an apically displaced, malformation of the TV with an "atrialized" portion of the RV and is highly variable in severity.
- Ebstein anomaly is surgically classified into four types:
  - Type I: Anterior TV leaflet large and mobile. Posterior and septal leaflets are apically displaced, dysplastic, or absent. Ventricular chamber size varies.
  - Type II: Anterior, posterior, and often septal leaflets are present but are small and apically displaced in a spiral pattern. Atrialized ventricle is large.
  - Type III: Anterior leaflet is restricted, shortened, fused, and chordae are tethered. Frequently, papillary muscles directly insert into the anterior leaflet. Posterior and septal leaflets are displaced, dysplastic, not reconstructable. Large atrialized RV.
  - Type IV: Anterior leaflet is deformed and displaced into the RVOT. Few to no chordae. Direct insertion of papillary muscle into valve is common. Posterior leaflet is absent or dysplastic. Septal leaflet is a ridge of fibrous material. Small atrialized RV.
- Associated defects include ASD or PFO (80% of patients), VSD, PS or pulmonary atresia, PDA, CoA, and 20% have accessory pathways (Wolff–Parkinson–White) and arrhythmias.[1,16]
- Pathophysiologic consequences depend on the severity of malformation, degree of TR or obstruction of the RVOT, and size of the RV cavity/amount of atrialized RV.

DIAGNOSIS

Clinical Presentation

- In children, earlier presentation is associated with worse outcome.
- Adults can present at any age and most commonly present with arrhythmia, exercise intolerance, or right heart failure.
- Sudden death can occur and has been attributed to atrial fibrillation with conduction through an accessory pathway or ventricular arrhythmias.
- Paradoxical embolism may occur and suggests the presence of a concomitant ASD.
- Systolic murmur of TR may be heard (holosystolic at left lower sternal border that increases with inspiration).

Diagnostic Testing

- Chest radiography: may or may not show cardiomegaly.
- ECG: RA enlargement as evidenced by tall Himalayan P waves, QR in V1 up to lead V4, RBBB, splintered QRS complex; accessory pathway is present in one-third of patients.
- TTE:
  - Diagnosis made with echo (apical displacement of septal tricuspid leaflet >8 mm/m² and the presence of redundant, elongated anterior leaflet and a septal leaflet tethered to the ventricular septum)
  - Also used to determine the degree of RAE, TR, and presence of associated defects

TREATMENT

Medications

Anticoagulation with warfarin is recommended if there is a history of paradoxical embolus or atrial fibrillation (Class I indication).

Surgical Management[1]

- Class I indications:
  - Repair or replace TV in Ebstein's anomaly if (along with ASD closure if present):
  - Symptoms or deteriorating exercise capacity
  - Paradoxical embolism
  - Progressive cardiomegaly on chest radiography
  - Progressive RV dilation or reduction of RV systolic function
  - Cyanosis
- Re-repair/replacement if
  - Symptoms, deteriorating exercise capacity, or New York Heart Association functional class III or IV
  - Severe TR after repair with progressive RV dilation, reduction RV systolic function, appearance/progression of atrial or ventricular arrhythmias.
  - If prosthetic valve is present, with evidence of significant prosthetic valve dysfunction.

Lifestyle/Risk Modification

- Endocarditis prophylaxis: warranted in cyanotic patients or those with a prosthetic valve.[1,3]
- Pregnancy: generally well tolerated, requires evaluation prior to pregnancy, risk of CHD in fetus is about 6%.[1]
- Activity:
  - Patients without cyanosis, normal RV size, and no tachyarrhythmias have no restrictions.
  - Moderate TR and no arrhythmia, Class IA low-intensity sports 36th Bethesda Conference (Table 35-2)[5]
  - Severe Ebstein anomaly, precluded until repair completed (then may participate in class IA if above limits are met)

Single Ventricle Disorders And Fontan Repair

GENERAL PRINCIPLES

- Includes multiple disorders characterized by one physiologically sized and functional ventricle: tricuspid atresia, mitral atresia, doublet-inlet left ventricle, single ventricle, hypoplastic RV, hypoplastic LV, and heterotaxy syndromes.[17]

- Generally, patients are grouped by physiology:
  - No pulmonary flow restriction:
    - Shunt is L-to-R shortly after birth.
    - Symptoms of heart failure ensue early.
    - End-stage uncorrected, pulmonary vascular disease present as an adult if patients do not succumb to congestive heart failure in early childhood.
  - Pulmonary flow restricted:
    - Cyanotic
    - Have a previous systemic-to-pulmonary shunt (i.e., modified Blalock-Taussig, central shunt, Waterston, Potts) to increase pulmonary flow.
    - Often have undergone a cavopulmonary connection or Fontan completion
    - (Table 35-4)
- There are multiple associated defects including, but not limited to valvular abnormalities, septal defects, coarctation, and great vessel anatomy.

DIAGNOSIS

- The pathophysiology and clinical presentation are primarily related to those of specific repair (Figure 35-4 and Table 35-4)
- Edema, effusions, and ascites are clues to a diagnosis of protein-losing enteropathy (PLE), which can be confirmed by low serum albumin and increased stool alpha-1-antitrypsin. PLE should prompt consideration for transplant.
- Arrhythmias (most common intra-atrial re-entrant tachycardia) should prompt evaluation of baffle, Fontan pathway, ventricular function, and electrophysiology evaluation.

TREATMENT

Medications

- Warfarin is indicated for atrial shunt, atrial thrombus, atrial arrhythmias, or a history of thromboembolic event (Class I indication).[17]
- Diuretics and angiotensin-converting enzyme inhibitors can be used to treat systemic ventricle dysfunction (Class IIa indication).[1]

Surgical Management[1]

- Re-operation in prior Fontan procedure (Class I indications):
  - Residual ASD with R-to-L shunt and symptoms/cyanosis
  - Hemodynamically significant systemic artery-to-PA shunt, residual surgical shunt, or residual ventricle-to-PA shunt not amenable to catheter-based intervention
  - Moderate to severe systemic AV valve regurgitation
  - >30 mmHg peak-to-peak subaortic obstruction
  - Fontan path obstruction
  - Venous collaterals or pulmonary arteriovenous malformations not amenable to catheter closure
  - Pulmonary venous obstruction
  - Rhythm disturbance requiring epicardial pacemaker
  - Creation or closure of fenestration not amenable to transcatheter intervention
- Re-operation in prior Fontan procedure (Class IIa indications):
  - Reoperation of atriopulmonary connection (traditional Fontan) to a modified version if the patient has recurrent arrhythmia.
  - Should be done with concomitant Maze procedure.
- Re-operation in prior Fontan procedure (Class IIb indications): heart transplant consideration in severe systemic ventricle dysfunction or PLE

TABLE 35-4   COMMON SURGICAL PROCEDURES IN PATIENTS WITH UNIVENTRICULAR HEART

Type of repair	Anatomy	Outcome	Complications
Systemic-to-pulmonary artery shunt (i.e., modified Blalock-Taussig)	Subclavian or carotid artery connection to right or main PA (now often a graft is used)	Allows for deoxygenated systemic blood to enter pulmonary circulation and palliate cyanosis before BDCPA and Fontan completion	Atrial arrhythmias secondary to systemic ventricular dilatation Falsely low blood pressure in the extremity near previous repair
Bidirectional cavopulmonary anastomosis (BDCPA, "bidirectional Glenn")	SVC is connected to the right and left pulmonary arteries in infancy/early childhood.	Venous return from upper extremities and head bypass the RV and go directly to the lungs. Blood from the IVC continues to enter the RV. This works to improve oxygen saturation.	Pulmonary arteriovenous fistulas develop and can cause cyanosis due to relatively more IVC than SVC flow.
BDCPA plus additional pulmonary flow	Includes a concomitant systemic-to-pulmonary shunt	Used to further increase systemic oxygenation (albeit with more load on the ventricle and SVC pressure)	Volume overload to the ventricle
Single ventricle repair (Fontan procedure/completions, direct atriopulmonary connection)	RA appendage is connected to the main PA shunting both SVC and IVC blood to the lungs.	Completes full systemic flow redirection to the pulmonary arteries Most patients of current adult age had this type of repair.	Atrial arrhythmias due to scarring of the atrium Protein-losing enteropathy Plastic bronchitis Thromboembolic events Chronic congestive hepatopathy Ventricular failure Systemic AV valve regurgitation

(Continued)

TABLE 35-4 COMMON SURGICAL PROCEDURES IN PATIENTS WITH UNIVENTRICULAR HEART *(Continued)*

Type of repair	Anatomy	Outcome	Complications
Modified Fontan	Extracardiac conduit: IVC → R PA/main PA via synthetic graft outside the RA Intra-atrial (lateral) conduit: IVC → R PA/main PA via partition in the RA Intracardiac lateral tunnel Fenestration between systemic venous path and LA	Creates a right-to-left shunt to reduce pressure in the systemic system, but results in hypoxia. Used once protein-losing enteropathy has developed	Same as with traditional Fontan except that arrhythmias and thromboembolic events less common
1.5 Ventricle repair	BDCPA + IVC flow directed to small pulmonary ventricle	Reduces systemic blood return to a small pulmonary ventricle	
2 Ventricle repair	Intraventricular or VSD patch placed to septate a common ventricle (or large VSD)	Separates systemic and pulmonic circulation	

IVC, inferior vena cava; SVC, superior vena cava; RA, right atrium; AV, arteriovenous; R, right; PA, pulmonary artery; VSD, ventricular septal defect.

Total extracardiac conduit fontan palliation of hypoplastic left heart

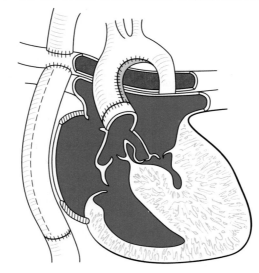

A

Tricuspid atresia palliation with bidirectional Glenn shunt

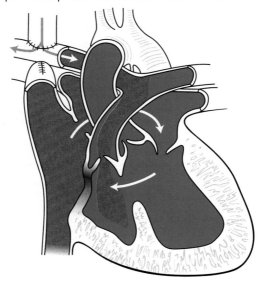

B

FIGURE 35-4. (**A**) Extracardiac Fontan procedure for hypoplastic left heart, resulting in a total cavopulmonary shunt (SVC and IVC into PA). (**B**) Bidirectional Glenn shunt (SVC to PA) in a patient with tricuspid atresia and an ASD.

Lifestyle/Risk Modification

- Endocarditis prophylaxis: warranted if prosthetic valve, recent repair (within 6 months), previous endocarditis, and in cases where endothelialization has not occurred on native or prosthetic grafts.[1,3]
- Pregnancy[1]:
  - Consultation in a center with expertise in adult CHD before pregnancy (Class I indication)
  - Full evaluation prior to conception
  - Risk is largely dictated by burden of arrhythmia, ventricular dysfunction, and presence or absence of PLE.
- Activity: diagnostic evaluation required prior to participation, Class IA low-intensity sports are recommended in absence of evaluation.[1]
- Thromboembolic prophylaxis: lifelong anticoagulation if the patient has a fenestration.

REFERENCES

1. Warnes, CA, Williams RG, Bashore TM, et al. ACC/AHA 2008 guidelines for the management of adults with congenital heart disease. Circulation 2008;118:e714-e833.
2. Webb G, Gatzoulis MA. Atrial septal defects in the adult: recent progress and overview. Circulation 2006;114:1645-1653.
3. Nishimura RA, Carabello BA, Faxon DP, et al. ACC/AHA 2008 guideline update on valvular heart disease: focused update on infective endocarditis. Circulation 2008;118:887-896.
4. Graham TP Jr, Driscoll DJ, Gersony WM. Task Force 2: congenital heart disease. J Am Coll Cardiol 2005;45:1326-1333.
5. Mitchell JH, Haskell W, Snell P, Van Camp SP. Task Force 8: classification of sports. J Am Coll Cardiol 2005;45:1364-1367.
6. Minette MS, Sahn DA. Ventricular septal defects. Circulation 2006;114:2190-2197.
7. Khairy P, Ouyang DW, Fernandes SM, et al. Pregnancy outcomes in women with congenital heart disease. Circulation 2006;113:517-524.
8. Schneider DJ, Moore JW. Patent ductus arteriosus. Circulation 2006;114:1873-1882.
9. Aboulhosn J, Child JS. Left ventricular outflow obstruction: subaortic stenosis, bicuspid aortic valve, supravalvular aortic stenosis, and coarctation of the aorta. Circulation 2006;114:2412-2422.
10. Schievink WI, Raissi SS, Maya MM, Velebir A. Screening for intracranial aneurysms in patients with bicuspid aortic valve. Neurology 2010;74:1430-1433.
11. Fernandes, SM, Sanders SP, Khairy P, et al. Morphology of bicuspid aortic valve in children and adolescents. J Am Coll Cardiol 2004;44:1648-1651.
12. Bonow RO, Carabello BA, Chatterjee K, et al. 2008 focused update incorporated into the ACC/AHA 2006 guidelines for the management of patients with valvular heart disease. J Am Coll Cardiol 2008;52:e1-e142.
13. Dillar GP, Gatzoulis MA. Pulmonary vascular disease in adults with congenital heart disease. Circulation 2007;115:1039-1050.
14. Bashore TM. Adult congenital heart disease: right ventricular outflow tract lesions. Circulation 2007;115:1933-1947.
15. Warnes CA. Transposition of the great arteries. Circulation 2006;114:2699-2709.
16. Attenhofer Jost CH, Connolly HM, Dearani JA, et al. Ebstein's anomaly. Circulation 2007;115:277-285.
17. Khairy P, Poirier N, Mercier LA. Univentricular heart. Circulation 2007;115:800-812.

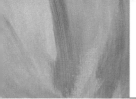

Cardiovascular Disease in Older Patients

36

Michael W. Rich

Introduction

GENERAL PRINCIPLES

Epidemiology

- The number of Americans aged 65 years or older will increase from approximately 40 million in 2010 to approximately 72 million in 2030. The most rapidly growing segment of the US population are individuals aged 75 or older.
- The prevalence of cardiovascular disease (CVD) increases progressively with age.[1] It exceeds 75% in men and women aged ≥80 years (Figure 36-1).[2]
- In the United States, 84% of all deaths attributable to CVD occur in people aged ≥65 years and 68% occur in people aged ≥75 years.
- People aged ≥65 years account for 63% of all CVD hospitalizations in the United States.
  - Over 50% of percutaneous and surgical revascularization procedures
  - 55% of defibrillator implantations
  - 80% of arterial endarterectomies
  - 86% of permanent pacemaker insertions

Pathophysiology

Effects of Aging on the Cardiovascular System[3,4]

- Aging is associated with diffuse changes throughout the cardiovascular system (Table 36-1).
- Resting cardiac performance (i.e., contractility and cardiac output) is generally preserved in healthy older individuals, but there is a progressive decline in cardiovascular reserve.
- As a result, the heart is less able to compensate in response to stress, both physiologic (e.g., exercise) and pathologic (e.g., acute coronary syndrome [ACS], pneumonia, or surgery).
- Older patients are at increased risk for complications, including ischemia, heart failure, arrhythmias, and death, in the setting of both cardiac and noncardiac illnesses and procedures.

Key Effects of Aging on Other Organ Systems

- Renal:
  - Decline in glomerular filtration rate (approximately 8 mL/minute/decade)
  - Decreased concentrating and diluting capacity
  - Impaired electrolyte homeostasis
- Pulmonary:
  - Decreased vital capacity
  - Increased ventilation/perfusion mismatching
- Hematologic:
  - Altered balance between thrombosis and fibrinolysis in favor of thrombosis
  - Increased risk of arterial (stroke, myocardial infarction [MI]) and venous thrombosis (deep vein thrombosis [DVT] and pulmonary embolism [PE])
  - Increased risk of hemorrhage, particularly with antiplatelet, anticoagulant, or fibrinolytic therapy

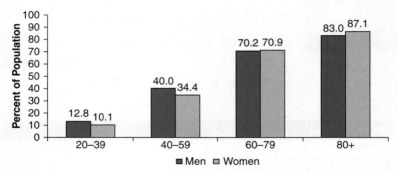

FIGURE 36-1. Prevalence of CVD in adults aged ≥20 by age and sex (National Health and Nutrition Examination Survey: 2007–2010). Data include coronary heart disease, heart failure, stroke, and hypertension. (From Go AS, Mozaffarian D, Roger VL, et al. Heart disease and stroke statistics—2013 update: a report from the American Heart Association. *Circulation* 2013;127:e6-e245, with permission.)

TABLE 36-1	PRINCIPAL EFFECTS OF AGING ON THE CARDIOVASCULAR SYSTEM
Effect	**Clinical implications**
Increased arterial stiffness	Increased afterload, systolic blood pressure, and pulse pressure
Impaired myocardial relaxation and increased myocardial stiffness	Impaired diastolic filling and increased risk for diastolic heart failure and atrial fibrillation
Impaired sinus node function and decreased conduction velocity in the AV node and infranodal conduction system	Increased prevalence of sick sinus syndrome, bundle branch block, and supraventricular and ventricular arrhythmias
Impaired responsiveness to β-adrenergic stimulation	Decreased maximum heart rate and cardiac output Impaired thermoregulation
Impaired endothelium-mediated vasodilation	Reduced maximum coronary blood flow, increased risk for demand ischemia and atherosclerosis
Decreased baroreceptor responsiveness	Increased risk for orthostatic hypotension, falls, and syncope

- Neurologic:
  - Decreased central nervous system (CNS) autoregulatory capacity (increased susceptibility to hypoperfusion)
  - Altered reflex responsiveness (increased risk of orthostasis and falls)
  - Impaired thirst mechanism (increased risk for dehydration)

- Musculoskeletal:
  - Osteopenia
  - Sarcopenia (loss of muscle mass and strength)
  - Joint stiffness/loss of flexibility
- Gastrointestinal:
  - Altered absorption and elimination of drugs
  - Altered hepatic metabolism of drugs

Cardiovascular Risk Factors

- Age itself is a potent risk factor for the development of CVD.
- Hypertension[5]:
  - Prevalence exceeds 70% in men and women aged >70 years.
  - Isolated systolic hypertension accounts for >90% of all hypertension after 75 years of age.
  - **Systolic blood pressure is the strongest independent risk factor for CVD in those aged >65 years.**
- Diabetes mellitus (DM):
  - Prevalence increases up to age 80.
  - Approximately 50% of all individuals with diabetes in the United States are aged ≥65 years.
  - **The attributable risk of diabetes to CVD is greater in patients aged ≥65 years than in younger individuals.**
  - Higher in women than in men
- Dyslipidemia:
  - In men total cholesterol levels increase until about age 70.
  - Women:
    - Total cholesterol levels rise rapidly after menopause.
    - Averages 15 to 20 mg/dL higher than in men after age 60.
    - High-density lipoprotein (HDL) cholesterol levels average about 10 mg/dL higher than in men throughout adult life.
  - **High total cholesterol to HDL-cholesterol ratios remain independently associated with coronary events among individuals aged ≥80 years.**
  - Strength of association of dyslipidemia with CVD declines with age.
- Tobacco:
  - Smoking prevalence declines with age, in part due to premature smoking-related deaths.
  - **Smoking cessation is associated with a marked reduction in CVD risk in all individuals.**
- Other risk factors:
  - The association between obesity and CVD risk in older adults is unclear. Mild-to-moderate obesity (BMI 30 to 40 kg/m^2) confers a more favorable prognosis in older patients with coronary artery disease (CAD) or heart failure (HF), the so-called **obesity paradox.**
  - **Physical inactivity** is associated with increased CVD risk and worse prognosis in individuals of all ages.
  - The clinical utility of C-reactive protein, B-type natriuretic protein, coronary artery calcium scores, ankle–brachial index, and carotid artery intima–media thickness in the routine assessment of CVD risk in older adults remains undefined.

DIAGNOSIS

The diagnosis of CVDs will be discussed in the following sections specific to those conditions.

TREATMENT

- Evidence base for managing older patients with CVD is severely limited as **this population has been markedly underrepresented in randomized clinical trials and observational studies**.
- Management is further complicated by the **high prevalence of comorbid conditions** that impact the benefit-to-risk ratio of diagnostic procedures and therapeutic interventions.
- **Management must be individualized**, with consideration to the nature and severity of the patient's cardiac and noncardiac conditions, psychosocial factors, and personal preferences, including the patient's perception of the importance of quality of life versus length of life.
- **Age alone is rarely a contraindication** to implementation of interventions that have a reasonable likelihood of improving quality and/or quantity of life.

Chronic Coronary Artery Disease

GENERAL PRINCIPLES

- A general discussion regarding chronic CAD can be found in Chapter 10.
- Autopsy studies indicate that up to 70% of adults aged ≥70 years have significant CAD, defined as ≥50% obstruction of one or more major coronary arteries.
- The prevalence of clinically significant CAD is approximately 22% in men and 13% in women aged ≥75 years.
- People aged ≥65 years account for approximately two-thirds of MIs in the United States, with 40 to 45% occurring in people aged ≥75 years.
- Women account for 26% of MIs in the 45- to 64-year age group, 35% of MI in the 65- to 74-year age group, and 55% of MI in the ≥75-year age group.
- Over 80% of deaths from MI occur in the 65- to 74-year age group, and approximately 60% occur in ≥75-year age group.

DIAGNOSIS

- Older patients are more likely to report exertional shortness of breath or fatigue that typical anginal symptoms.
- They have more extensive CAD at the time of diagnosis and there is a higher prevalence of left main and multivessel disease.
- **Exercise or pharmacological stress test is the initial diagnostic procedure of choice in older patients with stable symptoms**. An exercise test is preferred in patients who are able to exercise.
- The risk of coronary angiography increases slightly with age. The risk of major complications in experienced centers is <2%, even in nonagenarians.

TREATMENT

Medications

- Hypertension, dyslipidemia, and DM should be treated in accordance with published guidelines.
- Aspirin 75 to 325 mg daily is indicated in all CAD patients without contraindications.
- β-Blockers, calcium channel antagonists, long-acting nitrates, and ranolazine alone or in combination, to control anginal symptoms.

- β-Blockers are indicated in patients with prior MI or symptomatic HF with a left ventricular ejection fraction (LVEF) ≤40%.
- Angiotensin-converting enzyme (ACE) inhibitors, or angiotensin receptor blockers (ARBs) in ACE inhibitor intolerant patients, are indicated in patients up to age 85 with established CAD and an estimated GFR ≥30 mL/minute. They are also indicated in patients with an LVEF ≤40%.
- Smoking cessation with behavioral and/or pharmacological support should be provided as needed.

Surgical Management

- Indications for percutaneous coronary intervention (PCI) and coronary artery bypass graft (CABG) surgery are similar in older and younger patients.
  - There is improved quality of life in older patients whose symptoms fail to respond to aggressive medical therapy.
  - Risk of procedure-related complications increases with age.
- Up to 50% of older patients undergoing CABG experience postoperative cognitive decline that may persist for 3 to 6 months following surgery. A small percentage experience persistent cognitive impairment.
- Cardiac rehabilitation should be initiated prior to hospital discharge with subsequent referral to a structured rehabilitation program.

Acute Coronary Syndromes[6,7]

GENERAL PRINCIPLES

- General principles relating to CAD in other patients are presented in the Chronic Coronary Artery Disease section.
- A detailed discussion regarding ACS and acute MI can be found in Chapters 11 and 12.

DIAGNOSIS

- The likelihood of chest pain as a presenting symptom declines with age.
  - Shortness of breath is the most common presenting symptom in patients aged >80 years.
  - Approximately 20% of patients aged ≥85 years present with altered mental status, confusion, dizziness, or syncope.
- The initial ECG is more likely to be nondiagnostic due to higher prevalence of conduction abnormalities, left ventricular hypertrophy, prior MI, or paced rhythm.
- The proportion of patients with non-ST-segment elevation MI (NSTEMI) increases with age.
- Delays in presentation and diagnosis contribute to worse outcomes

TREATMENT

- In general, treatment is similar to that in younger patients.
- Age-related cardiovascular changes and comorbid conditions alter the benefit-to-risk analysis for virtually all interventions.

Medications

- Aspirin and β-blocker therapy unless there are contraindications.

- Addition of an ACE inhibitor or ARB is reasonable in elderly patients with adequate renal function (GFR ≥30 mL/minute) and heart failure or LV systolic dysfunction.
- Early initiation of a statin is reasonable.
- Indications for the use of adjunctive antithrombotic agents (i.e., heparin, low molecular heparin, bivalirudin, clopidogrel, prasugrel, fondaparinux, glycoprotein IIB/IIIA inhibitors, and emerging antithrombotic drugs) are similar to younger patients.
  ○ Adjustment for weight and renal function is essential to minimize the risk of hemorrhage.
  ○ Bleeding risk increases progressively with the number of antithrombotic agents administered.

Other Nonpharmacologic Therapies

- **Early reperfusion** (i.e., within 6 to 12 hours) in patients with STEMI is desirable.
- **Primary PCI is associated with more favorable outcomes** than fibrinolytic therapy (at least up to age 85).
- **Early invasive strategy in patients with NSTEMI/unstable angina is associated with lower mortality and reinfarction rates** than initial strategy of optimal medical therapy. Relatively few patients aged ≥80 years with significant comorbidities have been enrolled in these trials.
- Patients should be referred to a cardiac rehabilitation program if feasible.

Valvular Heart Disease

GENERAL PRINCIPLES

- A more general discussion of relevant valvular disease is found in Chapters 19 and 20.
- The incidence and prevalence of valvular heart disease increase with age.
- Aortic valve replacements and mitral valve repair or replacements are the second and third most common indications for open-heart surgery in older adults, respectively.
- **Aortic stenosis** (AS) is most commonly due to fibrosis and calcification of a previously normal aortic valve.
- **Mitral stenosis** (MS) is most commonly due to nonrheumatic calcification of the mitral valve annulus and subvalvular apparatus.
- **Aortic regurgitation** (AR) may be either acute or chronic. The most common etiologies include primary valve disease (e.g., coexisting AS or infective endocarditis) and diseases of the ascending aorta (e.g., aortic aneurysm or dissection).
- **Mitral regurgitation** (MR) may be acute or chronic. The most common etiologies of clinically significant MR include myxomatous degeneration of the valve, ischemic papillary muscle dysfunction, and annular dilatation due to ischemic or nonischemic dilated cardiomyopathy.

DIAGNOSIS

- Older patients with valvular disease present similarly to younger patient
- Older patients often present at a more advanced stage
- They often have preserved carotid upstrokes with severe AS in contrast to younger patients because of increased stiffness of the great vessels.

TREATMENT

- Indications for aortic valve replacement and mitral valve repair or replacement are similar to younger patients.
- Bioprosthetic valves are recommended ≥65 years of age.
- Mitral valve repair preferable to mitral valve replacement.
- Operative mortality for ≥80 years:
  - 3% to 10% for elective aortic valve procedures
  - 5% to 15% for elective mitral valve procedures
- There is an increased risk of perioperative complications.
- Length of hospital stay and recovery time tends to be longer.
- Long-term outcomes are generally favorable especially following aortic valve replacement for severe AS.
- Recent studies have demonstrated favorable outcomes following percutaneous aortic valve replacement in elderly patients considered to be at high operative risk.

Heart Failure[8]

GENERAL PRINCIPLES

The general discussion of HF is located in Chapters 14 and 15.

Epidemiology
- The incidence and prevalence of HF increase progressively with age and is projected to double over the next two decades.
- **HF is the leading cause of hospitalization and rehospitalization in older adults**.
- HF is a major cause of chronic disability and impaired quality of life in older individuals.
- The median age of patients hospitalized with HF in the United States is 75 years.
- Approximately two-thirds of deaths attributable to HF occur in individuals aged ≥75 years.
- Ten percent of people aged ≥80 years, half of whom are women, have HF.
- One-year mortality is 25% to 30%. Median survival is 2 to 3 years and 5-year survival is approximately 20% to 25%.

Etiology
- The etiology of HF in older patients is most often **multifactorial**.
- The most common antecedent condition is hypertension:
  - Principal cause in 60% to 70% of older women
  - Principal cause in 30% to 40% in older men and a similar percentage attributable to CAD
- Other common causes include valvular heart disease and nonischemic dilated cardiomyopathy.
- Less common causes include hypertrophic cardiomyopathy, restrictive cardiomyopathy (e.g., amyloidosis), and pericardial diseases.
- The prevalence of HF with preserved ejection fraction (HFPEF) increases with age:
  - Approximately 50% of all HF cases in patients aged ≥70 years.
  - More common in women than in men.

DIAGNOSIS

- HF in older patients is **more likely to present with atypical symptoms**, such as confusion, lethargy, irritability, anorexia, or gastrointestinal irregularities.

- Classical signs and chest radiographic findings of HF are both less sensitive and less specific.
- B-type natriuretic peptide (BNP) and *N*-terminal pro-BNP (nt-proBNP) levels increase with age; therefore, their specificity for diagnosing HF is reduced in older patients.
- Transthoracic echocardiography with color and spectral Doppler is indicated for newly diagnosed HF or an unexplained deterioration in clinical status.
- Stress testing followed by coronary angiography, if indicated, is appropriate for those with CAD who are suitable candidates for revascularization.

TREATMENT

- Older patients are more likely to have multiple comorbidities that may complicate therapy.
- Patients with advanced HF and anticipated life expectancy <6 months should be offered palliative care services and hospice.[9]
- Advance directive and assignment of durable power of attorney for health-care decisions should be encouraged for all due to the poor prognosis associated with HF in older patients.

Medications

- Pharmacotherapy of HF with reduced ejection fraction (systolic HF) is similar in older and younger patients.
- Older patients are at increased risk for adverse drug effects and interactions—slower dose titration and cautious addition of new medications is warranted.
- No pharmacologic agents have been shown to improve outcomes in patients with HFPEF. Treatment should focus on hypertension, decreased ischemic burden, rhythm or rate control (atrial fibrillation), and optimization of volume status with judicious diuretics use.
- Avoid nonsteroidal anti-inflammatory drugs (NSAIDs) in all HF patients. Adverse effects on renal function and tendency to promote sodium and water retention.

Other Nonpharmacologic Therapies

- Moderate dietary sodium restriction (1,500 mg per day)
- Limit excess fluid intake (>48 to 64 ounces per day)
- Regular exercise as tolerated (including flexibility, strengthening, and aerobic exercises)
- HF self-care education (e.g., daily weights, adherence to medications, and other recommended behaviors)
- Referral to a HF disease management program if available for patients with advanced HF (New York Heart Association Class III to IV)
- Implantable cardioverter-defibrillator (ICD) therapy in appropriately selected patients with systolic HF up to 80 years of age. The utility of ICDs in patients aged >80 years is uncertain.
- Cardiac resynchronization therapy (CRT) is a reasonable option in appropriately selected patients of advanced age (including ≥80 years) with persistent limiting symptoms despite optimal medical therapy.

Atrial Fibrillation[10]

GENERAL PRINCIPLES

- Atrial fibrillation (AF) is covered in detail in Chapter 26.
- The incidence and prevalence increase markedly with age:
  ○ Median age of patients with AF in the United States is 75 years.
  ○ Prevalence of about 10% in those aged ≥80 years

- The incidence of stroke attributable to AF also increases with age, accounting for 25% to 30% of strokes in those aged ≥80 years
- The risk of stroke in older patients with AF is higher in women than in men by a factor of 1.8.
- AF is also an independent risk factor for all-cause mortality.

DIAGNOSIS

- The most common symptoms of AF in older patients include palpitations, shortness of breath, and exercise intolerance.
- Many patients are asymptomatic while others develop acute HF and pulmonary edema, often associated with elevated troponin levels.
- Stroke, transient ischemic attack, or other thromboembolic event may be presenting symptom.
- Diagnostic evaluation should include ECG, serum electrolytes, thyroid function tests, and transthoracic echocardiography.

TREATMENT

- Principal goals of therapy are to **alleviate symptoms and minimize the risk of thromboembolic events**.
- **There is no benefit to restoring sinus rhythm over rate control on reducing stroke or mortality in AF patients with mild symptoms.**[11,12]
- Lenient rate control with resting heart rate up to 110 bpm as effective in controlling symptoms and reducing the risk of adverse events as more stringent rate control with resting heart rate <80 bpm.[13] It is also associated with fewer side effects.

Medications

Rhythm Control

- Rhythm control is appropriate for persistent moderate or marked symptoms despite measures to control heart rate.
- Amiodarone is the most effective agent for maintaining sinus rhythm but is associated with multiple limiting side effects in older patients.[14]
- Dronedarone has fewer side effects than amiodarone and is the only antiarrhythmic agent shown to reduce hospitalizations and mortality in patients with AF.[15] It is contraindicated in patients with significant HF.[16] Recent trial data have also cast doubt on its use in permanent AF.[17]

Anticoagulation

- Age ≥75 years is an independent risk factor for stroke.
- **Anticoagulation is indicated in all patients with paroxysmal or persistent AF in the absence of contraindications**.
- Warfarin reduces stroke risk by 60% to 70% in patients with nonvalvular AF.
- Dabigatran is a direct thrombin inhibitor that is at least as effective as warfarin in reducing the risk of ischemic stroke and is associated with a lower risk of intracranial hemorrhage.[18]
  - It does not require routine monitoring of the INR, significant dietary modifications, or interact with drugs metabolized by the CYP microsomal enzyme system.
  - Needs dose adjustment with CrCl <30 mL/minute.
- Rivaroxaban and apixaban are direct factor Xa inhibitor approved for nonvavlular atrial fibrillation.[19]
- Aspirin reduces stroke risk by 20% to 25% in AF patients aged <75 years but is ineffective in patients aged ≥75 years.

- Risk of falls is the most common reason for withholding warfarin therapy in older adults. The benefit of warfarin on stroke risk outweighs the potential bleeding risk associated with falls in the majority of cases.

Other Nonpharmacologic Therapies

- Limited data are available on the use of percutaneous catheter ablation of AF (i.e., pulmonary vein isolation) in older patients. The procedure appears to be less effective and associated with higher complication rates than in younger patients.
- The surgical Maze procedure is a reasonable option for treating symptomatic AF in older patients who require open-heart surgery for another indication (e.g., CABG, mitral valve surgery).

Ventricular Arrhythmias

- Ventricular arrhythmias are discussed in detail in Chapter 25.
- Increased ventricular ectopy is associated with increased mortality in older patients with structural heart disease.
- The diagnosis and management of ventricular arrhythmias is similar in older and younger adults.
- The indications for an ICD are similar in younger and older patients up to age 80 years.
- The value of ICDs in patients aged more than 80 years has not been established.

Bradyarrhythmias

- There is an increase incidence and prevalence of bradyarrhythmias and conduction disorders with increasing age. This is due to age-related changes in the sinus node, AV node, and infranodal conduction system.
- More than 75% of pacemaker recipients in the United States are aged ≥65 years and approximately 50% are aged ≥75 years.
- **Sick sinus syndrome** is manifested by resting sinus bradycardia, chronotropic incompetence (failure to increase heart rate commensurate with increased demands), sinus pauses, and/or sinus arrest.[20]
  - It is a common cause of dizziness, falls, near syncope, and syncope in older patients (see Chapter 6).
  - It accounts for up to 50% of pacemaker insertions in older adults.
- In general, the diagnosis and management of bradyarrhythmias and conduction disorders is similar in older and younger patients (see Chapter 25).
- Sick sinus syndrome is often associated with paroxysmal supraventricular tachyarrhythmias and treatment of the tachyarrhythmias may exacerbate the bradyarrhythmias (the tachy-brady syndrome) and necessitate pacemaker implantation.
- Symptomatic AV-nodal conduction abnormalities may require pacemaker insertion.
- Dual chamber pacing is associated with reduced incidence of AF and HF compared to single chamber ventricular pacemakers (VVI).
- Beneficial effects on mortality and stroke have not been demonstrated.

REFERENCES

1. Roger VL, Go AS, Lloyd-Jones DM, et al. Heart disease and stroke statistics—2011 update: a report from the American Heart Association. *Circulation* 2011;123:e18-e209.
2. Go AS, Mozaffarian D, Roger VL, et al. Heart disease and stroke statistics—2013 update: a report from the American Heart Association. *Circulation* 2013;127:e6-e245.
3. Lakatta EG, Levy D. Arterial and cardiac aging: major shareholders in cardiovascular disease enterprises: Part I: aging arteries: a "set up" for vascular disease. *Circulation* 2003;107:139-146.
4. Lakatta EG, Levy D. Arterial and cardiac aging: major shareholders in cardiovascular disease enterprises: Part II: the aging heart in health: links to heart disease. *Circulation* 2003;107:346-354.
5. Aronow WS, Fleg JL, Pepine CJ, et al. ACCF/AHA 2011 expert consensus document on hypertension in the elderly. *J Am Coll Cardiol* 2011;57:2037-2114.
6. Alexander KP, Newby LK, Cannon CP, et al. Acute coronary care in the elderly, part I: Non-ST-segment-elevation acute coronary syndromes. *Circulation* 2007;115:2549-2569.
7. Alexander KP, Newby LK, Armstrong PW, et al. Acute coronary care in the elderly, part II: ST-segment-elevation myocardial infarction. *Circulation* 2007;115:2570-2589.
8. Jugdutt BI. Heart failure in the elderly: advances and challenges. *Exp Rev Cardiovasc Ther* 2010;8:695-715.
9. Goodlin SJ. Palliative care in congestive heart failure. *J Am Coll Cardiol* 2009;54:386-396.
10. Fang MC, Chen J, Rich MW. Atrial fibrillation in the elderly. *Am J Med* 2007;120:481-487.
11. Van Gelder IC, Hagens VE, Bosker HA, et al. A comparison of rate control and rhythm control in patients with recurrent persistent atrial fibrillation. *N Engl J Med* 2002;347:1834-1840.
12. Wyse DG, Waldo AL, DiMarco JP, et al. A comparison of rate control and rhythm control in patients with atrial fibrillation. The Atrial Fibrillation Follow-up Investigation of Rhythm Management (AFFIRM) investigators. *N Engl J Med* 2002;347:1825.
13. Van Gelder IC, Groenveld HT, Crijns HJGM, et al. Lenient versus strict rate control in patients with atrial fibrillation. *N Engl J Med* 2010;362:1363-1373.
14. McNamara RL, Tamariz LJ, Segal JB, Bass EB. Management of atrial fibrillation: review of the evidence for the role of pharmacologic therapy, electrical cardioversion, and echocardiography. *Ann Intern Med* 2003;139:1018-1033.
15. Piccini JP, Hasselblad V, Peterson ED, et al. Comparative efficacy of dronedarone and amiodarone for the maintenance of sinus rhythm in patients with atrial fibrillation. *J Am Coll Cardiol* 2009;54:1089-1095.
16. Køber L, Torp-Pedersen C, McMurray JJ, et al. Increased mortality after dronedarone therapy for severe heart failure. *N Engl J Med* 2008;358:2678-2687.
17. Connolly SJ, Camm AJ, Halperin JL, et al. Dronedarone in high-risk permanent atrial fibrillation. *N Engl J Med* 2011;365:2268-2276.
18. Connolly SJ, Ezekowitz MD, Yusuf S, et al. Dabigatran versus warfarin in patients with atrial fibrillation. *N Engl J Med* 2009;361:1139-1151.
19. Patel MR, Mahaffey KW, Garg J, et al. Rivaroxaban versus warfarin in nonvalvular atrial fibrillation. *N Engl J Med* 2011;365:883-891.
20. Brignole M. Sick sinus syndrome. *Clin Geriatr Med* 2002;18:211-227.

Diabetes and Cardiovascular Disease

37

Ilia G. Halatchev and Ronald J. Krone

Diabetes And Coronary Artery Disease

GENERAL PRINCIPLES

Epidemiology

- Diabetes mellitus (DM) affects more than 10% of the population of the United States.
- Coronary artery disease (CAD) develops approximately 15 years earlier in DM.[1]
- Diabetics are two to four times more likely to have acute coronary syndrome (ACS).
- A contemporary meta-analysis of 37 studies showed that the risk of fatal coronary disease was higher in patients with diabetes (5.4% compared to 1.6%).[2]
- DM is CAD risk equivalent.[3-5]

Pathophysiology[6]

- The mechanism of endothelial damage and atheroma formation include endothelial dysfunction and enhanced thrombosis development, interaction with cellular inflammation, insulin resistance, and other genetic/environmental factors.
- Advanced glycation end-products contribute to dysfunctional high-density lipoprotein (HDL) which in turn results in increased atherogenesis.[7]
- There is increased risk of plaque rupture and subsequent thrombosis development with more lipid-rich tissue and macrophage infiltration in coronary atheromas.
- There is enhanced platelet aggregation and activation.
- Coronary collateral development is poor.

DIAGNOSIS

Clinical Presentation

- There is a spectrum of presenting symptoms of CAD ranging from none to stable angina, unstable angina, or acute myocardial infarction with no previous symptoms.
- Some diabetics have a blunted appreciation of myocardial ischemic pain due to autonomic denervation.
- Lack of symptoms contributes to delay in definitive treatment.
- The clinical severity and complications of acute myocardial infarction (AMI) are often greater and lead to a worse outcome than in nondiabetics.
- The incidences of heart failure (HF), acute pulmonary edema, cardiogenic shock, recurrent MIs, cardiac arrhythmias, and acute kidney injury are increased.

Diagnostic Testing

- The American College of Cardiology Foundation/American Heart Association (ACCF/AHA) guidelines regarding the diagnosis of CAD in asymptomatic patients with DM are as follows[8]:

- A **resting ECG** is reasonable for cardiovascular risk assessment in asymptomatic adults with diabetes (Class IIa, Level of Evidence: C).
- Measurement of **coronary artery calcium** (CAC) is reasonable for cardiovascular risk assessment in asymptomatic diabetics ≥40 years old (Class IIa, Level of Evidence: B).
- **Stress myocardial perfusion imaging** (MPI) may be considered when previous risk assessment testing suggests a high risk of CAD, such as a CAC score of ≥400 (Class IIb, Level of Evidence: C).[9-12]
- The diagnostic sensitivity and specificity of exercise ECG testing, exercise or pharmacologic stress MPI, and exercise/dobutamine echocardiography are similar for diabetics and nondiabetics.
- Stress MPI or echocardiography has higher sensitivity and specificity and prognostic value in DM compared with exercise ECG alone.
- Exercise stress is preferred because of the prognostic value.

TREATMENT

Medications

- Medical therapy is similar to that of the nondiabetic (see Chapters 11 and 12).
- Angiotensin-converting enzyme (ACE) inhibitors and angiotensin receptor blockers (ARBs):
  - ACC/AHA Class I indication
  - Reduce infarct size, limit ventricular remodeling, and reduce mortality
- Aldosterone antagonists: ACC/AHA Class I indication when ACS associated with left ventricular ejection fraction (LVEF) of ≤40% and serum creatinine of ≤2.5 mg/dL in men (or ≤2.0 mg/dL in women) and serum potassium of ≤5.0 meq/L
- Aspirin
- Glycemic control:
  - Insulin-based regimen to achieve and maintain glucose levels <180 mg/dL while avoiding hypoglycemia for patients with ST-segment elevation MI (STEMI) with either a complicated or uncomplicated course[13]
  - Strict glycemic control should be maintained after discharge with a goal HgbA1c of ≤7%.[14-16]
  - Fasting plasma glucose and HgbA1c should be routinely measured during hospitalization in nondiabetic patients with an acute MI.
    - Values that are elevated but do not meet the criteria for diabetes should be repeated after discharge.
    - If the diagnosis is confirmed, glycemic therapy should be started as early as possible.
- Glycoprotein (GP) IIb/IIIa inhibitors may have particular benefit in diabetic patients.[17-20]
- β-Blockers:
  - Previously not favored due to concerns of masking hypoglycemic symptoms or worsening glycemic control
  - Overall benefit has been found to be at least equivalent to or greater than that seen in nondiabetics.
- Statins[3,4]:
  - Drugs of choice for low-density lipoprotein cholesterol (LDL-C) lowering
  - Cholesterol levels should be reassessed after 2 to 3 months of therapy with a goal LDL-C of <70 mg/dL or 50% reduction from baseline
  - Addition of a second, nonstatin agent if further lowering needed
- Thienopyridine:
  - Clopidogrel or prasugrel
  - Prasugrel appears to have better efficacy and similar safety compared with clopidogrel in diabetics.[21,22]

Revascularization

- STEMI:
  - Primary percutaneous intervention (PCI) is associated with lower rates of death (9.4% vs. 5.9%), recurrent MI, and stroke compared with thrombolytic therapy.[23]
  - Despite revascularization after STEMI, diabetes is significantly more likely to have a fatal outcome, reinfarction, and stent thrombosis.[24]
- Unstable angina (UA)/non-STEMI (NSTEMI):
  - Early invasive evaluation followed by revascularization if appropriate
  - Higher rates of death, heart failure, recurrent MI, or stroke
- In-stent restenosis after PCI is related to smaller vessel caliber, greater length of the stented segment, and lower body mass index.
- Drug eluting stents (DESs) have lower rates of in-stent stenosis compared to bare metal stents (BMSs).[25,26] Those with insulin-requiring DM have a poorer outcome with PCI/DES than those with non–insulin-requiring DM.[27]
- Initial studies comparing percutaneous transluminal coronary angioplasty (PTCA) and CABG showed that all-cause mortality was significantly lower with CABG than PTCA at 4 years.[28]
- The BARI 2D study evaluated diabetic patients with stable ischemic heart disease[29,30]
  - Intensive medical therapy (IMT) with revascularization deferred versus revascularization initially with subsequent IMT for ischemic CAD
  - Revascularization by either PCI or CABG based on the judgment of the enrolling physicians.
  - No statistically significant differences in the rates of survival or freedom from major cardiovascular events (death, MI, or stroke) between revascularization and IMT
  - The PCI group had more subsequent procedures than the CABG group
  - The study was not designed to compare methods of revascularization.
- The randomized CARDia trial found no significant difference at 1 year of follow-up between PCI and CABG in the composite endpoint of rate of deaths/stroke/MI in symptomatic diabetics with multivessel or complex single vessel disease[31]
- After 5 years of follow-up the SYNTAX trial also found no significant difference in the composite of all-cause death/stroke/MI between PCI and CABG[32]
  - Diabetics treated with PCI did have significantly higher rates of repeat revascularizations compared to CABG (35.3% vs. 14.6%).
  - Diabetics with high SYNTAX scores (based on complexity of coronary lesions) had higher rates adverse events with PCI compared to CABG.
- In contrast, the FREEDOM trial did find a significantly higher rate of MI (at 5 years 13.9% vs. 6.0%) and all-cause mortality (16.3% vs. 10.9%) with PCI vs. CABG. The rate of stroke was higher in the CABG group (2.4% vs. 5.2%) but the composite endpoint (death/stroke/MI) still favored CABG (26.6% vs. 18.7%). There was no significant correlation with the SYNTAX score.[33]

Heart Failure in Diabetes

GENERAL PRINCIPLES

Definition

The term diabetic cardiomyopathy was introduced more than 30 years ago by Rubler and implies the presence of deleterious changes in heart muscle leading to systolic dysfunction and diastolic dysfunction in the absence of obstructive CAD.

Epidemiology

- The risk of HF is 2.4-fold higher in men and 5-fold higher in women.[34]
- The presence of DM predicts HD independent of coexisting hypertension or CAD.
- The incidence of heart failure after revascularization is also greater in diabetics.

Pathophysiology[35]

- Increased left ventricular mass and wall thickness
- Decline in ejection fraction and increase in diastolic diameter with aging
- Diastolic dysfunction
- Microscopic pathologic changes including myocardial fibrosis
- Depressed myocardial function from lipid deposition (lipotoxicity) related to elevated lipids and triglycerides and reduced ability to metabolize fatty acids[36-38]
- Impaired nitric oxide and vascular endothelial growth factor (VEGF) function

DIAGNOSIS

Clinical Presentation

- The clinical presentation of HF is similar to that of other kinds of cardiomyopathies.
- Symptoms and signs may be from either diastolic or systolic dysfunction.
- The level of urine microalbuminuria is proportional to the degree of cardiac diastolic dysfunction.[39] The presence of urine microalbuminuria may warrant echocardiography with pulsed-wave Doppler evaluation even in asymptomatic diabetic patients.

TREATMENT

- Glycemic control is important to prevent advancement from the early diastolic dysfunction to overt heart failure.
- ACE inhibitors or ARBs should be prescribed regardless of the degree of left ventricular dysfunction.
- β-Blockers prevent the remodeling process and shift myocardial metabolism from fatty acid to glucose, which may reduce lipotoxicity on cardiomyocytes. Carvedilol interferes less with glucose control than metoprolol.[40]
- Thiazolidinediones decrease myocardial fatty acid content and toxic metabolites and improve ventricular function.
  - They can cause fluid retention and thus are contraindicated in New York Heart Association (NYHA) functional class III or IV heart failure.
  - Rosiglitazone use should be limited to those patients who are unable to take pioglitazone.[41-43]
- Aldosterone antagonists have antifibrotic effects on the development of cardiomyopathy.
- Preliminary data with incretin-based therapies suggest that they may reduce cardiac risks.
- DM has been considered a relative contraindication for heart transplantation but diabetics should not be a priori excluded from consideration for transplant, particularly if they are free of significant diabetic complications.

Cardiac Risk Factor Reduction in Diabetes

- The approach to risk factor management is same as in persons with known CAD.
- Modifiable risk factors for CAD and HF in the diabetic patient include obesity, hypertension, dyslipidemia, smoking, and glucose control.
- Considerable evidence indicating that a substantial reduction in cardiovascular mortality achieved by multifactorial cardiac risk reduction.

- Aspirin is recommended for all patients with known coronary disease (75 to 162 mg daily) and as primary prevention for those at increased cardiovascular risk (10-year risk of cardiovascular event >10%).
- Hypertension: Pharmacologic treatment should be initiated in diabetics aged ≥18 years with to lower BP at SBP ≥140 mmHg or DBP ≥90mmHg and treat to goal SBP <140mmHg and goal DBP <90mmHg.[44,45]
- Dyslipidemia[3,4,14]:
  ○ Fasting lipid profile at least annually
  ○ New AHA/ACC Guidelines recommend the maximally tolerated moderate and intensive statin therapy for those >40 with diabetes mellitus even in absence of CAD. The intensity of the statin therapy is adjusted based on the overall risk of atherosclerotic cardiovascular disease (ASCVD).
  ○ The American Diabetes Association (ADA) recommends an LDL-C of <100 mg/dL as the primary goal even in the absence of known CAD.
  ○ Statin therapy should be initiated in patients aged >40 years without overt cardiovascular disease to achieve a reduction in LDL-C of 30% to 40%, regardless of baseline LDL-C levels.
- Glycemic control with goal HgbA1c ≤7%. HgbA1c should be checked at least twice yearly in patients with stable glycemic control and quarterly in patients with poor glycemic control.

REFERENCES

1. Booth GL, Kapral MK, Fung K, Tu JV. Relation between age and cardiovascular disease in men and women with diabetes compared with non-diabetic people: a population-based retrospective cohort study. *Lancet* 2006;368:29-36.
2. Huxley R, Barzi F, Woodward M. Excess risk of fatal coronary heart disease associated with diabetes in men and women: meta-analysis of 37 prospective cohort studies. *BMJ* 2006;332:73-78.
3. Third Report of the National Cholesterol Education Program (NCEP) Expert Panel on Detection, Evaluation, and Treatment of High Blood Cholesterol in Adults (Adult Treatment Panel III) final report. *Circulation* 2002;106:3143-3421.
4. Grundy SM, Cleeman JI, Merz CN, et al. Implications of recent clinical trials for the National Cholesterol Education Program Adult Treatment Panel III guidelines. *Circulation* 2004;110:227-239.
5. Juutilainen AS, Lehto S, Rönnemaa T, et al. Type 2 diabetes as a coronary heart disease equivalent: an 18-year prospective population-based study in Finnish subjects. *Diabetes Care* 2005;28:2901-2907.
6. Camici PG, Crea F. Coronary microvascular dysfunction. *N Engl J Med* 2007;356:830-840.
7. Ferretti GT, Bacchetti T, Nègre-Salvayre R, et al. Structural modifications of HDL and functional consequences. *Atherosclerosis* 2006;184:1-7.
8. Greenland P, Alpert JS, Beller GA, et al. 2010 ACCF/AHA guideline for assessment of cardiovascular risk in asymptomatic adults. *Circulation* 2010;122;e584-e636.
9. Young LH, Wackers FJ, Chyun DA, et al. Cardiac outcomes after screening for asymptomatic coronary artery disease in patients with type 2 diabetes: the DIAD study: a randomized controlled trial. *JAMA* 2009;301:1547-1555.
10. Miller TD, Rajagopalan N, Hodge DO, et al. Yield of stress single-photon emission computed tomography in asymptomatic patients with diabetes. *Am Heart J* 2004;147:890-896.
11. Rajagopalan N, Miller TD, Hodge DO, et al. Identifying high-risk asymptomatic diabetic patients who are candidates for screening stress single-photon emission computed tomography imaging. *J Am Coll Cardiol* 2005;45:43-49.
12. Upchurch CT, Barrett EJ. Clinical review: screening for coronary artery disease in type 2 diabetes. *J Clin Endocrinol Metab* 2012;97:1434-1442.
13. Ergelen M, Uyarel H, Cicek G, et al. Which is worst in patients undergoing primary angioplasty for acute myocardial infarction? Hyperglycaemia? Diabetes mellitus? Or both? *Acta Cardiol* 2010;65:415-423.
14. American Diabetes Association. Standards of medical care in diabetes—2013. *Diabetes Care* 2013;36:S11-S66.

15. Marso, SP, Kennedy KF, House JA, et al. The effect of intensive glucose control on all-cause and cardiovascular mortality, myocardial infarction and stroke in persons with type 2 diabetes mellitus: a systematic review and meta-analysis. *Diab Vasc Dis Res* 2010;7:119-130.

16. Montori VM, Fernandez-Balsells M. Glycemic control in type 2 diabetes: time for an evidence-based about-face? *Ann Intern Med* 2009;150:803-808.

17. Roffi M, Chew DP, Mukherjee D, et al. Platelet glycoprotein IIb/IIIa inhibitors reduce mortality in diabetic patients with non-ST-segment-elevation acute coronary syndromes. *Circulation* 2001;104:2767-2771.

18. Mehili J, Kastrati A, Schühlen H, et al. Randomized clinical trial of abciximab in diabetic patients undergoing elective percutaneous coronary interventions after treatment with a high loading dose of clopidogrel. *Circulation* 2004;110:3627-3635.

19. Kastrati A, Mehilli J, Neumann FJ, et al. Abciximab in patients with acute coronary syndromes undergoing percutaneous coronary intervention after clopidogrel pretreatment: the ISAR-REACT 2 randomized trial. *JAMA* 2006;295:1531-1538.

20. Angiolillo DJ. Antiplatelet therapy in diabetes: efficacy and limitations of current treatment strategies and future directions. *Diabetes Care* 2009;32:531-540.

21. Wiviott SD, Braunwald E, Angiolillo DJ, at al. Greater clinical benefit of more intensive oral antiplatelet therapy with prasugrel in patients with diabetes mellitus in the trial to assess improvement in therapeutic outcomes by optimizing platelet inhibition with prasugrel-Thrombolysis in Myocardial Infarction 38. *Circulation* 2008;118:1626-1636.

22. Angiolillo DJ, Badimon JJ, Saucedo JF, et al. A pharmacodynamic comparison of prasugrel vs. high-dose clopidogrel in patients with type 2 diabetes mellitus and coronary artery disease: results of the Optimizing anti-Platelet Therapy In diabetes MellitUS (OPTIMUS)-3 Trial. *Eur Heart J* 2011;32:838-846.

23. Timmer JR, Ottervanger JP, de Boer MJ, et al. Primary percutaneous coronary intervention compared with fibrinolysis for myocardial infarction in diabetes mellitus: results from the Primary Coronary Angioplasty vs Thrombolysis-2 trial. *Arch Intern Med* 2007;167:1353-1359.

24. De Luca G, Dirksen MT, Spaulding C, et al. Impact of diabetes on long-term outcome after primary angioplasty: insights from the DESERT cooperation. *Diabetes Care* 2013;36:1020-1025.

25. Maeng M, Jensen LO, Kaltoft A, et al. Comparison of stent thrombosis, myocardial infarction, and mortality following drug-eluting versus bare-metal stent coronary intervention in patients with diabetes mellitus. *Am J Cardiol* 2008;102:165-172.

26. Boyden TF, Nallamothu BK, Moscucci M, et al. Meta-analysis of randomized trials of drug-eluting stents versus bare metal stents in patients with diabetes mellitus. *Am J Cardiol* 2007;99:1399-1402.

27. Akin I, Bufe A, Eckardt L, et al. Comparison of outcomes in patients with insulin-dependent versus non-insulin dependent diabetes mellitus receiving drug-eluting stents (from the first phase of the prospective multicenter German DES.DE registry). *Am J Cardiol* 2010;106:1201-1207.

28. The BARI Investigators. Seven-year outcome in the Bypass Angioplasty Revascularization Investigation (BARI) by treatment and diabetic status. *J Am Coll Cardiol* 2000;35:1122-1129.

29. Boden WE, O'Rourke RA, Teo KK, et al. Optimal medical therapy with or without PCI for stable coronary disease. *N Engl J Med* 2007;356:1503-1516.

30. BARI 2D Study Group, Frye RL, August P, et al. A randomized trial of therapies for type 2 diabetes and coronary artery disease. *N Engl J Med* 2009;360:2503-2515.

31. Kapur A, Hall RH, Malik IS, et al. Randomized comparison of percutaneous coronary intervention with coronary artery bypass grafting in diabetic patients. 1-year results of the CARDia (Coronary Artery Revascularization in Diabetes) trial. *J Am Coll Cardiol* 2010;55:432-440.

32. Kappetein AP, Feldman TE, Mack MJ, et al. Comparison of coronary bypass surgery with drug-eluting stenting for the treatment of left main and/or three-vessel disease: 3-year follow-up of the SYNTAX trial. *Eur Heart J* 2011;32:2125-2134.

33. Farkouh ME, Domanski M, Sleeper FS, et al. Strategies for multivessel revascularization in patients with diabetes. *N Engl J Med* 2012;367:2375-2384.

34. Kannel WB, Hjortland M, Castelli WP. Role of diabetes in congestive heart failure: the Framingham study. *Am J Cardiol* 1974;34:29-34.

35. Boudina S, Abel ED. Diabetic cardiomyopathy revisited. *Circulation* 115:3213-3223.

36. Anderson EJ, Kypson AP, Rodriquez E, et al. Substrate-specific derangements in mitochondrial metabolism and redox balance in the atrium of the type 2 diabetic human heart. *J Am Coll Cardiol* 2009;54:1891-1898.

37. Borradaile NM, Schaffer JE. Lipotoxicity in the heart. *Curr Hypertens Rep* 2005;7:412-417.

38. Witteles RM, Fowler MB. Insulin-resistant cardiomyopathy: clinical evidence, mechanisms, and treatment options. *J Am Coll Cardiol* 2008;51:93-102.

39. Liu JE, Robbins DC, Palmieri V, et al. Association of albuminuria with systolic and diastolic left ventricular dysfunction in type 2 diabetes: the Strong Heart Study. *J Am Coll Cardiol* 2003;41:2022-2028.

40. Bakris GL, Fonseca V, Katholi RE, et al. Metabolic effects of carvedilol vs metoprolol in patients with type 2 diabetes mellitus and hypertension: a randomized controlled trial. *JAMA* 2004;292:2227-2236.

41. Graham DJ, Ouellet-Hellstrom R, MaCurdy TE, et al. Risk of acute myocardial infarction, stroke, heart failure, and death in elderly Medicare patients treated with rosiglitazone or pioglitazone. *JAMA* 2010;304:411-418.

42. Juurlink DN, Gomes T, Lipscombe LL, et al. Adverse cardiovascular events during treatment with pioglitazone and rosiglitazone: population based cohort study. *BMJ* 2009;339:b2942.

43. Simó R, Rodriguez A, Caveda E. Different effects of thiazolidinediones on cardiovascular risk in patients with type 2 diabetes mellitus: pioglitazone versus rosiglitazone. *Curr Drug Saf* 2010;5:234-244.

44. ACCORD Study Group. Effects of intensive blood-pressure control in type 2 diabetes mellitus. *N Engl J Med* 2010;362:1575-1585.

45. McBrien K, Rabi DM, Campbell N, et al. Intensive and standard blood pressure targets in patients with type 2 diabetes mellitus: systematic review and meta-analysis. *Arch Intern Med* 2012;172:1296-1303.

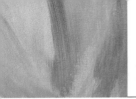

Cardiovascular Disease in Special Populations

38

Angela L. Brown and Jeffrey M.C. Lau

Cardiovascular Disease in Women

GENERAL PRINCIPLES

Epidemiology

- Cardiovascular disease (CVD) is the leading cause of death in women, accounting for one-third of all deaths in the United States. Forty-two million female Americans (34%) have CVD.[1]
- The incidence of CVD rises sharply after menopause to nearly equal that of men and women present approximately 10 years later in life than men.
- The clinical picture is different enough that the diagnosis is often delayed or even missed. Women (and their physicians) frequently attribute their chest pain to anxiety, stress, and other psychological problems, which further delays time to diagnosis.

Risk Factors

- The same risk factors for CVDs are present in both men and women.
- Certain risk factors—including diabetes, decreased high-density-lipoprotein cholesterol (HDL-C), elevated triglycerides, and depression—are associated with worse outcomes in women.[2]

Prevention

- Preventive measures for CVD in women are similar to those for men (Chapter 13).[3]
- Aspirin as primary prevention is sometimes recommended for men with a 10-year risk of >10% and for woman with risk of >20%, but this decision must be individualized and made on a case-by-case basis. Rates of serious vascular events are reduced but cardiovascular mortality does not appear to be significantly lessened.[3-5]
- The higher the global risk score the more beneficial aspirin is; however, the risk of aspirin use (gastrointestinal or intracranial bleeding) also increases with increasing global risk scores.

DIAGNOSIS

Clinical Presentation

- Chest pain in men is more predictive of coronary artery disease (CAD) than it is in women. A 60-year-old man with typical angina has a 90% chance of having obstructive CAD, whereas a woman presenting with the same chest pain has a 60% chance.[6,7]
- Women are more likely to present with atypical symptoms, including back, jaw, and neck pain, nausea and/or vomiting, dyspnea, palpitations, indigestion, dizziness, fatigue, loss of appetite, and syncope.[8]
  - Women present more often as stable angina rather than an acute ST-segment-elevation myocardial infarction (MI) (STEMI).

○ They have higher postrevascularization complication rates and higher in-hospital mortality with STEMI.

Diagnostic Testing

- Diagnostic testing in women is largely the same as in the general population (Chapter 10) but fewer women actually referred for testing.[9]
- Treadmill ECG exercise testing has a higher false-positive rate in women but a lower false-negative rate.
- Nuclear stress imaging is associated with breast tissue anterior attenuation artifacts, which may be mistaken for perfusion defects suggestive of ischemia.

TREATMENT

Medications

- Women are generally underrepresented in randomized trials of new therapies for CAD.
- Therapies used to treat CAD in men are equally efficacious in women.
- Women have a higher risk of bleeding complications from antiplatelet agents, anticoagulants, and thrombolytics. This is most likely due to failure to adjust dosage for smaller body size and advanced age.
- Hormone replacement therapy (HRT):
  ○ Early observational studies and initial data from the Heart and Estrogen/Progestin Replacement study (HERS) suggested protective effect of HRT on coronary heart disease (CHD) risk in postmenopausal women with established CAD.[10]
  ○ HERS II: Protective effects seen in the later years of the initial HERS trial did not persist over an additional 2.7 years of follow-up.[11]
  ○ **The Women's Health Initiative, a randomized trial that included 27,347 women, demonstrated an increased risk of CHD events in women treated with estrogen alone or estrogen plus progestin.**[12]
  ○ **The bottom line: HRT should not be prescribed for the purpose of reducing risk of CHD in women.**

Revascularization

- Success rates of coronary stenting and atherectomy appear similar in men and in women.
- Women are less likely than men to undergo coronary artery bypass grafting (CABG) and more likely to undergo percutaneous revascularization (PCI). This may be because of the higher prevalence of comorbidities and advanced age in the women presenting with CAD, and with this the perception of higher perioperative risk.

OUTCOME/PROGNOSIS

- **Prognosis of CAD is worse in women**, with higher mortality in the year following MI compared with men.
- Women have a greater likelihood of developing chronic heart failure (HF), having diabetes and/or hypertension, and being older at disease onset.

Physiologic Change in Pregnancy

- There are many normal physiologic changes that occur with pregnancy.
- In the fifth to sixth weeks of pregnancy, cardiac output begins to rise because of a 40% to 50% increase in blood volume. This is associated with an increase in left ventricular (LV) end-diastolic volume and atrial stretch.

- During the third trimester, cardiac output is approximately 7 L/minute and increases further to 10 to 11 L/minute during delivery. Arterial blood pressure remains unchanged and ventricular contractility despite a marked fall in vascular resistance.
- The pharmacokinetics of drugs administered during pregnancy are affected by a decrease in serum protein concentration, altered protein-binding affinity, as well as increased renal perfusion and liver metabolism.
- There is an increase in plasma catecholamines and adrenergic receptor sensitivity further increases cardiac demands.
- Most healthy women are able to meet these increased demands without difficulty.

Arrhythmias in Pregnancy

GENERAL PRINCIPLES

- Any arrhythmia can occur during pregnancy in women with and without known heart disease.
- Potential endogenous risk factors include anemia, hyperthyroidism, and electrolyte imbalances.
- Exogenous factors include tobacco, caffeine, medication side effects (such as tocolytics and oxytocins) and illicit drug use.
- These factors may exacerbate previously identified arrhythmias or initiate new arrhythmias.
- Fetal arrhythmias also occur and can carry a significant risk of morbidity and mortality, but this subject is beyond the scope of this chapter.

DIAGONSIS

- Presenting symptoms include palpitations, fatigue, dyspnea, chest pressure, dizziness, presyncope, or syncope.
- Onset, severity, frequency, and duration of symptoms, as well as a comprehensive physical examination and baseline ECG are essential to making the correct diagnosis.
- Differential diagnosis:
  - Sinus tachycardia is common, related to altered vascular resistance.
  - Atrial premature beats occur frequently and are benign.
  - Paroxysmal supraventricular tachycardia (SVT) is common and usually has a favorable outcome.
  - Atrial fibrillation/flutter (AF/AFl) is uncommon.
  - Ventricular tachycardia (VT) and ventricular fibrillation (VF) are rare and predominantly seen in women with structurally abnormal hearts.
  - Symptomatic bradycardia is rare and usually related to supine hypotensive syndrome of pregnancy. Uterus compresses the inferior vena cava and causes a paradoxic slowing of the sinus node.
  - Complete heart block is uncommon and temporary pacing may be required during delivery.

TREATMENT

Medications
- Antiarrhythmic agents can be safe to use during pregnancy but all cross the placenta.
- Treatment should be reserved for those with hemodynamic compromises, severe symptoms, or sustained arrhythmias.

Other Nonpharmacologic Therapy

- Vagal maneuvers, carotid massage, and Valsalva maneuver should be attempted (in the case of SVT) prior to medical therapy.
- Permanent pacemakers and internal defibrillators can be implanted during pregnancy if necessary; this is done either with echocardiographic guidance or with fluoroscopy, using a shield to protect the fetus.
- Algorithms for the management of narrow- and wide-complex tachyarrhythmias are shown in Figure 38-1.

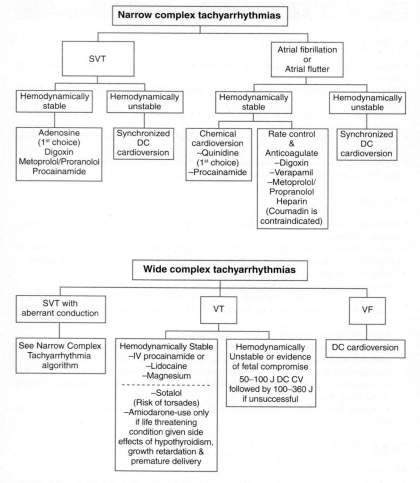

FIGURE 38-1. Tachycardia management in pregnancy. SVT, supraventricular tachycardia; DC, direct current; J, joules; VT, ventricular tachycardia; VF, ventricular fibrillation.

Hypertension in Pregnancy

GENERAL PRINCIPLES

Definition

- During pregnancy women may develop gestational hypertension with or without pre-existing hypertension.
- Pre-existing hypertension is defined as systolic blood pressure ≥140 mmHg and/or diastolic blood pressure ≥90 mmHg before the 20th week of pregnancy, or persistent hypertension after the 12th week postpartum.
- **Gestational hypertension** is hypertension diagnosed after the 20th week of pregnancy.
- Gestational hypertension accompanied by proteinuria and edema is **pre-eclampsia**.
- **Eclampsia** is defined as generalized convulsions and/or coma in the setting of pre-eclampsia, and requires emergent medical therapy with or without delivery.
- Pregnant women with uncomplicated gestational hypertension can be cared for solely by their gynecologist or family physician.
- Consultation with a cardiologist or hypertension specialist beneficial for high-risk patients such as those with congenital heart diseases, arrhythmia, difficult-to-control hypertension, or other pre-existing cardiac conditions.

Pathophysiology

- Maternal hypertension and pre-eclampsia are affected by maternal, fetal, and placental factors.
- Genetic predisposition, altered sensitivity of the renin–angiotensin system, abnormal placental vasculature development, proinflammatory state during pregnancy, dietary changes, and cytokine and immune modulations play a role in the process.

TREATMENT

- Multiple classes of antihypertensive medications have been shown to be reasonably safe for use during pregnancy.
- **The first-line agents are β-blockers, usually labetalol,** but other once-daily β-blockers such as extended release carvedilol and metoprolol may also be safely used.[13,14]
- Calcium channel blockers (CCBs) are in general safe during pregnancy.
- Methyl-dopa is very safe for pregnancy although it has mostly fallen out of favor.
- Intravenous β-blockers (labetalol, metoprolol, or esmolol) or hydralazine may be safely used for immediate reduction of blood pressure.[14]
- **Drugs to avoid include angiotensin-converting enzyme (ACE) inhibitors, angiotensin receptor blockers (ARBs), direct rennin inhibitors, and nitroprusside** (possible fetal cyanide poisoning).

Peripartum Cardiomyopathy

GENERAL PRINCIPLES

Definitions

- Peripartum cardiomyopathy (PPCM) is defined as LV systolic dysfunction presenting in the last month of pregnancy or the first 5 months postpartum.
- To meet the diagnostic criteria for PPCM, there must be no pre-existing LV dysfunction and no alternative etiology for the patient's HF.[15]
- It occurs in 1 in 3,000 to 4,000 pregnancies in the United States.

Etiology

- There are potential **viral etiology**, including coxsackievirus, parvovirus B19, adenovirus, and herpesvirus.
- Fetal microchimerism, in which fetal cells escape into the maternal circulation and induce an autoimmune myocarditis, has also been a suggested cause.
- The increased catecholamine release during pregnancy likely contributes to the pathogenesis of PPCM.
- There may be a potential role for abnormalities in oxidative stress.

Risk Factors

- Risk factors include advanced maternal age, multiparity, multiple pregnancy, preeclampsia, and gestational hypertension.
- There is a higher risk in African American women—confounded by the higher prevalence of hypertension and other cardiac comorbidities in this population.

DIAGNOSIS

Clinical Presentation

- PPCM may be difficult to recognize as dyspnea on exertion and lower extremity edema are common in late pregnancy.
- Cough, orthopnea, and paroxysmal nocturnal dyspnea are warning signs.
- Patients frequently present with New York Heart Association (NYHA) Class III and IV HF but can range from mild symptoms to sudden cardiac death as the initial presentation.
- Thromboembolic events (systemic and pulmonary emboli) may occur.
- Physical findings can include a displaced apical impulse and the murmur of mitral regurgitation (MR).

Diagnostic Testing

- Echocardiography[15]:
  - LV systolic dysfunction, with an ejection fraction <45%.
  - Fractional shortening <30%.
  - LV dilatation, although all four chambers may be dilated.
  - Functional MR is relatively common.
  - LV thrombus is common in patients with LVEF <35%.
- ECG: left ventricular hypertrophy (LVH) and ST-T-wave abnormalities.

TREATMENT[15]

- Afterload reduction: hydralazine and nitrates during pregnancy and ACE inhibitors in postpartum patient.
- β-Blockers to reduce the catecholaminergic tone, heart rate, the incidence of arrhythmia, and risk of sudden cardiac death. β-1-Selective blockers (metoprolol and atenolol) preferred to avoid peripheral vasodilation and uterine relaxation seen with β-2 blockade.
- Digoxin is safe during pregnancy and is used to augment contractility and rate control. Levels must be closely monitored.
- Diuretics are used for preload reduction and symptom relief.
- Anticoagulation in those with thromboembolism:
  - Heparin is required, followed by warfarin (postpartum).
  - The new reversible direct thrombin inhibitor dabigatran (pregnancy Class C) has been shown to cause adverse effects in animal fetuses with no human studies, and should be avoided prior to delivery.

OUTCOME/PROGNOSIS

- Prognosis with PPCM is better than that seen with nonischemic cardiomyopathies.
- Chance of complete recovery approaches 50%.[15]
- Extent of ventricular recovery at 6 months postdelivery predicts overall recovery and continued improvement has been seen 2 to 3 years after diagnosis.
- Subsequent pregnancies in patients with PPCM can be associated with significant deterioration in LV function and can result in death.
- Family-planning counseling is essential and women who do not recover LV function should be encouraged to consider forgoing future pregnancy.

Pregnant Women with Congenital Heart Diseases

GENERAL PRINCIPLES

- For a full discussion of this topic refer to Chapter 35.
- Advances in medical and surgical therapy have helped more patients with congenital heart disease survive to reproductive age.
- There are risks to both the mother and the fetus.
- A multidisciplinary approach with cardiology, obstetrics, and anesthesiology is needed to ensure a safe and successful pregnancy and delivery.
- Maternal cardiovascular risks include arrhythmia, stroke, HF, pulmonary edema, and death.
  - The risk is determined by a woman's ability to adapt to the physiologic stresses placed on her cardiovascular system during pregnancy.
  - The risks associated with different congenital conditions (Table 38-1) are determined by the patient's anatomy, previous operations, and hemodynamic status.[16]
- The risk of fetal adverse events is higher than that in the general population:
  - Includes intrauterine growth retardation, preterm birth, intracranial hemorrhage, and fetal loss.
  - Risks are higher in women with poor functional class, cyanotic heart disease, and LV outflow tract obstruction (LVOT).
  - Overall there is an approximate 3% to 7% risk that congenital heart disease will recur in the fetus but this varies by the specific condition, compared with a baseline risk of 0.8% in the general population.[17-19]

TREATMENT

- The level of care required during pregnancy depends on the severity of the patient's disease (Table 38-1).[16]
- Low-risk patients can receive care locally while moderate- to high-risk patients should be followed in a tertiary care facility.
- Highest risk patients may be hospitalized in the third trimester for bed rest, close monitoring, and oxygen if needed.
  - This includes women with Eisenmenger syndrome (or other forms of pulmonary hypertension), Marfan syndrome with an aortic root >4 cm in diameter, or severe LVOT obstruction.
  - These patients should be informed of the high risk of maternal morbidity and mortality and consider terminating the pregnancy.

TABLE 38-1	CONGENITAL HEART DISEASE IN PREGNANCY	
Lesion	**Potential risks**	**Recommendations**
Low risk		
Ventricular septal defects	Arrhythmia Endocarditis (if residual defect present)	Antibiotic prophylaxis if residual defect
Atrial septal defects	Arrhythmia Thromboembolic events	Thromboprophylaxis if on bed rest Consider low-dose aspirin
Repaired coarctation	Preeclampsia Aortic dissection Heart failure Endarteritis	β-Blockers for blood pressure control Elective C-section if aortic aneurysm or uncontrolled hypertension Antibiotic prophylaxis
Tetralogy of Fallot	Arrhythmia RV failure Endocarditis	Consider preterm delivery if RV failure Antibiotic prophylaxis
Moderate risk		
Mitral stenosis	Atrial fibrillation Thromboembolism Pulmonary edema	β-Blockers Low-dose aspirin Consider bed rest during third trimester with thromboprophylaxis Antibiotic prophylaxis
Aortic stenosis	Arrhythmia Angina Endocarditis LV failure	Bed rest during third trimester with thromboprophylaxis Consider balloon valvuloplasty for severe AS; cases of surgical AV replacement have also been reported in patients who are not candidates for balloon valvuloplasty Consider preterm delivery by C-section if cardiac decompensation Antibiotic prophylaxis

TABLE 38-1	CONGENITAL HEART DISEASE IN PREGNANCY (*Continued*)	
Lesion	**Potential risks**	**Recommendations**
Systemic right ventricle (corrected transposition of the great arteries)	RV dysfunction Heart failure Arrhythmia Thromboembolism Endocarditis	Regularly monitor rhythm Cardioversion if atrial flutter Stop ACE inhibitors, consider β-blockers Low-dose aspirin Antibiotic prophylaxis
Cyanotic lesions (without pulmonary hypertension)	Hemorrhage Thromboembolism Worsening cyanosis Heart failure Endocarditis	Consider bed rest and supplemental oxygen Thromboprophylaxis Antibiotic prophylaxis
Fontan-type circulation	Heart Failure Arrhythmia Thromboembolism Endocarditis	Consider low-molecular-weight heparin and aspirin throughout pregnancy Maintain filling pressures during delivery Antibiotic prophylaxis
High risk		
Marfan syndrome with dilated aortic root	Dissection of ascending aorta 30–50% mortality related to pregnancy	β-Blockers Elective C-section if aortic root >4.5 cm
Eisenmenger syndrome	Arrhythmia Heart failure Endocarditis	Consider termination Close cardiovascular monitoring, early bed rest, pulmonary vasodilators and supplemental oxygen Monitor 10 days postpartum

ACE, angiotensin-converting enzyme; AS, aortic stenosis; AV, aortic valve.

Modified from Uebing A, Steer PJ, Yentis SM, Gatzoulis MA. Pregnancy and congenital heart disease. *BMJ* 2006;332:401-406, with permission.

Safety of Cardiac Drugs Commonly Used during Pregnancy

REASONABLY SAFE[20]

- Adenosine:
  - Rapid action and short half-life, rapid metabolism reduces amount crossing the placenta.
  - First choice for acute SVT presentation.
  - No teratogenicity in second and third trimesters (unknown safety in first trimester).
  - Fetal heart rate monitoring recommended.
- β-Blockers:
  - Widely used in pregnancy to treat hypertension, hypertrophic cardiomyopathy, thyrotoxicosis, mitral stenosis, and fetal tachycardia.
  - Use leads to reduction in umbilical blood flow and increase in uterine contractility.
  - β-1-Selective agents (atenolol, metoprolol) may be preferable peripheral vasodilation and uterine relaxation.
- CCBs:
  - Widely used to treat fetal SVT and to prevent preterm delivery and preeclampsia.
  - Verapamil preferred for maternal and fetal SVT (acute and chronic).
  - Amlodipine and nifedipine are often used for maternal hypertension.
  - No teratogenicity but maternal/fetal hypotension, bradycardia, AV-nodal blockade, and decreased LV contractility reported.
  - IV verapamil associated with maternal hypotension and decreased uterine blood flow.
  - Excreted in breast milk.
- Digoxin:
  - Widely used for maternal/fetal arrhythmias, **safest antiarrhythmic agent at therapeutic doses**.
  - Freely crosses the placenta.
  - Digoxin levels decrease by up to 50% due to increase in renal excretion.
  - Digoxin toxicity associated with fetal loss.
- Flecainide:
  - Not widely used, no evidence of teratogenicity or fetal adverse effects.
  - Crosses placenta, but effectively excreted by fetal renal function.
  - Excreted in breast milk.
- Heparin:
  - AF/AFl for 3 weeks prior to cardioversion and 4 weeks postcardioversion.
  - Also used for mechanical valves or thromboembolism.
  - Unfractionated subcutaneous heparin preferred to low-molecular-weight heparin as the larger molecular weight decreases placental transfer.
- Lidocaine:
  - Crosses placenta but not known to increase fetal malformations.
  - Causes increase in myometrial tone, decrease in placental blow flow, and fetal bradycardia.
  - If fetus is acidotic, it can result in neonatal cardiac and central nervous system (CNS) toxicity.
  - Small amounts are excreted in breast milk.
- Mexiletine: similar to lidocaine.
- Procainamide: used frequently, no reports of teratogenicity in first trimester, limited data.
- Quinidine:
  - Used in pregnancy since the 1930s.
  - Adverse events are uncommon but include mild uterine contractions, premature labor, and neonatal thrombocytopenia.

○ Miscarriage and cranial nerve VII injury at toxic doses.
○ Low amounts in breast milk.

CARDIAC DRUGS NOT SAFE FOR USE IN PREGNANCY

- ACE inhibitors and ARBs: risk of neonatal renal failure, hypotension, renal tubular dysgenesis, intrauterine growth retardation, and decreased skull ossification.
- Amiodarone: may be used in life-threatening conditions but carries the risk of hypothyroidism and potential brain damage.
- Dabigatran.
- Dronedarone.
- Phenytoin.
- Spironolactone: amiloride preferred if a potassium-sparing diuretic is needed.
- Warfarin: there is some controversy regarding use during pregnancy and risks include skeletal and CNS malformations and intracranial hemorrhage.

Cardiovascular Issues in Minorities

- Over the last several decades, the population of the United States has become increasingly diverse, according to the 2010 U.S. census:
  ○ White/Caucasian American 72.4%
  ○ Hispanic/Latino 16.4%
  ○ African American 12.2%
  ○ Asian American 4.8%
  ○ American Indian/Alaskan native 0.9%
  ○ Two or more races 2.9%
- Studies have demonstrated a disparity between the levels of care and differences in outcomes. For example, minority populations are less likely to undergo PCI or CABG or to receive thrombolytic agents.[21]
- Many factors contribute to the disparities in patient care:
  ○ Health care delivery system with its lack of cultural awareness.
  ○ Communication and financial barriers.
  ○ Patient choice.
  ○ Variations in disease presentation.
  ○ Physician bias.
  ○ Concerns for deportation in the case of illegal immigrants.

African Americans

GENERAL PRINCIPLES

Epidemiology
- The leading cause of death among African Americans is CVD. And the death rate due to hypertension is much higher in African Americans than white Americans.[22]
- There is a higher prevalence of risk factors (hypertension, diabetes, obesity) in this population.
- African Americans receive less adequate care and are more likely to die from CVD than the general population.

Risk Factors
- Hypertension affects nearly 45% of African Americans (among the highest rates in the world), with much higher average blood pressures.[1]

- ○ Develop hypertension earlier in life, and it tends to be more severe.
- ○ Contributes to a higher risk of stroke, CVD, death from CVD, LVH, HF, and end-stage renal disease.
- ○ Hypertension remains undertreated in this population—only 45% have well-controlled hypertension, compared with 56% of whites.[23]
- Dyslipidemia is as common among African Americans as it is among whites but they tend to have lower mean LDL-C levels, lower small dense LDL-C levels, and higher HDL-C levels.

TREATMENT

- A multidrug regimen is reasonable in view of the increased incidence of end-organ disease.
- **Initial drugs of choice are the thiazide diuretic and CCBs for uncomplicated hypertension.**[24-27]
- ACE inhibitors and ARBs have renal and cardioprotective effects.[28]
- β-Blockers reduce arrhythmias and sudden cardiac death, particularly after an MI.
  - ○ Different β-blockers may have different effects in African Americans.
  - ○ Metoprolol, carvedilol, and propranolol decrease mortality and reduce hospitalizations.
  - ○ Bucindolol has not been shown to have a mortality benefit in African Americans.
- Fixed-dose combination isosorbide dinitrate/hydralazine in African Americans with stage III or IV HF (in addition to ACE-I or ARB)—the African American Heart Failure trial (AHeFT) found a 43% reduction in death from any cause, 33% relative risk reduction in hospitalization for CHF, and improved quality of life.[29]

Hispanic Americans

- CVD is the leading cause of death in the Hispanic population, accounting for about 40% deaths.
- Hispanic women are disproportionately obese with the highest incidence of the metabolic syndrome.
- Hispanic men have a high prevalence of CVD risk factors, including diabetes, hypertension, and physical inactivity.
- Hypertension awareness is lower and it is less likely to be detected, treated, and controlled.[30]
- Hispanics comprise only a small percentage of patients with acute decompensated HF despite the increased prevalence of risk factors in this population. They have worse outcomes compared with whites but better outcomes compared with African Americans.

Asian Americans

- Asian Americans have lower incidences of CVD than whites. Heart disease is second to cancer as the leading cause of death among Asians and Pacific Islanders, accounting for about a quarter of all deaths.
- Asians are less likely than white patients to undergo cardiac procedures.
- According to data released by American Heart Association (AHA) in 2013, 7.4% of Asian Americans have heart disease, 4.3% have CAD, and 18.7% have hypertension.[1]
- Tobacco use is low among Asian Americans (9.9%).
- The incidence of overweight (BMI 25 to 30 kg/m^2) and obese (BMI > 30 kg/m^2) Asian Americans in 2008 was 38%.

- Substantial differences of CVD patterns and genetics within the Asian American group:
  - Indian Americans have a higher rate of glucose intolerance, diabetes, and CAD.
  - Japanese men living in Hawaii have an increased risk of impaired glucose tolerance associated with a marked increase in thromboembolic and hemorrhagic stroke, CAD, sudden cardiac death, and all-cause mortality.
- Asian American has the highest incidences of Kawasaki disease, and predisposes the individual to develop myocarditis, pericarditis, and valvular heart disease.

Native Americans

- CVD is the leading cause of death among Native Americans and Alaska natives.
- Native Americans and Alaskan natives have the least understood CVD profile.
- There is a great deal of heterogeneity among the >500 tribes in the United States.
- According to AHA 2013 data, 12.7% of Native Americans or Alaskan Natives have heart disease vs. 11.1% of non-Hispanic whites.[1]
- Slightly more American Indian or Alaska Natives men smoke (24.6% vs. 23.9% of non-Hispanic whites) and about the same number of women smoke (20.7% vs. 20.9%).[1]
- Based on 2011 National Health Interview Survey statistics, 40.8% of American Indians or Alaskan Natives or obese vs. 27.2% if non-Hispanic whites.[1]
- Strong Heart Study:
  - Created in the 1980s as a five-phase, longitudinal demographic study to investigate the prevalence and genetics of CVD in Native Americans, three of the five phases have been completed.
  - Incidences of diabetes and obesity are high among Native Americans, **the highest incidences of diabetes among all race groups**, 2.3 times higher than non-Hispanic whites.[31]
  - Native Americans suffer disproportionately from sudden cardiovascular death and sequelae of metabolic syndrome.
  - CVD risk calculator similar to the Framingham risk score is available on line (http://strongheart.ouhsc.edu/CHDcalculator/calculator.html, last accessed 10/9/13).
  - Phases 4 and 5 of the Strong Heart Study will look at the genetic linkage analysis and correlate this with imaging studies (i.e., carotid Doppler and echocardiography).

Chemotherapy-Induced Cardiomyopathy

GENERAL PRINCIPLES

Classification

- Anthracyclines (e.g., doxorubicin, epirubicin, idarubicin, and daunorubicin): associated with both early (≤1 year) and late (>1 year following treatment) cardiotoxicity.
- Trastuzumab (Herceptin): humanized monoclonal antibody used either alone or in combination with anthracyclines for the treatment of HER-2-positive metastatic breast cancer.
- Other chemotherapies: BCR-ABL inhibitors (e.g., imatinib), microtubule-targeting drugs (e.g., taxane), mitoxantrone, vinca alkaloids, alkylating agents (e.g., cyclophosphamide).
- Several other classes of chemotherapeutic agents are known to cause MI or myocarditis including antimetabolites such as 5-FU, and anti-angiogenic agents such as bevacizumab.

Epidemiology

- The reported incidence of CHF related to anthracycline treatment ranges from 1.6% to 2.8%. Up to 57% of long-term survivors have been found to have cardiac abnormalities, including both symptomatic and asymptomatic LV dysfunction.
- In the National Surgical Breast and Bowel Project (NSABP), trastuzumab in combination with anthracyclines plus cyclophosphamide plus paclitaxel (standard therapy) was associated with a 4.1% incidence of cardiac events, HF, and cardiac death, compared with 0.8% incidence seen when the latter agents used without trastuzumab.[32]
- In a meta-analysis of randomized trials of trastuzumab, the incidence of HF was five times higher.[33]

Pathophysiology

- The proposed mechanism for anthracycline-induced cardiotoxicity involves myocyte damage from free radicals that form from ferrous complexes.
- The mechanism of trastuzumab-related cardiomyopathy remains unclear. It does not appear to be cumulative or dose related.

Risk Factors

- Risk factors for the development of anthracycline-induced cardiomyopathy include age > 50 years and treatment with >200 mg/m^2 doxorubicin.
- Risk factors for developing trastuzumab-related cardiomyopathy include older age, exposure to anthracyclines, previous cardiac disease, HF, LV dysfunction, and hypertension.

Prevention

- Randomized trials have shown cardioprotection with the coadministration of dexrazoxane, an iron chelator, which may interfere with the efficacy of the anthracyclines. Pooled results, however, do not allow for a clear evidence-based recommendation.[34,35]
- Liposomal encapsulated doxorubicin has been formulated, in which the drug is sequestered from organs with tight capillary junctions like the heart; this may also offer some cardioprotection.
- Slow infusion rate may reduce the incidence of cardiomyopathy.

DIAGNOSIS

- Anthracyclines:
  - Baseline ECG and evaluation of resting LV function by radionuclide gated blood pool imaging prior to initiating treatment.
  - Require routine monitoring of LV function during and after treatment.
- Trastuzumab:
  - Prior to receiving, patients should undergo evaluation of LV function, preferably by radionuclide imaging.
  - Risk–benefit analysis should occur before initiating therapy with LVEF <40%.
  - EF should be monitored every 4 to 6 weeks during treatment.
    - If the LVEF falls by more than 10% or to less than 40% or if symptoms of CHF develop, trastuzumab should be discontinued.
    - Resumed only if the EF improves to ≥40% and symptoms resolve.
- Myocardial biopsies are generally not indicated before or after chemo-induced cardiomyopathy.

TREATMENT

- Similar to that of HF due to other causes and with proper management may improve.
- Associated with a high incidence of tachycardia.
- Trastuzumab-induced cardiomyopathy appears to be more reversible than that seen with anthracyclines.

Stent Thrombosis in Chemotherapy Patients

- Endothelialization of the internal lumen of a coronary stent is necessary to protect against thrombotic stent occlusion.
- Patients who receive chemotherapy and require stent placement may have delayed neointimalization.
- Important issues include:
  - Timing of discontinuation of antiplatelet agents in the setting of delayed neointimalization process by chemotherapy.
  - Thrombocytopenia induced by chemotherapy in those who receive drug-eluting stents.
  - Hypercoagulability associated with cancer and risk for subacute or late stent thrombosis.
- Consultation with the patient's oncologist should be made prior to any percutaneous coronary revascularization.
- **Bare metal stents should be favored over drug eluting stents to reduce the time necessary for dual antiplatelet therapy.**[36]

HIV AND CAD

- There is a higher incidence of CAD and MI in HIV patients taking antiretroviral therapy (ART) compared with general population.[37]
- Some ART regimens worsen the atherogenic profile.[38,39]
- HIV itself is associated with the development of metabolic derangements, including dyslipidemia, insulin resistance, and central obesity.
- It is not clear whether the higher incidence is due to (1) the viral infection and inflammatory response, (2) metabolic derangement from ART, or (3) environmental and behavioral factors.[40]
- Atherosclerotic changes caused by HIV virus include endothelial dysfunction, inflammation (with increased levels of C-reactive protein [CRP], tumor necrosis factor [TNF], and γ-interferon), increased platelet adhesion due to elevated von Willebrand factor, and hypercoagulability secondary to decreased levels of protein S.
- HIV patients are more likely to present with single-vessel disease.
- Treatment is similar to those without HIV but there are many drug–drug interactions (Table 38-2).

Pericarditis/Myocarditis and HIV

- Pericardial disease used to be common in HIV patients before the advent of ART. Incidence of pericardial effusions and pericarditis has declined since ART. Larger effusions leading to cardiac tamponade are uncommon.
- Etiologies of pericarditis include tuberculosis, *Staphylococcus* and *Streptococcus*, and lymphoma and Kaposi sarcoma.[41,42]

TABLE 38-2	DRUG INTERACTIONS IN THE HIV PATIENT		

Drug	Mechanism/ adverse reaction	Drugs to avoid	Alternative Rx
Protease inhibitors (ritonavir, atazanavir, saquinavir)	Inhibit metabolism by cytochrome P450 system Risk of myopathy, rhabdomyolysis	Statins— simvastatin and lovastatin	Pravastatin or fluvastatin (not metabolized by P450)
Protease inhibitors	Decrease concentrations of PIs	St. John wort	Atorvastatin at reduced dose
Phosphodiesterase 5 inhibitors (sildenafil, tadalafil, vardenafil)	Increased side effects, including hypotension, vision changes, priapism	Protease inhibitors	
Atazanavir	Prolongs PR interval	Caution if conduction disease, avoid β-blockers, nondihydropyridine CCBs, and digoxin	
Protease inhibitors (fosamprenavir, nelfinavir, ritonavir, saquinavir)	Inhibit CYP3A	Antiarrhythmic drugs (amiodarone, quinidine, flecainide, propafenone)	
Protease inhibitors	Increased risk of ergot toxicity, including peripheral vasospasm and limb ischemia	Ergots	

- Pericardiocentesis is essential for diagnosis and to guide therapy and is obviously indicated if hemodynamic compromise. Treatment depends on the cause. Corticosteroids may be appropriate for some patients. Definitive drainage may be required for some effusions.
- The incidence of myocarditis has decreased significantly with the advent of ART. Typically the cause is unknown, possibly due to HIV itself. Other causes included toxoplasmosis, aspergillosis, histoplasmosis, tuberculosis, cryptococcosis, cytomegalovirus, and herpes simplex virus.

HIV-Associated Cardiomyopathy

- LV systolic dysfunction detected by echocardiography is no uncommon in HIV patients. Most will be asymptomatic but a few will have clinically significant cardiomyopathy.
- Since ART, the incidence of HIV-related cardiomyopathy has declined.
- The exact mechanism is unclear but may include direct cardiotoxicity of the HIV virus, cardiotoxicity of ART (particularly zidovudine [infrequently used currently] through cardiac mitochondrial toxicity), IV drug and other substance abuse (especially alcohol), increased cytokine activity, nutritional deficiencies, and opportunistic infections.[42]
- Response to the treatment of HIV-induced cardiomyopathy may be complicated by the presence of opportunistic infections, autoimmune response to the HIV, and the cardiotoxic effects of ART.

Endocarditis in HIV

- HIV by itself is not a risk factor for infective endocarditis (IE) but is an independent risk factor for IE in IV drug abusers.[42,43]
- Long-term indwelling central venous, lower CD4 counts, and higher viral loads are risk factors. The incidence has decreased since the introduction of ART.[43]
- *Staphylococcus aureus* is the most common causative organism and *Streptococcus viridans* is also common.
- Recurrence and mortality at 1 year are relatively high, 16% and 52%, respectively.[43]
- Treatment is essentially the same as for those without HIV.
- Noninfectious thrombotic endocarditis may also occur in HIV patients.

Cardiac Tumors in HIV

- The most common causes of cardiac tumors in HIV patients are Kaposi sarcoma and B-cell lymphoma.
- Kaposi sarcoma can cause widespread mucocutaneous disease but is usually otherwise asymptomatic. It can involve the pericardium, epicardium, and myocardium. An effusion may be present. The incidence has decreased markedly with ART.
- B-cell lymphomas can cause primary or secondary cardiac tumors that are usually located in the right atrium. They may be aggressive tumors. Symptoms and signs can include those of HF, atrioventricular (AV) block, or other conduction abnormalities caused by myocardial infiltration, VT, and pericardial effusion.
- Patients with cardiac B-cell lymphomas should be monitor for arrhythmias caused by tumor necrosis in response to chemotherapy.

HIV and Pulmonary Hypertension

- The incidence of primary pulmonary hypertension (PPH) is 0.5% in HIV patients compared with 1 to 2 per million in the general population.[42,44]
- The role of human herpesvirus 8 (HHV-8), the causative agent for Kaposi sarcoma, remains to be proven.
- There may be a confounding contribution of foreign materials (i.e., talc) in IV drug abusers who develop PPH and of prior pulmonary infections.
- Echocardiography and right heart catheterization are diagnostic.

- Histopathology reveals plexogenic arteriopathy similar to the PPH seen in non-HIV patients.
- Therapy is similar to that in the non-HIV population including CCBs, diuretics, anticoagulation, prostacyclin analogs, phosphodiesterase inhibitors, and the endothelin antagonist bosentan.
- Prognosis is poor and the effect of ART is unknown but may be improving.[45]

REFERENCES

1. Go AS, Mozaffarian D, Roger VL, et al. Heart disease and stroke statistics—2013 update: a report from the American Heart Association. *Circulation* 2013;127:e6-e245.
2. Huxley R, Barzi F, Woodward M. Excess risk of fatal coronary heart disease associated with diabetes in men and women: meta-analysis of 37 prospective cohort studies. *BMJ* 2006;332:73-78.
3. Mosca L, Banka CL, Benjamin EJ, et al. Evidence-based guidelines for cardiovascular disease prevention in women: 2007 update. *Circulation* 2007;115:1481-1501.
4. Antithrombotic Trialists' (ATT) Collaboration. Aspirin in the primary and secondary prevention of vascular disease: collaborative meta-analysis of individual participant data from randomised trials. *Lancet* 2009;373:1849-1860.
5. Seshasai SR, Wijesuriva S, Sivakumaran R, et al. Effect of aspirin on vascular and nonvascular outcomes: meta-analysis of randomized controlled trials. *Arch Intern Med* 2012;172:209-216.
6. Pryor DB, Harrell FE Jr, Lee KL, et al. Estimating the likelihood of significant coronary artery disease. *Am J Med* 1983;75:771-780.
7. Castelli WP. Epidemiology of coronary heart disease: the Framingham study. *Am J Med* 1984;76:4-12.
8. Patel H, Rosengren A, Ekman I. Symptoms in acute coronary syndromes, does sex make a difference? *Am Heart J* 2004;148:27-33.
9. Daly C, Clemens F, Lopez Sendon JL, et al. Gender differences in the management and clinical outcome of stable angina. *Circulation* 2006;113:490-498.
10. Hulley S, Grady D, Bush T, et al. Randomized trial of estrogen plus progestin for secondary prevention of coronary heart disease in postmenopausal women. Heart and Estrogen/progestin Replacement Study (HERS) Research Group. *JAMA* 1998;280:605-613.
11. Grady D, Herrington D, Bittner V, et al. Cardiovascular disease outcomes during 6.8 years of hormone therapy. Heart and Estrogen/Progestin Replacement Study Follow-up (HERS II). *JAMA* 2002;288:49-57.
12. Manson LE, Hsia J, Johnson KC, et al. Women's Health Initiative Investigators: Estrogen plus progestin and risk of coronary heart disease. *N Engl J Med* 2003;349:523-534.
13. Yakoob MY, Bateman BT, Ho E, et al. The risk of congenital malformations associated with exposure to β-blockers early in pregnancy: a meta-analysis. *Hypertension* 2013;62:375-381.
14. Committee on Obstetric Practice. Committee Opinion no. 514: emergent therapy for acute-onset, severe hypertension with preeclampsia or eclampsia. *Obstet Gynecol* 2011;118:465-468.
15. Elkayam U. Clinical characteristics of peripartum cardiomyopathy in the United States: diagnosis, prognosis, and management. *J Am Coll Cardiol* 2011;58:659-670.
16. Uebing A, Steer PJ, Yentis SM, Gatzoulis MA. Pregnancy and congenital heart disease. *BMJ* 2006;332:401-406.
17. Burn J, Brennan P, Little J, et al. Recurrence risks in offspring of adults with major heart defects: results from first cohort of British collaborative study. *Lancet* 1998;351:311-316.
18. Siu SC, Sermer M, Colman JM, et al. Prospective multicenter study of pregnancy outcomes in women with heart disease. *Circulation* 2001;104:515-521.
19. Gill HK, Splitt M, Sharland GK, Simpson JM. Patterns of recurrence of congenital heart disease: an analysis of 6,640 consecutive pregnancies evaluated by detailed fetal echocardiography. *J Am Coll Cardiol* 2003;42:923-929.
20. Fishman WH, Elkayam U, Aronow WS. Cardiovascular drugs in pregnancy. *Cardiol Clin* 2012;30:463-491.
21. Lillie-Blanton M, Maddox TM, Rushing O, Mensah GA. Disparities in cardiac care: rising to the challenge of Healthy People 2010. *J Am Coll Cardiol* 2004;44:503-508.
22. Gadegbeku CA, Lea JP, Jamerson KA. Update on disparities in the pathophysiology and management of hypertension: focus on African Americans. *Med Clin North Am* 2005;89:921-933.

23. Hajjar I, Kotchen TA. Trends in prevalence, awareness, treatment, and control of hypertension in the United States, 1988-2000. *JAMA* 2003;290:199-206.

24. Brewster LM, van Montfrans GA, Kleijnen J. Systematic review: antihypertensive drug therapy in black patients. *Ann Intern Med* 2004;141:614-627.

25. ALLHAT Officers and Coordinators for the ALLHAT Collaborative Research Group. Major outcomes in high risk hypertensive patients randomized to angiotensin converting enzyme inhibitor or calcium channel blocker vs diuretic: The Antihypertensive and Lipid-Lowering Treatment to Prevent Heart Attack Trial (ALLHAT). *JAMA* 2002;288:2981-2997.

26. Wright JT Jr, Dunn JK, Cutler JA, et al. Outcomes in hypertensive black and nonblack patients treated with chlorthalidone, amlodipine, and lisinopril. *JAMA* 2005;293:1595-1608.

27. Flack JM, Sica DA, Bakris G, et al. Management of high blood pressure in Blacks: an update of the International Society on Hypertension in Blacks consensus statement. *Hypertension* 2010;56:780-800.

28. Jamerson K, Weber MA, Bakris GL, et al. Benazepril plus amlodipine or hydrochlorothiazide for hypertension in high-risk patients. *N Engl J Med* 2008;359:2417-2428.

29. Taylor N, Ziesche S, Yancy C, et al. Combination of isosorbide dinitrate and hydralazine in blacks with heart failure. *N Engl J Med* 2004;351:2049-2057.

30. Egan BM, Zhao Y, Axon RN. US trends in prevalence, awareness, treatment, and control of hypertension, 1988-2008. *JAMA* 2010;303:2043-2050.

31. Indian Health Service. Department of Health and Human Services. www.ihs.gov. Last Accessed 10 October 2013.

32. Tan-Chiu E, Yothers G, Romond E, et al. Assessment of cardiac dysfunction in a randomized trial comparing doxorubicin and cyclophosphamide followed by paclitaxel, with or without trastuzumab as adjuvant therapy in node-positive, human epidermal growth factor receptor 2-overexpressing breast cancer: NSABP B-31. *J Clin Oncol* 2005;23:7811-7819.

33. Moja L, Tagliabue L, Balduzzi S, et al. Trastuzumab containing regimens for early breast cancer. *Cochrane Database Syst Rev* 2012;4:CD006243.

34. Smith LA, Cornelius VR, Plummer CJ, et al. Cardiotoxicity of anthracycline agents for the treatment of cancer: systematic review and meta-analysis of randomised controlled trials. *BMC Cancer* 2010;10:337.

35. Van Dalen EC, Caron HN, Dickinson HO, Kremer LC. Cardioprotective interventions for cancer patients receiving anthracyclines. *Cochrane Database Syst Rev* 2011;6:CD003917.

36. Krone RJ. Managing coronary artery disease in the cancer patient. *Prog Cardiovasc Dis* 2010;53:149-156.

37. Currier JS, Taylor A, Boyd F, et al. Coronary heart disase in HIV-infected individuals. *J Acquir Immune Defic Syndr* 2003;33:506-512.

38. DAD Study Group. Class of antiretroviral drugs and the risk of myocardial infarction. *N Engl J Med* 2007;356:1723-1735.

39. Bavinger C, Bendavid E, Niehaus K, et al. Risk of cardiovascular disease from antiretroviral therapy for HIV: a systematic review. *PLoS One* 2013;8:e59551.

40. Boccara F, Lang S, Meuleman C, et al. HIV and coronary heart disease: time for a better understanding. *J Am Coll Cardiol* 2013;61:511-523.

41. Gowda RM, Khan IA, Mehta NJ, et al. Cardiac tamponade in patients with human immunodeficiency virus disease. *Angiology* 2003;54:469-474.

42. Khunnawat C, Mukerji S, Havlichek D Jr, et al. Cardiovascular manifestations in human immunodeficiency virus-infected patients. *Am J Cardiol* 2008;102:635-642.

43. Gebo KA, Burkey MD, Lucas GM, et al. Incidence of, risk factors for, clinical presentation and 1-year outcomes of infective endocarditis is an urban HIV cohort. *J Acquir Immune Defic Syndr* 2006;43:426-432.

44. Sitbon O, Lascoux-Combe C, Delfraissy JF, et al. Prevalence of HIV-related pulmonary arterial hypertension in the current antiretroviral therapy era. *Am J Respir Crit Care Med* 2008;177:108-113.

45. Degano B, Guillaume M, Savale L, et al. HIV-associated pulmonary arterial hypertension: survival and prognostic factors in the modern therapeutic era. *AIDS* 2010;24:67-75.

Index

Page numbers followed by *f* refer to figures; page numbers followed by *t* refer to tables.